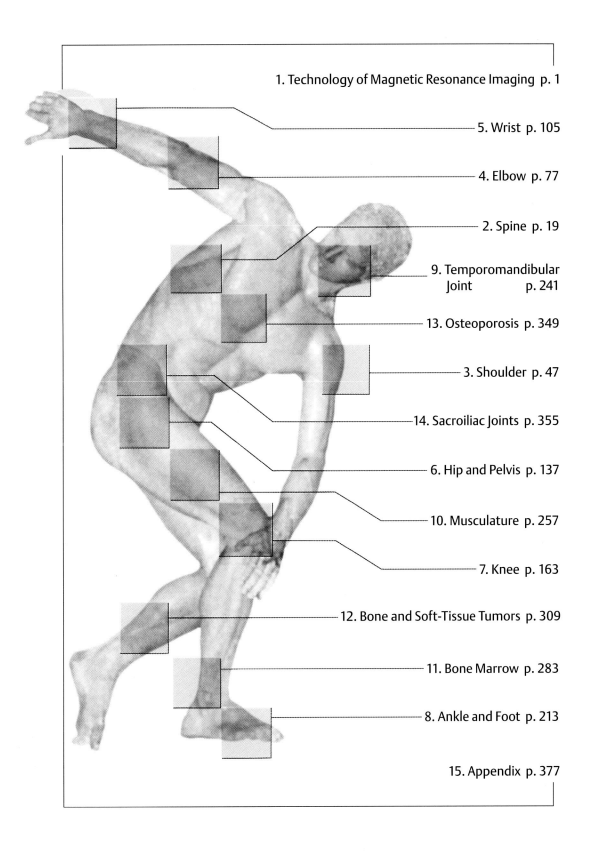

MRI of the Musculoskeletal System

Martin Vahlensieck, M.D.
Medical Faculty
University of Bonn
Bonn, Germany

Harry K. Genant, M.D.
Professor of Radiology
Medicine, Epidemiology,
and Orthopedic Surgery
Department of Radiology
University of California
San Francisco, USA

Maximilian Reiser, M.D.
Professor and Director
Institute of Diagnostic
Radiology
Großhadern Clinic
Munich, Germany

With contributions by

M. Bollow
J. Braun
B. M. Eitel
R. Fischbach
H. K. Genant
J. Gieseke
S. Grampp
A. Heuck
J. O. Johnston

P. Lang
G. Layer
G. Lutterbey
M. Reiser
P. Schnarkowski
A. Stäbler
M. Steinborn
F. Träber
M. Vahlensieck

Translated by Peter Winter, M.D.

898 illustrations
48 tables

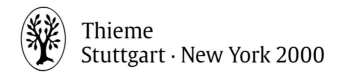

Thieme
Stuttgart · New York 2000

Die Deutsche Bibliothek – CIP-Einheitsaufnahme

MRI of the musculoskeletal system : 48 tables / Martin
Vahlensieck ... With contributions by M. Bollow ...
Transl. by Peter Winter. – Stuttgart ; New York ;
Thieme, 2000
  Dt. Ausg. u.d.T.: MRT des Bewegungsapparats

This book is an authorized and adapted translation of
the 1st German edition published and copyrighted 1997
by Georg Thieme Verlag, Stuttgart, Germany. Title of the
German edition: MRT des Bewegungsapparats

© 2000 Georg Thieme Verlag,
Rüdigerstraße 14, D-70469 Stuttgart, Germany
Thieme Medical Publishers, Inc., 333 Seventh Avenue,
New York, N.Y. 10001

Typesetting by Druckhaus Götz GmbH,
D-71636 Ludwigsburg
(CCS-Textline [Linotronic 630])
Printed in Germany by Offizin Andersen Nexö, Leipzig

ISBN 3-13-116571-5 (GTV)
ISBN 0-86577-875-2 (TNY)   1 2 3 4 5 6

Preface to the English Translation

Following the success of the original German edition of this book, it was only a matter of time until an English edition was necessary. Vahlensieck and Reiser have done an excellent job of reviewing the latest developments and techniques for the use of this relatively new, and still very exciting technology. No doubt this book will contribute to the increased clinical use of MRI, as well as to further technical research.

It has been an honor to be involved in this translation of this fine book. I would like to thank my colleague, Dr Andrew Grainger for the time and effort he put into reviewing and revising the draft of the translation. His careful reading and thoughtful revisions contributed greatly to the quality of this edition.

San Francisco, Summer 1999   *Harry K Genant*

Preface

In only a few years, MRI has become an established method in the diagnostic evaluation of musculoskeletal disorders, largely replacing conventional tomography, computed tomography, and nuclear medicine, and often providing information not previously available. MRI is still developing rapidly, with improved image displays and shorter acquisition times. In addition to technological advances, accumulated experience and a better understanding of the development of many diseases continue to enhance the diagnostic utility of MRI.

This book provides an overview of the application of MRI in the evaluation of the joints, including the temporomandibular joints, spine, bone marrow, and musculature. The principles of the available technologies, including opposed-phase echo technique, fast STIR sequence, and muscle spectroscopy, are also discussed. Because of the rapid developments in this field, the presented material might not always reflect the latest developments but should still provide adequate guidance for most clinical situations. Separate chapters cover the MRI findings observed in various conditions affecting the sacroiliac joints and the interesting findings when MRI is applied to the study of osteoporosis.

We wish to thank all the contributing authors for their cooperation and commitment, and we are indebted to the staff of Thieme for their professional guidance.

We hope that all physicians involved in musculoskeletal imaging will find this book helpful in applying MRI to the benefit of their patients.

Bonn/München, Summer 1999   *Martin Vahlensieck*
Maximilian Reiser

Contributors' Addresses

Matthias Bollow, M.D.
Institute of Radiographic
Diagnostics
Charité University Clinic
Berlin, Germany

Jürgen Braun, M.D.
Benjamin Franklin University Clinic
Rheumatology Section
Department of General Internal
Medicine and Nephrology
Free University of Berlin
Berlin, Germany

Beate M. Eitel, M.D.
Institute of Radiologic Diagnostics
Ludwig Maximilians University
Clinic
Munich, Germany

Roman Fischbach, M.D.
Institute and Clinic of Radiologic
Diagnostics
University of Cologne
Cologne, Germany

J. Gieseke
Philips Medical Systems
Hamburg, Germany

Stephan Grampp, M.D.
Radiodiagnostics Section
University Clinic Vienna
Vienna, Austria

Andreas Heuck, M.D.
University Clinic Großhadern
Institute of Radiologic Diagnostics
Munich, Germany

James O. Johnston
Clinical Professor of
Orthopedic Surgery
University of California
San Francisco
San Francisco, CA, USA

Phillip Lang, M.D.
Department of Radiology
University of California
Musculoskeletal Section
San Francisco
San Francisco, CA, USA

Günter Layer, M.D.
University Clinic for Radiology
Bonn, Germany

Götz Lutterbey, M.D.
University Clinic for Radiology
Bonn, Germany

P. Schnarkowski, M.D.
Radiotherapy and Radio-oncology
Section
Hanover Medical University
Hanover, Germany

Axel Stäbler, M.D.
Großhadern Clinic
Institute of Radiologic Diagnostic
Munich, Germany

M. Steinborn
Großhadern Clinic
Institute of Radiologic Diagnostics
Munich, Germany

F. Träber, M.D.
Radiologic University Clinic
Bonn, Germany

Peter Winter, M.D.
Clinical Assistant Professor
University of Illinois
College of Medicine at Peoria
Peoria, IL, USA

Contents

1 Technology of Magnetic Resonance Imaging 1

M. Vahlensieck, F. Träber, and J. Gieseke

2 Spine 19

G. Lutterbey and G. Layer

3 Shoulder 47

M. Vahlensieck

4 Elbow 77

B. M. Eitel and P. Schnarkowski

5 Wrist 105

A. Stäbler and M. Vahlensieck

6 Hip and Pelvis 137

M. Reiser and A. Heuck

7 Knee 163

M. Reiser and M. Vahlensieck

8 Ankle and Foot 213

M. Steinborn and M. Vahlensieck

9 Temporomandibular Joint   **241**
R. Fischbach

10 Musculature   **257**
M. Vahlensieck and G. Layer

11 Bone Marrow   **283**
M. Vahlensieck and G. Layer

12 Bone and Soft-Tissue Tumors

309

P. Lang, M. Vahlensieck, J. O. Johnston, and H. K. Genant

13 Osteoporosis   349

S. Grampp, M. Vahlensieck, P. Lang, and H. K. Genant

14 Sacroiliac Joints   355

M. Bollow and J. Braun

15 Appendix   377

M. Vahlensieck

Index   385

Technology of Magnetic Resonance Imaging

M. Vahlensieck, F. Träber and J. Gieseke

Introduction

This chapter will present the fundamental physics underlying the techniques used for magnetic resonance imaging (MRI) as applied to the musculoskeletal system. The discussion will be clinically oriented and focused on how the different techniques affect image contrast, signal-to-noise ratio, application and practicality. Readers who wish to learn more about the physics and techniques of imaging with magnetic resonance should refer to the appropriate literature.

To produce a magnetic resonance signal, the patient is placed in a strong external magnetic field (B_o). This outer magnetic field aligns the tissue's protons, which can be pictured as small magnets with their magnetic fields randomly oriented, parallel to the strong field (longitudinal magnetization M_z). When a suitable high frequency pulse (90 degree pulse) is applied, the magnetic fields of the protons change their orientation, with the change measurable as so-called transverse magnetization (M_{xy}). After the high frequency (radio frequency [RF]) pulse is turned off, the magnetic fields of the protons return to their original orientation parallel to the outer magnetic field. The transverse magnetization rapidly decays (free induction decay, FID) at a rate dependent on the homogeneity of the external magnetic field and on the tissue itself. This time for decay is given by the constant T_2^* (star) known as the effective T_2 time. Because of the rapid decay, measurement of the signal can only be made for a short time. To resolve this, further suitable RF pulses (180 degree pulses) can be applied producing additional signals. These are known as spin echoes (SE) and can be thought of as echoes of the original signal. They gradually decrease in intensity with time and the time constant for this decay is called the spin–spin or T_2 relaxation time. This decay is no longer dependent on external magnetic field heterogeneities and reflects only the intrinsic properties of the tissue being imaged. A second parameter characteristic to each tissue is the time for longitudinal magnetization to return after the 90 degree pulse has been applied. This is given by the T_1 time constant and the time is referred to as the spin-lattice or T_1 relaxation time. The final signal intensity detected by the MRI scanner is determined both by the T_1 and T_2 relaxation times, and also by the number of mobile protons present in the tissue. This third characteristic is known as the proton density.

To determine the spatial position of any unit (voxel) of tissue from which the signal is received, linear magnetic gradients are applied along the three axes. These are known as the slice, frequency, and phase-encoding gradients, and spatially encode the signal from each voxel with a characteristic frequency and phase. This spatial encoding assigns the magnetic resonance signal its spatial location, ultimately leading to the formation of a gray scale matrix. The gray scale position of each pixel is based on the signal intensity received from each voxel. The contribution made by these three factors to the image is determined by the parameters selected by the operator. In a T_1-weighted sequence, for instance, the parameters are selected to emphasize the differences in T_1 relaxation time between the different tissues being studied. The choice of sequences performed depends on the clinical question being asked.

The two most important parameters varied to alter the contrast weighting are the repetition time (the time between 90 degree pulses [TR]) and the echo time (the time between the 90 degree pulse and the detection of the spin echo [TE]).

Spin-Echo (SE) Sequences

■ T_1-weighted Sequences

T_1-weighted SE sequences have a repetition time shorter than the T_1 relaxation time of the tissue (TR < 700 ms) and a short echo time (TE < 20 ms). They are the basis of MR imaging of the connective tissue and musculoskeletal system. Fat and paramagnetic substances, such as some breakdown products of blood, exhibit a high signal intensity, muscles and most pathologic processes an intermediate signal intensity, and cortical bone and calcifications a low signal intensity. This sequence is less susceptible to artifacts and possesses a high signal-to-noise ratio. It is a helpful sequence for anatomical orientation and proves particularly useful for the identification of fat and hematoma. A T_1-weighted SE image should be part of any examination protocol.

■ Proton Density-weighted Sequences

Proton density-weighted SE sequences have a repetition time much longer than the T_1 relaxation time (TR < 1800 – 3000 ms) and a short echo time (TE 10 – 20 ms). These sequences are less important in MR imaging of the connective tissue and musculoskeletal system.

■ T₂-weighted Sequences

T_2-weighted SE sequences are produced by long T_1 relaxation times (TR < 1800–3000 ms) and long echo times (TE 80–120 ms). Fat and muscle are less signal intense than on T_1-weighted images. In contrast, fluid and most pathologic changes are of high signal intensity. Initially, this was the most important sequence for depicting pathologic changes. T_2 sequences are particularly susceptible to artifacts induced by motion or pulsation and are very time consuming. Today, essentially T_2-weighted images can be attained with other less time intensive techniques, such as fast (or turbo) spin-echo sequences and gradient echo sequences. These advanced imaging techniques have largely displaced the conventional SE sequences and will be described in more detail.

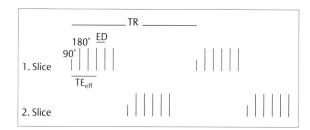

Fig. 1.**1**   Simplified scheme of the TSE sequence. Several echos of constant distance are produced by 180 degree impulses during the repetition time interval after the 90 degree pulse. The echo time determining the contrast is in the middle of the echo train and is referred to as effective echo time. By using the multi-slice technique, several slices can be interrogated at different times (for instance, two slice cases as illustrated here).
ED = echo distance
TR = repetition interval
TE_eff = effective echo time

Fast (or Turbo) Spin Echo (TSE) Sequences, RARE

Fast spin echo sequences have evolved from rapid acquisitions with relaxation enhancement (RARE) (16) and from multiple-echo multiple-shot sequences (MEMS) (22). They are essentially SE sequences with multiple spin echoes within the repetition time (TR interval), creating the echoes by an echo train of 180 degree pulses (Fig. 1.1). These are based on standard spin-echo sequences, but multiple echoes are obtained by the application of a train of 180 degree pulses within a single repetition time. Each echo is then separately phase encoded so multiple data for the spatial encoding process can be acquired in a single TR. In comparison to conventional SE sequences, the acquisition time is reduced by a factor corresponding to the number of 180 degree pulses per excitation (echo train length [ETL], turbo factor [TF]). The distance between the echo pulses is referred to as echo spacing (ES). While the echo train length can be arbitrarily selected between 3 to 128, an echo train length of 3 to 16 is characteristically used for examinations of the connective tissue and musculoskeletal system. The image contrast is determined by the echoes of the low order phase encoding, expressed as effective echo time.

The maximum echo train length (achieving the shortest acquisition time) is not feasible for all examinations. In bone marrow imaging, for instance, the fat signal can become unusually intense in comparison with conventional SE sequences because of spin coupling, effective rephasing and magnetization transfer effects. This phenomenon is more pronounced with shorter echo spacing and a low magnetic field strength.

The time saved by the shortened acquisition time of fast echo sequences can also be used to improve resolution or signal-to-noise ratio, or both, while maintaining an acceptable acquisition time. Using conventional sequences, comparable images can only be achieved with relatively long acquisition times (25 minutes and more).

The fast spin-echo sequence images have a few peculiarities that are relevant to the musculoskeletal system. Fat appears bright on fast echo sequence images compared with conventional SE. This can interfere with the detection of pathological processes in the immediate vicinity of fatty tissue, primarily in the extremities. Depending on the clinical question, this potentially undesirable side effect can be ameliorated by shortening the echo train length, with correspondingly less time saving, or by frequency-selective fat suppression (47) (Fig. 1.**2**). Another aspect of fast spin-echo sequences is the decreased sensitivity to susceptibility effects and, especially with a high echo train length, some blurring (rippling) of the images (43).

Fast spin-echo sequences showed good results in musculoskeletal MR imaging in a comparison with conventional spin-echo sequences (50), and fast SE sequences, particularly when combined with fat suppression techniques, are now widely used in place of conventional T_2 SE sequences.

Gradient-Echo (GRE) Sequences

Rather than using 180 degree rephasing pulses, the gradient-echo sequence produces the image-forming signal by *gradient reversal*. Furthermore, reducing the flip angles can change the image contrast. Three parameters must be considered in gradient-echo imaging: repetition time, echo time, and flip angle. Gradient-echo sequences permit markedly shorter acquisition times than spin-echo techniques.

Gradient echo sequences employ rephasing gradients in place of the 180 degree rephasing pulses

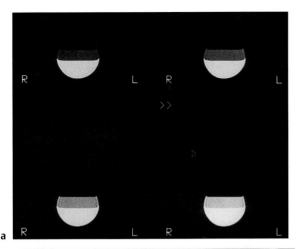

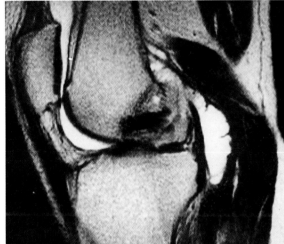

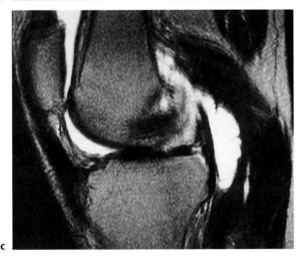

Fig. 1.**2a–c** **a** TSE sequences of a fat-water phantom with TR = 3000, TE$_{eff}$ = 100 msec. Fat above, NaCl solution below. Same window setting. Left above ETL = 3, right above ETL = 6, left below ETL = 9, right below ETL = 12. The signal intensity clearly increases with increasing ETL. **b** The TSE sequence of the knee with TR = 3000 msec, TE$_{eff}$ = 100, ETL = 12. **c** ETL = 3, same window setting. Large Baker cyst, joint effusion. With an ETL of 3, the fluid-to-fat contrast is higher.

ETL = echo train length (number of echoes)

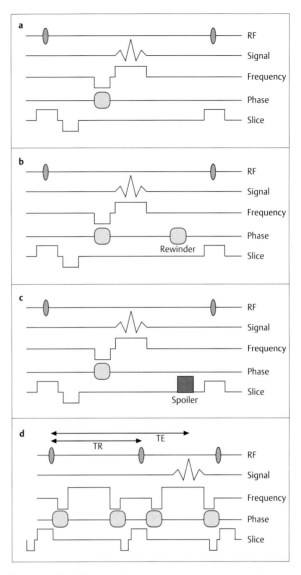

Fig. 1.**3a–d** Scheme of four basic GRE sequences. **a** Simple GRE sequence. **b** Steady state GRE. **c** Spoiled GRE. **d** Contrast enhanced GRE. The upper line represents the excitation radiofrequency, the second line the corresponding received signal, the third line the frequency encoding gradient and fifth line the slice gradient.

RF = radiofrequency pulse
TE = echo time
TR = repetition time interval

that are used in spin echo imaging. In addition flip angles of less than 90 degrees are used. These two factors allow the use of shorter TRs than are possible with spin-echo imaging, and result in shorter image acquisition times.

Four GRE techniques can be distinguished (7) (Fig. 1.**3**):

The most **basic gradient echo technique** (Fig. 1.**3a**) fundamentally corresponds to a SE sequence, except for the missing 180-degree rephasing pulse. This is one of the earliest techniques and is degraded by many artifacts. It is rarely used today.

The **steady-state GRE sequences** (Fig. 1.**3b**) produce a steady state of longitudinal and transverse magnetization of the tissue. This steady state is maintained through the application of a so-called rewinder gradient. Image contrast depends on the ratio or mixed weighting of the T_2 and T_1 relaxation times. This only applies to intermediate flip angles (10–40 degrees), short repetition times (<250 msec) and short echo times (<18 msec). The image contrast for small flip angles (<5 degrees) has a proton density weighting regardless of the GRE technique used. A large flip angle (>40 degrees) results in a dominant T_2 weighting and long echo times in T_2^* weighting (effective T_2), producing a contrast proportional to free induction decay (FID).

The **spoiled GRE technique** is based on the destruction of the residual transverse magnetization by a so-called spoiler gradient or high frequency pulse (Fig. 1.**3c**).

Since the transverse magnetization does not reach a steady state, the tissue contrast depends on T_1 relaxation time and produces a T_1-weighted image. With extreme flip angles or long echo times, the above mentioned factors do have an effect on image weighting. With a long TR (>250 msec) complete dephasing of transverse spins can occur (TR is now longer than T_2) eliminating the need for a spoiler gradient.

The **contrast-enhanced GRE** technique samples the echo that is induced by the second 90 degree RF pulse within an acquisition sequence. It is basically a spin echo (SE), but with the difference that no separate 180 degree RF pulse is applied and a gradient reversal is used instead. The nominal echo time of this technique is longer than its repetition time. Because of the strong T_2 contrast, the term contrast-enhanced GRE was given to this sequence (Fig. 1.**3d**). Since this technique passes over late spin echo, its signal-to-noise ratio (SNR) is low. The contrast-enhanced GRE technique has not proved useful in routine applications.

Table 1.**1** shows a summary of the image contrast of the different gradient-echo sequence techniques. Different manufacturers use their own nomenclature. The most important acronyms are listed in Table 1.**2**.

A common feature of all GRE sequences is that, in contrast to the SE sequences, the gradient rephasing of

Table 1.1 Simplified guidelines for achieving specific contrast with GRE sequences

Rho	small flip angle
T_1	large flip angle
T_2	CE-GRE
Mixed (T_2/T_1)	steady state with short TE
T_2^*	long TE

Rho	= proton density
T_1	= T_1 relaxation time
T_2	= T_2 relaxation time
Mixed	= contrast depending on T_2/T_1
T_2^*	= effective T_2 relaxation time
TE	= echo time
CE-GRE	= contrast-enhanced GRE

the signal serves to correct phase shifts induced by the gradient itself. This contributes to the image contrast. In particular, it increases the expression of susceptibility artifacts with longer echo times as well as the sensitivity to the different phase encoding of fat and water protons. The difference in the phases of fat and water is based on the difference between the resonance frequency of these signal components (Fig. 1.**4**). The phase of the particular component depends on the echo time and, depending on the relative phase of the two components, an image can be in-phase, out-of-phase or in opposed-phase, with adding of the in-phase and subtraction of the opposed-phase signal intensities (Fig. 1.**5**). Pixels containing a certain ratio of fat and water protons exhibit oscillating signal intensities related to the echo times. A 1 : 1 ratio and an echo time in opposed-phase can extinguish the signal, referred to as etching artifact or chemical shift of the second kind. The oscillation period between in-phase and opposed-phase echo times is proportionate to the difference between the resonance frequency Δ_f of fat and water (3.2–3.5 ppm) and therefore also depends on the magnetic field strength (period in msec = $1000/\Delta_f$). The oscillation period is about:

- 19.7 msec for 0.35 T($\Delta_f \approx 51$ Hz)
- 13.8 msec for 0.5 T($\Delta_f \approx 72$ Hz)
- 6.9 msec for 1.0 T($\Delta_f \approx 144$ Hz)
- 4.6 msec for 1.5 T($\Delta_f \approx 271$ Hz).

With longer echo times, the oscillation period for fat and other composite tissues increasingly deviates from

Table 1.2   Acronyms for the four basic GRE techniques from several manufacturers

Manufacturer	Basic GRE types	Spoiled GRE	Steady-state GRE	Contrast-enhanced GRE
Siemens	–	FLASH	FISP	PSIF
Picker	FE	PSR	FAST	CE-FAST
Philips	–	CE-FFE T_1	FFE	CE-FFE T_2
GRE	MPGR	SPGR	GRASS	SSFP
Toshiba	PFI	–	FE	–
Elscint	–	SHORT	F-SHORT	E-SHORT

the theoretical values of the dual water–methylene complex since these tissues have additional resonance peaks (e.g., protons adjacent to double bindings, methylene and carboxyl groups) that can lead to inaccuracies (Fig. 1.**6**). For this reason, different MR units have to be calibrated individually for optimal opposed-phase echo times.

Opposed-phase GRE-images are highly sensitive to visualizing hematopoietic bone marrow (20) and pathologic bone marrow lesions (Fig. 1.**7**).

Because of the high signal intensity, steady-state GRE sequences have proved useful for the acquisition of three-dimensional data sets with subsequent *multiplanar reformatting*, especially for the evaluation of joints. Spoiled GRE with short repetition times (TR = 40–50 msec), short echo times (TE = 5–10 msec) and intermediate flip angle (Θ = 30–60 degree) combined

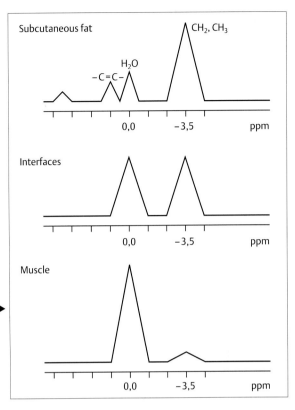

Fig. 1.**4** Diagram of the proton spectrum of subcutaneous fat ▶ and musculature. Pixels along the interface between fat and water show about equal contribution of both components.
C = C-   = double binding predominantly in unsaturated fatty acids
H_2O = water
CH_2, CH_3 = methylene and methyl groups
ppm   = parts per million

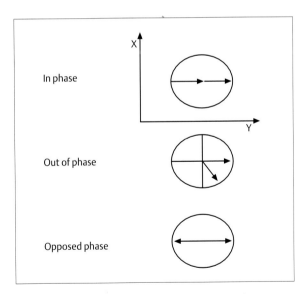

Fig. 1.**5** Signal vectors of fat and water in the XY planes in GRE sequences. Different phases of the fat and water vectors with different echo times. For pixels with fat and water components the signal intensities are added in-phase and subtracted in opposed-phase.

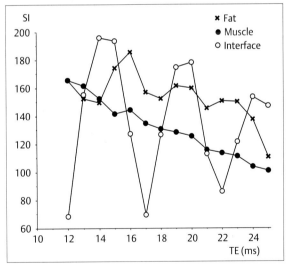

Fig. 1.**6** Signal intensities of fat, muscle, and fat–muscle interface in relation to an echo time of 1.5 T for GRE sequences. Muscle shows no signal oscillation and fat only minor oscillation. The interface exhibits a marked signal oscillation at a slightly different oscillation frequency. This difference can be explained by the spectra (see Fig. 1.**4**) since the spectrum of subcutaneous fat has several peaks (multiple component system) and not just two major peaks (two component system) as found, for instance, in pixels along the interface. The signal maximum is referred to as in-phase and the minimum of opposed-phase echo time.
SI = signal intensity
TE = echo time

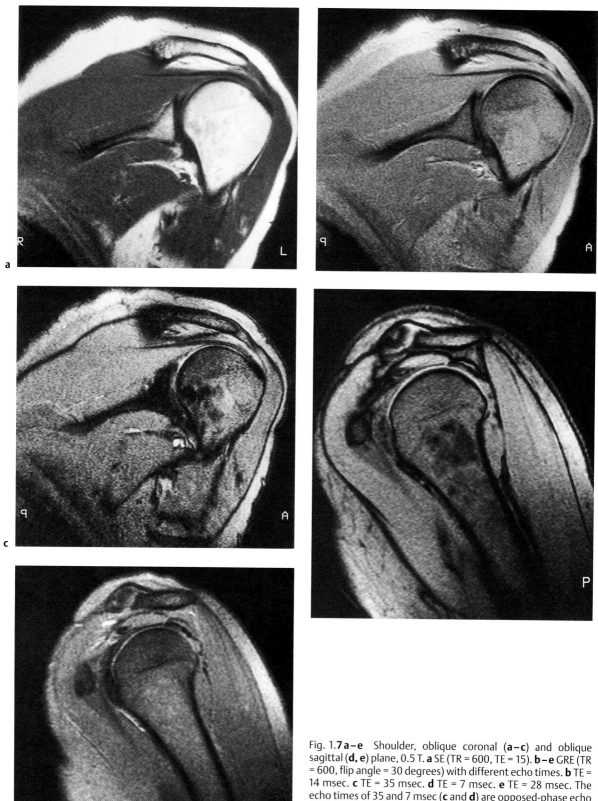

Fig. 1.**7 a–e** Shoulder, oblique coronal (**a–c**) and oblique sagittal (**d, e**) plane, 0.5 T. **a** SE (TR = 600, TE = 15). **b–e** GRE (TR = 600, flip angle = 30 degrees) with different echo times. **b** TE = 14 msec. **c** TE = 35 msec. **d** TE = 7 msec. **e** TE = 28 msec. The echo times of 35 and 7 msec (**c** and **d**) are opposed-phase echo times with low signal intensity of the hematopoietic bone marrow and signal-void fat–muscle interface (etching artifact). With 14 and 26 msec, fat and water protons are in-phase (**b** and **e**).

with fat suppression is useful for *visualizing cartilage.* Spoiled or steady-state GRE sequences with long repetition times (TR = 450 – 600 msec), two echo times (short in-phase echo, long out-of phase echo) and medium flip angle (Θ = 25 – 30 degree) have generally proved useful for the evaluation of the musculoskeletal system (dual echo GRE) (Fig. 1.**7**) (39). The short echo produces a strong signal for visualizing the anatomy and the second echo a strong $T_2{}^*$ contrast for detecting pathologic changes. We have found this sequence useful for routine examinations of the musculoskeletal system as long as the interpretation accounts for peculiarities of the GRE images, such as increased susceptibility effects, especially of the second echo, and dephasing effects, which can cause an apparent magnification of calcifications or disk prolapses.

Ultra-Fast MR Techniques

In the recent past, numerous new sequences with very short acquisition times have been proposed (Table 1.**3**), some of which are still under investigation. In the musculoskeletal system, the high temporal resolution achieved with ultra-fast MR sequences can be used for cinematic motion analysis of the joints (see below) and for dynamic contrast-enhanced imaging.

Low Field Strength Imaging

A low magnetic field strength is used with dedicated extremity MRI systems, which image the extremity of interest by placing it within the magnetic bore while the rest of the body remains outside the field. Images obtained with a low magnetic field strength have a lower signal-to-noise ratio, which may necessitate longer imaging times and decrease spatial resolution. The longer imaging times are partially offset by the gain in acquisition time due to shorter T_1 values at lower field strength. Furthermore, contrast-to-noise ratio, which is clinically more relevant since it determines the conspicuity of the lesions, does not decrease significantly with a low magnetic field strength (4 a). Low field strengths are less susceptible to magnetic heterogeneity, but diminish spectral separation (chemical shift) and restrict spectral suppression.

Table 1.**3**   Fast GRE sequences

Sequence	Abbreviation	Acquisition time per slice
Fast GRE	TFE, Snapshot GRE, Turbo FLASH	1 – 4 sec
GRE and SE	GRASE	300 – 100 msec
Echo planar sequence	EPI	50 – 100 msec

Though dedicated extremity MRI systems with a low field strength are increasingly finding use in the armamentarium of musculoskeletal imaging, at the present time the clinical performance of low field strengths is still awaiting the assessment of diagnostic parameters, including sensitivity, specificity and receiver-operating characteristic curve analysis.

◼ Fat Suppression

Fat suppression sequences are useful in detecting subtle bone and soft tissue injuries as well as inflammatory changes and masses (A), which otherwise might be obscured by a relatively high signal from fat. The fat signal can be suppressed by various techniques, each with its advantages and disadvantages (4 b).

Dixon fat suppression. This method takes advantage of the chemical shift of fat and water protons, and pure fat and pure water images can be acquired by the different echo times. It is susceptible to magnetic field heterogeneities and is rather time consuming since it requires a minimum of two data acquisitions. For special questions in the evaluation of bone marrow disorders, it can be used to quantify the fat and water content. It has not become established in routine imaging and is virtually never used today.

Chemical shift or frequency-selective saturation. The fat protons can be saturated by a frequency-selective saturation pulse immediately before the echo-imaging pulse sequence. Since the subsequent signal no longer contains any component from fat protons, fat no longer contributes to the image formation. The frequency-selective pulse can be combined with any sequence. This technique can be used for special clinical questions, such as the differentiation of fat-containing tumor components from blood. It provides an excellent contrast for the visualization of cartilage (Fig. 1.**8**). The use of fat saturation is particularly advantageous in conjunction with fast spin echo T_2-weighted sequences where fat otherwise is of higher intensity than is seen with conventional SE T_2-weighted imaging. Another important role for fat saturation is its use with intravenous gadolinium enhanced T_1-weighted images where areas of enhancement may otherwise be obscured by adjacent high intensity fat. Similarly it is helpful in conjunction with T_1 images acquired after intra-articular gadolinium instillation in direct MR arthrography. If used in the shoulder, it increases sensitivity for detecting rotator cuff tears.

Fat suppression techniques have not been found useful for routine examinations of juxta-articular soft tissues (46).

Short T_1 inversion recovery (STIR). The inversion recovery sequence consists of an inverting 180 degree pulse that precedes the signal producing 90 degree and 180 degree pulses. The time to inversion between the

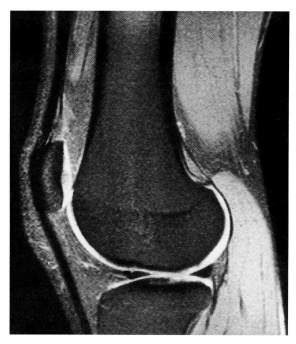

Fig. 1.**8**   Knee, sagittal plane. The SE sequence (TR = 600, TE = 15) with selective fat suppression, 1.5 T. Especially high signal intensity of the cartilage.

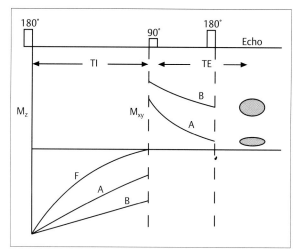

Fig. 1.**9**   STIR sequence. Schematic diagram of the longitudinal magnetization after the 180 degree inversion pulse and transverse magnetization of fat (F) after the 90 degree pulse in tissue with short T_1 and T_2 relaxation time (A) and in tissue with long T_1 and T_2 relaxation time (B). Fat has no longitudinal magnetization and produces no signal during the subsequent course of the sequence. At the time of the 90 degree pulses, tissue A has a lower longitudinal magnetization than tissue B and shows a faster decay of transverse magnetization, resulting in a signal intensity that is higher for B than for A. This is called additive T_1/T_2 contrast. It explains the high sensitivity of STIR sequences for detecting edema and other pathologic conditions.

A   = tissue with short T_1 and T_2 relaxation time
B   = tissue with long relaxation times
F   = fat
TE   = echo time
TI   = inversion time
M_z = longitudinal magnetization
M_{xy} = transverse magnetization

inverting 180 degree pulse and the 90 degree pulse affects the image contrast and is referred to as tau. By selecting a short tau (dependent on the external magnetic field strength), such that the longitudinal magnetization of fat has decayed to 0 at the time the 90 degree pulse is applied (the so-called null point), the signal from fat is eliminated (Fig. 1.**9**).

Inversion recovery sequences are sensitive to both long T_1 and T_2 times and have an additive effect. This enables the visualization of pathologic changes, such as edema or tumor, with better contrast (48).

Numerous studies have supported the superiority of such a sequence for disorders of the musculoskeletal system. Bone marrow edema or soft tissue infections can be delineated with exquisite contrast. The acquisition time can be shortened by modifying STIR, such as shortening of the repetition and inversion times (fast STIR) (48) (Fig. 1.**10**), or by combining it with the turbo technique (TSE-STIR).

While STIR images have excellent contrast, they suffer from a low signal-to-noise ratio. It is a potentially misleading disadvantage that STIR is not specific for fat. Signal tissue with a T_1 signal similar to that of fat will also be suppressed. In particular this includes structures that have been enhanced with gadolinium. This makes the STIR sequence inappropriate for use following administration of i.v. gadolinium. Furthermore, tissue with a short T_1 and tissue with a long T_1 may have the same signal intensity. The advantage of STIR is its insensitivity to magnetic field inhomogeneity and its suitability for low-field-strength magnets.

Opposed-phase Imaging. This technique is based on the phase differences of the magnetization vector in the transverse plane (25 b, 5 a). Because of the different resonance frequencies of fat protons and water protons, the phase relative to each other changes with time after excitation. The signals can be sampled when they are in-phase or in opposed-phase, with the signal intensity additive for in-phase signals and subtractive for opposed-phase signals. By selecting the appropriate echo time, the sampled signal can be lowered by the signal from the fatty tissue.

The fat suppression of the opposed-phase technique is most suitable for imaging tissues with similar amounts of fat and water. Opposed-phase imaging is fast and readily available, but generally applicable only to gradient-echo sequences. After administration of contrast material, enhancement can be undetectable or cause a paradoxical increase in fat suppression (25 a).

Water excitation. This is a new technique that uses combinations of radio frequency pulses to excite water only, with the spins of the fatty protons left in equi-

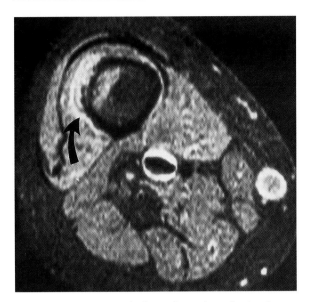

Fig. 1.10 Metastasis to the femur from a bronchoalveolar carcinoma. Fast STIR sequence with 0.5 T (TR = 1000 msec, TI = 100 msec, TE = 15). In addition to the signal-intense osseous component, the extraosseous component and the cortical erosion are visualized. Signal-intense peritumorous reactive zone (arrow).

librium and without producing a signal (14). This technique is still under investigation.

Contrast Enhancement, Dynamic Enhanced Imaging

Routine intravenous application of gadolinium-containing contrast agents is not part of the diagnostic evaluation of the musculoskeletal system, but a few indications have become established, such as the assessment of chronic inflammatory conditions and the differentiation between liquid and solid components and between edema and infiltration in primary and secondary musculoskeletal tumors (33, 36). However the use of dynamic enhancement studies may be required to distinguish edema from infiltration since only edema will enhance with intravenous gadolinium (8, 20a, 36).

Dynamic Gd-DTPA-enhanced MR imaging with fast GRE sequences can assist with the differentiation between malignant and benign tumors (8). The qualitative lesion specification was not impressive in a pilot study for characterization of musculoskeletal masses (25), and dynamic enhancement has not found a place in the routine evaluation of musculoskeletal neoplasms.

Direct MR Arthrography

The direct intra-articular injection of an 1 : 250 diluted Gd-DTPA solution distends the joint capsule and outlines the intra-articular structures. Gadolinium arthro-

graphy has been found to improve the assessment of several conditions, such as rotator cuff tears, avulsions of the glenoid labrum or cartilaginous defects of the knee (17, 31). Improved visualization of the intra-articular structures can also be achieved by capsular distension after intra-articular injection of a normal saline solution (so-called saline arthrography). Since either method of direct arthrography is invasive and time consuming, it should be used selectively and added only when conventional MRI is inconclusive.

Indirect MR Arthrography

An arthrographic effect can also be achieved with joint fluid enhancement following intravenous injection of Gd-DTPA. The T_1-weighted signal intensity in the joint fluid increases due to intra-articular diffusion of intravascular Gd-DTPA. This method is referred to as indirect MR arthrography since no articular puncture is required. The intra-articular diffusion is slow and the maximal enhancement is attained after 1 hour. Exercising the joint (for about 5 – 10 minutes) can markedly increase the intra-articular passage of Gd-DTPA (51) (Fig. 1.11). The enhancement is most apparent with fat suppression and the paramagnetically sensitive T_1 sequences (Fig. 1.12). The Gd-DTPA is injected in a concentration of 0.1 mmol/kg body weight.

MR arthrography has been used in the evaluation of the knee (6), ankle and shoulder (41, 51 – 54). It has been found superior to conventional MRI in evaluating menisci, surgically altered menisci and disks, and possibly also in staging osteochondritis dissecans (51). Indirect MR arthrography does not distend the joint

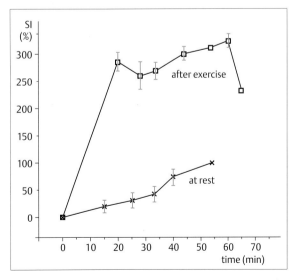

Fig. 1.11 Indirect MR arthrography. Signal intensity in the joint space of the ankle after IV injection of 0.1 mmol/kg Gd-DTPA. Slow increase in signal at rest. Rapid and more intense increase after exercise (10 minute walk).

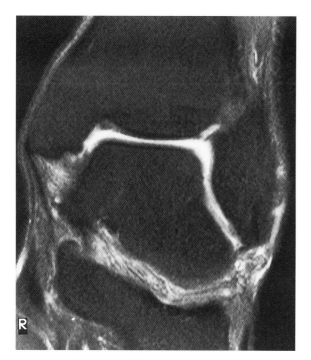

Fig. 1.**12** Indirect MR-arthrography (0.1 mmol/kg Gd-DTPA, 10 minute joint motion, chemical shift fat suppression, TR = 600, TE 20, SE sequence) of the ankle. High signal visualization of the joint space. Moderate signal intensity of the cartilage. Subtle irregularities along the cartilage of the fibulotalar articulation.

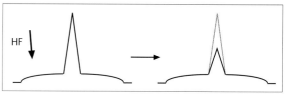

Fig. 1.**13** Saturation of the broad resonance signal of the protons bound to macromolecules with resultant reduction of the resonance signal of the free protons by magnetization transfer. RF = radio frequency pulse

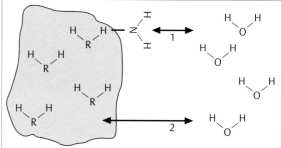

Fig. 1.**14** Chemical exchange (1) and dipolar coupling (2) between protons bound to macromolecules (left) and free protons (right).

capsule. The distension of the joint capsule occurring with direct arthrography has proved advantageous in the evaluation of numerous conditions, such as injuries of the glenoid labrum of the shoulder. Extra-articular enhancement of bursae and tendon sheaths observed on indirect MR arthrography should not be mistaken for extra-articular extension of contrast medium. Such misinterpretations can be avoided with experience, and bursal enhancement may even prove to be advantageous (for instance, in the evaluation of superior rotator cuff of the shoulder). Especially on delayed images, the vascular enhancement is markedly less pronounced than the intra-articular enhancement.

Magnetization Transfer Contrast (MTC)

In addition to the resonance peak for the protons of unbound water, the proton spectrum of biologic tissues has a broad-based flat resonance corresponding to protons bound to macromolecules. Conventional MR imaging uses the peak of the unbound protons. If the broad base of the bound protons is saturated, the resonance peak of the unbound protons changes without any direct effect on the unbound protons (Fig. 1.13). This process constitutes a shortening of the longitudinal magnetization, the so-called magnetization transfer, and, to a lesser degree, a shortening of the T_1 relaxation

time of the water proton peak, the so-called cross relaxation. The visible changes of the proton peak can be attributed to the chemical interaction between the freely moving and immobile protons along the compartmental interfaces (Fig. 1.14).

Two methods can be used to achieve magnetization transfer contrast (MTC): on-resonance or off-resonance. The *on-resonance* method applies special composite pulses to saturate the bound protons (H_b). Each composite pulse consists of a series of individual pulses that are equal in length but different in phase. The individual pulses have the resonance frequency of the mobile water protons (H_f) (Fig. 1.15). Short pulses cancel the saturation effects on the mobile protons due to phase reversal of the high frequency and long T_2 relaxation time, without any direct effect on the longitudinal magnetization. Because of the long T_2 time, the magnetization of the bound protons relaxes during the pulsed excitation. The alternating phases of the pulses prevent a complete restoration of the initial condition of the magnetization of the bound protons. This induces a magnetization transfer. Such a composite pulse is referred to as binomial pulse. Each pulse in the group must be short to avoid direct saturation of the mobile protons (for instance, 0.9 msec with an excitation angle of 180–390 degrees). A composite pulse characteristically consists of 2, 4, or 8 elements with alternating phases. The phase is indicated by + 1 and – 1 (also by 1 and a dash over the 1, respectively) corresponding to the cos 0 degree = 1 and cos 180 degree = – 1.

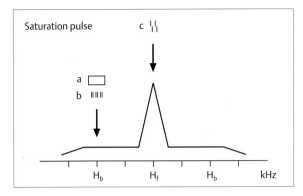

Fig. 1.**15** Techniques of producing magnetization transfer contrast.
a Continuous wave off-resonance pulse. **b** Pulsed off-resonance pulse. **c** composite pulse on resonance pulse.
H_b = pool of bound protons
H_t = pool of free protons

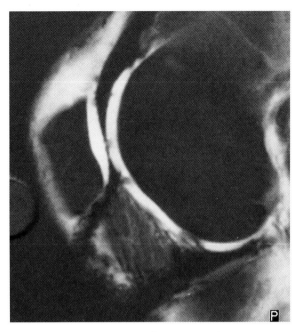

Fig. 1.**16** Magnetization transfer contrast subtraction image of the knee. Good visualization of superficial lesions of the cartilage. Tissue without magnetization transfer contrast is seen as black structures.

The *off-resonance* method saturates the pool of bound protons with a high frequency pulse, with the frequency 1–20 kHz below or above the resonance frequency of the mobile water protons (for instance, – 1.5 kHz frequency shift with a pulse length of 50 msec and an excitation angle of 1770 degrees). This results in the desired interaction between the compartments of mobile and bound protons. *Continuous wave* off-resonance MTC imaging refers to a very long (20–4000 msec), low energy ($B_1 \approx 9\,\mu T$) pulse and *pulsed* off-resonance MTC imaging to several short (1–9 msec), high energy (B_1 20 μT) pulses (Fig. 1.**15**).

Both MTC techniques afford a sharp contrast that is largely independent of the magnetic field strength (56). To generate MTC images, the above mentioned pulses can be combined with any conventional MR sequence, though the best contrast is achieved with GRE sequences.

The image contrast generated in this way differs from the contrast based on different relaxation times and proton densities. Muscle, cartilage, tendon, and cerebral parenchyma are tissues with a strong magnetization transfer effect, which can be quantified and expressed as MT ratio. Fat and water lack a magnetization transfer effect (Table 1.**4**). This method could be found to enhance cartilage lesions and intrasubstance degeneration in vitro (49), but clinical experience with

this image contrast is still limited. Subtracting the MTC image from an image without MTC furnishes an image with signal intensities proportional to the magnetization transfer effect (*MTC subtraction*), which visualizes superficial lesions of the cartilage very well (Fig. 1.**16**) (42). MTC suppresses the magic angle phenomenon seen in tendons obliquely oriented to the direction of the magnetic field (Fig. 1.**17**). The MTC of cartilaginous tumors does not differ substantially from that of other tumors (Fig. 1.**18**). The high MTC of scar tissue might harbor the potential of advancing the search for recurrent tumor. No real difference in MTC is found between benign and malignant tumors (48) (Table 1.**5**). In addition, MTC can enhance MR angiography by suppressing the background signal.

Tabelle 1.**4** Average MT ratio of different tissue of the musculoskeletal system of healthy subjects (n = 9) in % ± standard deviation. 1.5 T, GRE sequence TR = 400 msec, TE = 10 msec, flip angle = 30 degrees, off-resonance pulse (frequency shift -1.5 kHz, pulse length 50 msec, excitation angle = 1770 degree). Fibrous connective tissue = menisci, patellar ligament, glenoid labrum, biceps tendon, rotator cuff, ulnar disc, flexion tendons.

Tissue	Fibrous connective tissue	Cartilage	Muscle	Subcutaneous fat	Fatty bone marrow	Water
MT ratio	45 ± 6	50 ± 6	54 ± 8	0.3 ± 6	3 ± 5	−1.5 ± 4

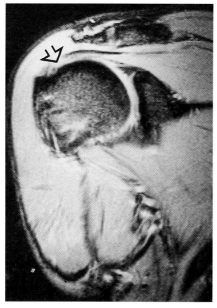
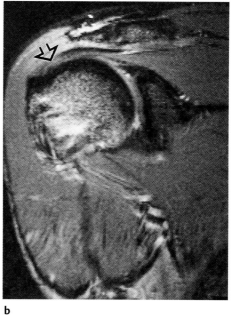

a   b

Fig. 1.**17 a, b**   Shoulder, oblique coronary plane. **a** GRE sequence (TR = 600 msec, TE = 18 msec, flip angle = 30 degrees). **b** Magnetization transfer contrast sequence with same parameters and window setting otherwise. Clear signal reduction of the artificially signal increase of the rotator cuff (magic angle phenomenon) caused by magnetization transfer contrast (arrow).

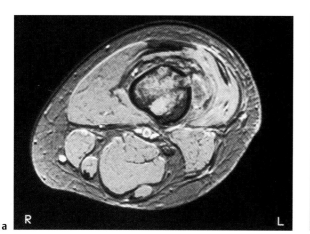
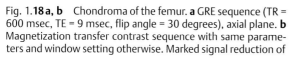
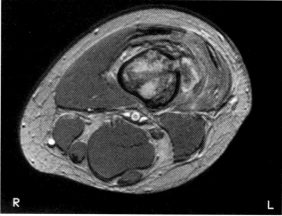

a   b

Fig. 1.**18 a, b**   Chondroma of the femur. **a** GRE sequence (TR = 600 msec, TE = 9 msec, flip angle = 30 degrees), axial plane. **b** Magnetization transfer contrast sequence with same parameters and window setting otherwise. Marked signal reduction of muscle with contrast reversal of the fatty tissue, moderate signal reduction of the tumor. Cortical defect and muscle changes following biopsy.

Table 1.**5**   Average MT ratio of different diseases of the musculoskeletal system in % $\pm$ standard deviation. 1.5 T, GRE sequence TR = 400 msec, TE = 10 msec, flip angle = 30 degrees, off-resonance pulse (frequency shift -1.5 kHz, pulse length 50 msec, excitation angle = 1770 degree)

Entity	Benign tumors	Malignant tumors	Scars	Chondroid producing tumors	Ganglions	Bone cysts
MT ratio	26 $\pm$ 15	22 $\pm$ 6	39 $\pm$ 16*	29 $\pm$ 5	25 $\pm$ 1.5	13 $\pm$ 1*

* Significant difference

Diffusion-weighted and Perfusion-weighted Imaging

Diffusion-weighted imaging uses MRI to image and measure molecular diffusion. Diffusion images are obtained by applying two or more MR sequences that are identical except for different weighting to diffusion, i.e., to translational molecular motion.

Perfusion-weighted imaging is based on the contribution of microcirculation to signal attenuation. Some perfusion imaging methods are equivalent to conventional approaches by using paramagnetic susceptibility contrast agents. Other methods use the natural sensitivity of the flowing blood as internal marker, measuring the dephasing of the spin of the protons moving in a magnetic field gradient.

Both methods have found considerable interest in the research community and have already been applied to functional brain imaging. They have not yet found clinical applications in musculoskeletal MRI.

MR Angiography

The inflow of a bolus of unsaturated blood introduces a higher signal intensity than that of the surrounding stationary tissue. This time-of-flight effect may be utilized for angiographic visualization. The intravascular signal can also be altered by turbulent flow as well as by magnetic susceptibility and spin saturation. At certain sites, such as bifurcations, flow separation can lead to circular flow with a longer residence time in the vascular volume. This phenomenon produces undesirable partial spin saturation and a secondary decrease in signal intensity (10).

The visualization of vascular malformations tumor-feeding vessels is a relatively rare indication for MR angiography. With few exceptions, the vessels of the lower extremities can be adequately visualized. The blood flow is pulsatile with an extreme velocity range to the point of flow reversal with subsequent signal losses in small confined regions. Since the total diameter of all individual vessels added together is rather large, the flow in small caliber vessels might be too slow for a signal not obscured by the saturation effects. Overcoming this problem is only possible by improving the resolution at the expense of a reduced signal intensity and a considerably prolonged acquisition time. Surface coils can ameliorate the problem of signal reduction but do not eliminate it. Furthermore, pulsation often gives rise to displacement and local turbulence with signal loss. These artifacts can be mistaken for stenosis or thrombosis.

The gated inflow method is an elegant approach to circumvent the image deterioration caused by pulsatile flow (5, 12). This method synchronizes the data acquisition with the cardiac cycle. This is accomplished by selecting a gate of slow flow and consequently less artifactual variations in the EKG determined RR interval. The data are acquired over a number of cardiac cycles only during the selected gate until the data set is complete. The optimal delay of the gate relative to the R peak depends on the anatomical site of the vascular region of interest. The width of the gate also effects the image quality (Fig 1.**19**). For artifact-free visualization, the gate should encompass 70–80% of the RR-interval for the carotid arteries and 25–30% for the arteries of the lower leg (37). The gated-inflow technique suppresses the artifacts caused by retrograde or pulsatile flow and, furthermore, produces a sharper vascular outline.

The second technique used for MR angiography makes use of the flow-induced phase shift between blood and stationary tissue and is referred to as *phase contrast angiography*. Its value in the evaluation of the vessels of the extremities has not yet been definitively assessed.

Relaxometry, Relaxation-Time Maps

Determining the relaxation times, referred to as relaxometry, generally cannot enhance the specificity of MRI and plays no role in the routine diagnostic evaluation of the musculoskeletal system. For follow-up examinations of diffuse infiltrative disorders, it can be beneficial to measure the T_1 times to reveal interval changes since measurable changes of the relaxation times often do not translate into visible intensity changes of the signal. The relaxation times can be pictorially displayed, with the degree of brightness proportionate to measured times. Such displays are referred to as relaxation-time maps or T_1- and T_2-maps.

Three-dimensional Reconstruction

The three-dimensional reconstruction of two-dimensional images can be advantageous for certain conditions of the musculoskeletal system (44). These conditions include comminuted fractures and fractures of regions with a complex anatomy, such as the skull base or facial bones. This facilitates the planning of surgical reconstruction. Other applications include volumetric rendering of tumors to monitor the effect of radiotherapy and chemotherapy. Two basic techniques for the three-dimensional reconstruction can be identified:

- *Surface rendering*, simulating a virtual light source that illuminates the surface of the object, and
- *Volume rendering*, simulating a virtual light source that transmits the object (Fig. 1.**20**). A combination of both techniques (*hybrid rendering*) yields the best three-dimensional impression (45).

The three-dimensional presentation of CT data uses a threshold classification by setting a density value of a pixel (i.e., bone) for the three-dimensional display.

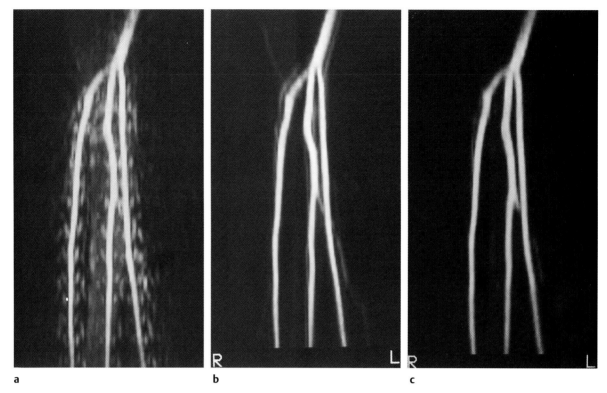

a   b   c

Fig. 1.**19a–c**   Arterial MR angiography of the lower leg with EKG-gated inflow, maximum intensity projection. TR = 23 msec, TE = 6.9 msec, flip angle = 60 degrees, signal acquisition = 1, matrix 128 × 256, FOV = 161 × 230 mm², 61 4 mm sections overlapping by 0.5 mm, caudal saturation, heart rate between 55 and 60/min. **a** Without EKG gating, acquisition time 2 min 18 s. **b** With EKG gating, data acquisition 500 msec with a delay of 150 msec after the R wave, acquisition time 5 min 7 s. **c** As in **b** but with smaller gate of 250 msec, acquisition time 8 min 7 s. Marked reduction of the artifacts with gating. With shorter gate (**c**) less pronounced pulsation artifacts, but longer acquisition time.

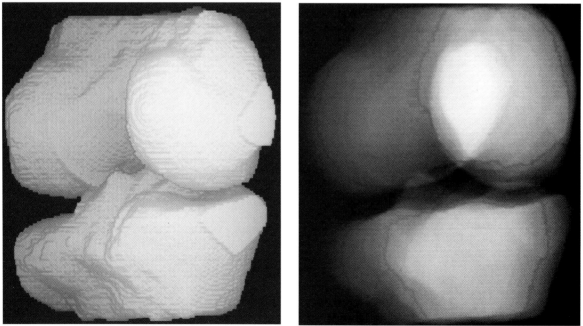

a   b

Fig. 1.**20a, b**   Three-dimensional visualization of MR data of the knee. **a** Surface rendering technique. **b** Volume rendering technique.

Fig. 1.**21** Knee, axial plane: Visualized planes of radial acquisition.

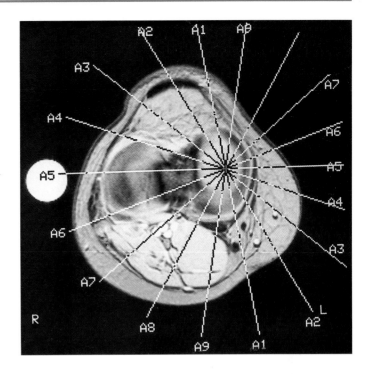

More complicated approaches are necessary for the three-dimensional presentation (segmentation) of MR data since the signal intensities can be quite dissimilar in the same tissue and tissues not intended to be displayed can show signal intensities similar to the object to be rendered three-dimensionally. For instance, subcutaneous fat and bone marrow can display a similar signal intensity. Thresholding alone would not be adequate for the segmentation of MR data. A combination of segmentation by thresholding and manual selection is generally applied (44). This requires the object designated for three-dimensional rendering to be manually extracted from the image display of the MR data. This is very time-consuming and error-prone. The three-dimensional visualization of MR data of the musculoskeletal system has not yet proved useful in daily clinical practice.

Multiplanar Reformation, Radial Acquisition

Multiplanar reformatting. The data set of an MR image sequence can be post-processed to obtain reformatted images in different planes, analogous to the re-formation of CT data. While the re-formation does not alter the image contrast, the spatial resolution of the reformatted images is related to the parameters of the original data set. If the voxel dimensions of the original data set are unequal (*anisotropic data set*), the spatial resolution of the reformatted images differs from the original image. If the voxel dimensions are equal (*isotropic data set*), the original image and reformatted image have identical spatial resolution. Computing the isotropic

data set from a large field of view at a high resolution, as in the case of a knee joint, is rather time consuming even when 3-D-transformed GRE sequences are used. Furthermore, most clinical questions require T_1- and T_2-weighted images. The generation of an isotopic data set with subsequent reformatting cannot be recommended for MRI of the musculoskeletal system. Reformatting of anisotopic data sets with inferior resolution of the computed images can be used to illustrate the extent of large tumors and to monitor the effect of therapy.

Radial Acquisition. This technique consists of a radial sequence of images, programmed to rotate at increments of several degrees around a central axis (27) (Fig. 1.**21**). Radial acquisition applied to the knee and shoulder failed to establish any advantage over standard image sections. This technique has not found a place in routine MRI evaluation of the musculoskeletal system.

Magnetic Resonance Spectroscopy (MRS) and Spectroscopic Imaging (SI)

Magnetic resonance spectroscopy is a time consuming, complicated technique that has still not entered the routine diagnostic armamentarium. Since it can provide specific metabolic information, it can be expected to advance and may play a role in the diagnostic evaluation of the musculoskeletal system in the future. Research in this area is intensive and promising results are on the horizon.

The technique gives information on tissue metabolism and biochemistry. It allows the estimation of different levels of molecules in the tissue under investigation. The technique is based on the subtle differences in resonant frequencies between protons or certain atoms depending on the molecule to which they are attached. These differences result from the differing magnetic environments created by the molecule to which the proton or atom is bound. Other than hydrogen, the most frequently studied atoms are phosphorus (^{31}P) and carbon (^{13}C).

Phosphorus spectroscopy is a particularly promising technique in musculoskeletal radiology since phosphorus is an important constituent of many of the metabolites in muscle. The technique allows the levels of these different metabolites in a tissue to be estimated. Anaerobic metabolites such as lactic acid can be assessed using hydrogen spectroscopy. In vivo levels of ^{13}C are low, making acceptable spectra more difficult to obtain. However, tracer studies have been performed with enriched ^{13}C-labeled glucose to determine the turnover rate of intermediary metabolites.

Cinematic Examinations

In numerous painful conditions of the joint, symptoms are only elicited if the joint is in a certain position. Conventional radiography can address these conditions by obtaining functional views. Functional MRI of the joint links the advantages of sectional imaging with functional assessment of the joint. An added benefit is the concurrent evaluation of the soft tissues that interact with the joint. Three different techniques can be applied for cinematic MRI.

- Static images are obtained with the joint in various positions and are reviewed in *cine mode*. These techniques require positioning devices that restrict the movement to a specified plane. MR images are obtained with the joint kept in the positioning device in a defined position. Usually, conventional SE or GRE sequences are selected, and the acquisition times are relatively long. Experience with this approach has been gathered for almost all major joints and the cervical spine. Nonferromagnetic positioning devices designed for the various joints, such as TM joint, knee, hand and ankle, are not commercially available everywhere and most published articles report the experience gathered with self-made devices (38). Movement of the joint is rather restricted in a closed MR unit and only a small range of the joint motion can be assessed. Open units allow a considerably wider range of motion and can examine shoulder, elbow and hip (24).
- *Motion-triggered* image acquisition during continuous motion. The joint moves and data acquisition is triggered by a pneumatic sensor, analogous to the respiratory and EKG gating for spatial localization for the suppression of motion artifacts (23). This technique can be combined with GRE or rapid GRE sequences.

- With very fast sequences, such as GRE, TSE, GRASE or EPI, functional imaging can be obtained in quasi real time. These techniques are under development and can be expected to improve cinematic examinations to the point of MR 'fluoroscopy'. This will lead to broader clinical indications.

Since articular incongruence due to imbalanced muscular contraction can predispose to dislocations and uneven cartilage wear, active-movement kinematic MRI with exercise (gated real-time examination) is a sensitive way of tracking joint movements (39, 40).

Cinematographic MR imaging has been performed in various regions. Cinematographic MR imaging of the cervical spine has provided relevant information of the impingement of the spinal cord (28). Specially designed positioning devices permit imaging in various degrees of flexion (26).

Positional changes of the periarticular soft tissues of the *shoulder* have been studied during rotation with the help of positioning devices specially designed for the shoulder (24). A possible application of the cinematography of the shoulder joint is the evaluation of the motion of the glenoid labrum in cases of suspected partial tears, especially, in detecting otherwise hard to diagnose superior or posterior partial tears. MR arthrography of the glenohumeral joint with the shoulder in external rotation optimizes the visualization of the biceps–labral complex (19a). Abduction with external rotation is the best position for evaluating the inferior glenohumeral ligament and anterior capsular attachment (19a). Open MR units are highly suitable for examining the shoulder in abduction and adduction, which is especially valuable in the assessment of position-dependent narrowing of the subacromial space in impingement syndrome.

Cinematographic examination of the *TM joints* is conducted with a positioning device that blocks the joints at specified mouth openings. The static images obtained at incremental mouth openings can be reviewed in cine mode. This technique can be applied to assess position-dependent disorders, such as lateral deviation, asymmetric movements or partial subluxation (38).

The *Wrist* and *ankle* have also been evaluated for motion studies, with ulnar and radial abduction of the wrist and dorsal and plantar flexion of the ankle. Cinematography can be conducted for carpal instability and position-dependent compression syndromes (38).

The most extensive experience has been with cinematography of the *knee*. This will be described in detail in Chapter 7.

References

A   ACR Standards 1998, p.427
1   Bachert, P., M. E. Bellemann, G. Layer, T. Koch, W. Semmler, W. J. Lorenz: In vivo 1 H, 31 P-(1 H) and 13 C-(1 H) magnetic resonance spectroscopy of malignant histiocytoma and skeletal muscle tissue in man. NMR Biomed. 5 (1992) 161 – 170
2   Bachert-Baumann, P., F. Ermark, H. J. Zabel, R. Sauter, W. Semmler, W. J. Lorenz: In vivo nuclear Overhauser effect in 31 P-(1 H) double-resonance experiments in a 1,5 T whole-body MR system. Magn. Reson. Med. 15 (1990) 165 – 172
3   Bárány, M., P. N. Venkatasubramanian, E. Mok, I. M. Siegel, E. Abraham, N. D. Wycliffe, M. F. Mafee: Quantitative and qualitative fat analysis in human leg muscle of neuromuscular diseases by 1H MR-spetroscopy in vivo. Magn. Reson. Med. 10 (1989) 210 – 226
4   Bendall, M. R., D. T. Pegg: Uniform sample excitation with surface coils for in vivo spectroscopy by adiabatic rapid half passage. J. Magn. Reson. 67 (1986) 376 – 381
4a Butt, B. K., D. E. Lee: The impact of field stength on image quality in MRI. J. Magn. Reson. Imaging 6 (1996) 57 – 62
4b Default, E. M., L. Betran, G. Johnson, J. Rosseau, X. Marchandise, A. Cotton: Fat suppression in MR imaging: Techniques and Pitfalls. RadioGraphics 19 (1999) 373 – 382
5   DeGraaf, R. G., J. P. Groen: MR angiography with pulsatile flow. Magn. Reson. Imag. 10 (1992) 25 – 34
5a Disler, D. G., T. R. McClauley, L. M. Ratner, C. D. Kesack, J. A. Cooper: Im-phase and out-of-phase imaging of bone marrow: prediction of neoplasia based on the detection of coexistent fat and water. Amer. J. Roentgenol. 169 (1997) 1071 – 1077
6   Drapé, J. L., P. Thelen, P. Gay-Depassier, O. Silbermann, R. Benacerraf: Intraarticular diffusion of Gd-DOTA after intravenous injection in the knee: MR imaging evaluation. Radiology 188 (1993) 277 – 234
7   Elster, A. D.: Gradient-echo MR imaging: techniques and acronyms. Radiology 186 (1993) 1 – 8
8   Erlemann, R., M. Reiser, P. E. Peters, P. Vasallo, P. Nommensen, R. Kusnierz-Glaz, R. Ritter, A. Roessner: Musculoskeletal neoplasms: static and dynamic Gd-DTPA-enhanced MR imaging. Radiology 171 (1989) 767 – 773
9   Frahm, J., H. Bruhn, M. L. Gyngell, K. D. Merbold, W. Hänicke, R. Sauter: Localized high resolution proton NMR spectroscopy using stimulated echos: initial applications to human brain in vivo. Magn. Reson. Med. 9 (1989) 79
10 Gieseke, J., B. Ostertun, L. Solymosi, F. Träber, P. van Dijk, M. Reiser: MR-Arterio und Venographie: Strategien zum Einsatz von 2D- und 3D-Inflow Verfahren. Biomed. Techn. 35 (1990) 247 – 248
11 Gordon, R. E., P. E. Hansley, D. Shaw, D. G. Gadian, G. K. Radda, P. Styles, P. J. Bore, L. Chen: Localization of metabolites using 31 P topical magnetic resonance. Nature 287 (1980) 736
12 Groen, J. P., R. G. DeGraaf, P. van Dijk: MR angiography based on inflow. Proc. SMR M 7 (1988) 906
13 Haase, A., J. Frahm, W. Hänicke, D. Mattei: 1H NMR chemical shift selective (CHESS) imaging. Phys. Med. Biol. 30 (1989) 341
14 Harms, S. E., D. P. Flaming, K. L. Hesley et al.: MR imaging of the breast with roatating delivery of excitation off resonance: clinical experience with pathologic correlation. Radiology 187 (1993) 493 – 501
15 Heerschap, A., P. R. Luyten, J. I. van der Heiden, P. Oosterwald, J. A. denHollander: Broatband proton decoupled natural abundance 13C NMR spectroscopy of humans at 1,5 T. NMR Biomed. 2 (1989) 124 – 132
16 Hennig, J., A. Nauerth, H. Friedburg: RARE imaging: a fast imaging method for clinical MR. Magn. Reson. Med. 3 (1986) 823 – 833
17 Hodler, J., S. Kursunoglu-Brahme, S. J. Snyder, V. Cervilla, R. P. Karzel, M. E. Schweitzer, B. D. Flannigan, D. Resnick: Rotator cuff disease: assessment with MR arthrography versus standard MR imaging in 36 patients with arthroscopic confirmation. Radiology 182 (1992) 431 – 436
18 Kimmich, R., G. Schnur, D. Hoepfel, D. Ratzel: Volume selective multi-pulse spinecho spectroscopy and selective supression of spectral lines. Phys. Med. Biol. 32 (1987) 1335 – 1343
19 Kuhl, C. K., G. Layer, F. Träber, S. Ziers, W. Block, M. Reiser: 31P exercise MR spectroscopy in mitochondrial encephalomyopathy: correlation with clinical findings. Radiology 192 (1994) 223 – 230
19a Kwak, S. M., R. R. Brown, D. Trudell, D. Resick, Glenohumeral joint: comparison of shoulder positions at MR arthrography. Radiology 208 (1998) 375 – 380.
20 Lang, P., R. Fritz, M. Vahlensieck, S. Majumdar, Y. Berthezene, S. Grampp, H. K. Genant: Residuales und rekonvertiertes hämatopoetisches Knochenmark im distalen Femur – Spinecho und gegenphasierte Gradientenecho-MRT. Fortschr. Röntgenstr. 156 (1992) 89 – 95
20a Lang, P., G. Honda, T. Roberts, M. Vahlensieck, J. O. Johnston, W. Rosenau, A. Mathur, C. Peterfy, C. A. Gooding, H. K. Genant: Musculoskeletal neoplasm: perineoplastic edema versus tumor on dynamic postcontrast MR images with spatial mapping of instantaneous enhancement rates. Radiology 197 (1995) 831 – 839
21 Luyten, P. R., A. J. H. Marien, W. Heindel, P. H. J. van Gerwen, K. Herholz, J. A. denHollander, G. Friedmann, W. D. Heiss: Metabolic imaging of patients with intracranial tumors: H-1 MR spectroscopic imaging and PET. Radiology 176 (1990) 791 – 799
22 Mehlkopf, A. F., P. van der Meulen, J. Smidt: A multiple-echo and multiple-shot sequence for fast NMR Fourier imaging. Magn. Reson. Med. 1 (1984) 295 – 297
23 Melchert, U. H., C. Schröder, J. Brossmann, C. Muhle: Motion triggered cine MR imaging of active joint movement. Magn. Reson. Imag. 10 (1992) 457 – 460
24 Minami, M., K. Yoshikawa, Y. Matsuoka, Y. Itai, T. Kokubo, M. Iio: MR study of normal joint function using a low field strength system. J. Comput Assist Tomogr 15 (1991) 1017 – 1023
25 Mirowitz, S. A., W. G. Totty, J. K. T. Lee: Characterization of muskuloskeletal masses using dynamic Gd-DTPA enhanced spin-echo MRI. J. Comput. assist. Tomogr. 16 (1992) 120 – 125
25a Mitchell, D. G., A. H. Stolpen, E. S. Siegelmann, L. Bolinger, E. K. Outwater: Fatty tissue on opposed-phase MR images: paradoxical suppression of signal intensity by paramagnetic contrast agents. Radiology 198 (1996) 351 – 357
25b Mitchell, D. M., I. Kim, T. S. Chang, et al.: Chemical shift phase-difference and suppression magnetic resonance imaging technique in animals, phantoms, and human fatty liver. Invest. Radiol. 26 (1991) 1041 – 1052
26 Muhle, C., U. H. Melchert, J. Brossmann, C. Schröder, J. Wiskirchen, M. Heller: Positionsgestell zur kinematographischen MRT der Halswirbelsäule. Fortschr. Röntgenstr. 162 (1995) 252 – 254
27 Munk, P. L., R. G. Holt, C. A. Helms, H. K. Genant: Glenoid labrum: preliminary work with use of radial-sequence MR imaging. Radiology 173 (1989) 751 – 753
28 Nägele, M., W. Koch, B. Kaden, B. Wöll, M. Reiser: Dynamische Funktions-MRT der Halswirbelsäule. Fortschr. Röntgenstr. 157 (1992) 222 – 228
29 Noggle, J. H., R. E. Schirmer: The Nuclear Overhauser Effect. Academic, San Diego 1971
30 Ordidge, R. J., A. Connelly, J. Lohman: Image-selective in-vivo spectroscopy (ISIS). J. Magn. Reson. 66 (1986) 283 – 294
31 Palmer, W. E., J. H. Brown, D. I. Rosenthal: Rotator cuff: evaluation with fat-suppressed MR arthrography. Radiology 188 (1993) 683 – 687
32 Patt, B. D., D. Sykes, T1 water eliminated Fourier transform NMR spectroscopy. J. chem. Phys. 56 (1972) 3182 – 3184
33 Reiser, M., W. Wiesmann, R. Erlemann, A. Härle, K. Bohndorf, P. Wuismann, V. Kunze, P. E. Peters: Computertomographie und magnetische Resonanztomographie bei Weichteiltumoren. Orthopäde 17 (1988) 134 – 142

34 Schick, F., H. Bongers, W. I. Jung, B. Eismann, M. Skalej, H. Einsele, O. Lutz, C. Claussen: Proton relaxation times in human red bone marrow by volume selective magnetic resonance spectroscopy. Appl. Magn. Reson. 3 (1992) 947–963

35 Schick, F., H. Bongers, W. I. Jung, M. Skalej, O. Lutz, C. Claussen: Volume-selective proton MRS in vertebral bodies. Magn. Reson. Med. 15 (1992) 207–217

36 Seeger, L. L., B. E. Widoff, L. W. Bassett, G. Rosen, J. Eckardt: Preoperative evaluation of osteosarcome: value of Gadopentetate Dimeglumine-enhanced MR imaging. Amer. J. Roentgenol. 157 (1991) 347–351

37 Seelos, K., A. von Smekal: MR angiography in congenital heart disease. Amer. J. Roentgenol. 172 (1992) 118 (abstr.)

38 Shellock, F. G., J. H. Mink, A. Deutsch, B. D. Pressman: Kinematic magnetic resonance imaging of the joints: techniques and clinical applications. Magn. Reson. Quart. 7 (1991) 104–135

39 Shellock, F. G., J. H. Mink, A. Deutsch, T. K. F. Foo: Kinematic magnetic resonance imaging of the patellofemoral joint: comparison of passive positioning and active movement techniques. Radiology 184 (1992) 574–577

40 Shellock, F. G., A. L. Deutsch, J. Fox, T. Molnar, R. Ferkel: Effect of a patellar realignment brace on patellofemoral relationships: evaluation with klinematic MR imaging. JMR 4 (1994) 590–594

41 Sommer, T., M. Vahlensieck, T. Wallny, E. Keller, G. Lutterbey, C. Kuhl, H. Schild: Indirekte MR Arthrographie in der Diagnostik von Verletzungen des Labrum glenoidale. Fortschr. Röntgenstr. 164 (1996) 9

42 Träber, F., W. A. Kaiser, G. Layer, C. Kuhl, M. Reiser: Magnetic resonance spectroscopy of skeletal muscle. Front. Europ. Radiol. 9 (1993) 23–43

43 Träber, F., W. Block, G. Layer, J. Gieseke, H. Schild: Chemical shift selective determination of 1H relaxation times in human bone marrow by fat-suppressed Turbo Spin Echo (TSE) in comparison to MR spectroscopic methods. Proc. SMR 2 (1994) 1246

44 Vahlensieck, M., P. Lang, W. P. Chan, S. Grampp, H. K. Genant: Three-dimensional reconstruction part I: applications and techniques. Europ. Radiol. 2 (1992) 503–507

45 Vahlensieck, M., P. Lang, W. P. Chan, S. Grampp, H. K. Genant: Three-dimensional reconstruction part II: optimisation of segmentation and rendering of MRI. Europ. Radiol. 2 (1992) 508–510

46 Vahlensieck, M., S. Majumdar, P. Lang, H. K. Genant: Shoulder MRI: routine examinations using gradient recalled and fat-saturated sequences. Europ. Radiol. 2 (1992) 142–147

47 Vahlensieck, M., K. Seelos, J. Gieseke, M. Reiser: Turbo (Fast) Spin-Echo bei 0,5 T: Einfluß der Echodistanz und Echozahl auf den Bildkontrast. Fortschr. Röntgenstr. 158 (1993) 260–264

48 Vahlensieck, M., K. Seelos, F. Träber, J. Gieseke, M. Reiser: Magnetresonanztomographie mit schneller STIR-Technik: Optimierung und Vergleich mit anderen Sequenzen an einem 0,5-Tesla-System. Fortschr. Röntgenstr. 159 (1993) 288–294

49 Vahlensieck, M., F. Dombrowski, C. Leutner, U. Wagner, M. Reiser: Magnetization Transfer Contrast (MTC) and MTC-subtraction enhances cartilage lesions and intrasubstance degeneration in vitro. Skelet. Radiol. 23 (1994) 535–539

50 Vahlensieck, M., P. Lang, K. Seelos, D. Yang-Ho Sze, S. Grampp, M. Reiser: Musculoskeletal MR imaging: Turbo (Fast) Spin-Echo versus Conventional Spin-Echo and Gradient-Echo imaging at 0,5 Tesla. Skelet. Radiol. 23 (1994) 607–610

51 Vahlensieck, M., T. Wischer, A. Schmidt, K. Steuer, T. Sommer, E. Keller, J. Gieseke, M. Reiser, H. Schild: Indirekte MR-Arthrographie: Optimierung der Methode und erste klinische Erfahrung bei frühen degenerativen Gelenkschäden am oberen Sprunggelenk. Fortschr. Röntgenstr. 162 (1995) 338–341

52 Vahlensieck, M., T. Sommer, H. H. Schild: Rotator cuff tears: value of indirect MR-Arthrography. Radiology 201 (1996) 156 (abst.)

53 Vahlensieck, M., C. G. Peterfy, T. Wischer, T. Sommer, P. Lang, U. Schlippert, H. K. Genant, H. H. Schild: Indirect MR-Angiography: Optimization and Clinical applications. Radiology 200 (1996) 249–254

54 Vahlensieck, M., T. Sommer: Indirekte MR-Arthrographie der Schulter: Alternative zur direkten MR-Arthrographie? Radiologe 36 (1996) 960–965

55 Vahlensieck, M., F. Träber, R. DeBoer, U. Schlippert, H. Schild: Magnetization-Transfer-Contrast (MTC): Vergleich maligner und benigner Erkrankungen des Stütz- und Bewegungsapparates. Radiologe 35 (1995) 100 (abst.)

56 Vahlensieck, M., F. Träber, B. Kreft, G. Layer, R. DeBoer, H. Schild: Magnetization-Transfer-Contrast (MTC): Comparison of on- and off-resonance techniques at 0,5 and 1,5 Tesla. Europ. Radiol. 5 (1995) 74 (abst.)

Spine
G. Lutterbey and G. Layer

Anatomic Basis

The spine is formed by seven cervical vertebrae, twelve thoracic vertebrae, five lumbar vertebrae and five additional vertebrae that are fused with the costal remnants to constitute the sacrum. Rudimentary vertebrae that make up the coccyx terminate the spine (Figs. 2.**1** – 2.**3**).

All vertebrae have a common basic form, regionally modified by the particular load carried by that region. The vertebral body, which is attached to the intervertebral disk with its superior and inferior end plates, occupies the largest part of each vertebra. A pair of pedicles projects posteriorly from the vertebral body to form the base for the vertebral arch. Each pedicle is constricted in the middle, creating an articular notch as part of the intervertebral foramen. An articular process arises superiorly and inferiorly from each pedicle. These superior and inferior articular processes form an articulation between the vertebrae. The transverse processes project laterally where the laminae begin and the spinous process arises posteriorly where the laminae join to complete the vertebral arch. The vertebral arch encloses the spinal canal, which has openings for the spinal nerve on either side between two vertebrae, the intervertebral foramina (Fig. 2.**4**).

The vertebral bodies increase in height in the craniocaudal direction. The movements of the different

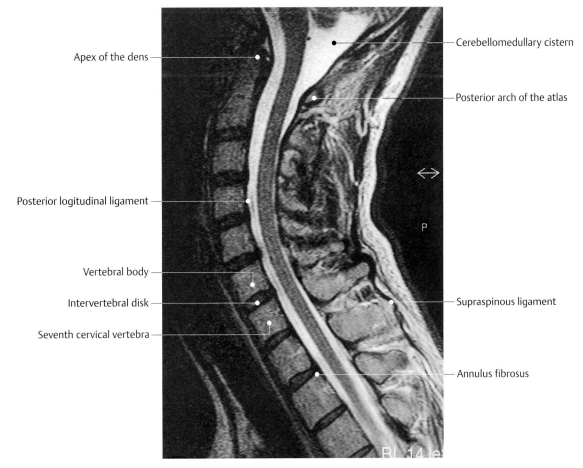

Apex of the dens

Posterior logitudinal ligament

Vertebral body

Intervertebral disk

Seventh cervical vertebra

Cerebellomedullary cistern

Posterior arch of the atlas

Supraspinous ligament

Annulus fibrosus

Fig. 2.**1**   T$_2$-weighted SE sequence, sagittal section of the cervical spine.

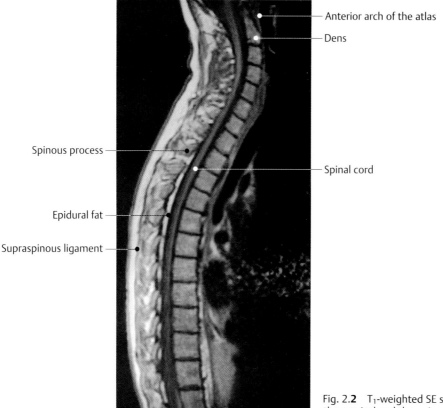

Anterior arch of the atlas

Dens

Spinous process

Spinal cord

Epidural fat

Supraspinous ligament

Fig. 2.**2**   T$_1$-weighted SE sequence, sagittal section of the cervical and thoracic spine with a 'synergy coil.'

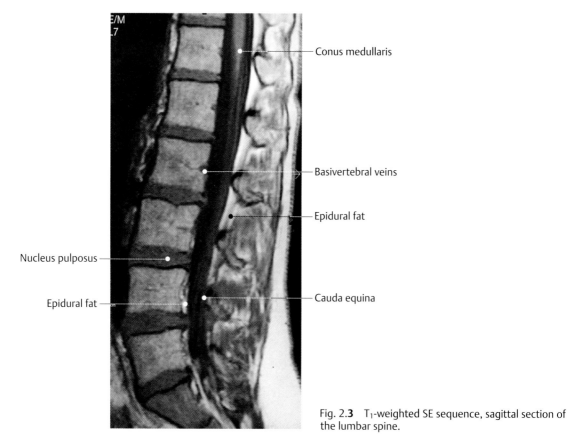

Conus medullaris

Basivertebral veins

Epidural fat

Nucleus pulposus

Epidural fat

Cauda equina

Fig. 2.**3**   T$_1$-weighted SE sequence, sagittal section of the lumbar spine.

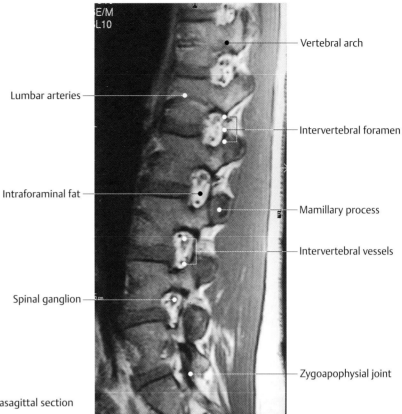

Lumbar arteries

Intraforaminal fat

Spinal ganglion

Vertebral arch

Intervertebral foramen

Mamillary process

Intervertebral vessels

Zygoapophysial joint

Fig. 2.4   T$_2$-weighted SE sequence, parasagittal section of the lumbar spine.

spinal regions are influenced by the form and orientation of the articular surfaces. The articular surfaces of the cervical spine are flat and inclined 45° from the horizontal plane following an anterosuperior to posteroinferior orientation. The articular surfaces of thoracic spine are frontally oriented. In the lumbar region, the sagittaly oriented articular surfaces markedly limit any rotation and almost exclusively permit only flexion and extension.

The first two cervical vertebrae, which support the load of the head and allow movements like a ball and socket joint, assume a special role in the discussion of the vertebrae (Fig. 2.5). The first vertebral body (atlas) deviates from the basic vertebral form in that it lacks a body. The space normally taken by the vertebral body is occupied by the dens. The dens is posteriorly contained by the transverse ligament, which protects the medulla from injuries of the moving dens. Axis and occipital bone are joined by an articulating system that consists of six small individual articulations.

The length and configuration of the spine, as well as its function, are determined significantly by the connecting ligaments and the intervertebral disks, as well as by the osseous structures. All disks added together constitute about one fourth of the entire length of the spine. In the thoracolumbar spine the thickness of the disks decreases craniocaudaly. The slight wedging of the disks markedly contributes to the curvature of the spine. Each disk consists of a gelatinous nucleus, the nucleus pulposus, which is surrounded by laminated fibrous tissue, the annulus fibrosus. The firm attachment of the annulus fibrosus to the hyaline cartilage covering the vertebral end plates constitutes a synchondrosis. The nucleus pulposus is under constant high pressure and its role consists of keeping the vertebral bodies apart. It is confined by the annulus fibrosus and the anterior and posterior longitudinal ligaments. The ligamenta flava, which connect the laminae of adjacent vertebrae, primarily consist of elastic fibers and owe their name to the yellow color of these fibers. The spinous processes are connected with each other by the supraspinal ligament and the interspinal ligaments (Fig. 2.1).

Examination Protocol for MRI

In general, the spine is examined in segments, guided by the presenting symptom. It is less common to screen the entire spine, but this is indicated whenever metastatic infiltrations are suspected. In this situation, the largest field of view should be selected for the sagittal view, to encompass the medullary spaces of the cervical, thoracic and lumbar spine. These examinations are performed with the body coil or with special rectangular or phase-array coils (Fig. 2.2).

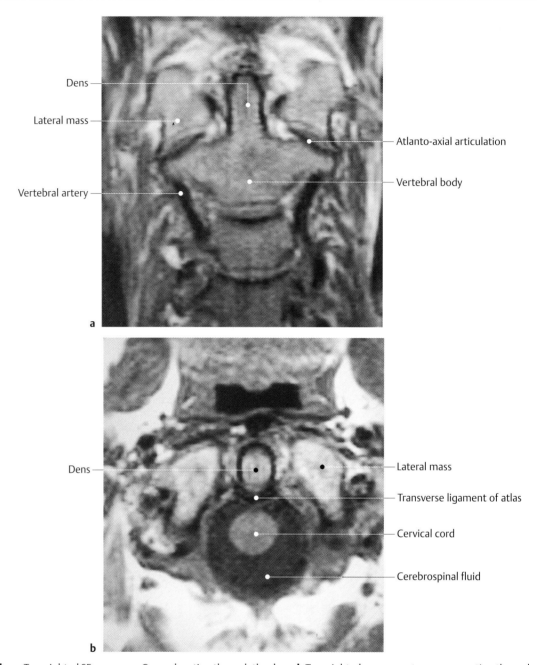

Fig. 2.**5 a, b**   **a** T$_1$-weighted SE sequence. Coronal section through the dens. **b** T$_1$-weighted sequence, transverse section through atlas and axis at the level of the dens.

Alternatively, individual segments of the spine can be examined with flexible surface or rectangular coils. The field of view is variable and is about 180 mm for the cervical and lumbar spine and 360 mm for the thoracic spine.

Sagittal sections are mandatory for MR imaging of the spine, complemented by axial sections through the area of interest. Coronal sections are only occasionally needed (Figs. 2.**6** and 2.**7**).

A section thickness of 3–4 mm has proved to be useful since it is a satisfactory compromise between spatial resolution and signal-noise ratio for modern MRI units and properly designed coils.

Matrix and the number of excitations should be in a reasonable relationship to the total examination time. Individual sequences exceeding 5 minutes negate the apparent advantages of higher matrix resolution or signal intensity by adding motion artifacts.

Selection of the sequences has to be guided by the question asked. T$_1$-weighted SE sequences provide a good anatomic display and should be part of every examination. However, the dual echo technique of SE

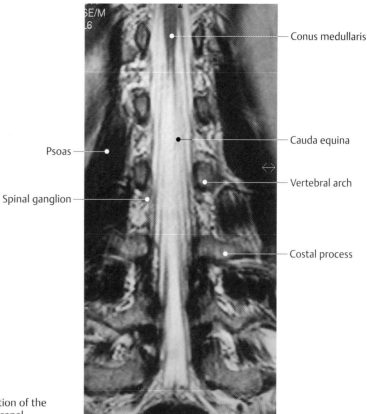

Conus medullaris

Cauda equina

Psoas —

Vertebral arch

Spinal ganglion —

Costal process

Fig. 2.**6**   T₂-weighted sequence. Coronal section of the lumbar spine through the plane of the spinal canal.

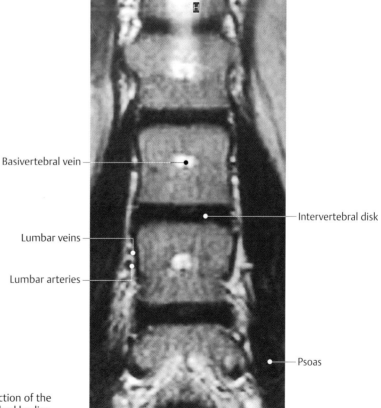

Basivertebral vein —

Intervertebral disk

Lumbar veins —

Lumbar arteries —

Psoas

Fig. 2.**7**   T₂-weighted sequence. Coronal section of the lumbar spine through the plane of the vertebral bodies.

sequences (proton density and T_2-weighted images) has lost its importance through the introduction of TSE sequences (see Chapter 1). In the spine, the proton density images rarely add relevant information and generally can be omitted.

T_2-weighted TSE sequences are marked by a crisp contrast, a better signal-to-noise ratio and a shorter examination time. They have essentially replaced the conventional SE sequence. However, the achieved contrast can make it difficult to distinguish fluid, such as CSF, from fat and areas of necrosis or edema which also appear high in signal intensity (Figs. 2.**6** and 2.**7**).

T_2-weighted GE sequences are helpful when evaluating post-traumatic changes since they detect hemosiderin deposits due to their sensitivity to susceptibility effects. The very same susceptibility effects seen on these sequences can overestimate degenerative changes and spinal stenosis. Fast GRE sequences are used for functional imaging in real time. Fat suppression using STIR or frequency-selective fat saturation can be added (see Chapter 1).

Both sequences allow the visualization of minor injuries with bone marrow edema.

Opposed-phase GRE sequences with or without enhancement are recommended for detection of malignant bone marrow infiltrates. They have the best signal-to-noise ratio for differentiating malignant bone marrow infiltrates from healthy red or yellow bone marrow.

Intravenous contrast enhancement is generally used for the evaluation of tumor infiltrates or inflammatory changes and in postsurgical changes where it might improve the differentiation of recurrent or residual disk from a scar, at least in advanced stages.

Degenerative Conditions of the Spine

■ Spondylosis Deformans

Spondylosis deformans is characterized by the formation of anterior or lateral osteophytes, or both, along the margin of the vertebral bodies. The osteophytes may contain bone marrow and thus share its signal pattern. Strictly osseous osteophytes are characterized by the extreme short T_2 times of cortical bone and have a low signal intensity on all sequences (Fig. 2.**8**). They are best appreciated on GRE sequences. Susceptibility artifacts, however, might overestimate the extent of the osseous changes.

■ Degenerative Bone Marrow Changes

The diagnostic evaluation of degenerative changes of the spine demands an understanding of the abnormalities induced in the bone marrow of the affected vertebral body. These degenerative marrow changes adjacent to the end plates are invisible on conventional radiographs or CT, but have been described on MRI in up

to 50% of patients with degenerative disk disease. Modic (26) distinguishes three types of change which are generally band-like (Fig. 2.**9**):

- Type 1: Replacement of the adjacent bone marrow by vascularized fibrous tissue (with gadolinium enhancement) with increased signal intensity on the T_2-weighted image and decreased signal intensity on the T_1-weighted image (Fig. 2.**10**).
- Type 2: Replacement of the adjacent bone marrow by abundant fat with increased signal intensity on the T_1-weighted image and moderately hyperintense to isointense signal intensity on the T_2-weighted image (depending on the selected sequence) (Fig. 2.**11**).
- Type 3: Increasing sclerosis and cicatrization of the bone marrow with a decrease signal intensity in all sequences.

The types are not always clearly distinguishable from each other and frequently coexist. A systematic review of consecutive patients referred for lumbar spine MR imaging revealed type 2 change in 16% of the patients. Histologic specimens demonstrated yellow marrow adjacent to the end plates. This conversion of red to yellow bone marrow is attributed to chronic repetitive micro traumas associated with degenerative disk disease. These changes remain stable over several years and do not have the tendency to involve the entire vertebral

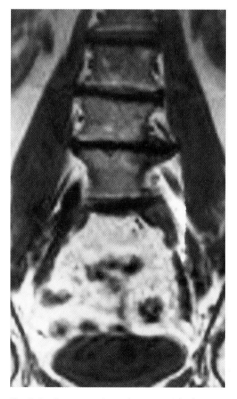

Fig. 2.**8** Degenerative change with large spondylophyte, L3/L4 vertebral body on the left. T_1-weighted SE sequence (500/15) coronal. The osseous appositions are of low signal intensity.

Fig. 2.**9** Differential diagnosis of degenerative and inflammatory changes of vertebral bodies and interposed disk, following the classification proposed by Modic (26).

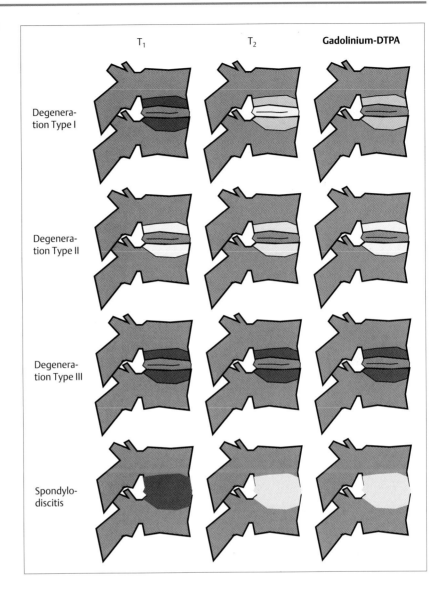

body. Fractures or vertebral compressions secondary to these bone marrow changes alone were not observed. The changes of the less frequent type 1 (4%) can pose differential diagnostic problems since they might be interpreted as osseous metastases in patients with known malignancy. Cases with such signal changes along the end plates should be followed expectantly since these changes generally convert to the aforementioned increased signal intensity on the T_1-weighted image. The transient decrease in signal intensity of the bone marrow on the T_1-weighted image observed with degenerative disk disease corresponds histologically to vascular granulation tissue with multiple small blood vessels. When the degenerative process becomes more chronic and stable, a change with fatty replacement can be expected. The time interval of the underlying investigations was up to 18 months. Because of the few patients studied longitudinally, the evolving bone marrow

degeneration that accompanies disk degeneration cannot yet be definitively answered.

Differential diagnoses. The degenerative vertebral changes of type 1 can resemble a spondylodiskitis (Fig. 2.**10**), though the inflammatory changes in the latter produce an increased signal intensity in the disk and enhance more than a tear of the annulus fibrosus. Furthermore, the interface between disk and adjacent vertebral body is indistinct with infection. Pathologic changes in the surrounding tissues are rare in case of degeneration.

Vertebral hemangiomas, which represent benign vascular tumors and are found in about 11% of all autopsies, are to be distinguished from degenerative disease type 2 (Fig. 2.**12**). Their predisposition for the spine and the differential diagnostic implications justify their special mention. Histopathologically, they represent

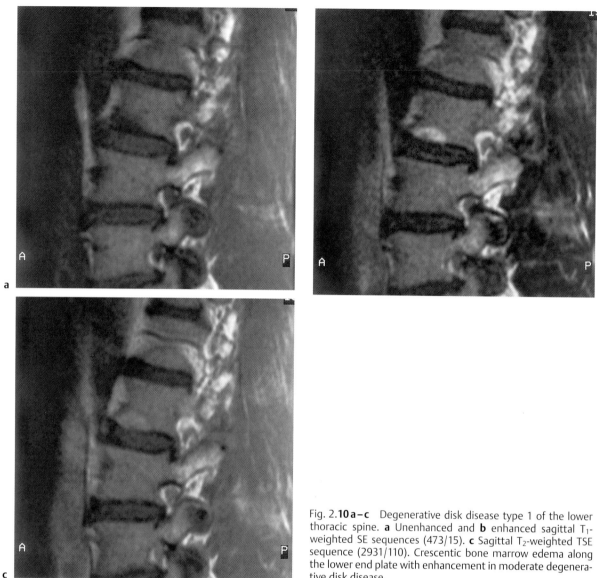

Fig. 2.**10 a–c** Degenerative disk disease type 1 of the lower thoracic spine. **a** Unenhanced and **b** enhanced sagittal T_1-weighted SE sequences (473/15). **c** Sagittal T_2-weighted TSE sequence (2931/110). Crescentic bone marrow edema along the lower end plate with enhancement in moderate degenerative disk disease.

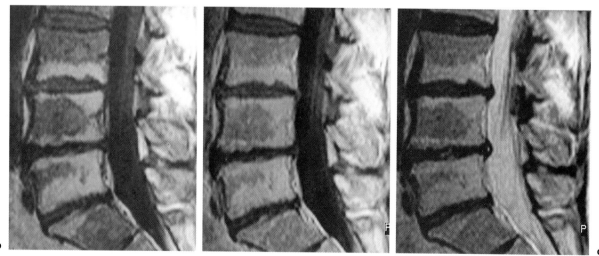

Fig. 2.**12 a,b** Hemangioma, T8 vertebral body. **a** sagittal T_1-weighted SE sequence (500/15) and **b** T_2-weighted TSE sequence (3000/90). Centrally in the vertebral body, sharply demarcated lesion of the bone marrow with increased signal intensity on both sequences.

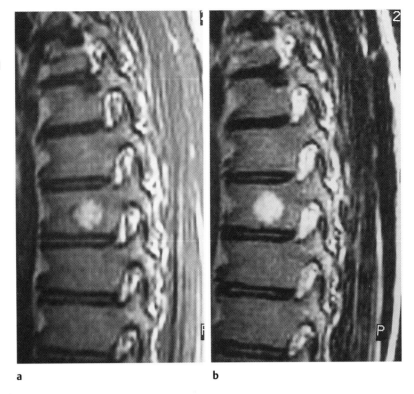

a   b

thin-walled blood-filled vessels and sinusoids, surrounded by endothelium and interspersed with longitudinally osseous trabeculae. They have a characteristic and well-known appearance on plain radiographs and CT (Fig. 2.**13**), and also produce a characteristic finding on MR. They are well demarcated and can occupy the entire vertebral body in the sagittal section or form a round, punched-out lesion. Characteristically, hemangiomas are of very high signal on both T_1-weighted and T_2-weighted images. Comparison of chemical shift images with histologic sections has demonstrated that the typical signal pattern is caused by extraosseous fat components. The differential diagnosis should not be a problem as long as these characteristic findings are kept in mind. A malignancy can be excluded on the basis of the high signal observed in hemangiomas on the T_1-weighted images. Degenerative osseous changes are band-like, less well demarcated and of lower signal intensity.

■ Disk Degeneration

The healthy disk undergoes a physiologic aging process. Similar to hyaline cartilage, the nucleus pulposus con-

tains collagen fibers of type II and large amounts of proteoglycans with the propensity to bind water. This accounts for the high signal intensity on the T_2-weighted images. The nucleus pulposus is surrounded by the concentric lamellae of the fibrocartilaginous annulus fibrosus, which are interconnected by a network of collagenous fibers. The content of type I collagen increases centrifugally resulting in a low signal intensity of the peripheral components on T_1 and T_2 weighting. Sharpey's fibers attach the periphery of the disk to the ring epiphysis of the vertebral body. The annulus fibrosus, which is frequently thinner dorsally, is firmly attached to the anterior and posterior longitudinal ligaments.

Up to the second year of life, the disk receives its nutrients through vessels. Thereafter, it becomes completely avascular and is exclusively nourished through diffusion. Only pathologic processes can induce the ingrowth of secondary vessels. Furthermore, repetitive micro traumas and biochemical processes contribute to the aging process. By the time of adolescence, a band that is low signal on all sequences appears in the nucleus pulposus in each T weighting, presumably corresponding to invaginated inner lamellae of the annulus fibrosus.

Aging induces various MRI findings. In particular, the T_2-weighted images show the dehydration of the nucleus pulposus as decrease in signal intensity. In advanced age, the entire disk is exclusively composed of fibrous cartilage and elicits a very low signal intensity. Furthermore, annular tears appear. They are of high sig-

◄ Fig. 2.**11 a–c** Degenerative disk disease type 2 at L3 to S1. **a** Unenhanced, and **b** enhanced sagittal T_1-weighted SE sequences (473/15) as well as **c** sagittal T_2-weighted TSE sequence (2931/110). Band-like increase in signal intensity along the end plates without discernible enhancement.

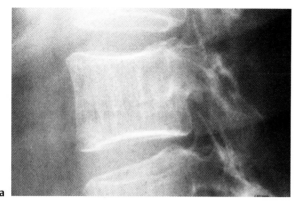

a

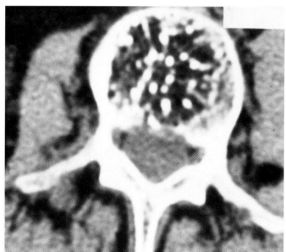

b

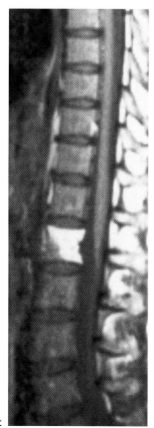

Fig. 2.**13 a–c** Hemangiomatous vertebral body. **a** Lateral radiograph. Increased longitudinal trabecular markings. **b** CT. Increased fat content and transversely dissected thickened longitudinal trabeculation. **c** MRI. T$_1$-weighted SE sequence. The increased fat content causes an increased signal intensity of the hemangiomatous body.

c

nal on T$_2$ images. When vascularized tissue extends into these tears, which can be concentric, radial and transverse in orientation, they are of high signal intensity on T$_1$-weighted images after administration of Gd-DTPA. Annular tears predispose to protrusion and prolapse of disk material. Similar to CT and conventional radiographs, MRI can exhibit a *vacuum phenomenon* in the affected disk. This phenomenon reflects a nitrogen-rich accumulation of gas, caused by a negative pressure in the disk and poor resorption because of absent vascularization.

Gaseous inclusions appear as a signal void on all sequences and must be differentiated from calcifications and chemical shift artifacts. At this stage of degeneration, the height of the disk is invariably decreased.

■ Disk Herniation

A very important aspect of degenerative disk disease is the displacement of portions of the nucleus pulposus through the annulus fibrosus. The terminology relating to disk herniation is difficult. The following nomenclature has been proposed by the North American Spine Association (Fig. 2.**14**):

Bulge. This refers to a concentric extension of the disk beyond the vertebral margin.

Protrusion. This represents a broad-based, frequently somewhat eccentric extension of the degenerated disk beyond the vertebral margin in the presence of an intact annulus fibrosus and longitudinal ligament. The protrusion can be anterior, posterior, or lateral.

Extrusion. If part of the nucleus pulposus extends through the annulus fibrosus, it produces a focal convex extension of the disk beyond the vertebral margin. The extrusion can be central, paracentral, lateral, and far lateral. Depending on the location there may be corresponding predominantly radicular or myelopathic symptoms.

If the outer layer of the annulus fibrosus and the longitudinal ligament remain intact, a band of low signal intensity on T$_1$-weighted and T$_2$-weighted images is seen between the extruded disk and the epidural fat. The delineation of the band varies depending on the residual water content of the disk, and on the surrounding structures, which may show the high signal intensity of the epidural fat on T$_1$-weighted images and a myelographic effect on the T$_2$-weighted images. If the extrusion extends beyond the outer fibers of the annulus fibrosus and through the longitudinal ligament (Fig. 2.**15**), it can exhibit a circumferential narrowing where it passes through the ligamentous structures. These transligamentous extrusions are often small. Dural penetration is rare. The majority of disk protrusions and extrusions exhibit a low signal intensity on all sequences.

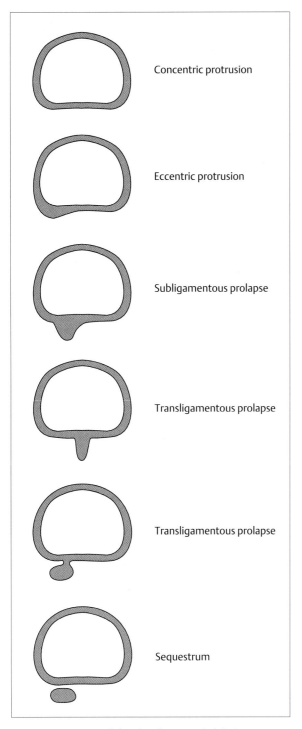

Fig. 2.**14**   Diagram of the classification of disk degeneration with protrusion or prolapse.

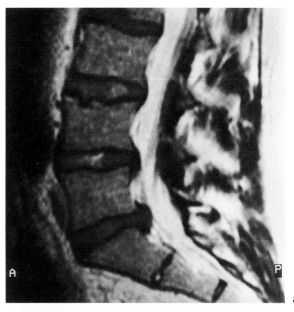

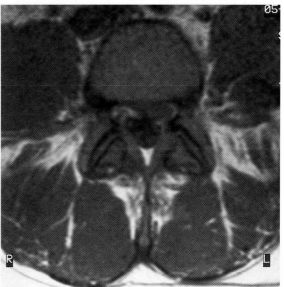

Fig. 2.**15 a, b**   Left mediolateral disk prolapse with compression of the left S1 root and encroachment on the left lateral recess. **a** sagittal and **b** transverse T_1-weighted SE sequence (545/15).

Sequestration. If continuity with the disk is lost, the herniated disk has become sequestered (Fig. 2.**16**). The sequestrum can be anterior or posterior to the longitudinal ligament and may migrate, usually in the caudal direction. On T_2-weighted images, the sequestrum can often be of higher signal intensity than the parent disk, ascribed to neovascularity with increased fluid content. This might also explain peripheral enhancement of sequestrations.

Schmorl's nodes (Fig. 2.**17**). These represent small intramedullary herniations of disk material through the end plates. They have the same signal pattern as the adjacent disk and occasionally enhance.

The assessment of the disk herniation must also consider indirect signs and sequelae, such as efface-

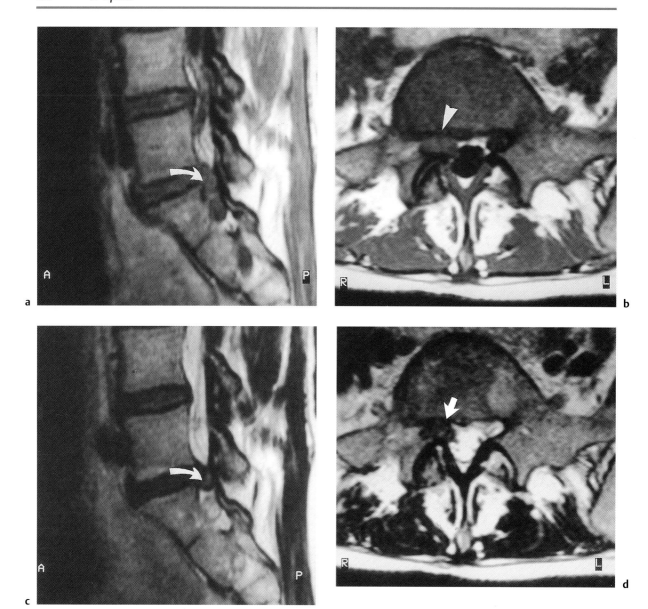

Fig. 2.**16a–d**   Right mediolateral sequestered disk prolapse L5/S1. **a** sagittal and **b** transverse T$_1$-weighted SE sequence (500/15). **c** sagittal and **d** transverse T$_2$-weighted SE sequence (3000/110). The prolapse has formed a sequester caudally and encroaches on the right neural foramen (arrow).

ment of epidural fat, compression of the dural sac and cord, displacement and swelling of the nerve roots, narrowed neural foramina and congested plexus veins.

Degenerative disk herniation often occurs in patients of middle age. It is less frequent in older age since the disk is completely fibrosed by that time. Approximately 90% of all disk herniations occur at the L4/L5 and L5/S1 segments. About 10% are at L3/4; they are less frequent in the upper lumbar spine.

Thoracic and cervical disk herniations are less frequent than lumbar herniations. Since the anatomic structures are smaller, thinner sections have to be obtained. The use of 3D sequences is advantageous.

Because of the thoracic kyphosis, the position of the spinal cord in the bony canal is more anterior at this level, and the anterior epidural space is relatively small, and even small prolapses can induce myelopathic changes (Fig. 2.**18**). Approximately 90% of the cervical disk herniations occur at the C5/6 and C6/7 segments. Central prolapses are commoner in the cervical spine than in the lumbar and thoracic spine. Since in the cervical region the fat-containing epidural space is very small and the epidural vascular network quite extensive, administration of Gd-DTPA for T$_1$-weighted images can be beneficial for the preoperative delineation of a prolapse.

Fig. 2.**17 a, b** Schmorl's node of the superior end plate of the L1 vertebral body following remote Scheuermann's disease. **a** sagittal T_1-weighted SE sequence (500/20) after IV Gd-DTPA. **b** sagittal T_2-weighted TSE sequence (2880/90). Almost centrally located intramedullary indentation of vertebral end plate, of low signal intensity comparable to the intensity of the surrounding disk tissue even after IV Gd-DTPA.

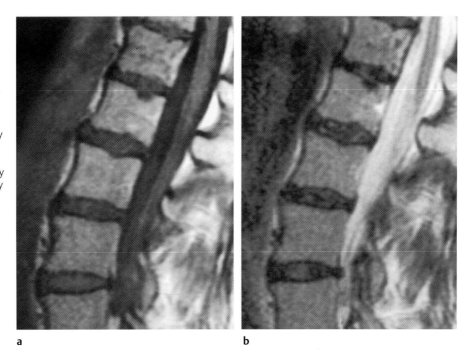

a b

Changes seen on MRI are only relevant with corresponding clinical findings. Teresi (47) conducted a study on 100 neurologically asymptomatic patients with degenerative changes. Significant disk space narrowing occurred in 24% of patients aged 45–54 years and 67% of patients older than 64 years. Disk protrusion was seen in 20% of patients in the younger age group and in 57% of patients in the older age group. Compression of the dural sac with displacement of the spinal cord was observed in 16% of the patients younger than 64 years and in 26% of those older than 64 years. Cord compression was observed in only 7% of the patients. No obliteration of the intraforaminal fat was seen in any of these asymptomatic patients.

The close spatial relationship of the prolapse to the nerve roots, spinal ganglia and spinal nerves of the affected segments explains the clinical findings. The clinically pertinent anatomy at the level of the lumbar spine is illustrated in Fig. 2.**19** and schematized in the corresponding diagram. The central, intraforaminal or extraforaminal location of the extrusion determines whether the extrusion causes a myelopathy or radiculopathy at one or several segmental roots.

Differential diagnosis. Small *extradural tumors* can mimic a disk prolapse. They frequently enhance, however, and are often of higher signal intensity on T_2-weighted sequences. The same distinguishing feature applies to *epidural abscesses* and *hematomas*. Nonsequestered prolapses are always at the level of, and in continuity with, the disk they are originating from. *Synovial cysts* of the facet joints also are of higher signal intensity than disk prolapses on T_2-weighted images, but lack enhancement. With hemorrhage or calcifications, the signal pattern can resemble that of a prolapse. In these cases, CT frequently can detect blood or calcium.

■ Spinal Stenosis and Cervical Myelopathy

Congenital spinal stenoses, such as achondroplasia, are less common than acquired stenoses. The stenosis can affect the spinal canal, neural foramina and lateral recesses, with corresponding radiculopathic and myelopathic complaints clinically. It is to be expected that even a minimal change, for instance a disk protrusion, can cause a critical stenosis in a borderline spinal canal. In the lumbar spine, the AP diameter of the osseous spinal canal at the level of the disk should not be less than 15 mm, the interpeduncular distance at the level of the recess at least 18 mm and the recesses themselves 4–5 mm in AP diameter (Fig. 2.**20**).

Acquired spinal stenosis is most frequently caused by degenerative changes (Fig. 2.**21**). In addition to the osteophytes of spondylosis deformans and altered disks, osteoarthritic changes are seen at the facet joints and hypertrophic changes at the ligamenta flava. The arthrotic changes of the facet joints are analogous to those of other joints: joint space narrowing, cortical erosions, and hypertrophic bone formation at the articular margins. Moreover, inflammatory changes, such as joint effusion as well as synovial proliferation and synovial cysts, are found around the facet joints.

The specific conditions that can narrow the spinal canal, such as pannus around the dens in rheumatoid arthritis, ankylosing spondylitis and intraspinal tumors, will be discussed in the appropriate chapters.

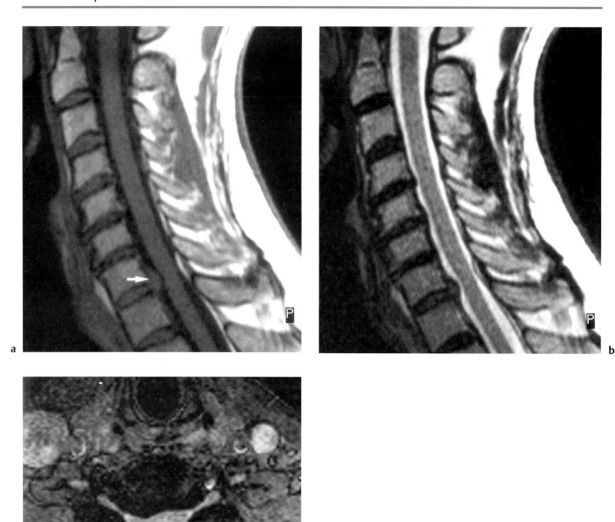

a

b

c

Fig. 2.**18 a–c** Right paracentral disk prolapse at C7/T$_1$. **a** sagittal T$_1$-weighted SE sequence (401/15). **b** sagittal T$_2$-weighted TSE sequence (2500/120). **c** transverse GRE sequence (TR = 593 msec, TE = 35 msec, flip angle = 60 degree). The GRE sequences show the indentation of the dural sac and the encroachment of the right neural foramen. The spinal cord is not affected.

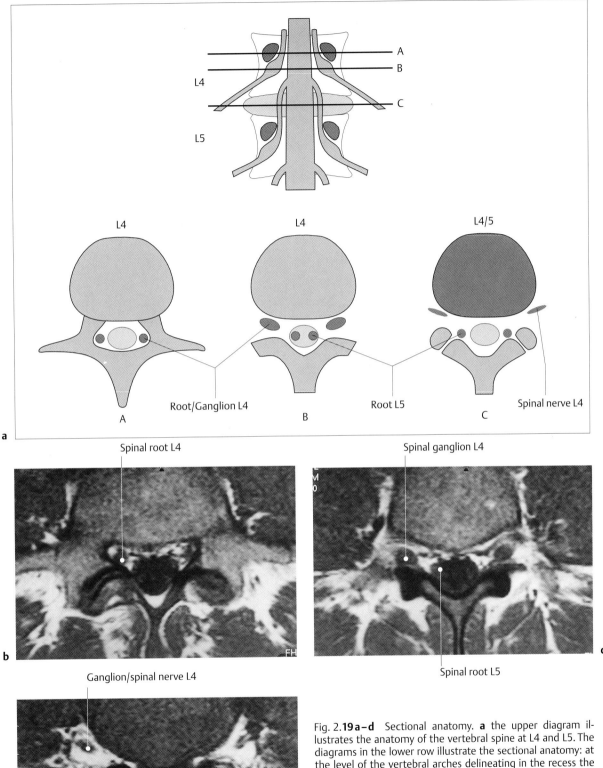

Fig. 2.**19a–d** Sectional anatomy. **a** the upper diagram illustrates the anatomy of the vertebral spine at L4 and L5. The diagrams in the lower row illustrate the sectional anatomy: at the level of the vertebral arches delineating in the recess the nerve root of the segment of one level above (A); at the level of the upper aspect of the neural foramen delineating the ganglion of the nerve root one level above (B); and at the level of the intervertebral disk delineating the spinal nerve two levels above lateral to the neural foramen and lateral to the dural sac the nerve root one level above. **b–d** T$_1$-weighted SE sequences at comparable levels (**b** corresponds to A, **c** to B, and **d** to C).

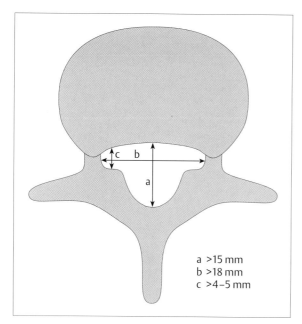

Fig. 2.**20**   Measurements of the lumbar vertebrae.

a >15 mm
b >18 mm
c >4–5 mm

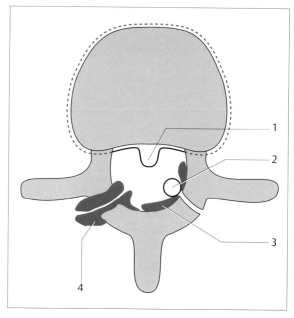

Fig. 2.**21**   Synopsis of the degenerative stenosis of the spinal canal.
1 = prolapse
2 = synovial cyst
3 = hypertrophic ligamenta flava
4 = arthrosis of the facet joints

Spondylitis and Spondylodiskitis

Characteristically, infection of the spine affects both the intervertebral disk and vertebral body. It is for this reason that the term spondylodiskitis is used and a distinction is no longer made between the more or less synonymously used terms of spondylitis, diskitis, and vertebral osteomyelitis.

Infectious pathways of spondylodiskitis:

- hematogenous spread,
- spread by continuity (e.g., retrograde abscess),
- percutaneous spread (e.g., trauma, surgery).

Hematogenous infection is the commonest cause of a spondylodiskitis. Typical organisms are *Staphylococcus aureus*, *Streptococcus*, *Enterobacter aerogenes*, *Klebsiella*, *Pseudomonas*, and acid fast bacilli. In adults, the vertebral body is primarily infected, followed by spread of the infection through the end plates and adjacent disk into other vertebral bodies. In the child, the primary infection can be in the disk because of the persistent blood supply of the disk at that age.

MRI diagnosis. MRI plays an important role in the early diagnosis of a spondylodiskitis since conventional radiographs and CT can be unremarkable at that stage. Clinical and laboratory findings are generally nonspecific. For the MRI diagnosis of a spondylodiskitis, the signal pattern of the vertebral bodies and the disks, as well as the pattern of involvement, are indicative. The typical T_1-weighted image (Fig. 2.**22**) demonstrates a markedly decreased bone marrow signal caused by bone marrow edema and hyperemia. The vertebral body shows an increased signal on the T_2-weighted images. Administration of Gd-DTPA causes enhancement. Involvement of the adjacent disk is characteristic, with increased signal intensity on the T_2-weighted image and contrast enhancement in the late stage. Additional findings of disk involvement are loss of height, deformity, obliteration of the intranuclear cleft, and blurring of the vertebral end plates (Fig. 2.**9**). Characteristically, adjacent vertebral bodies are involved with sparing of the posterior vertebral aspects. However, there may be early involvement of the posterior vertebral elements and paraspinal soft tissues in spondylodiskitis following surgery or penetrating injury. Only 30% of acute cases show deformity of the vertebral body and involvement of the epidural space. Paravertebral granulation tissue is found in around 20% of cases.

Tuberculous spondylodiskitis. This condition deserves special consideration. While pyogenic spondylodiskitis has a predilection for the lower lumbar spine, tuberculous infection most frequently affects the thoracolumbar transition. Another peculiarity of tuberculous spondylitis is the frequent and extensive destruction of the vertebral body, leading to a deformity of the spine in 25% of cases. Moreover, paraspinal abscesses are invari-

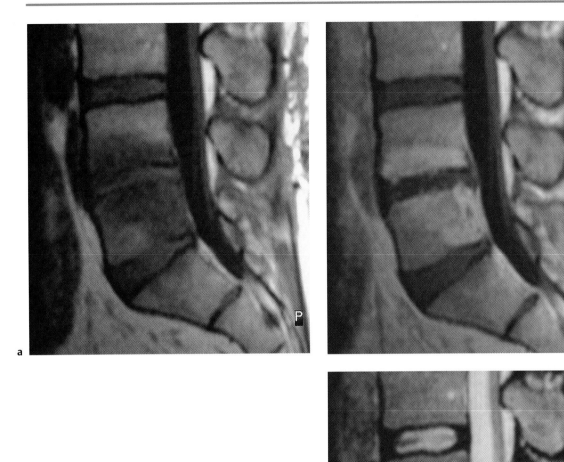

Fig. 2.**22a–c** Spondylodiskitis after nucleotomy L4/L5. Unenhanced **a** and enhanced **b** T_1-weighted sequence (474/15). **c** sagittal T_2-weighted TSE sequence (2931/110). Partial involvement of the vertebral bodies adjacent to the disk. Contrast enhancement in the disk and affected bone marrow space.

ably found and the epidural space is involved in 68% of the cases. A characteristic feature of tuberculous infections is that they may affect several levels (skip lesions).

Brucellosis. Focal infection of the vertebral body with *Brucella* should also be mentioned because of a few typical changes. Characteristically, this infection involves the anterior margins of the end plates of the lower lumbar vertebral bodies, in particular the L4 vertebral body. The disks herniate through the well-de-

marcated end plates, resembling the findings of Schmorl's nodes. A vacuum phenomenon is frequently observed within the disk, which is otherwise rare with spondylodiskitis.

Differential diagnosis. Atypical cases can pose differential diagnostic problems:

- An *acute osteoporotic fracture* may exhibit a signal pattern similar to that of an infection because of bone marrow edema, but contrary to an infection, the disk has a lower signal on the T_2-weighted image. If vessels have grown into the degenerated disk, however, the T_2-weighted image and IV Gd-DTPA are of little value in the differential diagnosis.
- *Neoplastic bone marrow infiltration* exhibits the same signal and enhancement pattern as found in an infection. Concurrent neoplastic involvement of the disk is rare. Furthermore, posterior elements and disseminated vertebral involvement is considerably more frequent with malignancy. Neoplastic bone marrow infiltration involves the entire vertebral body and, in the case of an associated fracture, invariably causes convex bulging of the posterior vertebral border into the spinal canal. Osteoporotic fractures often only lead to posterior displacement of individual bone fragments. After IV Gd-DTPA, the osteoporotic vertebral body is isodense with the healthy vertebral body, while the neoplastically infiltrated vertebral body frequently exhibits a heterogeneous and intense enhancement.

Naturally, the appearance of a spondylodiskitis can vary from the findings just described, depending on the organism and stage of the infection. In particular, mixed infections and infections superimposed on vertebral neoplasms can be hard to classify.

Traumatic Changes of the Spine

Despite increased availability of MRI scanners, performing emergency MRI has to be selective. MRI is time consuming and may delay crucial therapeutic measures. Furthermore, the magnetic field might interfere with the equipment needed for maintaining the vital functions. CT still remains the preferred method for the evaluation of bony injury in acutely traumatized patients.

Nevertheless, MRI has its place in the evaluation of acute trauma in view of its superior delineation of any involvement of the cord, which is found in about 20% of spinal injuries caused by motor vehicle accidents, falls from a height, and sports injuries.

The important questions to be addressed are whether a *fracture* is present and whether it is *stable*. MRI cannot determine stability using the biomechanical concept of three weight-bearing columns as proposed by Holdsworth (18) and Dennis (7). A fracture is considered unstable when all three columns or the middle column and one neighboring column are disrupted. The anterior column is formed by the anterior longitudinal ligament and anterior two-thirds of the vertebral body including the disk, the middle column by the posterior third of the vertebral body including the annulus fibrosus, and the posterior longitudinal ligament. The posterior column is formed by the posterior arch, including facet joints, and by the posterior ligaments. Only the posterior column and spinal canal are well seen at MRI. CT has become the modality of choice for the detection and evaluation of fractures and fracture-dislocations.

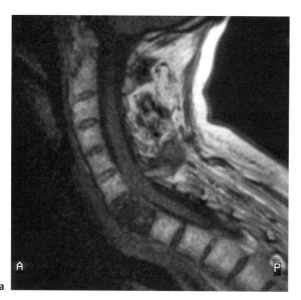

a

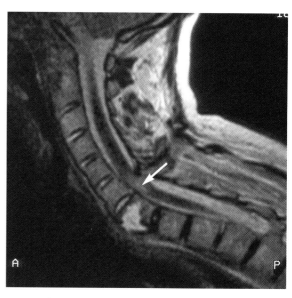

b

Fig. 2.**23 a, b** Post-traumatic fracture of C7. **a** sagittal T_1-weighted SE sequence (427/16) and **b** T_2-weighted TSE sequence (2700/120). Destruction of the vertebral body and massive bone marrow edema. In addition, osseous encroachment on the spinal canal at the level of C6 dorsally. Evidence of cord contusion with focally increased signal intensity on the T_2-weighted image at this level (arrow).

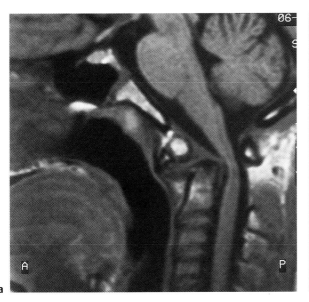

a

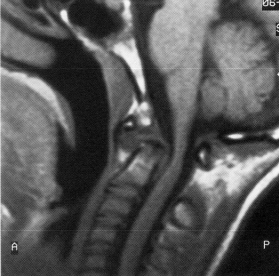

b

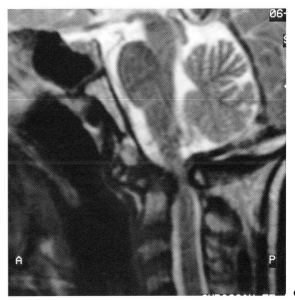

c

Fig. 2.**24 a–c** Dens fracture with detached proximal fragment. T$_1$-weighted SE sequence (500/13) in **a** flexion and **b** extension. **c** sagittal T$_2$-weighted TSE sequence (32 268/110). Sliding of the atlas with severe compression of the craniocervical transition.

■ Injuries of the Vertebral Body

MRI has advantages in assessing segments of the spine that are not easily evaluated by conventional radiography and are rather frequently injured on the basis of the vector diagram of the traumatic forces. This applies to the cervicothoracic transition (Fig. 2.**23**) and dens (Fig. 2.**24**), while the thoracolumbar transition is generally well assessed radiologically. CT allows a detailed visualization of the osseous structures, but is limited by only covering a small volume of interest.

According to Anderson and D'Alonzo (1), three types of dens fractures can be distinguished:

- Type I is rare and constitutes an oblique fracture through the upper part of the odontoid process. It is stable.

- Type II is the most common type and represents a fracture through the base of the dens. In general, these fractures are unstable and must be treated surgically.
- Type III is actually a fracture through the body of the atlas and generally does well with conservative treatment.

Since many fractures are horizontally oriented, MRI with its inherent multiplanar visualization has a decisive advantage over CT, which requires reformatting to delineate this manifestation of trauma adequately. Foregoing the re-formation entails the risk of overlooking fracture lines because of partial volume effect.

Moreover, the sagittal MRI sections provide a more comprehensive visualization of the compression of additional vertebral bodies than all other imaging modalities. Sequence selection does not play an important role in the diagnostic evaluation of acute conditions. The T_2-weighted spin-echo sequences reveal the anatomy together with the severity of the spinal canal involvement since CSF, cord, osseous cortex, and ligamentous apparatus are clearly delineated. T_2-weighted gradient echo sequences demarcate intraspinal hemorrhages from the surrounding normal structures by susceptibility effects, and T_1-weighted spin-echo and STIR sequences show bone marrow edema rather well. The age of a hemorrhage can be derived from the relative signal intensities of the T_1- and T_2-weighted images. Acute hemorrhages are very sensitively detected by

fluid attenuated inversion recovery (FLAIR) sequences since they display CSF and blood at high signal intensity.

■ Ligamentous Instability

While osseous injuries are clearly delineated by CT, ligamentous injuries are better detected by MRI because of its superior soft tissue contrast. Within the first weeks after the trauma, lesions of high-signal intensity, which interrupt the low signal intensity of the normal ligamentous structure, are especially well visualized on T_2-weighted images. These high signals correspond to small areas of hemorrhage or post-traumatic edema or

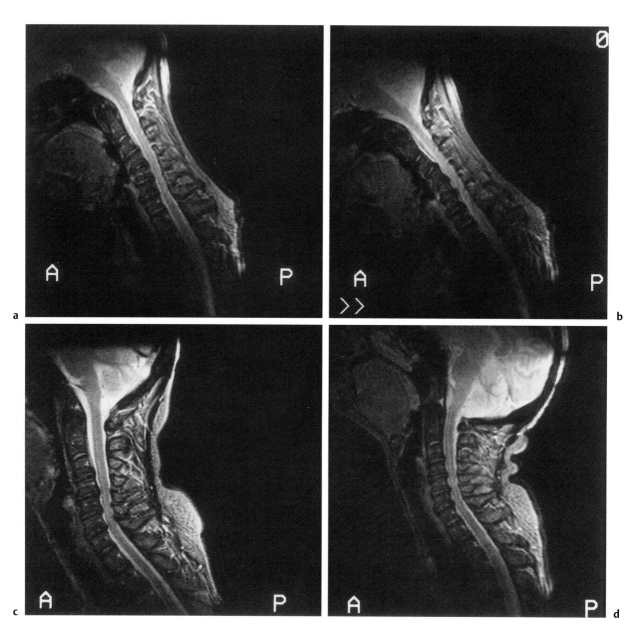

Fig. 2.**25 a–d**   Functional MR images of the cervical spine to assess position-related cervical myelopathy. **a** and **b** T_2-weighted GRE sequence (TR = 400 msec, TE = 12 msec, flip angle = 15 degree) of maximal flexion and extension. **c** and **d** images obtained in extension show string of pearl-like indentations of the spinal cord caused by osteophytes.

both. If radiographic examinations have excluded osseous injuries, functional views of the spinal region in question can be added. These views are very sensitive for the detection of segmental instability (Fig. 2.**25**). Rapid gradient-echo sequences have proved useful and allow acquisition almost in real time, especially in the cervical spine. Systems with an open magnet of low field strength are most suitable for such examinations.

■ Cord Injuries

While myelo-CT used to be the gold standard for detecting acute spinal injuries, such as epidural hematoma, pseudomeningocele, nerve root tears or cord compression, it is increasingly being replaced by MRI.

Traction injuries can disrupt dural or cordal structures. In either case, the MR images detect asymmetric accumulation of blood or CSF or both, replacing the expected soft tissue structures regardless of whether the underlying cause is a root tear or a pseudomeningocele (Fig. 2.**26**).

MRI is particularly advantageous for detecting contusions of the cord with impaired microcirculation of the cord and resultant edema or hematomyelia. Intramedullary edema is sensitively detected as increased signal on T_2-weighted images. The cord shows a transient enhancement after IV Gd-DTPA as a manifestation of the impaired blood–CSF barrier. Extent and duration of the enhancement do not follow a characteristic pattern. Intramedullary hematomas have a time-dependent signal pattern on MRI and are as characteristic as soft tissue bleedings in other locations. The extent of medullary edema and hematomyelia can be used to predict the clinical course. Areas of ischemia and infarction caused by medullary perfusion deficits exhibit a low signal on the T_1-weighted image and a high signal on the T_2-weighted image. Syringomyelia can be the sequela of a remote trauma, and is well shown on MRI.

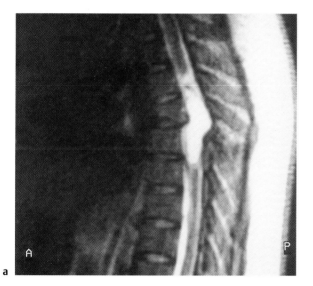

a

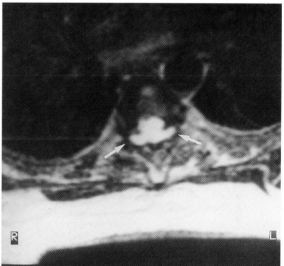

b

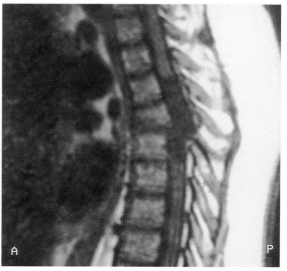

c

Fig. 2.**26 a–c** Total dissection of the spinal cord due to traumatic spondylolisthesis. **a** sagittal T_1-weighted TSE sequence (2700/150). **b** transverse and **c** sagittal T_1-weighted SE sequence (400/18).
The transverse section shows the empty nerve root (arrows).

Postoperative Changes of the Spine

Evaluating postsurgical changes rests on knowing the surgical procedures and any possible deviations from the standard surgical approach as well as the date of the surgery. Furthermore, obtaining the history of the complaints before and after the surgery can be helpful.

■ Laminectomy

Laminectomy removes the lamina of the vertebral arch, including the attached ligamentum flavum (Fig. 2.**27**). The extent of the surgical defect in the vertebral arch is variable. Partial removal of the lamina is called laminotomy (Fig. 2.**28**). This operation serves as osseous decompression and as surgical access route to the spinal canal. The absence of a vertebral arch is easily recog-

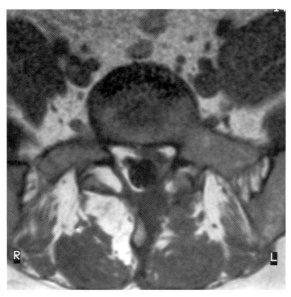
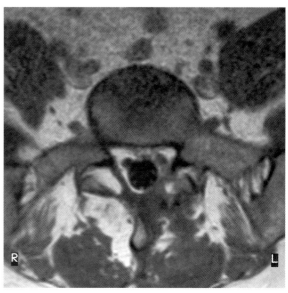

a   b

Fig. 2.**27 a, b**   Status post left hemilaminectomy. **a** transverse unenhanced and **b** enhanced T₁-weighted SE sequences. Marked enhancement of anterior epidural scar tissue. No evidence of a recurrent prolapse. The posterior scar tissue characteristically enhances less than the anterior scar tissue.

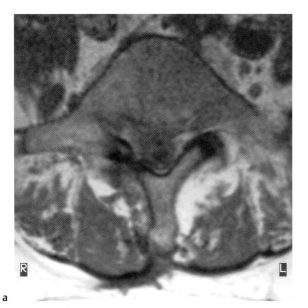
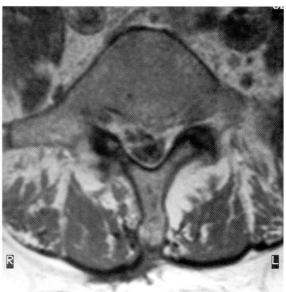

a   b

Fig. 2.**28 a, b**   Status post right laminotomy. **a** unenhanced and **b** T₁-weighted SE sequence (550/17). In contrast to the laminectomy, only a portion of the lamina has been removed.

nized on sagittal and transverse sections. The surgical defect presents as absence of the osseous structures and asymmetry of the muscle-fat layer, which is less demarcated on the affected side. The defect fills with scar tissue, which exhibits a signal pattern related to the time elapsed since the surgery. New scars have a higher signal intensity than musculature on the T_2-weighted image and clearly enhance. Moreover, the signal pattern is determined by the postsurgical edema and blood residues at the surgical site and can be quite variable and heterogenous. Fresh granulation tissue can have a space-occupying effect, while scar tissue contracts with a tendency for compensatory widening of the dural sac. It takes about six months until the postsurgical changes reach their final stage. Other postsurgical findings consist of a traumatically altered musculature and enhancement of the intervertebral joints and decompressed nerve roots. Some surgeons use fat to cover the surgical defect, which is clearly recognized by the sharp outline and fat-equivalent signal pattern. The impaired stability following the laminectomy can lead to degenerative changes of the intervertebral joints.

■ Diskectomy

Diskectomy consists of the more or less complete removal of the disk using a posterior or anterior approach. The posterior access route through a laminectomy is most frequently followed. Postoperatively, scar tissue can be detected in the anterior epidural space, displaying intermediate signal intensity on the T_1-weighted image and high signal intensity on the T_2-weighted image for several weeks. This scar tissue extends to the remnant of the resected disk and is initially indistinguishable from it because of the absence of the annulus fibrosus and its low signal intensity. The anterior epidural scar frequently keeps its space-occupying effect and increased signal intensity on the T_2-weighted image for a longer period of time than the scar in the posterior soft tissues. Usually after two to six months, the epidural scar has a lower signal intensity on the T_2-weighted image than the disk remnant, which at that time has formed a new annulus fibrosus posteriorly. In the early postsurgical period, IV Gd-DTPA can assist to demarcate the strongly enhancing scar tissue from surrounding structures, but the value of MRI must still be considered limited for up to six weeks after the surgery because of the surgically induced edema and hematoma. Even enhancement of the end plates must be considered a normal postsurgical finding. In 18.5% of patients with a normal postoperative course and no signs of infection after disk surgery, a focal decrease in signal intensity was observed on the T_1-weighted images with enhancement after IV Gd-DTPA.

Residual or recurrent prolapse and hypertrophic epidural scar are frequent causes of the failed back surgery syndrome (FBSS), which is observed in 25 to 40% of patients after back surgery. The need to distinguish between the two is obvious since the prolapse, in contrast to the scar, is amenable to surgical correction. Removing scar tissue can elicit a renewed abundance of scar tissue. In 70 to 80% of the cases, prolapse and scar are distinguishable by morphologic criteria. The prolapse follows the same signal pattern observed in the original disk, is frequently connected to it and has a space-occupying effect. It is polypoid to lobulated and relatively well demarcated. If several months have passed since the surgery, the annulus fibrosus, together with the posterior longitudinal ligament, demarcates the prolapse from the epidural space by a low-signal band. The anterior epidural scar tissue is indistinctly outlined and exhibits a heterogenous and variable signal pattern. It is easy to recognize an old scar that exhibits a low signal on all image sequences and pulls the dural sac toward it. However, a scar can also have a space-occupying effect and a sequestered prolapse a variable signal pattern. To distinguish between a prolapse and scar, enhanced images after IV Gd-DTPA must often be obtained. Scar tissue can show enhancement as long as 20 years after the surgery. Disk tissue enhances faintly only 30–45 minutes after IV Gd-DTPA. The tissue differentiation approaches 100% with a properly timed assessment (6 to 10 minutes after the injection) of the enhancement.

■ Surgical Fusion

Several surgical approaches can be followed and, depending on the indication, are combined with other surgeries, such as a diskectomy. Frequently, an osseous fragment taken from another part of the patient's body (*autograft*) or from another person (*allograft*) are inserted into the disk space for stabilization. The osseous graft can be taken from the iliac wing or a long tubular bone. The autograft includes the bone marrow, and spongiosa and cortex can be identified. The allograft is processed and bone marrow removed. It has a low signal intensity on all sequences. Most artificial implants, such as acrylic cement, are also of low signal intensity. Frequent sequelae of surgical fusion are disk degenerations that can progress to a prolapse and osseous changes in adjacent segments (incidence about 25% after two years) that can lead to spinal stenosis. Furthermore, osseous deformities with malalignment and spondylolisthesis can develop. The low signal intensity of osseous changes consisting exclusively of dense bone are less well appreciated by MRI than by conventional radiography. Osteophytes and autologous implants frequently contain bone marrow, which is of high signal intensity on T_1-weighted images. MRI is better suited for evaluating the *stability* of fusions as long as the time interval between surgery and MRI exceeds six to twelve months. At that time, postsurgical repair is completed and a biomechanical balance has been achieved. Bands of increased signal seen on the T_2-weighted sequences in the segments of the surgical site together with decreased signal on the T_1-weighted sequences favor an unstable fusion. Analogous to the bone marrow of the type 1 degenerative changes, these signal changes reflect bone marrow edema, aseptic inflammatory changes, reactive hyperemia and micro fractures due to biomechanical stress. Stable fusion rarefies the trabecular pattern with incorporation of fatty bone marrow, identified as high signal intensity on the T_1-weighted images and as intermediate signal intensity on the T_2-weighted images. This signal pattern is also found adjacent to the end plates and resembles a type 2 bone marrow reaction of disk degeneration. Furthermore, similar bone marrow changes are found after chemonucleolysis with chymopapain since the treated disk undergoes an accelerated aging process.

Several postsurgical changes and complications should be mentioned here. Lateral osseous *spinal stenosis* is responsible for 50 to 60% of the cases with FBSS. The height of the intervertebral disk space is decreased after diskectomy, leading to narrowing of the intervertebral foramina. Moreover, surgical fusion leads to degenerative osseous changes due to imbalanced strain on the intervertebral joints and, if the fusion is unstable, to *pseudoarthrosis*. MRI shows obliteration of the infraforaminal epidural fat. The osteophyte formation itself can be quite variable (see above).

Spinal surgery can damage the dura, potentially leading to a *pseudomeningocele* by forming a fibrous capsule in the tissue around a CSF leak. Alternatively, an

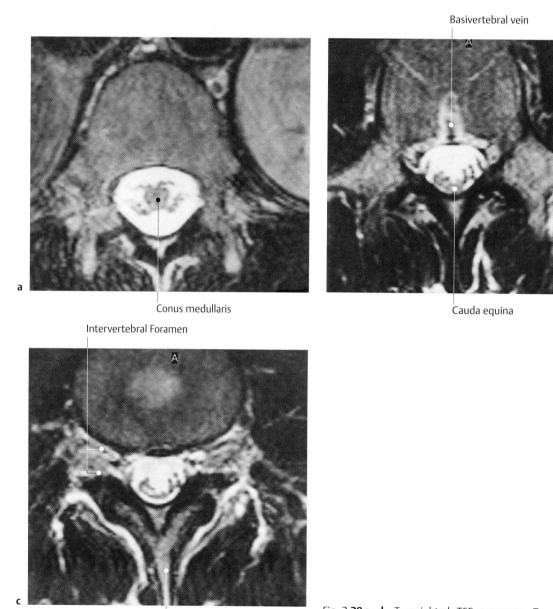

Fig. 2.**29 a–d** T_2-weighted TSE sequence. Transverse sections at the level of **a** T12, **b** L2, **c** L3, and **d** L5.

Fig. 2.**29 d**

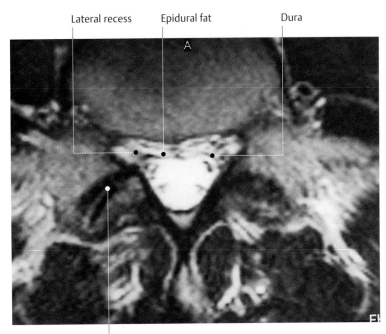

Lateral recess   Epidural fat   Dura

Zygoapophysial joint

arachnoid herniation might be present and contain the extravasated CSF. Such herniations generally exhibit a CSF signal, but can have a different signal or a fluid–fluid level because of intermixed blood products or inspissated CSF due to encapsulation. In these cases, differentiation from an epidural abscess is difficult and myelography might be necessary.

Intraspinal infections can lead to *arachnoiditis*. Because of its multifarious presentation by MRI, its interpretation rests on cognizance of the normal arrangement of the filum terminale and its normal variants. The normal MRI findings are shown in Fig. 2.**6** and Fig. 2.**29** and the most frequent variants in Fig. 2.**30**. The arachnoiditis produces intraspinal inflammatory space-occupying lesions with moderate enhancement and obliteration of the spinal canal. Its differentiation from a neoplastic growth is not always possible by MRI. In the lower spine, neural fibers can aggregate to form nodular structures that are centrally located in the dural sac. Conversely, the fibers can adhere along the outline

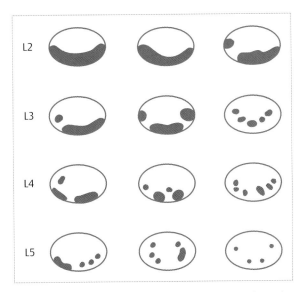

Fig. 2.**30** Anatomic variants of the filum terminale. Schematic drawing of axial sections through the healthy lumbar spine at the levels L2 to L5 (according to Modic). The dural sac is shown with three normal but different distributions of the nerve roots, to be differentiated from asymmetric distribution due to inflammatory adhesions (Fig. 2.**31**).

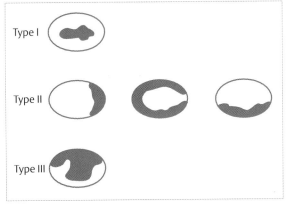

Fig. 2.**31** Arachnoiditis. Asymmetric distribution of the nerve roots in the lumbar dural sac caused by adhesions in arachnoiditis. The inflammatory adhesions can be primarily centrally (type I), peripherally (type II) or diffusely (type III) throughout the dural sac.

of the spinal canal to create the finding of an empty dural sac, as illustrated in Fig. 2.**31**. Postoperative *hematomas* are generally seen as well-demarcated lesions at the surgical site, without space-occupying effect and with a high signal on T_1- and T_2-weighted images. The signal pattern can be altered by various decay products of hemoglobin, water content and any fibrotic transformation. Inconclusive findings have to be followed with serial examinations.

References

1 Anderson, L. D., R. T. D'Alonzo: Fractures of the odontoid process of the axis. J. Bone Jt Surg. 56-A (1974) 1663

2 Baker, L. L., S. B. Goodman, I. Perkash, B. Lane, D. R. Enzmann: Benign versus pathologic compression fractures of vertebral bodies: assessment with conventional spin-echo, chemical-shift, and STIR MR imaging. Radiology 174 (1990) 495–502

3 Boden, S. D., D. O. Davis, T. S. Dina, G. P. Parker, S. O'Malley, J. L. Sunner, S. W. Wiesel: Contrast-enhanced MR Imaging performed after successfull lumbar disk surgery: prospective study. Radiology 182 (1992) 59–64

4 Bundschuh, C. V., M. T. Modic, J. S. Ross et al: Epidural fibrosis and recurrent disc herniationi in the lumbar spine: assessment with magnetic resonance. Amer. J. Neuroradiol. 9 (1988) 169–178

5 Castillo, M., J. A. Malko, J. C. Hoffmann Jr.: The bright intervertebral disk: an indirect sign of abnormal spinal bone marrow on T1-weighted MR Images. Amer. J. Neuroradiol. 11 (1990) 23–26

6 Cuénod, C. A., J.-D. Laredo, S. Chevret, B. Hamze, J.-F. Naori, X. Chapaut, J.-M. Bondeville, J.-M. Tubiana: Acute vertebral collapse due to osteoporosis or malignancy: appearance on unenhanced and Gadolinium-enhanced MR Images. Radiology 199 (1996) 541–549

7 Dennis, F.: The three column spine and its significance in classification of acute thoracolumbar spinal injuries. Spine 8 (1983) 817–831

8 De Roos, A., H. Kressel, C. Spritzer, M. Dalinka: MR imaging of marrow changes adjacent to end plates in degenerative lumbar disk disease. Amer. J. Roentgenol. 149 (1987) 531–534

9 Djukic, S., M. Vahlensieck, M. Resendes, H. K. Genant: The lumbar spine: postoperative magnetic resonance imaging. Bildgebung 59 (1992) 136–146

9a Flanders, A. E., C. M. Spettell, L. M. Tartaglino, D. P. Friedman, G. J. Herbison: Forecasting motor recovery after cervical spinal cord injury: value of MR Imaging. Radiology 201 (1996) 649–655

10 Forristall, R. M., H. O. Marsh, N. T. Pay: Magnetic resonance image and contrast CT of the lumbar spine: comparison of diagnostic methods and correlation with surgical findings. Spine 13 (1988) 1049–1054

11 Fox, J. L., W. L. Werner, D. C. Rennan, H. J. Manz, D. J. Won, O. Al-Metty: Central spinal cord injury: magnetic resonance imaging confirmation and operative considerations. Neurosurgery 22 (1988) 340–347

12 Grand, C. M., W. O. Bank, D. Baleriaux, C. Matos, M. Levivier, J. Brotchi: Gadolinium enhancemant of vertebral endplates following lumbar disc surgery. Neuroradiology 35 (1993) 503–505

13 Grenier, N., R. I. Grossmann, M. L. Schiebler, B. A. Yeager, H. I. Goldberg, H. Y. Kressel: Degenerative lumbar disk disease: pitfalls and usefulness of MR imaging in detectioini of vacuum phenomenon. Radiology 164 (1987) 861–865

14 Hackney, D. B., R. Asato, P. M. Joseph et al.: Hemorrhage and edema in acute spinal cord compression: demonstration by MR imaging. Radiology 161 (1986) 387–390

15 Haddad, M. C., H. S. Sharif, O. A. Aideyan, D. C. Clark, M. S. Al Shahed, Z. G. Quereshi, M. Y. Aabed, B. Sammak, T. M. Bay-

doun, J. S. Ross, H. J. Bloem: Infection versus neoplasm in the spine: differentiation by MRI and diagnostic pitfalls. Europ. Radiol. 3 (1993) 439–446

16 Hajek, P. C., L. L. Baker, J. E. Goobar, D. J. Sartoris, J. R. Hesselink, P. Haghighi, D. Resnick: Focal fat deposition in axial bone marrow: MR characteristics. Radiology 162 (1987) 245–249

17 Hochhauser, L., S. A. Kieffer, E. D. Cacayorin, G. R. Petro, W. F. Teller: Recurrent postdiskectomy low back pain: MR-surgical correlation. Amer. J. Roentgenol. 51 (1988) 755–760

18 Hodsworth, F.: Fractures, dislocations and fracture dislocations of the spine. J. Bone Jt Surg. 52-A (1970) 1534–1551

19 Johnson, M. H., S. H. Lee, T. H. Liu: Magnetic Resonance Imaging of degenerative disorders of the spine. In Bloem, J. L., D. J. Sartoris: MRI and CT of the Muskuloskeletal System: a Text-Atlas. Williams & Wilkins, Baltimore 1992 (pp. 544–563)

20 Kalfas, I., J. Wilberger, A. Goldberg, E. R. Prostko: Magnetic Resonance Imaging in acute spinal cord trauma. Neurosurgery 23 (1988) 295–299

21 Lang, P., N. Chafetz, H. K. Genant, J. M. Morris: Lumbar spinal fusion assessment of functional stability with Magnetic Resonance Imaging. Spine 15 (1990) 581–588

22 Li, K. C., P. Y. Poon: Sensitivity and specifity of MRI in detecting spinal cord compression and in distinguishing malignant from benign compression fractures of vertebrae. Magn. Reson. Imag. 6 (1988) 547–556

23 Masaryk, T. J., M. T. Modic, M. A. Geisinger, J. Standefer, R. W. Hardy, F. Boumphrey, M. Duchesneau: Cervical myelopathy: a comparison of Magnetic Resonance and Myelography. J. Comput. assist. Tomogr. 10 (1986) 184–194

24 Mirvis, S. E., F. H. Geisler, J. J. Jelinek, J. N. Joslyn, F. Gellad: Acute cervical spine trauma: evaluation with 1.5-T MR Imaging. Radiology 166 (1988) 807–816

25 Modic, M. T., D. H. Feiglin, D. W. Piraino, F. Boumphrey, M. A. Weinstein, P. M. Duchesneau, S. Rehm: Vertebral osteomyelitis: assessment using MR. Radiology 157 (1985) 157–166

26 Modic, M. T., P. M. Steinberg, J. S. Rosek, T. J. Masaryk, J. R. Cartez: Degenerative disk disease: assessment of changes in vertebral body marrow with MR-Imaging. Radiology 166 (1988) 193–199

27 Naul, L. G., G. J. Peet, W. B. Maupin: Avascular necrosis of the vertebral body: MR Imaging. Radiology 172 (1989) 2219–2222

28 Roosen, N., T. Kahn, M. Messing, R. P. Trappe, U. Moedder, E. Lins, W. J. Bock: Gadolinium-DTPA-enhanced MRI of the asymptomatic postdiscectomy lumbar spine: early postoperative results. Neuroradiology 33, Suppl. (1991) 99–100

29 Ross, J. S. et al: Gadolinium DTPA-enhanced MR imaging of the postoperative lumbar spine: time course and mechanism of enhancement. Amer. J. Roentgenol. 152 (1989) 825–834

30 Ross, J. S.: Magnetic Resonance assessment of the postoperative spine. Radiol. Clin. N. Amer. 29 (1991) 793–8085

31 Ross, J. S., J. Masaryk, M. T. Modic: Postoperative cervical spine: MR assessment. J. Comput. assist. Tomogr. 11 (1987) 955–963

32 Ross, J. S., T. J. Masaryk, M. T. Modic, H. Bohlman, R. Delamater, G. Wilber: Lumbar spine: postoperative assessment with surface-coil MR Imaging. Radiology 164 (1987) 851–860

33 Ross, J. S., J. Masaryk, M. T. Modic, J. R. Carter, T. Mapstone, F. H. Dengel: Vertebral hemangiomas: MR Imaging. Radiology 165 (1987) 165–169

34 Ross, J. S., T. J. Masaryk, M. T. Modic et al.: Magnetic Resonance Imaging of lumbar arachnoiditis. Amer. J. Neuroradiol. 8 (1987) 885–892

35 Ross, J. S., R. Delamater, M. G. Hueftle et al.: Gadolinium-DTPA-enhanced MR Imaging of the postoperative lumbar spine: time course and mechanism of enhancement. Amer. J. Neuroradiol. 10 (1989) 37–46

36 Ross, J. S., M. T. Modic, T. J. Masaryk et al.: Assessment of extradural degenerative disease with Gd-DTPA-enhanced MR Imaging: correlation with surgical and pathologic findings. Amer. J. Neuroradiol. 10 (1989) 1243–1249

37 Schinco, F. P., L. E. Ladaga, J. D. Dillon: Distinguishing between scar and recurrent herniated disk in postoperative patients: value of contrast-enhanced CT and MR-Imaging. Amer. J. Neuroradiol. 11 (1990) 949–958

38 Schnarkowski, P., W. Weidenmaier, A. Heuck, M. F. Reise: MR-Funktionsdiagnostik der Halswirbelsäule nach Schleudertrauma. Fortschr. Röntgenstr. 162 (1995) 319–324

39 Schüller, H., M. Reiser: Magnetic Imaging and Computed Tomography of the spinal trauma. In Bloem, J. L., D. J. Sartoris: MRI and CT of the Muskuloskeletal System: a Text-Atlas. Williams & Wilkins, Baltimore 1992 (pp. 564–579)

40 Smoker, W. R. K., W. D. Keyes, V. D. Dunn, A. H. Menezes: MRI versus conventional radiologic examinations in the evaluation of the craniovertebral and cervicomedullary junction. Radiographics 6 (1986) 953

41 Sotiropoulos, S., N. T. Chafetz, P. Lang et al.: Differentiation between postoperative sear and recurrent disk herniation: prospective comparison of MR, CT and contrast-enhanced CT. Amer. J. Neuroradiol. 10 (1989) 639–643

42 Stäbler, A., K. Krimmel, M. Seiderer, Ch. Gärtner, S. Fritsch, W. Raum: Kernspintomographische Differenzierung osteoporotisch- und tumorbedingter Wirbelkörperfrakturen. Fortschr. Röntgenstr. 157 (1992) 215–221

43 Steiner, von H.: MR-Tomographie nach lumbalen Bandscheibenoperationen: differentialdiagnostische Möglichkeiten durch Gd-DTPA. Fortschr. Röntgenstr. 151 (1989) 179–185

44 Stoker, D. J.: Imaging of spinal disorders. Curr. Opin. Radiol. 2 (1990) 691–696

45 Tanaka, Y., T. Inoue: Fatty marrow in the vertebrae a parameter for hematopoietic activity in the aged. J. Gerontol. 31 (1976) 527–532

46 Tarr, R. W., L. F. Drolshagen, T. C. Kerner, J. H. Allen, C. L. Partain, E. A. James: MR Imaging of recent spinal trauma. J. Comput. assist. Tomogr. 11 (1987) 412–417

47 Teresi, L., R. B. Lufkin, M. A. Reicher, B. J. Moffit, F. V. Vinuela, G. M. Wilson, J. R. Bentson, W. N. Hanafee: Asymptomatic degenerative disk disease and spondylosis of the cervical spine: MR Imaging. Radiology 164 (1987) 83–88

48 Yu, S., L. A. Sether, P. S. P. Ho, M. Wagner, V. M. Haughton: Tears of the anulus fibrosus: correlation between MR and patho logic findings in cadavers. Amer. J. Neuroradiol. 9 (1987) 367–370

49 Yu, S., V. M. Haughton, K. L. Lynch, K. Ho, L. A. Sether: Fibrous structure in the intervertebral disc. correlation of MR appearance with anatomic sections. Amer. J. Neuroradiol. 10 (1989) 1105–1110

50 Yuh, W. T. C., C. K. Zachar, T. J. Barloon, Y. Sato, W. J. Sickels, D. R. Hawes: Vertebral compression fractures: distinction between benign and malignant causes with MR-Imaging. Radiology 172 (1989) 215–218

Shoulder

M. Vahlensieck

Introduction

As a ball-and-socket joint, the shoulder is a common site of chronic complaints. It is not unusual for the shoulder pain in young athletes to have no corresponding radiographic changes. The clinical evaluation can be complemented by a variety of imaging procedures, among which MRI has evolved as a procedure of high diagnostic value. This increasing role for MRI of the shoulder has been well documented in numerous review papers (3, 21, 27, 33, 49, 56, 58, 63, 68). This chapter will present the anatomy and pathologic changes as displayed by MRI as well as the role of MRI in the diagnostic evaluation of the shoulder joint.

Examination Technique

■ Patient Positioning

The patient is examined supine in the head first position. The patient should rest comfortably to reduce motion artifacts during the examination. A generous use of supporting pillows and other means can be helpful. To avoid respiratory artifacts, the arm to be examined should not be placed on the abdomen. It should be kept in *external rotation or a neutral position*. Internal rotation should be avoided since it overlaps the tendons of the rotator cuff and surrounding soft tissues, making assessment difficult and potentially leading to misinterpretations (9). The shoulder to be examined can be stabilized with sand bags to avoid minor movements. Suppression of respiratory artifacts is generally unnecessary. For patients with very *broad shoulders*, it may be necessary to position the patient obliquely by elevating the opposite shoulder. This will move the side in question toward the isocenter of the magnetic field and improve the image quality.

■ Surface Coil

To achieve an adequate signal, the shoulder is examined with a surface coil. A flexible or a rigid ring coil has proved useful. Rectangular coils can be used as well.

■ Sequences and Parameters

The imaging protocol should begin with fast T_1-weighted images in the *coronal plane* (SE), using a large field of view (FOV) and a body coil. These images serve as a pilot view to compare the distribution of the bone marrow signal between both sides and to select the appropriate high resolution sequences for the symptomatic shoulder. The first high resolution sequence is performed in the *axial plane*. It is important to assure an adequate resolution and the inclusion of the acromioclavicular articulation. To achieve an optimal resolution, the FOV should be confined to the area to be examined, as necessary for all high-resolution MRI examinations, and should be between 140 and 180 mm². Because of the signal-to-noise ratio, this measurement is determined by the magnetic field strength of the MR system. The section thickness should not exceed 4 mm. Based on theoretical and practical considerations, a dual echo steady state GRE sequence with an in-phase first echo has proved useful (57). The first short echo produces a good anatomic visualization and the second later echo the desired T_2 or T_2^* weighting (see Chapter 1). Axial images are best suited for disease processes of the glenoid labrum and the long biceps tendon. The images obtained with these sequences through the supraspinatus muscle are used to plan both subsequent sequences (Fig. 3.**1**), an oblique coronal T_1-weighted SE sequence and an oblique coronal dual echo steady state

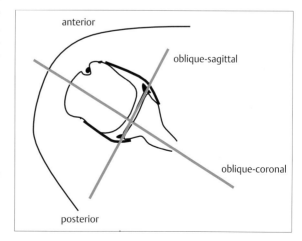

Fig. 3.**1** Transverse schematic drawing of the shoulder illustrating the oblique sagittal and oblique coronal planes.

GRE sequence. This plane is at an angle of about 45 degrees to the coronal plane and consequently parallel to the main orientation of the supraspinatus muscle. It is the only plane that requires a T_1-weighted sequence. The SE sequence facilitates the detection of susceptibility artifacts and hemorrhage as well as bone marrow infiltrates. Oblique coronal images are best suited for the evaluation of the rotator cuff and the subacromial-subdeltoid bursa. The examination is completed with a dual echo steady state GRE sequence in the *oblique sagittal* plane. This plane is perpendicular to the oblique coronal plane and suitable for the evaluation of the outer rotator cuff and the supraspinatus outlet.

When evaluating the bone marrow for edema or tumor infiltration, a *STIR sequence* or possibly a fast STIR (FSTIR) should be added. These sequences have the benefit of additive T_1 and T_2 contrast as well as the visualization of fat against a background void of any signal and therefore are extremely sensitive to the detection of intramedullary processes (see Chapter 1).

■ Special Examination Techniques

Fat suppression. This can improve the delineation of the tendons or capsular structures of the shoulder (34). It reduces artifacts caused by chemical shift and eliminates interference from adjacent fat-containing tissues and tendons or musculature. The clinical routine has proved that the sensitivity of detecting soft tissue lesions is not higher in comparison with T_2^*-weighted GRE sequences and that fat suppression does not have to be used routinely (57).

Acquisition of a three-dimensional data set. The acquisition of a three-dimensional data set with subsequent *multiplanar reformatting* has been advocated. In some circumstances, where an isotropic data set has been obtained, the multiplanar reformatting allows visualization of anatomical structures such as the coracoacromial ligament that may not be well seen on standard sections. However, the use of these sequences needs to balanced by some limitations.

The contrast comprises a mixed weighting of T_1 over T_2 if the three-dimensional steady state GRE sequence with short TR and TE is employed. This lacks important criteria for image interpretation, such as the signal pattern of T_1 and T_2 weighting, and can result in interpretative errors. Moreover, the resolution of the reformatted sections is only identical with the original data set if it is isotropic (see Chapter 1). Generating a high resolution isotropic data set of the shoulders is very time consuming and, in the end, no time saving is achieved in comparison with conventional methods because of the additional long reconstruction times. Further disadvantages include the vulnerability of GRE sequences to magnetic field heterogeneity and to susceptibility effects such as those seen between trabecular bone and adjacent bone marrow. GRE sequences are also more vulnerable to magic angle effects because of the need to employ a short TE. This may lead to the false positive diagnosis of rotator cuff pathology (see below).

Special methods. Special methods, such as the *radial sequence* with its radial rather than parallel acquisition of the planes (37), or the three-dimensional (3-D-rendering), which is even more time consuming, have not proved useful in routine clinical application.

ABER position. The ABER position refers to the position of the patient's arm, which is placed in **AB**ducted and **E**xternal **R**otation. This is achieved by placing the patient's hand behind the head. Sections are then obtained in an oblique axial plane aligning them with the long axis of the humerus on a coronal localizer. Several advantages have been found with the use of this technique. The undersurface of the supra- and infraspinatus tendons is well shown and visualization of subtle undersurface tears is improved. Furthermore, the technique has been found to be helpful in visualizing the anteroinferior glenoid labrum and associated inferior glenohumeral ligament which is under tension in this position. The evaluation of these structures is important when assessing the shoulder for causes of instability since they act as important static stabilizers of the joint (54a).

MR arthrography. This can markedly improve the detection rate of partial tears of the articular surface of the rotator cuff, in particular with the aid of fat suppression (20, 45). Furthermore, diagnosing lesions of the glenoid labrum can be improved by MR arthrography (14, 46). This is performed by injecting 10–15 ml of a 1:250 diluted Gd-DTPA solution (corresponding to 0.002 mmol/ml Gd-DTPA) into the joint, followed by T_1-weighted imaging with fat suppression. While this technique has the disadvantage of converting a non-invasive procedure into an invasive one, many centers now feel that the advantages justify its use. This is particularly the case for the investigation of shoulder instability in younger patients where labral abnormalities are suspected. In such cases MR arthrography may be the investigation of choice. In older patients, where chronic instability generally results from a different pattern of underlying abnormality, or where rotator cuff lesions are the primary concern, conventional MRI is probably adequate. This technique may be combined with the ABER position described above.

Indirect MR arthrography following intravenous injection and joint movements can be seen as an alternative (27a, 56b, 65a) (see Chapter 1).

Cinematic examination. This method is feasible with fast GRE sequences. Clinical applications have not yet been established (5).

Anatomy

■ General Anatomy

In the shoulder girdle, humerus and scapula articulate, forming the glenohumeral joint, as well as acromion and clavicle, forming the acromioclavicular joint. The articular surface of the glenoid fossa covers only one-third of the articular surface of the humerus. The area of contact is extended by a fibrocartilaginous rim (*glenoid labrum*). The joint capsule is reinforced anteriorly by the three glenohumeral ligaments (superior, middle, and inferior). Two variable outpouchings of the joint capsule above and below the middle glenohumeral ligament are known as the superior and inferior subscapular recesses.

The joint is surrounded by a fibrous envelope formed by the tendons of four muscles (*rotator cuff*). The multigastric subscapularis passes anteriorly, the digastric supraspinatus superiorly, and infraspinatus and teres minor posteriorly. It has only been discovered recently, partly by MRI, that the supraspinatus muscle consists of two parts (Fig. 3.**5**) (61). The spatial relationship of the supraspinatus muscle to the surrounding tissues is of great importance for pathologic alterations of the rotator cuff. The undersurface of the acromion, the

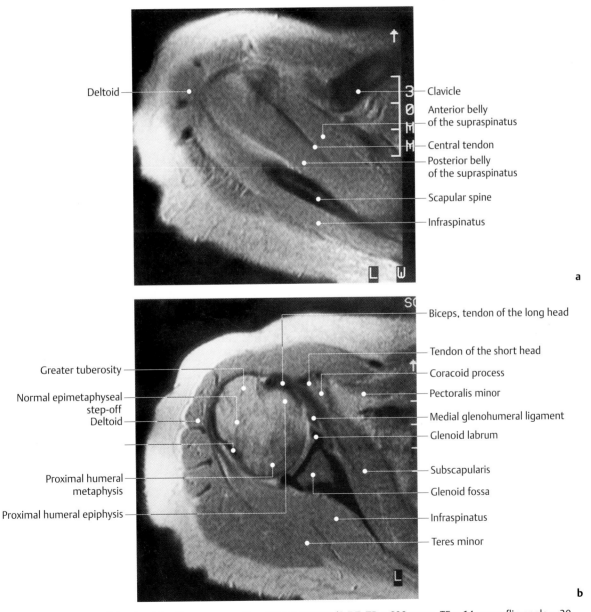

Deltoid — Clavicle — Anterior belly of the supraspinatus — Central tendon — Posterior belly of the supraspinatus — Scapular spine — Infraspinatus

a

Greater tuberosity — Biceps, tendon of the long head — Tendon of the short head — Coracoid process — Normal epimetaphyseal step-off — Pectoralis minor — Deltoid — Medial glenohumeral ligament — Glenoid labrum — Subscapularis — Proximal humeral metaphysis — Glenoid fossa — Proximal humeral epiphysis — Infraspinatus — Teres minor

b

Fig. 3.**2a–c** Anatomy of the shoulder. Transverse section. GRE sequence (0.5 T, TR = 600 msec, TE = 14 msec, flip angle = 30 degrees).

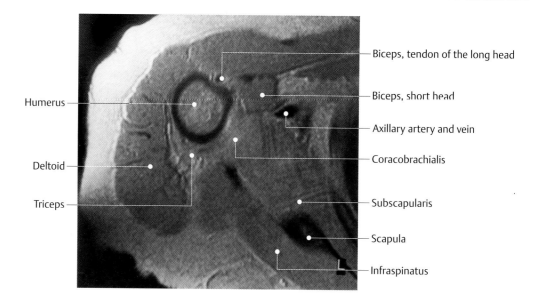

Fig. 3.**2c**

Structures labeled: Humerus, Deltoid, Triceps, Biceps, tendon of the long head, Biceps, short head, Axillary artery and vein, Coracobrachialis, Subscapularis, Scapula, Infraspinatus

Table 3.**1**   Important anatomic structures of the shoulder, arranged according to the most suitable MR imaging plane

Axial	Oblique coronal	Oblique sagittal
Supraspinatus muscle	Supraspinatus tendon	Rotator cuff
Glenoid labrum	Infraspinatus tendon	Coracoacromial ligament
Joint capsule	Subacromial bursa	Acromion
Glenohumeral ligaments	Acromioclavicular joint	
Biceps tendon	Superior labrum and biceps anchor	

coracoacromial ligament and acromioclavicular joint form the supraspinatus outlet or *coracoacromial arch* (39). The proximal tendon of the long head of biceps has a complex and variable insertion. The insertion sites include the superior glenoid tubercle and superior glenoid labrum. Fibrous slips also extend to the posterior and anterior labrum and the joint capsule. The tendon curves anteriorly through the joint to the intertubercular sulcus of the humerus where it is enclosed by a tendon sheath. The short head of the biceps arises from the coracoid apex together with the coracobrachialis. The subacromial-subdeltoid bursa lies superficial to the rotator cuff beneath the acromioclavicular joint and the deltoid muscle. It does not normally communicate with the glenohumeral joint. It is the largest bursa of the body and consists of a subacromial compartment and a subdeltoid compartment, which are demarcated by an indentation. In 10% of the cases, the subacromial-subdeltoid bursa communicates beneath the coracoid process with the subcoracoid bursa. A wedge-shape *intra-articular disk* projects into the acromioclavicular joint from the upper part of the articular capsule.

■ Specific MR Anatomy and Variants

Figs. 3.2– 3.4 illustrate the most important structures of the shoulder in the three imaging planes: axial, oblique coronal, and oblique sagittal. Table 3.**1** assigns the relevant anatomic structures to the plane most suitable for their visualization.

Fig. 3.**3a–c**   Anatomy of the shoulder. Oblique coronal sec- ▶ tion. GRE sequence (1.5 T, TR = 550 msec, TE = 15 msec, flip angle = 30 degrees).

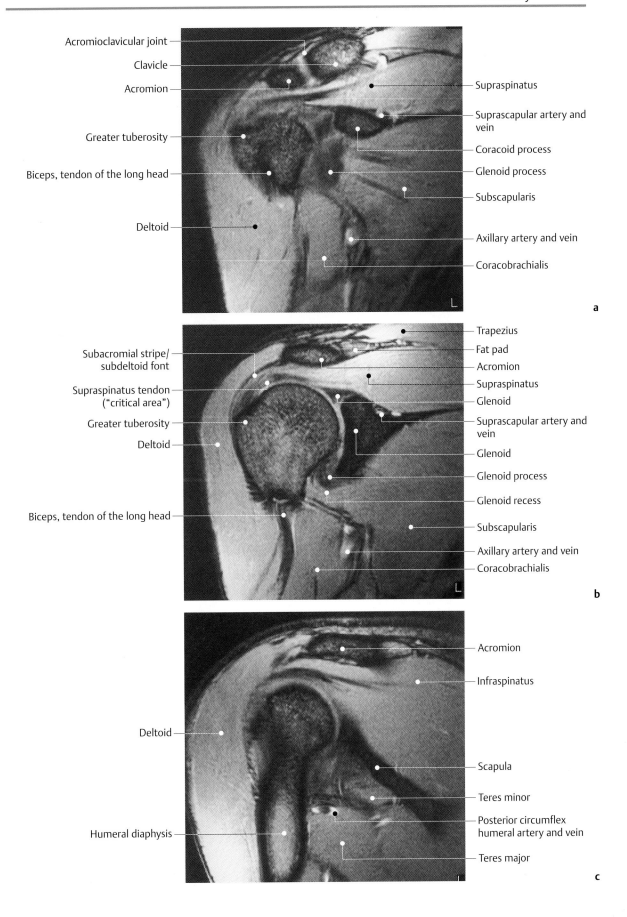

Acromioclavicular joint —
Clavicle —
Acromion —

Greater tuberosity —

Biceps, tendon of the long head —

Deltoid —

— Supraspinatus
— Suprascapular artery and vein
— Coracoid process
— Glenoid process
— Subscapularis
— Axillary artery and vein
— Coracobrachialis

a

Subacromial stripe/ subdeltoid font —
Supraspinatus tendon ("critical area") —
Greater tuberosity —
Deltoid —

Biceps, tendon of the long head —

— Trapezius
— Fat pad
— Acromion
— Supraspinatus
— Glenoid
— Suprascapular artery and vein
— Glenoid
— Glenoid process
— Glenoid recess
— Subscapularis
— Axillary artery and vein
— Coracobrachialis

b

Deltoid —

Humeral diaphysis —

— Acromion
— Infraspinatus
— Scapula
— Teres minor
— Posterior circumflex humeral artery and vein
— Teres major

c

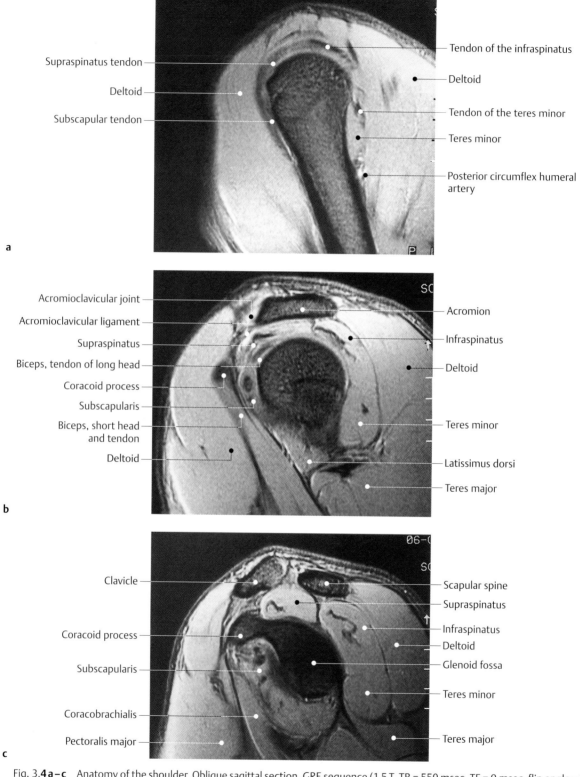

Fig. 3.**4 a–c**   Anatomy of the shoulder. Oblique sagittal section. GRE sequence (1.5 T, TR = 550 msec, TE = 9 msec, flip angle = 30 degrees).

Axial plane. The *supraspinatus muscle*, which runs at an approximate 40 degree angle to the coronal plane, is well delineated on the axial plane (Fig 3.**2**). The centrally located tendon accepts fibers of the anterior and posterior muscle belly and assumes an eccentric course at an angle of 50 degrees within the muscle fibers (Fig. 3.**5**). Both muscle bellies as well as the eccentric strong tendon insert at the greater tuberosity. In more than 80% of the cases, the central tendon also inserts at the lesser tuberosity as well as at the intertubercular ligament (61). Identifying the supraspinatus muscle serves to set up the oblique coronal and oblique sagittal sections. It does not matter whether a 40 or 50 degree angulation is selected for the oblique coronal sections (60). The subscapularis is best shown in this plane.

The axial sections delineate the *anterior* and *posterior glenoid labrum* well as low-signal, structures. They cap the cortical surfaces of the scapula as well as the high-signal hyaline articular cartilage. The labrum can have numerous variants and may not be visualized in up to 8% of normal cases (31, 32, 41) (Fig. 3.**6**). The morphologic variants affect the anterior labrum. Anteriorly and posteriorly, the labrum usually has a triangular configuration, but variations in the shape are seen, the most frequent being a rounded appearance. The labral variants are predominantly observed in the upper anterior portion (up to 10% of the cases), where the labrum can be separated from the osseous glenoid fossa (the so-called sublabral foramen) or may be completely absent (partial labral aplasia). Either normal variant can be mistaken for a tear by arthroscopy or imaging (Fig. 3.**7**) (56a). Areas of focal and linear increase in signal intensity have been described within the labrum of patients without known trauma or complaints This is in part explained by the magic angle effect seen in sections of the labrum orientated at 55 degrees to the main magnetic field. A similar effect is seen in the menisci of the knee. In addition, residual vascularization may account for this appearance. These signals should not be mistaken for a tear.

The *joint capsule* can be well evaluated on axial images. The insertion of the anterior capsule at the glenoid labrum is quite variable and can be classified into *three types* (52) (Figs. 3.**8** and 3.**45**). A recess between scapula

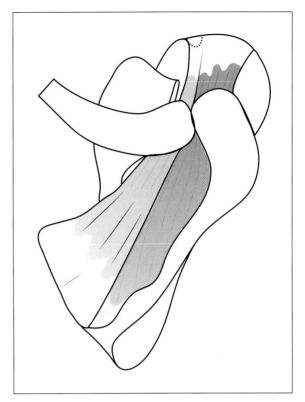

Fig. 3.**5**   Schematic drawing of the supraspinous fossa seen from above. The supraspinatus consists of two muscle bellies and has a central, eccentrically located tendon.

and anterior capsule should not hastily be interpreted as capsular separation. The diagnosis has to rest on the history and clinical examination. A proximal insertion at the scapular neck (type III) is considered a predisposition to an anterior shoulder dislocation. The anterior joint capsule is strengthened by three ligaments, the *glenohumeral ligaments*. They extend obliquely from the anterior glenoid margin to the humeral head. Between the ligaments are two openings of the joint capsule, which communicate with the superior and inferior subscapular recesses of the joint capsule. The superior glenohumeral ligament is small and thin

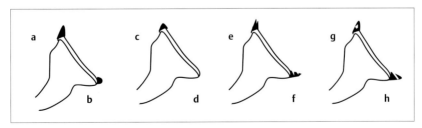

Fig. 3.**6**   Schematic drawing of the transverse section. Morphologic variants of the glenoid labrum with relative distribution in percentage for the anterior labrum. **a** triangular with line of increased signal intensity along the hyalin articular cartilage (50%). **b** rounded (20%). **c** comma-shaped flattened (7%). **d** absent (3%). **e** cleaved (15%). **f** notched (8%). **g** central increase in signal intensity. **h** linear increase in signal intensity. The posterior labrum generally exhibits a triangular or rounded form.

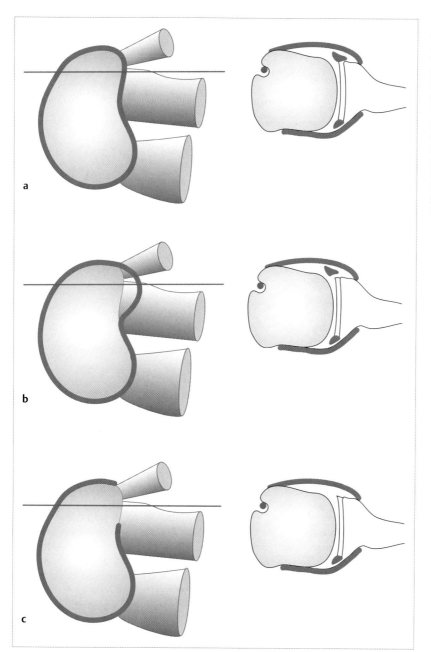

Fig. 3.**7 a – c**   Morphologic variants of the glenoid labrum in the upper anterior aspect. Left: orthograde view of the glenoid fossa with glenoid labrum and the three glenohumeral ligaments. Right: corresponding transverse MR images through the upper portion of the glenoid fossa (level marked by line on orthograde view). **a** Normal finding. **b** So-called sublabral foramen through the partially absent labral attachment to the glenoid fossa. **c** Partial labral aplasia. These normal variants should not be mistaken for labral avulsions.

and not always seen on MRI. The middle glenohumeral ligament is rather strong and is regularly delineated as a signal-free, band-like formation. Since it follows an oblique course relative to the axial plane, it is often only partially seen (Fig. 3.**2 b**). A well described variant is a thickened, prominent middle glenohumeral ligament in combination with an attenuated or absent anterosuperior glenoid labrum. This is known as the Buford complex.

The inferior glenohumeral ligament comprises an anterior and posterior band, with the axillary recess of the joint capsule arising between these two bands. The three glenohumeral ligaments actually represent thick-

enings of the anterior joint capsule. They usually arise from the anterior aspect of the glenoid including the labrum and are best seen when the joint capsule is distended with fluid, or at MR arthrography. In up to 15 % of cases, variations are observed in the ligamentous anatomy. Additional oblique images obtained in the ABER position may assist in the visualization of the anteroinferior glenoid labrum and the inferior glenohumeral ligamentous complex. In this position the tension produced may distract an otherwise undetectable anterior labral tear (54 a).

The *long biceps tendon* as well as its *sheath* are also best assessed in the axial plane. The tendon extends

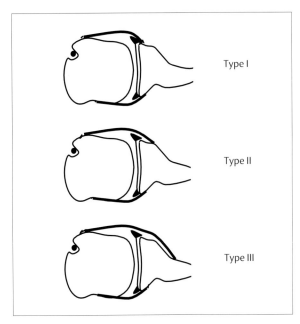

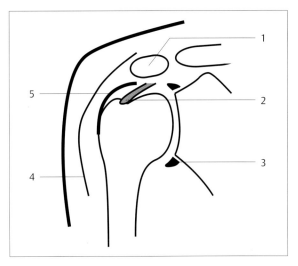

Fig. 3.**9**   Oblique coronal plane.
1 = Acromion
2 = Supraspinatus tendon
3 = Inferior glenoid labrum
4 = Deltoid fat stripe
5 = Fat stripe of the subacromial-subdeltoid bursa

Fig. 3.**8**   Schematic drawing of the transverse plane. Variations in configuration of the scapular insertion of the anterior joint capsule. The capsule inserts at the base of the glenoid labrum in type I, more medially in type II and along the glenoid neck in type III. The type III capsular insertion predisposes the shoulder to dislocate and should not be mistaken for a traumatic capsular detachment. A traumatic detachment of the capsule can be mistaken for a type III capsular insertion.

through the glenohumeral joint as well as through the bicipital sulcus, an osseous groove in the anterior humeral shaft. Within the sulcus, the tendon is surrounded by a tendon sheath, which communicates with the joint. Anteriorly, the sulcus is covered by the transverse ligament. The tendon is seen as a round, signal-free structure in the intertuberculous sulcus. Even in healthy individuals, it can be surrounded by a small amount of fluid (23).

Oblique coronal plane. This plane (Figs. 3.**3** and 3.**9**) is well suited for evaluating the insertion of the supraspinatus muscle at the greater tuberosity. The fibroconnective tissue of the tendons is generally shown as low signal on all sequences. Pathologic changes are characterized by increased signal intensity, but an increase in signal intensity can be observed near the insertion of the supraspinatus tendon in 80% of the cases without further evidence of traumatic or degenerative alteration of the rotator cuff (Fig. 3.**3b**). This increased signal, which is especially conspicuous on T_1-weighted and proton density images and characteristically does not further increase in intensity on T_2–weighted images, may result from a variety of causes. The increased signal may be focal or linear in shape and has a superior, central or inferior location within the tendon (43). In some cases the appearance may represent early myxoid degeneration which may relate to the poor vascularity

of this zone (the 'critical zone') (51). This appearance may be seen in asymptomatic young volunteers and is therefore presumably not age related. Other causes of this appearance include interposition of the tendon fibers with fat or connective tissue and partial volume averaging of adjacent muscle fibers (60). It is now recognized that in many cases this phenomenon is the result of the so-called 'magic angle' effect related to the orientation of the tendon in the main magnetic field (11).

It is known that anisotropic tissues, such as hyaline or collagen fibers, change their relaxation times if their longitudinal microfibrils are at a certain angle to the magnetic field. This angle was found experimentally to be 55 degrees and is referred to as the *magic angle*. This phenomenon also explains signal abnormalities found in other tendons and cartilages without documented pathology (see Appendix, section 1).

Another important structure to be evaluated in the oblique coronal plane is the *subacromial-subdeltoid bursa*. The bursa itself is normally invisible, but it is surrounded by extrasynovial fat that is identifiable by MRI in up to 70% of cases. The thickness of this peribursal fat plane correlates positively with the patient's age and weight and negatively with athletic activity and muscle mass (35). It is visualized as a stripe of high-signal intensity on T_1-weighted images (Fig. 3.**10**). Displacement and obliteration of the fat stripe and fluid accumulation within the bursa can serve as diagnostic criteria for various diseases (59).

The *acromioclavicular joint* is also best evaluated in the oblique coronal plane. The position of the articular disk and the width of the joint capsule are clearly de-

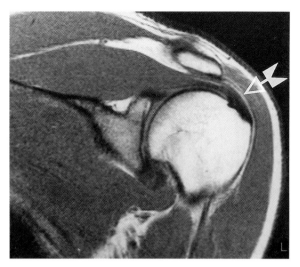

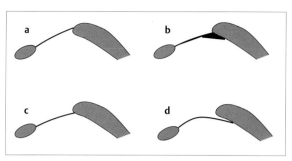

Fig. 3.**12 a–d**   Variants of the acromial attachment of the coracoacromial ligament. **a** Attachment at the tip of the acromion (approximately 10%). **b** Attachment at the base and undersurface of the acromion (approximately 20%). **c** Attachment at the base of the acromion (approximately 50%). **d** Attachment at the undersurface of the acromion (approximately 20%).

Fig. 3.**10**   Oblique coronal T₁-weighted SE image with visualization of the fat stripe of the subacromial-subdeltoid bursa as line of high signal (arrow). (0.5 T, TR = 600 msec, TE = 20 msec).

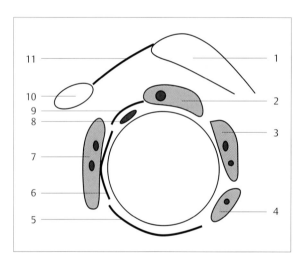

Fig. 3.**11**   Schematic drawing of the shoulder in the oblique coronal plane corresponding to Fig. 3.**4 b**.
1 = Acromion
2 = Supraspinatus muscle
3 = Infraspinatus muscle
4 = Teres minor muscle
5 = Inferior glenohumeral ligament
6 = Middle glenohumeral ligament
7 = Subscapularis muscle
8 = Long biceps tendon
10 = Coracoid process
11 = Coracoacromial ligament

lineated. Changes of the acromioclavicular joint are relevant in context with the impingement syndrome of the supraspinatus muscle (62 a).

Oblique sagittal plane. This plane is relevant for the assessment of the entire *rotator cuff* (Figs. 3.**4** and 3.**11**). The characteristic arrangement of four rotators around the glenoid process and humeral head lead to easy identification of the individual muscles and any tears involving their tendons.

The *coracoacromial arch* also can be evaluated in this plane. This arch is formed by the coracoid process, coracoacromial ligament and acromion. The *coracoacromial ligament* is inconsistently visualized as a linear signal void. The acromial attachment of the ligament is variable and four different types can be identified (16) (Fig. 3.**12**). The *acromion* varies in shape and position and these morphologic variants play an important role in the development of the shoulder impingement syndrome. Bigliani's classification, which describes the shape of the acromial undersurface, is frequently used (3 a). Type I has a flat or straight undersurface, type II a smooth, curved undersurface closely paralleling the superior humeral head in the oblique sagittal plane, and type III an anteroinferior hook shape of the undersurface. Type III is less common than types I and II, but is more often associated with a rotator cuff tear than the other types. Furthermore, a shallow slope is more often associated with a tear than a steep slope (Figs. 3.**13** and 3.**16**) (2, 4, 36). The normal acromial slope in this plane is between 10 and 40 degrees.

Occasionally, the *coracohumeral ligament* is visible in the oblique sagittal plane (Fig. 3.**14**). If a joint effusion is present or MR arthrography is performed, the insertion of the glenohumeral ligaments at the glenoid labrum can be identified (Fig. 3.**15**).

Fig. 3.**13 a–d** Morphologic and positional variants of the acromion in the oblique sagittal plane. The slope angle can be steep (**a**) or shallow (**b**). The undersurface of the acromion can be flat (**a** and **b**), curved (**c**) or hook-shaped (**d**). Shallow slope and hooked shape form a markedly narrowed supraspinatus outlet with the risk of an impingement.

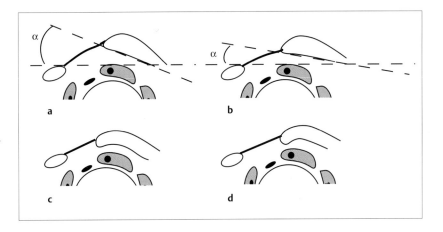

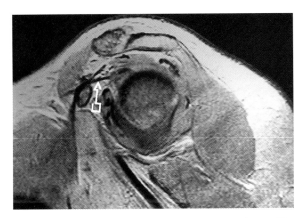

Fig. 3.**14** Oblique sagittal section. GRE sequence (0.5 T, TR = 600 msec, TE = 14 msec, flip angle = 30 degrees). Clear delineation of the coracohumeral ligament (arrow) beneath the coracoacromial ligament.

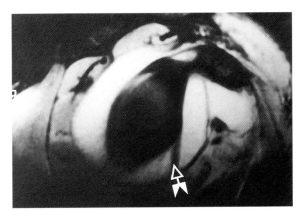

Fig. 3.**15** Oblique sagittal section. GRE sequence (1.5 T, TR = 550 msec, TE = 30 msec, flip angle = 25 degrees). Clear delineation of the attachment of the inferior glenohumeral ligament at the glenoid labrum (arrow).

Disorders of the Rotator Cuff

■ Impingement

According to Neer, tendons of the rotator cuff are subject to mechanical stress by repetitive impingement from compression against the acromion, leading to mucoid degeneration and subsequent tendon tear (38, 40). Neer considers impingement lesions in three progressive stages:

- Stage I: Reversible edema and hemorrhage
- Stage II: Fibrosis and tendinitis
- Stage III: Osseous changes and tendon tears.

The supraspinatus tendon is most commonly affected. Mechanical impingement of the rotator cuff tendons may have a variety of causes, many of which can be identified by MRI (53).

The *causes* include:

- hooked acromion (Fig. 3.**16**)
- flat undersurface of the acromion (Fig. 3.**17**)

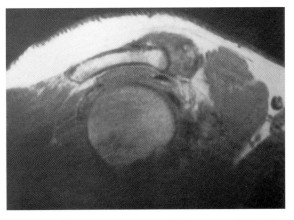

Fig. 3.**16** Oblique sagittal section. GRE sequence (0.5 T, TR = 1800 msec, TE = 20 msec). Hooked acromion with impingement of the supraspinatus.

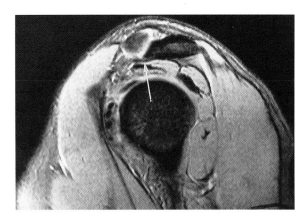

Fig. 3.**17**   Oblique sagittal section. GRE sequence (1.5 T, TR = 600 msec, TE = 14 msec, flip angle = 30 degrees). Flat acromion (arrow) with impingement of the supraspinatus by the shallow acromial slope.

- subacromial and acromioclavicular spurs (Fig. 3.**18**)
- thickened coracoacromial ligament
- capsular hypertrophy of the acromioclavicular joint (Fig. 3.**19**).

The MR findings of impingement are a compressed rotator cuff at the site of mechanical entrapment and thinning of the surrounding fat planes (16). Since the MR findings do not correlate closely with the clinical findings, they must be interpreted in the context of the clinical history.

■ **Degeneration, Tendinitis**

Chronic degenerative tendinitis and microhemorrhage. Histologic examination of the tendons shows some degree of mucoid degeneration seen on MRI as increased signal intensity without altered contour of the rotator cuff (26). The increased signal intensity can be especially appreciated on T_1-weighted and proton-density images, without further increased intensity on T_2-weighted images. Calcifications in chronic tendinitis (tendinitis calcarea) appear as signal void and can cause severe susceptibility artifacts, particularly on GRE images with long echo times (Fig. 3.**20**).

Acute tendinitis. Because of the associated edema, the tendon is swollen and exhibits an increased signal intensity on the T_2-weighted images. It is frequently accompanied by bursitis with a bursal effusion of high signal intensity on the T_2-weighted images.

■ **Partial-Thickness Tear**

Partial-thickness tears of the rotator cuff secondary to an impingement syndrome or trauma can become visible by MRI as focal contour defect or increased signal intensity on the T_2-weighted images (Fig. 3.**21**) or both. In general, superior and inferior tears cannot be reliably distinguished. Because of artifactually increased signal intensity in this region, false positive findings are common. MRI generally cannot distinguish chronic and acute inflammatory changes of the rotator cuff from partial tears. Direct or indirect MR arthrography can improve the sensitivity and specificity in the detection of

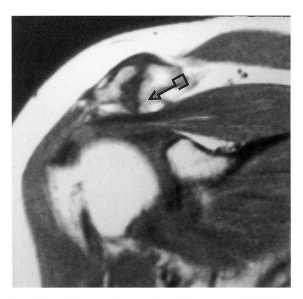

Fig. 3.**18**   Oblique sagittal section. GRE sequence (0.5 T, TR = 600 msec, TE = 20 msec). Degenerative osteoarthritis with osteophytic impingement of the supraspinatus (arrow).

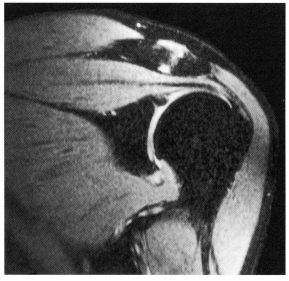

Fig. 3.**19**   Oblique sagittal section. GRE sequence with fat suppression (1.5 T, TR = 600 msec, TE = 20 msec, flip angle = 25 degrees). Effusion in the acromioclavicular joint with bulging joint capsule and mild impingement of the supraspinatus .

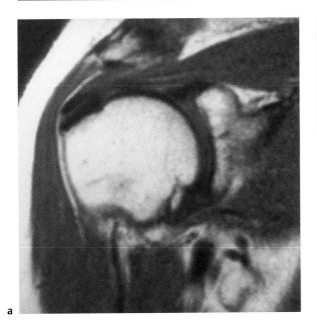

a

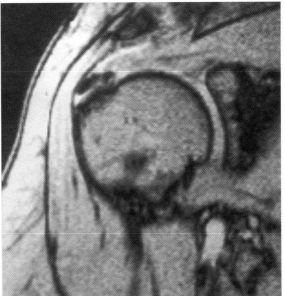

b

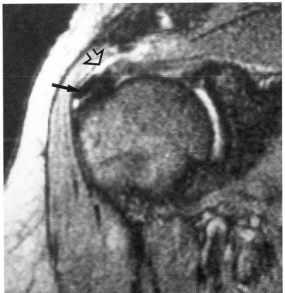

c

Fig. 3.**20 a – c** Oblique sagittal section. Calcifying tendinitis. **a** SE sequence (1.5 T, TR = 600 msec, TE = 20 msec). **b** GRE sequence, first echo (1.5 T, TR = 600 msec, TE = 7 msec, flip angle = 30 degrees). **c** GRE sequence, second echo (TE = 36 msec). The calcific deposit appears larger on the image with the longer echo time because of susceptibility artifacts (arrow). Concomitant effusion in the subacromial bursa (open arrow).

partial tears of the articular (under) surface of the tendon.

■ Full-Thickness Tear

A full-thickness tear of the rotator cuff causes a gap in the tendon, with the signal pattern of the gap related to the age of the tear:

Acute tear. In addition to edema, the gap fills with fluid and exhibits a low signal intensity on T_1-weighted and high signal intensity on T_2-weighted images (Figs. 3.**22** and 3.**23**). Since the rotator cuff is fused to the subacromial-subdeltoid bursa, the tear generally extends into the bursa and causes a massive bursal effusion (54).

This effusion is well seen as a high-signal structure on T_2-weighted images. Extensive tears can even continue into the unattached bursal wall as well as into the acromioclavicular capsule to cause an effusion of the acromioclavicular joint (the so-called 'geyser' sign). Furthermore, these findings are frequently accompanied by a large effusion of the glenohumeral joint (Fig. 3.**24**).

Old tear. The defect can fill with granulation tissue (covered rupture) and no longer displays the signal pattern of edema and fluid. It remains isointense or may become hypointense on T_2-weighted images (47). In these cases the articular and bursal effusion seen in acute cases may have largely resolved. These features

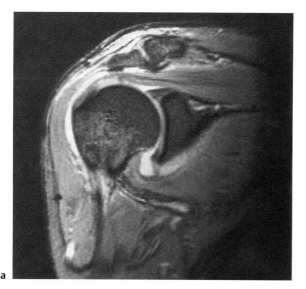

a

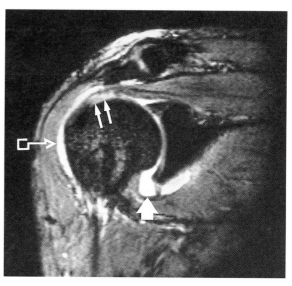

b

Fig. 3.**21a, b**   Oblique sagittal section. Partial-thickness tear of the supraspinatus (small arrows). **a** GRE sequence, first echo (1.5 T, TR = 600 msec, TE = 13 msec, flip angle = 25 degrees).

b Second echo (TE = 30 msec). The contrast increases with longer echo times (more T₂ weighting). Joint effusion (arrow), fluid in the subacromial-subdeltoid bursa (open arrow).

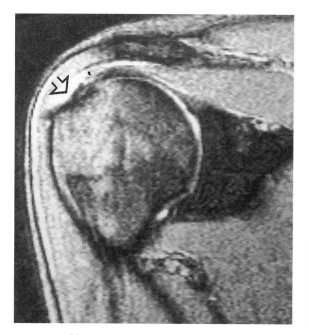

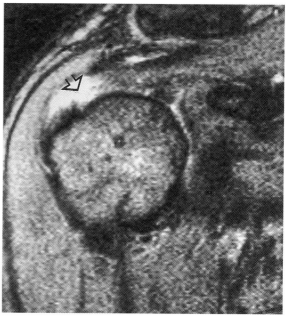

Fig. 3.**22**   Oblique sagittal section. GRE sequence (0.5 T, TR = 600 msec, TE = 36 msec, flip angle = 30 degrees). Rupture of the supraspinatus. Increased signal intensity and gap in the supraspinatus tendon (arrow).

Fig. 3.**23**   Oblique sagittal section. GRE sequence (0.5 T, TR = 600 msec, TE = 35 msec, flip angle = 30 degrees). Large defect showing increased signal intensity in the supraspinatus tendon (arrow). Frayed tendon margins.

make chronic tears difficult to diagnose at MRI. In particular, a confident distinction from chronic tendinitis may be impossible.

Disuse or lost muscular function following extensive chronic tears frequently causes fatty muscular *atrophy*, seen as characteristic linear and focal increase in signal intensity within the muscle on T₁-weighted images (Fig. 3.**24**).

Tears of the supraspinatus muscle occur most frequently as part of the impingement syndrome, whereas tears of the infraspinatus and subscapularis are less frequent and usually are traumatic in origin (Figs. 3.**25** and 3.**26**).

Mechanical impingement constitutes the most common cause of rotator cuff tears and, according to Neer, is responsible in more than 90% of cases (38).

Fig. 3.**24 a, b**   Oblique sagittal section. Large defect in the supraspinatus tendon. Retraction of the muscle belly with fatty atrophy (black arrow). Joint effusion (open arrow). Fluid in the acromioclavicular joint (white arrow). **a** SE sequence (1.5 T, TR = 600 msec, TE = 20 msec). **b** GRE sequence (TR = 600 msec, TE = 35 msec, flip angle = 30 degrees).

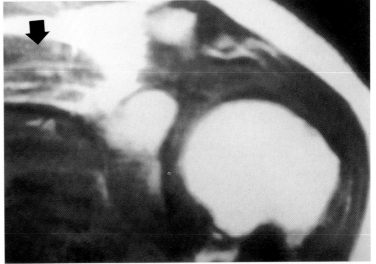

a

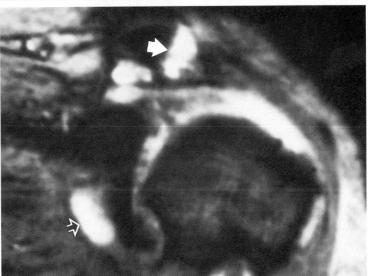

b

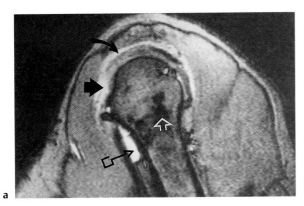

a

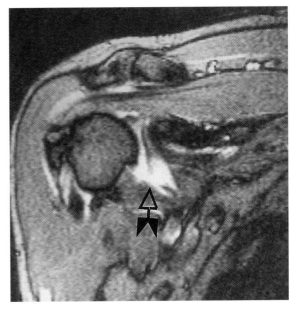

b

Fig. 3.**25 a, b**   Rupture of the subscapular tendon. **a** oblique sagittal section. GRE sequence (0.5 T, TR = 600 msec, TE = 35 msec, flip angle = 30 degrees). High signal defect in the subscapular tendon (arrow), joint effusion, here seen in the biceps sheath (open arrow), fluid in the subacromial bursa (curved arrow), hematopoietic bone marrow (open white arrow). **b** oblique sagittal section. GRE sequence (0.5 T, TR = 600 msec, TE = 35 msec, flip angle = 30 degrees). Defect extending into the muscle belly of the subscapularis (arrow).

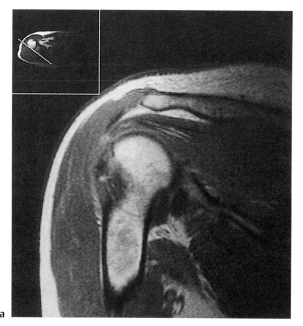

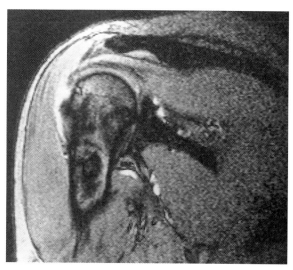

a   b

Fig. 3.**26 a, b**   Rupture of the infraspinatus tendon. **a** Oblique sagittal section. SE sequence (0.5 T, TR = 600 msec, TE = 20 msec). Heterogeneous signal in the rotator cuff. Inset of a transverse image showing the level of the section. Differentiating between infra- and supraspinatus tears can be difficult. The inset showing the imaging plane assists in the differentiation. **b** Oblique sagittal section. GRE sequence (TR = 600 msec, TE = 35 msec, flip angle = 30 degrees). High signal defect in the infraspinatus tendon. Fluid in the subacromial-subdeltoid bursa.

Trauma or overuse with degeneration are less frequent causes. The location predisposed for degeneration is the so-called critical zone of the supraspinatus tendon, a round area of reduced vascular supply a few centimeters away from the osseous insertion of the tendon (48).

MRI has proved a highly sensitive method for the detection of full-thickness tears. The sensitivity has been found to be 80 – 100 % and the specificity higher than 90 %, comparable to the results of conventional arthrography (13, 22, 67). Because of a more comprehensive visualization of the rotator cuff, MRI is superior to sonography (6). As already mentioned, the sensitivities and specificities are considerably less for partial tears, chronic covered small tears and chronic tendinitis.

While conventional MRI is accurate for the diagnosis of full thickness tears, where the distinction between a full thickness and partial thickness tear is difficult MR arthrography is often helpful. This is particularly the case when the abnormal signal is seen to contact the underside of the tendon (45).

MRI can assist in planning the surgical repair of tears by revealing the condition of the edges of the torn tendon, the extent of retraction or the presence of fatty atrophy.

Table 3.**2** summarizes the diagnostic criteria of the pathologic findings and artifacts at the insertion of the supraspinatus muscle.

◼ Enthesopathy

Degenerative changes of the teno-osseous transition must be distinguished from impingement. Excessive stress affecting the tendon at its osseous insertion seems to play the dominant role rather than impingement. This leads to subchondral cyst formation in the greater tuberosity, seen as low signal intensity on the T_1-weighted images (Fig. 3.**29**) and high signal intensity on the T_2-weighted images. These may be in continuity with the surface of the humeral head. Findings of enthesopathy and impingement of the subacromial space frequently coexist.

Table 3.**2** Signal pattern and other diagnostic criteria of the insertion of the supraspinatus tendon on MRI

T₁ ⟶ T₂		Finding	Diagnosis	Neer	Zlatkin	Possible additional findings
		F: normal C: regular S: none	normal tendon		0	
		F: normal C: regular S: mildly increased	acute tendinitis	1	1	thickened tendon, bursitis with joint effusion
		F: normal, thin C: regular S: similar	chronic tendinitis, degeneration, artifact	2	1	chronic bursitis with thick wall, thinned tendon
		F: thin C: irregular (superiorly or inferiorly) S: similar	old tear with scar, artifact		2	chronic bursitis
		F: thin C: irregular (superiorly or inferiorly) S: mildly increased	partial-thickness tear		2	bursal and joint effusion
		F: variable C: defect S: similar	old tear with scar	3	3	tendon and muscle retraction, fatty muscle degeneration, upward humerus displacement
		F: variable C: defect S: mildly increased	full-thickness tear	3	3	tendon and muscle retraction, bursal and joint effusion

F = form, **C** = contour, **S** = signal pattern of T₂-weighted images in comparison with T₁-weighted images, **Neer** = Neer classification, **Zlatkin** = Zlatkin

Disorders of the Biceps Muscle

Fluid in the sheath of the long head of the biceps muscle occurs with an effusion of the glenohumeral articulation as well as with tendinitis of the bicipital tendon. On the axial T₂-weighted images, such a fluid accumulation is seen as a round structure of high signal intensity, anterior to the humerus (Fig. 3.**27**). The tendon of the long head of the biceps muscle is delineated centrally within the effusion as a small round signal void. In case of *tendinitis*, the signal intensity of the tendon is increased, best appreciated on the T₂-weighted images.

Tendinitis of the long bicipital tendon frequently accompanies the impingement syndrome of the rotator cuff.

Tears of the long biceps tendon cause the central round signal void in the bicipital sulcus to disappear, which is referred to as the 'empty sulcus' (Fig. 3.**28**). An extensive effusion of the tendon sheath might be present. Occasionally, the superior tendon segment can be identified within the joint.

A tear of the transverse ligament can be directly visualized by MRI as long as the resolution is adequate. The axial sections show a discontinuity of the ligament that is normally seen as signal-void on all sequences. A

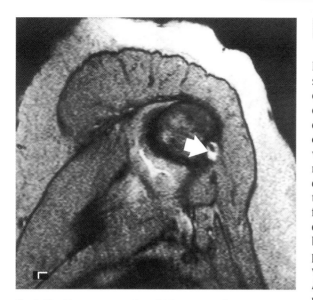

Fig. 3.**27**   Transverse section. GRE sequence (0.5 T, TR = 600 msec, TE = 35 msec, flip angle = 30 degrees). Fluid accumulation in the biceps tendon sheath (arrow) together with a joint effusion.

torn transverse ligament can lead to a medial *subluxation* of the long bicipital tendon. MRI displays an 'empty sulcus' and a subluxated tendon in the typical position anterior to the tendon of the subscapularis muscle. Tears of the transverse ligament are frequently associated with subscapularis tendon tears. In this case the biceps tendon may become displaced deep to the subscapularis (8, 12). If biceps subluxation is associated with shoulder dislocation, the biceps tendon may lie in such a position as to block reduction. In this case surgical intervention is required (1).

Disorders of the Remaining Musculature

Muscle atrophy reduces the muscle mass with compensatory fat deposition. This leads to characteristic streaks of increased signal intensity within the affected muscle on the T_1-weighted images. Such a fatty *atrophy* can develop with inactivity, especially in the presence of obesity (Fig. 3.**29**), and with shoulder girdle dystrophy, which may be generalized or confined to individual muscles (Fig. 3.**30**). If individual muscles are involved, denervation atrophy must be considered and the anatomic region traversed by the nerve supplying the affected muscle must be scrutinized for a tumor. Atrophy of the infraspinatus muscle, for instance, can be caused by a space-occupying lesion in the posterior supraspinous fossa, especially in the spinoglenoid notch, with involvement of the distal suprascapular nerve. Atrophy of the supraspinatus muscle and infraspinatus muscle can be caused by a space-occupying lesion in the anterior supraspinous fossa with involvement of the proximal suprascapular nerve (15). Paralabral cysts account for the majority of lesions found in this region (Fig. 3.**31**). They have a low signal intensity on T_1-weighted images and a high signal intensity on T_2-weighted images, and can be septated. They show rim enhancement and may be associated with a labral tear. Compression of the axillary nerve can lead to selective atrophy of the teres minor muscle or deltoid muscle or both (29).

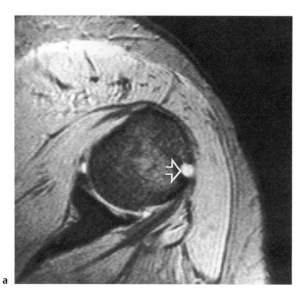

a

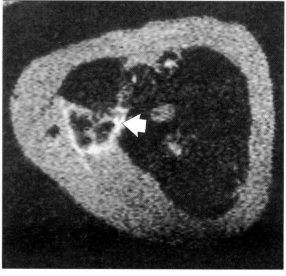

b

Fig. 3.**28 a, b**   Rupture of the tendon of the long biceps head. **a** Transverse section. GRE sequence (1.5 T, TR = 600 msec, TE = 13 msec, flip angle = 30 degrees). Fluid in the bicipital sulcus without biceps tendon ('empty sulcus') (arrow).

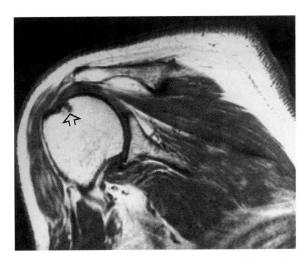

Fig. 3.**29** Oblique sagittal section. SE sequence (1.5 T, TR = 600 msec, TE = 20 msec). Intramuscular lines of increased signal intensity secondary to deposits of fat in obesity. Cystic resorption in the humeral head as manifestation of supraspinatus enthesopathy.

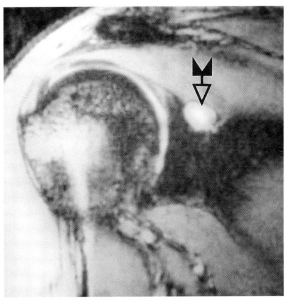

Fig. 3.**31** Oblique sagittal section. GRE sequence (1.5 T, TR = 600 msec, TE = 25 msec, flip angle = 30 degrees). High signal ganglion in the supraspinous fossa (arrow).

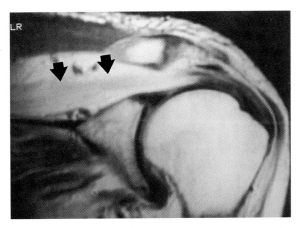

Fig. 3.**30** Oblique sagittal section. SE sequence (1.5 T, TR = 600 msec, TE = 20 msec). Marked increase in signal intensity in the supraspinatus due to fatty atrophy (arrows).

Disorders of the Subacromial-Subdeltoid Bursa

Inflammation of the subacromial-subdeltoid bursa frequently accompanies the impingement syndrome as well as a glenohumeral arthritis. Bursal inflammation can be an isolated finding. Acute *bursitis* presents as bursal effusion, which is of low signal intensity on T_1-weighted and of high signal intensity on T_2-weighted images (Fig. 3.**32**). The amount of accumulated fluid determines the configuration of the bursa and the peribursal fat plane, which is delineated as a high-signal stripe on the T_1-weighted images (Fig. 3.**33**). This stripe is *laterally displaced* with small effusions, as encountered frequently with impingement syndrome and iso-

lated bursitis. Larger effusions also displace the inferior portions of the bursa lateral to the humeral shaft, causing the fat stripe to assume a *teardrop configuration* (Fig. 3.**38**). Such large bursal effusions are frequently observed with glenohumeral arthritis as a manifestation of chronic polyarthritis. Extension of the inflammatory changes into the peribursal tissues (*peribursitis*) obliterates the peribursal fat stripe due to infiltration of the fatty tissue layers. This finding is frequently observed in association with a rotator cuff tear. A solely mechanical bursal destruction found with extensive rotator cuff tears can also obliterate the fat stripe. When applying this diagnostic sign, it must be considered that the peribursal fat stripe is weight-dependent and already absent in about 30% of healthy subjects (35). Therefore, an obliterated fat stripe is only a reliable indicator for a rotator cuff lesion or bursitis if the obliteration has evolved since preceding examinations.

The fat stripe around the subacromial-subdeltoid bursa and its pathologic changes can occasionally be identified on conventional radiographs (64, 65).

Normally, the fatty tissue is asymmetrically distributed in the bursal wall and more abundant in the superficial wall. This accounts for the single fat stripe seen in healthy individuals. The fibrous proliferation of chronic inflammation also increases the fatty tissue in the articular wall of the bursa and, if the bursa becomes fluid-distended, the oblique coronal sections can display two fat stripes (*double fat stripe*) (59).

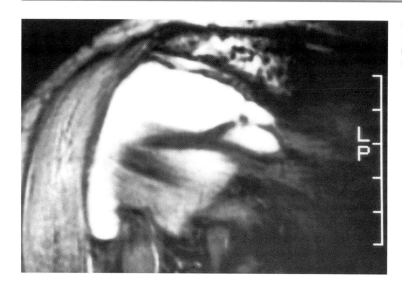

Fig. 3.**32** Oblique sagittal section. GRE sequence (1.5 T, TR = 600 msec, TE = 25 msec, flip angle = 30 degrees). Large effusion in the subacromial-subdeltoid bursa.

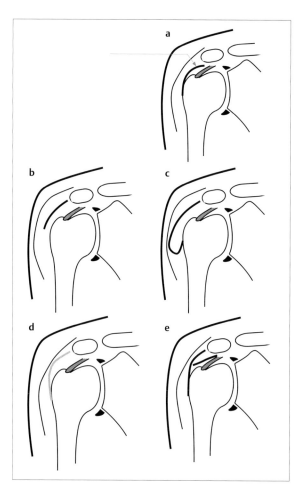

Fig. 3.**33 a–e** Schematic drawing of the fat stripe of the subacromial-subdeltoid bursa as seen in the oblique coronal plane. **a** Normal findings (arrow). **b** Laterally displaced due to small bursal effusion. **c** 'Teardrop' configuration due to large effusion. **d** Obliteration due to inflammation or rupture. **e** Double fat stripe due to chronic inflammation.

Disorders of the Glenoid Labrum and the Joint Capsule

Traumatic lesions of the labrum comprise partial-thickness tears, full-thickness tears and full-thickness tears with labral detachment. Partial tears are identified by MRI as increased signal intensity within the signal void of the labrum. Additional morphologic changes are a round configuration and cleft formation (Fig. 3.**34**). These changes are independent of the sequence and are best seen on axial sections. Reducing the section thick-

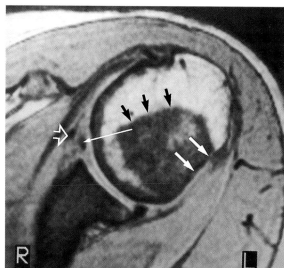

Fig. 3.**34** Transverse section. GRE sequence (0.5 T, TR = 600 msec, TE = 9 msec, flip angle = 30 degrees). Partial avulsion of the glenoid labrum with deformity and separation from the base (long arrow). No dislocation. Medial glenohumeral ligament (open arrow), hematopoietic bone marrow in the metaphysis (black arrow), normal wavy con tour at the meta-/epiphyseal junction (white arrows), no Hill–Sachs deformity.

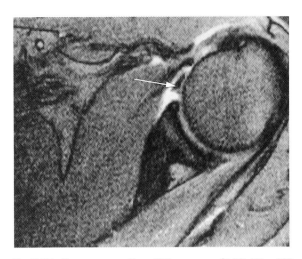

Fig. 3.**35** Transverse section. GRE sequence (0.5 T, TR = 600 msec, TE = 35 msec, flip angle = 30 degrees). Avulsion of the anterior glenoid labrum with anterior displacement (arrow).

ness to 1 mm can increase the diagnostic accuracy. Full-thickness tears can lead to labral detachment and, if the labral fragment is displaced, can be reliably diagnosed (Fig. 3.**35**). A tear of the anteroinferior labrum is called a Bankart lesion. An associated avulsion fracture of the glenoid is referred to as osseous Bankart lesion. Since the Bankart lesion ruptures the anterior scapular periosteum, labrum and attached ligaments become displaced anterior to the glenoid rim. The anterior labroligamentous periosteal sleeve avulsion (ALPSA) lesion is similar to the Bankart lesion but has an intact anterior scapular periosteum and allows medial displacement and inferior rotation of the labroligamentous structures.

The MRI findings of the labral tears can be divided into four stages:

- Stage I shows a basal increase in signal intensity in continuity with the articular surface of the labrum as evidence of a partial tear.
- Stage II shows a basal increase in signal intensity in continuity with the articular and non-articular surface of the labrum without dislocation of the labral fragment as evidence of a complete tear.
- Stage III shows a basal increase in signal intensity with dislocation of the labral fragment as evidence of a complete tear with dislocation.
- Stage IV shows a labral dislocation with avulsion of the capsule from the glenoid neck.

Stages I and II can be treated conservatively and stages III and IV require surgical intervention by arthroscopy.

When using this categorization, it must be kept in mind that the signal pattern of stage I often cannot be distinguished from basal signal changes found in normal variants. Furthermore, the variants of capsular insertion can make a reliable differentiation of stage III and IV impossible. Follow-up examinations can assist in deciding between trauma and normal variants.

Because of the numerous normal variants morphologic criteria for the evaluation of the labrum have some limitations. For the detection of labral tears, MRI only achieves a sensitivity between 45% and 85% (17, 42), with the location of the tear determining the actual sensitivity. Predicting anterior lesions is considerably more accurate than predicting posterior, inferior and especially superior lesions (19, 28). Axial images demonstrate the anterior and posterior labral tears to best advantage and oblique coronal images are best for superior and inferior labral tears.

The superior labral tear with anterior and posterior extension (so-called SLAP lesions) can be classified into four types, depending on the extent (21 a) (Fig. 3.**36**).

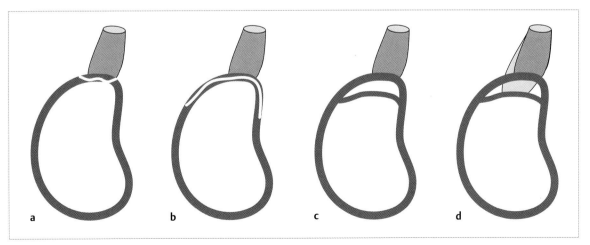

Fig. 3.**36 a–d** Schematic drawing of injuries to the superior glenoid labrum with anteroposterior extension (SLAP lesions). Schematic rendering of the orthograde view of the glenoid fossa with insertion of the long biceps tendon (above). **a** Tear in the region of biceps insertion at the glenoid fossa and glenoid labrum. **b** Capacious anterior (left) and posterior (right) extension of the tear (type II). **c** Bucket-handle tear (type III). **d** Bucket-handle tear with involvement of the biceps tendon (partial tear) (type IV).

- Type I lesions are characterized by a tear confined to the region inferior to the insertion of the biceps tendon at the glenoid fossa.
- Type II lesions demonstrate more anterior and posterior extension.
- Type III lesions involve partial intra-articular extension of the detached labral fragment (so-called bucket-handle tears),
- Type IV lesions are bucket-handle tears with involvement of the long biceps tendon, showing a partial longitudinal tear. This type of labral tear is commonly associated with a torn rotator cuff.

The detection rate of labral tears is considerably higher with direct or indirect MR arthrography (Fig. 3.**37**), and increasingly centers are using these techniques as the first step for the investigation of chronic instability.

In habitual shoulder dislocation, MRI can reveal the underlying condition or its sequelae or both. The anterior and posterior labrum can be deformed or the labrum may be completely absent. The Hill–Sachs deformity is marked by a notch defect of the humeral head. A separation of the anterior joint capsule from the scapular neck can be the cause or result of the instability. It is important to recognize signs of multidirectionality of the instability when planning the surgical approach to habitual shoulder dislocations. Correction by anterior capsulorrhaphy alone can promote frequent posterior dislocations after surgery.

Glenoid labral cysts are believed to be post-traumatic, analogous to the mechanism underlying meniscal cysts of the knee. They frequently coexist with glenoid labral tears (55). Labral cysts have a decreased signal intensity on T_1-weighted and increased signal intensity on T_2-weighted images. Lines of decreased signal intensity caused by septations are frequently observed. The cysts are observed as cystic masses with slight ballooning of the labrum. They can prolapse

through labral tears and appear as space-occupying perilabral lesions (55), which are characteristically located posterosuperiorly, posteroinferiorly and anterosuperiorly. Such cysts are often identified on MRI by their connection to the parent cyst or underlying labral tear.

Glenohumeral Arthritis and Other Conditions of the Synovial Membrane

So far, MRI has not played a major role in the diagnostic evaluation of *arthritis*, despite its ability to display both osseous and soft tissue changes including any cartilage destruction and the extent of any joint effusion. With the help of these findings, the degree of articular destruction can be accurately determined and the treatment planning improved.

Osseous erosions are displayed as cortical defects and are more readily detected by MRI than by conventional radiography (25). The signal intensity of the erosions is low on T_1-weighted images and high on T_2-weighted images. Active *pannus* formation also appears as low signal intensity on T_1-weighted images and as high signal intensity on T_2-weighted images. Since fluid has a longer T_2 relaxation time than pannus, effusion can be distinguished from active pannus on heavily T_2-weighted sequences. Moreover, pannus enhances after IV contrast medium. Inactive fibrous pannus is of low signal intensity on all sequences, approaching the intensity of muscle.

Tears of the rotator cuff or tendon of the long biceps head characteristically accompany chronic polyarthritis (Fig. 3.**38**). These tears have the same MR findings as the tears occurring without arthritis. Muscular atrophy, bursitis, and tendinitis are additional associated changes.

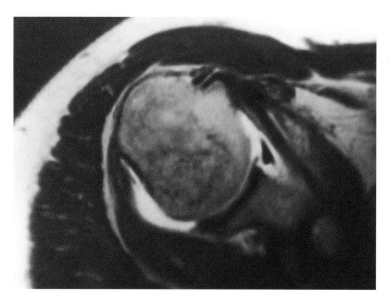

Fig. 3.**37**   Transverse section. SE sequence after intra-articular injection of contrast medium (MR arthrography) (1.5 T). Avulsion of the anterior glenoid labrum with lateral and posterior displacement.

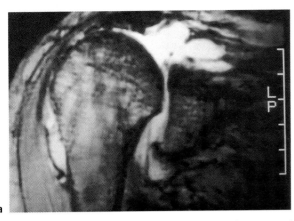

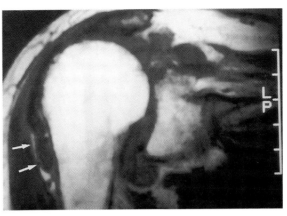

a

b

Fig. 3.**38 a, b** Glenohumeral arthritis as manifestation of chronic polyarthritis with rotator cuff tear and large joint effusion. Oblique sagittal section. **a** T$_1$-weighted SE sequence (1.5 T, TR = 600 msec, TE = 20 msec). **b** GRE sequence (TR = 600 msec, TE = 35 msec, flip angle = 30 degrees). The extensive fluid accumulation in the subacromial-subdeltoid bursa produces a teardrop-like displacement of the bursal fat stripe (arrow).

A rare disease of the shoulder is post-traumatic osteolysis of the clavicle, constituting a destruction of the distal clavicular end induced by synovial proliferation secondary to acute or chronic trauma. The clinical findings include a painful swelling and crepitation. On the T$_1$-weighted images, these synovial proliferations are heterogenous with the signal partially increased and partially decreased in intensity (10). The acromioclavicular joint space appears widened.

Hemosiderin deposits as found with pigmented villonodular synovitis or hemophilic arthropathy cause focally decreased signal intensity in the joint, which is best seen on T$_2$-weighted images. Calcified or ossified loose bodies, as found with *synovial chondromatosis*, also present as low signal intensity or signal void on all sequences.

In 50% of the cases, avascular necrosis is accompanied by a *joint effusion*. During the course of the disease, the osseous structures collapse and reactive fibrosis and sclerosis develop, depicted as decreased signal intensity on all sequences. MRI is considered the most sensitive method for the detection of avascular osteonecrosis.

Humeral head compression fractures following shoulder dislocation are seen on axial images as irregularity along the circumference of the humeral head and, depending on the severity, present as a notch defect or just as flattened contour (Fig. 3.**40**). Acute compression fractures are also accompanied by bone marrow edema, seen as increased signal intensity on the T$_2$-weighted images. The lesions can be quantified by the angular circumferential involvement:

Osseous Disorders

Avascular osteonecrosis of the humeral head has the same diagnostic criteria as osteonecrosis of the femoral head. The T$_1$-weighted images display a focal or band-like subchondral decrease in signal intensity. The low-signal band frequently surrounds a high signal center attributed to normal fatty bone marrow (Fig. 3.**39**). On the T$_2$-weighted images, a band-like decrease in signal intensity is often seen alongside a band-like increase in signal intensity. This is referred to as the ›double line sign‹ and considered pathognomonic for osteonecrosis. The decreased signal intensity corresponds to sclerosis and the increased signal intensity to a reactive region between viable and necrotic bone marrow. The disease is frequently bilateral. The risk factors include:

- corticosteroid therapy
- alcoholism
- trauma
- sickle cell anemia.

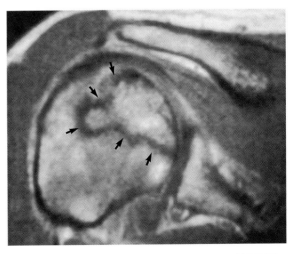

Fig. 3.**39** Oblique sagittal section. SE sequence (1.5 T, TR = 600 msec, TE = 20 msec). Avascular osteonecrosis with high-signal subchondral center and surrounding low-signal band-like zone (arrow).

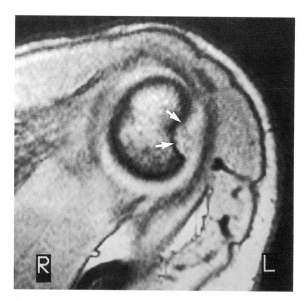

Fig. 3.**40** Transverse section. GRE sequence (0.5 T, TR = 600 msec, TE = 9 msec, flip angle = 30 degrees). Posterolateral indentation of the humeral head following shoulder dislocation. Hill–Sachs defect, II (arrows).

- up to 30 degrees of the circumference: grade I,
- between 30 and 60 degrees of the circumference: grade II, and
- exceeding 60 degrees of the circumference: grade III.

A distinction is made between superior compression fracture after inferior dislocation, posterolateral compression (*Hill–Sachs lesion*) after anterior dislocation and anteromedial compression (*reverse Hill–Sachs lesion*) after posterior dislocation.

By using the clock face as a reference, and with the bicipital sulcus at 12 o'clock, the location of the Hill–Sachs lesion ranges from 3 to 5 o'clock on the left and from 7 to 9 o'clock on the right. Using a section thickness of 4–5 mm, all fractures are seen on the two uppermost sections distal to the top of the humeral head. They must be distinguished from the anatomic indentation at the posterolateral portion of the humerus, which always begins on more distal axial sections of the humerus at or below the coracoid process (Fig. 3.**34**) (50). MR imaging detects Hill–Sachs lesions with a sensitivity of 97% (66). The same sensitivity can be achieved with conventional radiography when special views are obtained.

The visualization of inflammatory and traumatic lesions of the skeleton by MRI is presented in Chapter 11.

Tumors

For the diagnostic evaluation of tumors, MRI can provide information on the tumor size, infiltration into the articular soft tissues and the presence of any joint effusion. The different tumor categories are discussed in Chapter 12.

Post-Therapy Findings

Painful rotator cuff impingement syndromes are frequently treated with *injections* of corticosteroids or local anesthetics or both. On the T_2-weighted image, these injections can induce focally increased signal intensity in the rotator cuff that should not be mistaken for a localized inflammation (24). Occasionally, the subacromial-subdeltoid bursa is injected and can mimic a bursal effusion. At least two weeks should elapse between injection of such preparations and MRI examination.

Surgical procedures for a torn rotator cuff include tendon-to-tendon repair, tendon-to-bone repair and closing the defect with autografts or allografts. The impingement syndrome can be treated surgically with acromioplasty, which can be combined with bursectomy, or with an incision of the coracoacromial ligament. Surgery for recurrent shoulder dislocations due to instability should stabilize the glenohumeral joint. Several methods are available, such as reinforcement of the anterior capsule (Putti-Platt), bone graft insertion (Eden-Hybbinette), transfer of the subscapular muscle (Magnuson-Stack) and coracoid transposition (Bristow-Helfer). Recurrent or persistent complaints after shoulder surgery represent a frequent problem (up to 25% of the cases) and are caused by tendinitis, new full-thickness or partial-thickness tear of the rotator cuff, persistent impingement and others. These postoperative conditions must be distinguished from the usual postoperative appearance.

The MRI of the postoperative shoulder shows a loss of the periarticular soft tissue layers due to scarring or resection (Fig. 3.**41**). The peribursal fat stripe can no

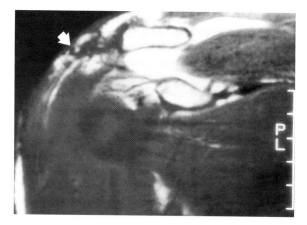

Fig. 3.**41** Oblique sagittal section. SE sequence (1.5 T, TR = 600 msec, TE = 20 msec). Status post shoulder surgery with loss of the regular cutaneous layers (arrow). The subacromial-subdeltoid bursa is partially resected.

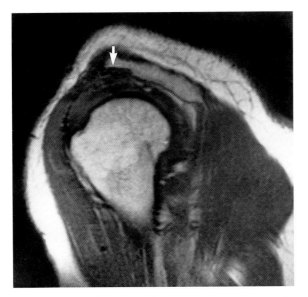 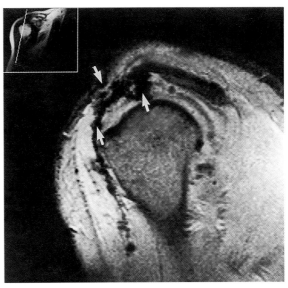

Fig. 3.**42 a, b**   Oblique sagittal section. Status post acromio-plasty. **a** SE sequence (1.5 T, TR = 600 msec, TE = 20 msec). Defect and step deformity of the acromion (arrow). Smooth re-section margin. **b** GRE sequence (TR = 600 msec, TE = 14 msec, flip angle = 30 degrees). Multifocal signal extinction due to metallic and osseous fragments (arrows).

longer serve as diagnostic finding since the bursa has been removed. A small persistent bursal effusion, which is frequently seen after surgical intervention, should not be mistaken for a bursitis or indirect sign of a recurrent bursal effusion (44). Furthermore, bony and metallic fragments characteristically can induce susceptibility artifacts that appear as multiple signal voids and are most conspicuous on GRE sequences with long echo times (Fig. 3.42).

The Eden-Hybinette procedure, which consists of a bone graft inserted into the anteroinferior glenoid rim, is depicted on MRI as localized scar tissue with a low signal intensity on all sequences (Fig. 3.43). The scar tissue is presumably induced by the bone graft and prevents a recurrent anterior dislocation by extending the anterior glenoid labrum.

Acromioplasty alters the configuration of the acromion and decreases its signal intensity on T_1-weighted and T_2-weighted images, presumably due to

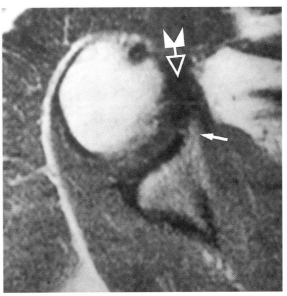

a

b

Fig. 3.**43 a, b**   Transverse section. **a** SE sequence (1.5 T, TR = 600 msec, TE = 20 msec). Status post Eden-Lange-Hybinette surgery. Bone graft fused with the glenoid process (small arrow). Low-signal scar tissue anteriorly (large arrow). **b** schematic drawing of the transverse plane of the normal shoulder (left) and of a shoulder following bone grafting with delineation of a ventral scar (right) (›doorstop sign›).

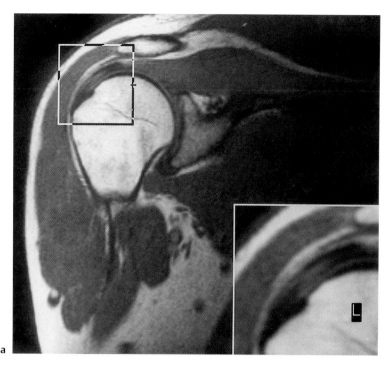

a

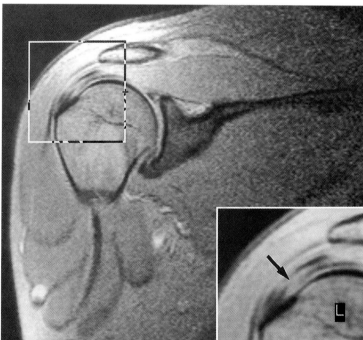

b

Fig. 3.**44 a–c**   Oblique sagittal section.
a SE sequence (0.5 T, TR = 600 msec,
TE = 20 msec). **b** GRE sequence, first echo
(TR = 600 msec, TE = 14 msec, flip angle =
30 degrees).

sclerosis and fibrosis. Tendon repair generally leads to persistent increase in signal intensity in the tendon on the T_1-weighted and proton density images, with the signal unchanged or more intense on T_2-weighted images (44). This signal pattern is indistinguishable from that found in recurrent or partial tear and makes it difficult, if not impossible, to diagnose either condition. In tendon-to-bone repair, the humeral head shows a trough of low signal intensity on all sequences.

Pitfalls in Interpreting the Images

A field orientation artifact with increased signal intensity in the tendons of the rotator cuff, especially the one observed in the supraspinatus tendon, should not be misinterpreted as tendinitis or partial tear (Fig. 3.**44**). The increased signal probably depends on the orientation of anisotropic tissue in the main mag-

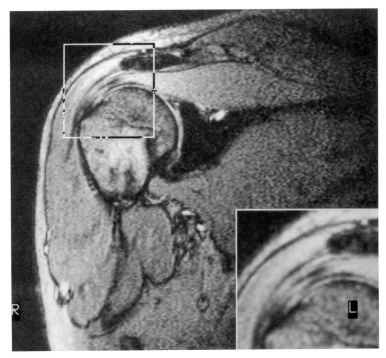

Fig. 3.**44c**　second echo (TE = 35 msec). T₁-weighted image and first GRE image show an increased signal along the course of the supraspinatus tendon, without further increase in intensity with increased T₂ weighting in the second echo (arrow). This most likely reflects an artifactual increase in signal intensity and not a partial-thickness tear or tendinitis.

netic field (see Appendix) and is most pronounced on T_1-weighted and proton-density images. The presence of any increased signal intensity on the $T_2{}^*$-weighted or T_2-weighted images, which is an established sign of a rotator cuff lesion, should help to avoid this misinterpretation.

The numerous morphologic variants of the glenoid labrum should be known to avoid interpreting them as tears. The hyaline cartilage, which is of high-signal intensity, lies between glenoid labrum and cortical bone, which are of low signal intensity, and this anatomic interposition might be mistaken for a basal tear of the labrum (Fig. 3.**45**). Furthermore, the close vicinity of the glenoid labrum to the medial glenohumeral ligament can cause a linear increase in signal intensity that should not be interpreted as labral tear (30).

Axial sections occasionally show a morphologic variant of the posterolateral contour of the humeral head that should not be mistaken for a Hill–Sachs lesion (Fig. 3.**34**) (18).

Fluid accumulation in the subscapular recess should not be misinterpreted as a ruptured capsule with extension of fluid into the soft tissues (Fig. 3.**46**). The recess can extend a considerable distance anteriorly and may even 'saddlebag' over the subscapularis to lie in the subcoracoid space.

A small amount of fluid in the tendon sheath of the tendon of the long biceps head is normal and should not be called a pathologic effusion. Moreover, a branch of the anterior circumflex humeral artery may mimic a fluid accumulation adjacent to the biceps tendon sheath in the bicipital groove on axial GRE sections (23).

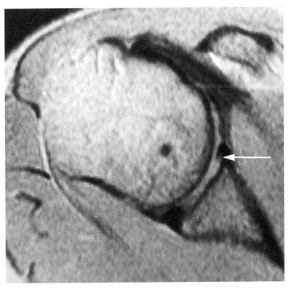

Fig. 3.**45**　Transverse section. GRE sequence (0.5 T, TR = 600 msec, TE = 14 msec, flip angle = 30 degrees). The anterior glenoid labrum exhibits an increased signal at its base representing the hyaline articular cartilage (arrow). This finding should not be mistaken for a labral avulsion. Type I joint capsule with insertion of the capsule at the anterior labrum.

A signal increase in the rotator cuff or a fluid accumulation in the subacromial-subdeltoid bursa induced by therapeutic injections should not be misinterpreted as a pathologic finding.

The proximal humerus metaphysis invariably harbors hematopoietic bone marrow, which has a lower

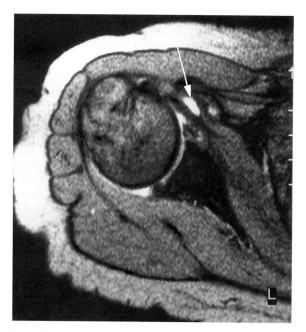

Fig. 3.**46** Transverse section. GRE sequence (0.5 T, TR = 600 msec, TE = 35 msec, flip angle = 30 degrees). Joint effusion with fluid in the subcoracoid recess. This finding should not be mistaken for a capsular tear (arrow).

signal intensity than fat on the T_1-weighted images. This normal bone marrow pattern should not be mistaken for an infiltrative process of the humerus (Fig. 3.**34**).

Clinical Relevance of MRI and Comparison with Other Imaging Modalities

Conventional radiography remains essential for the initial diagnostic evaluation of the shoulder. MRI and conventional radiography can be considered complementary modalities, wherein each technique has distinct advantages and limitations (7). In particular, calcifications and cortical abnormalities are better delineated on plain films than on MR images. Table 3.**3** should serve as a guideline for the contribution of MRI in comparison with other imaging methods to the sequential evaluation of various disorders of the shoulder. Availability and costs of the various methods are not taken into consideration.

Tabelle 3.**3** The role of the various imaging methods in the sequential diagnostic evaluation of the shoulder as related to the suspected diagnosis

	Radiography	Sonography	Arthrography	CT	Arthro-CT	MRI	Arthro-MR
Impingement	1	2	4			3	4
Instability		1			2		2
Bursitis/Tendinitis	2	1					
Tumors	1	(2)				2	
Osteonecrosis	1					2	
Arthritis	1	2					
Adhesive capsulitis			1				2
Muscular dystrophies		(1)					
Trauma							
• fracture	1			2			
• dislocation	1				2		
• marrow edema						1	
• capsular tear			1				
• biceps tendon tear/ dislocation		1					

1   = Method should be performed first
2 – 4 = Method should be performed sequentially if uncertainty remains

Literatur

1 Allard, J. C., J. Bancroft: Irreducible posterior dislocation of the shoulder: MR and CT findings. J. Comput. assist. Tomogr. 15 (1991) 694–696

2 Aoki, M., S. Ishii, M. Usui: The slope of the acromion and rotator cuff impingement. Orthop. Trans. 10 (1986) 228

3 Beyer, D., W. Steinbrich, G. Krestin, J. Koebke, B. Kummer, J. Bunke: MR des Schultergelenkes mit Oberflächenspulen bei 1,5 Tesla: Anatomie und mögliche klinische Anwendungen. Fortschr. Röntgenstr. 146 (1987) 294–299

3a Bigliani, L. U., et al.: The morphology of the olecranon and its relationship to rotator cuff tears. Orthop. Trans. 10 (1986) 216

4 Bigliani, L. U., D. S. Morisson: The Morphology of the acromion and its relationship to rotator cuff tears. Orthop. Trans. 10 (1986) 228

5 Bonutti, P. M., J. F. Norfray, R. J. Friedman, B. M. Genez: Kinematic MRI of the shoulder. J. Comput. assist. Tomogr. 17 (1993) 666–669

6 Burk, D. L., D. Karasick, A. B. Kurtz, D. G. Mitchell, M. D. Rifkin, C. L. Miller, D. W. Levy, J. M. Fenlin, A. R. Bartolozzi: Rotator cuff tears: prospective comparison of MR imaging with arthrography, sonography and surgery. Amer. J. Roentgenol. 153 (1989) 87–92

7 Burk, D. L., D. Karasick, D. G. Mitchell, M. D. Rifkin: MR imaging of the shoulder: correlation with plain radiography. Amer. J. Roentgenol. 154 (1990) 549–553

8 Cervilla, V., M. E. Schweitzer, C. Ho, A. Motta, R. Kerr, D. Resnick: Medial dislocation of the biseps brachii tendon: appearance at MR imaging. Radiology 180 (1991) 523–526

9 Davis, S. J., L. M. Teresi, W. G. Bradley, J. A. Ressler, R. T. Eto: Effect of arm rotation on MR imaging of the rotator cuff. Radiology 181 (1991) 265–268

10 Erickson, S. J., J. B. Kneeland, R. A. Komorowski, G. J. Knudson, G. F. Carrera: Posttraumatic osteolysis of the clavicle: MR features. J. Comput. assist. Tomogr. 14 (1990) 835–837

11 Erickson, S. J., I. H. Cox, J. S. Hyde, G. F. Carrera, J. A. Strandt, L. D. Estkowski: Effect of tendon orientation on MR imaging signal intensity: a manifestation of the „magic angle" phenomenon. Radiology 181 (1991) 389–392

12 Erickson, S. J., S. W. Fizgerald, S. F. Quinn, G. F. Carrera, K. P. Black, T. L. Lawson: Long bisipital tendon of the shoulder: normal anatomy and pathologic findings on MR imaging. Amer. J. Roentgenol. 158 (1992) 1091–1096

13 Evancho, A. M., R. G. Stiles, W. A. Faiman, S. P. Flower, T. Macha, M. C. Brunner, L. Fleming: MR imaging diagnosis of rotator cuff tears. Amer. J. Roentgenol. 151 (1988) 751–754

14 Flannigan, B., S. Kursunoglu-Brahme, S. Snyder, R. Karzel, W. DelPizzo, D. Resnick: MR arthrography of the shoulder. Amer. J. Roentgenol. 155 (1990) 829–832

15 Fritz, R. D., C. A. Helms, L. S. Steinbach, H. K. Genant: Suprascapular nerve entrapment: evaluation with MR imaging. Radiology 182 (1992) 437–444

16 Gagey, N., E. Ravaud, J. P. Lassau: Anatomy of the Acromial Arch: Correlation of anatomy and magnetic resonance imaging. Surg. radiol. Anat. 15 (1993) 63–70

17 Garneau, R. A., D. L. Renfrew, T. E. Moore, G. Y. El-Khoury, J. V. Nepola, J. H. Lemke: Glenoid labrum: evaluation with MR imaging. Radiology 179 (1991) 519–522

18 Heuck, A., M. Appel, E. Kaiser, K. Lehner, G. Luttke: Magnetresonanztomographie (MRT) der Schulter: Möglichkeiten der Überinterpretation von Normalbefunden. Fortschr. Röntgenstr. 152 (1990) 587–594

19 Hodler, J., S. Kursunoglu-Brahme, B. Flannigan, S. J. Snyder, R. P. Karzel, D. Resnick: Injuries of the superior portion of the glenoid labrum inviluing the insertion of the biceps tendon: MR imaging findings in nine cases. Amer. J. Roentgenol. 159 (1992) 565–568

20 Hodler, J., S. Kursunoglu-Brahme, S. J. Snyder, V. Cervilla, R. P. Karzel, M. E. Schweitzer, B. D. Flannigan, D. Resnick: Rotator cuff disease: assessment with MR arthrography versus standard MR imaging in 36 patients with arthroscopic confirmation. Radiology 182 (1992) 431–436

21 Holt, R. G., C. A. Helms, L. Steinbach, C. Neumann, P. L. Munk, H. K. Genant: Magnetic resonance imaging of the shoulder: rationale and current applications. Skelet. Radiol. 19 (1990) 5–14

21a Hunter, J. S., D. J. Blatz, E. M. Escobedo: SLAP lesions of the glenoid labrum: CT arthrographic and arthroscopic correlation. Radiology 184 (1992) 513–518

22 Iannotti, J. P., M. B. Zlatkin, J. L. Esterhai, H. Y. Kressel, M. K. Dalinka, K. P. Spindler: Magnetic resonance imaging of the shoulder. J. Bone Jt Surg. 73-A (1991) 17–29

23 Kaplan, P. A., K. C. Bryans, J. P. Davick, M. Otte, W. W. Stinson, R. G. Dussault: MR imaging of the normal shoulder: variants and pitfalls. Radiology 184 (1992) 519–524

24 Kieft, G. J., J. L. Bloem, P. M. Rozing, W. R. Obermann: Rotator cuff impingement syndrome: MR imaging. Radiology 166 (1988) 211–214

25 Kieft, G. J., B. A. C. Dijkmans, J. L. Bloem, H. M. Kroon: Magnetic resonance imaging of the shoulder in patients with rheumatoid arthritis. Ann. rheum. Dis. 49 (1990) 7–11

26 Kjellin, I., C. P. Ho, V. Cervilla, P. Haghighi, R. Kerr, C. T. Vagness, R. J. Friedman, D. Trudell, D. Resnick: Alterations in the supraspinatus tendon at MR imaging: correlation with histopathologic findings in cadavers. Radiology 181 (1991) 837–841

27 Kursunoglu-Brahme, S., D. Resnick: Magnetic resonance imaging of the shoulder. Radiol. Clin. N. Amer. 28 (1990) 941–954

27a Kwak, S. M., R. R. Brown, D. Trudell, D. Resnick: Glenohumeral joint: comparison of shoulder positions at MR arthrography, Radiology 208 (1998) 375–380

28 Legan, J. M., T. K. Burkhard, W. B. Goff, Z. N. Balsara, A. J. Martinez, D. D. Burks, D. A. Kallman, T. J. O'Brien: Tears of the glenoid labrum: MR imaging of 88 arthroscopically confirmed cases. Radiology 179 (1991) 241–246

29 Linker, C. S., C. A. Helms, R. C. Fritz: Quadrilateral space syndrome: findings at MR imaging. Radiology 188 (1993) 675–676

30 Liou, J. T., A. J. Wilson, W. G. Totty, J. J. Brown: The normal shoulder: common variations that simulate pathologic conditions at MR imaging. Radiology 186 (1993) 435–441

31 McCauley, T. R., C. F. Pope, P. Jokl: Normal and abnormal glenoid labrum: assessment with multiplanar Gradient-Echo MR imaging. Radiology 183 (1992) 35–37

32 McNiesh, L. M., J. J. Callaghan: CT Arthrography of the shoulder: variations of the glenoid labrum. Amer. J. Roentgenol. 149 (1987) 963–966

33 Meyer, S. J. F., M. K. Dalinka: Magnetic resonance imaging of the shoulder. Semin. Ultrasound 11 (1990) 253–266

34 Mirowitz, S. A.: Normal rotator cuff: MR imaging with conventional and fat-suppression techniques. Radiology 180 (1991) 735–740

35 Mitchell, M. J., G. Causey, D. P. Berthoty, D. J. Sartoris, D. Resnick: Peribursal fat plane of the shoulder: anatomic study and clinical experience. Radiology 168 (1988) 699–704

36 Morrison, D. S., L. U. Bigliani: The clinical significance of variations in acromial morphology. Orthop. Trans. 11 (1987) 234–244

37 Munk, P. L., R. G. Holt, C. A. Helms, H. K. Genant: Glenoid labrum: preliminary work with use of radial-sequence MR imaging. Radiology 173 (1989) 751–753

38 Neer, C.: Impingement lesions. Clin. Orthop. 173 (1982) 70–77

39 Neer, C. S.: Shoulder Reconstruction. Saunders, Philadelphia 1990

40 Neer, C. S., R. P. Welsh: The shoulder in sports. Orthop. Clin. N. Amer. 8 (1977) 583–591

41 Neumann, C. H., S. A. Petersen, A. H. Jahnke: MR imaging of the labral capsular complex: normal variations Amer. J. Roentgenol. 157 (1991 a) 1015–1021

42 Neumann, C. H., S. A. Petersen, H. H. Jahnke, L. S. Steinbach, F. W. Morgan, C. Helms, H. K. Genant, T. E. Farley: MRI in the evaluation of patients with suspected instability of the shoulder Joint including a comparison with CT-arthrography. Fortschr. Röntgenstr. 154 (1991 b) 593 – 600

43 Neumann, C. H., R. G. Holz, L. S. Steinbach, A. H. Jahnke, S. A. Petersen: MR imaging of the shoulder: appearance of the supraspinatus tendon in asymptomatic volunteers. Amer. J. Roentgenol. 158 (1992) 1281 – 1287

44 Owen, R. S., J. P. Iannotti, J. B. Kneeland, M. K. Dalinka, J. A. Deren, L. Olega: Shoulder after surgery: MR imaging with surgical validation. Radiology 186 (1993) 443 – 447

45 Palmer, W. E., J. H. Brown, D. I. Rosenthal: Rotator cuff: evaluation with fat-suppressed MR arthrography. Radiology 188 (1993) 683 – 687

46 Palmer, W. E., J. H. Brown, D. I. Rosenthal: Labral-ligamentous complex of the shoulder: evaluation with MR arthrography. Radiology 190 (1994) 645 – 651

47 Rafii, M., H. Firooznia, O. Sherman, J. Minkoff, J. Weinreb, C. Golimbu, R. Gidumal, R. Schinella, K. Zaslav: Rotator cuff lesions: signal patterns at MR imaging. Radiology 177 (1990) 817 – 823

48 Rathbun, J. B., I. MacNab: The microvascular pattern of the rotator cuff. Jt Bone J. Surg. 52-B (1970) 541 – 553

49 Reiser, M., R. Erlemann, G. Bongartz, T. Pauly, V. Kunze, H. Mathiass, P. E. Peters: Möglichkeiten der Magnetischen Resonanz Tomographie (MRT) in der Diagnostik des Schultergelenkes. Radiology 28 (1988) 79 – 83

50 Richards, R., D. J. Sartoris, M. N. Pathria, D. Resmick: Hill-Sachs lesion and normal humeral groove: MR imaging features allowing their differentiation. Radiology 190 (1994) 665 – 668

51 Rothman, R. H., W. W. Parke: The vascular anatomy of the rotator cuff. Clin. Orthop. 41 (1965) 176

52 Rothman, R. H., R. B. Marvel, R. B. Heppenstall: Anatomic considerations in the glenohumeral Joint. Orthop. Clin. N. Amer. 6 (1975) 341 – 352

53 Seeger, L. L., R. H. Gold, L. W. Basset, H. Ellman: Shoulder impingement syndrome: MR findings in 53 shoulders. Amer. J. Roentgenol. 150 (1988) 343 – 347

54 Strizak, A. M., T. L. Danzig, D. W. Jackson, G. Greenway, D. Resnick, T. Staple: Subacromial bursography: an anatomical and clinical study. J. Bone Jt Surg. 64-A (1982) 196 – 201

54a Tirman, P. F. J., F. W. Bost, L. S. Steinbach et al.: MR arthrography depiction of tears of the rotator cuff: Benefit of abduction and external rotation of the arm. Radiology 192 (1994) 851

55 Tirman, P. F. J., J. F. Feller, D. L. Janzen, C. G. Peterfy, A. G. Bergman: Association of glenoid labral cysts with labral tears and glenohumeral instability: radiologic findings and clinical sigificance. Radiology 190 (1994) 653 – 658

56 Tsai, J. C., M. B. Zlatkin: Magnetic resonance imaging of the shoulder. Radiol. Clin. N. Amer. 28 (1990) 279 – 291

56a Tuite, M. J. J. F. Orwin: Anterosuperior labral variants of the shoulder: appearance on gradient-recalled-echo and fast spin-echo MR Images. Radiology 199 (1996) 537 – 540

56b Vahlensieck, M., T. Sommer: Indirekte MR Arthographie der Schulter: Alternative zur direkten MR-Arthographie? Radiologie 36 (1996) 960 – 965

57 Vahlensieck, M., S. Majumdar, P. Lang, H. K. Genant: Shoulder MRI: routine examinations using gradient recalled and fat-saturated sequences. Europ. J. Radiol. 2 (1992) 142 – 147

58 Vahlensieck, M., M. Resendes, H. K. Genant: MRI of the shoulder. Imaging 59 (1992) 123 – 132

59 Vahlensieck, M., M. Resendes, P. Lang, H. Genant: Shoulder MRI: The subacromial-subdeltoid bursa fat stripe in healthy and pathologic conditions. Europ. J. Radiol. 14 (1992) 223 – 227

60 Vahlensieck, M., M. Pollack, P. Lang, S. Grampp, H. K. Genant: Two segments of the supraspinatus muscle: cause of high signal in the supraspinatus critical zone on MRI? Radiology 186 (1993) 449 – 454

61 Vahlensieck, M., K. van Haack, H. M. Schmidt: Two portions of the supraspinatus muscle: a new finding about the muscles macroscopy by dissection and magnetic resonance imaging. Surg. radiol. Anat. 16 (1994) 101 – 104

62 Vahlensieck, M., F. Möller, M. Nägele, U. van Deimling: Habituelle Schulterluxation: Kernspintomographie nach Knochenspansplastik. Zbl. Radiol. 150 (1994) 210

62a Vahlensieck, M., E. Wiggert, U. Wagner, H. M. Schmidt, H. Schild: Subacromial fat pad. Surg. Radiol. Anat. 18 (1996) 33 – 36

63 Vestring, T., G. Bongartz, W. Konermann, R. Erlemann, G. Reuther, W. Krings: Stellenwert der Magnetresonanztomographie in der Diagnostik von Schultererkrankungen. Fortschr. Röntgenstr. 154 (1991) 143 – 149

64 Weston, W. J.: The enlarged subdeltoid bursa in rheumatoid arthritis. Brit. J. Radiol. 42 (1969) 481 – 486

65a Willemsen, U., E. Wiedemann, U. Brunner, R. Scheck, T. Pfluger, G. Kueffer, K. Hahn: Prospective evaluation of MR arthography performed with high-volume intraarticular saline enhancement in patients with recurrent anterior dislocations of the shoulder. AJR 170 (1998) 79 – 84

65 Weston, W. J.: The Subdeltoid bursa. Aust. Radiol. 17 (1973) 214 – 215

66 Workman, T. L., T. K. Burkhard, D. Resnick, W. B. Goff, Z. N. Balsara, D. J. Davis, J. M. Lapoint: Hill-Sachs lesions: comparison of detection with MR imaging, radiography and arthroscopy. Radiology 185 (1992) 847 – 852

67 Zlatkin, M. B., M. A. Reicher, L. E. Kellerhouse, M. McDade, L. Vetter, D. Resnick: The painful shoulder: MR imaging of the glenohumeral joint. J. Comput. assist. Tomogr. 12 (1988) 995 – 1001

68 Zlatkin, M. B., J. P. Iannotti, M. C. Roberts, J. L. Esterhai, M. K. Dalinka, H. Y. Kressel, J. S. Schwartz, R. E. Lenkinski: Rotator cuff tears: diagnostic performance of MR imaging. Radiology 172 (1989) 223 – 229

4 *Elbow*

B. M. Eitel and P. Schnarkowski

Introduction

The proliferation of recreational sport and the popularity of sport disciplines involving batting and throwing have increased the number of patients with acute and chronic functional disorders of the elbow. The different mechanical forces acting on the complicated anatomic structure can induce a variety of symptoms. The elbow consists of three separate joint compartments with different planes of movements and is surrounded by muscles, tendons and ligaments. It is often difficult to examine the complicated osseous and soft tissue anatomy with conventional radiography. The advantages of MRI will be shown in comparison to other methods available for imaging the elbow. The increasing role of MRI in diagnostic imaging of the elbow is also reflected in the current literature (10, 11, 12, 13, 14, 23, 24). MRI was rarely applied to the elbow when it was introduced for the evaluation of joints in 1983 and, for a long time, experience in diagnosing pathologic processes in the elbow region was sparse (3, 8, 9, 21). Since then, however, MRI has become an established modality for investigating complaints related to the elbow.

Examination Technique

■ Patient Positioning

Suitable surface coils are now available. With appropriate positioning of the elbow, which can be placed at the side of the body or over the head (if the shoulder is freely movable), sections along the various articulating planes with good contrast visualization of the soft tissues can be obtained. The patient's position is determined by the available equipment. It should be kept in mind that the patient is more comfortable supine than prone and that the prone position is subject to frequent motion artifacts. In the body coil, the arm has to be elevated above the head, which can be achieved only with an essentially unrestricted range of motion at both shoulder and elbow. It is more comfortable to place the arm along the body with the lower arm in pronation and the palm of the hand resting on the thigh, particularly for longer examinations. Cushions for shoulder and head and a pad underneath the relevant limb improve the patient's compliance and lower the rate of motion artifacts. The overhead position allows the

elbow to be positioned nearer to the isocenter of the magnetic field. This results in more homogeneous fat suppression when chemical fat presaturation sequences are used. The elbow can be positioned with the arm overhead if the patient is placed in an oblique position. However this may lead to further discomfort and increase the likelihood of motion artifact. One study suggests that motion artifacts occur in around 25% of cases when the patient is turned into the oblique position and/or the elbow is placed above the head (2). Whenever the overhead position is used the hand should be immobilized. The design of the MRI gantry limits certain positions, in particular for obese patients. In the majority of cases, it will be most suitable to position the patient supine with the elbow in pronation along the body (4). To encompass the entire elbow, a small off-center field of view (FOV) with a surface coil must be available. When imaging the common flexor and extensor origins for insertional tendinopathy (epicondylitis), the use of coronal images with 20 degrees of elbow flexion has been advocated (5 a). This allows better visualization of the common tendons on coronal sequences. An alternative is a 20 degree posterior oblique coronal plane with the elbow in full extension. This may prove useful when small coils, such as the wrist coil, which prevent the acquisition of images in flexion, are used or when restricted movement of the elbow prevents flexion images being obtained. Alternatively, the elbow can be examined with partial flexion in an extremity coil such as a knee coil. With the elbow in a splint or kept in flexion, a shoulder coil can be used. Applying a pair of surface coils is another measure to offer more comfort to the patient during the examination. Since examinations of the elbow can last up to one hour, anything that might irritate the patient should be avoided. Claustrophobic patients should be adequately premedicated. The patient should be free from any pain (4), should not be thirsty, and should have emptied the bladder prior to the examination.

■ Coils

For the examination of the elbow, additional surface coils have been found advantageous. They improve signal-to-noise ratio and spatial resolution. They come in various forms and can be both flat and circular, with a diameter of 8 or 16 cm, or rectangular. Flexible coils are also available. Surface coils are placed over the region to be examined and image the underlying volume close to the surface. A circular surface coil, for instance, encompasses the region it covers and has a regional sensitivity corresponding to its radius.

■ Sequences and Parameters

In the majority of cases, the examination begins with a coronal survey view. SE sequence, large field of view (320–400 mm) and 256 × 128 image matrix are used to obtain 1 cm thick sections. The imaging time is about $^1/_2$ minute. Numerous disorders of the elbow can be detected on transverse T_1-weighted and T_2-weighted images. The transverse sections are generally obtained with T_2-weighted sequences because of their excellent soft tissue contrast. The selection of the initial sections is guided by the size of the suspected lesion and the region to be imaged. Using a field of view of 160 mm × 240 mm and a 256 × 256 or 256 × 192 image matrix, the transverse T_2-weighted images take about 9 minutes. Fast T_2-weighted sequences, such as FSE or TSE sequences, reduce the examination times to 5 minutes. These sequences should be followed by a T_1 sequence in the transverse, coronal, or sagittal plane, depending on the clinical symptoms, the anatomic structures to be imaged and the finding on the preceding transverse images. The field of view and the matrix size remain the same as used for the T_2-weighted sequences. The imaging time is about 2–5 minutes.

STIR sequences are best for disclosing small lesions, especially in the bone marrow. STIR sequences take about 25% less time than T_2-weighted sequences, although a T_2 sequence with fat saturation does provide an alternative to the STIR sequence. Though STIR sequences have a relatively poor signal-to-noise ratio owing to the suppression of the fat signal, pathologic structures frequently are better recognized due to the additive T_1 weighting and T_2 weighting (7), with an achieved contrast ratio of lesion to fat of 18 : 1 and of lesion to musculature of 12 : 1. GRE sequences with reduced flip angle and short repetition times (RT) are especially suitable for investigating joint lesions in the different articulating planes. Static GRASS sequences are suitable for examinations of the vascular system (2). It should be emphasized that the protocol of sequences and planes used is usually dictated by the clinical problem to be solved, and the anatomy to be demonstrated (see Table 4.**1**).

■ Special Examination Techniques

The STIR sequences and the chemical shift technique have already been mentioned. The GRE sequences have the capability of three-dimensional display. Cinematic examinations of the elbow with fast GRE sequences are under investigation and have not yet been introduced clinically.

Dynamic sequences with IV contrast medium can be helpful for evaluating the activity of inflammatory or tumorous processes.

Anatomy

■ General Anatomy

The elbow comprises three parts:

- humeroulnar articulation,
- humeroradial articulation,
- radioulnar articulation.

All three articulations communicate with each other and are surrounded by one capsule. They are stabilized by the radial and ulnar collateral ligaments. Moreover, the radial head is encircled by the annular ligament and held against the ulna. Both the coronoid process and the ulnar collateral ligament are crucial for the stability of the elbow. Flexion is achieved by the brachialis, biceps and brachioradialis, and extension by the triceps and anconeus. Pronation is accomplished by the pronator quadratus and pronator teres, and supination by the supinator and biceps muscle. The muscles acting on the elbow can be divided into four groups:

- the anterior group: the biceps and brachialis,
- the lateral group: the supinator, brachioradialis, and carpal extensors,
- the medial group: the pronator teres, carpal flexors, and palmaris longus,
- the posterior group: the triceps and anconeus.

The brachial artery is the major artery. It is anterior to the brachialis and medial to the biceps, and branches immediately below the elbow into ulnar and brachial arteries. The major nerves traversing the elbow region are:

- the median nerve, which is anterior to the brachialis,
- the radial nerve, which passes the elbow between brachialis and brachioradialis,
- the ulnar nerve, which passes behind the medial epicondyle.

The extensors arise from the lateral epicondyle and the flexors from the medial epicondyle. This is of particular relevance for the insertional tendinopathies (tennis and golfer's elbow). The groove for the ulnar nerve on the medioposterior surface of the humerus accounts for the frequently encountered entrapment syndrome of the ulnar nerve. Furthermore, the bicipital aponeurosis is important, extending from the tendon of the biceps brachii medially and distally and crossing the brachial artery and median nerve. In the cubital fossa, which is demarcated laterally by the brachioradialis and medially by the pronator teres, the biceps tendon is lateral, the brachial artery next to it, and the median nerve medial. The radial artery generally is a direct continuation of the brachial artery and the ulnar artery arises from the main artery at an right angle. The lateral cephalic vein and the medial basilic vein are the superficial veins of the elbow. The median nerve perforates the pronator teres and the ulnar artery passes under the ulnar head of the pronator teres. With the elbow extended, the medial epicondyle, lateral epicondyle, and olecranon are on the same horizontal line, and with the elbow flexed, they form the corners of an equilateral triangle. The humeroulnar joint is a hinge joint, with the trochlear notch containing a smooth ridge, which glides in a groove of the humeral trochlea. The extended elbow forms a physiologic cubitus valgus with an angle of 85 degrees. The articulating surfaces of the radial head and capitellum (radiohumeral articulation) as well as the surfaces of the proximal radiohumeral joint are only partially congruent. The annular ligament of the radius encircles the radial head and arises anteriorly and posteriorly at the radial notch of the ulnar. It measures about 10 mm in width and changes its form with the rotation of the radial head.

The articulating surfaces are covered by hyaline cartilage. The joint capsule is thin anteriorly and ventrally, and receives deep fibers from the brachialis anteriorly and from the anconeus posteriorly. Laterally, the joint capsule is reinforced by the collateral ligaments, which passively hold the joint together. The internal joint capsule forms synovial folds over extrasynovial fat in the olecranon, radial, and coronoid fossae. A meniscus-like fold of firm consistency projects into humeroradial articulation. Bursae occur at the olecranon, both humeral epicondyles and radial head. Additional bursae can be observed under the extensor carpi radialis brevis as well as under the anconeus. Several normal anatomical variants exist that may lead to potential pitfalls in the interpretation of the elbow examination. These are discussed at the end of the chapter.

■ Specific MRI Anatomy

The sections of the elbow are obtained in the coronal (Figs. 4.**1**– 4.**3**), sagittal (Figs. 4.**4**– 4.**6**), and transverse (Figs. 4.**7**– 4.**9**) planes. Since the elbow is a hinge joint, optimal positioning of the transverse and coronal sections requires full extension of the joint. In the sagittal plane, the anatomic structures are also well identified with the joint in flexion. This plane is therefore always indicated whenever full extension of the joint is impossible. The recommended sections are listed in Table 4.**1**.

When imaging the common extensor and flexor origins for epicondylitis, a 20-degree posterior oblique coronal plane may also prove useful.

Signal intensities. The different signal intensities of the various tissues are listed in Table 4.**2**. A SE sequence with relative T_1 weighting yields the best contrast for soft tissues, articular cartilage, and bone marrow. Fat produces an intense signal and appears white on the images. Musculature has a less intense signal and is dark gray. Cortical bone, fibrous cartilage, capsule ligamentous structures, and tendons are of low signal intensity and appear as black areas. The bone marrow contains a large amount of fat, which appears white on MRI, but 'bands' of low signal intensity, which correspond to epiphyseal cartilage (growth plates) or its remnants, can be observed. On the T_2-weighted images, fat and fluid exhibit a high signal intensity.

Joint capsule. It is generally not visualized unless it is thickened or effusion is present secondary to synovitis. Normally, it is difficult to separate the capsule from the brachialis anteriorly and from the triceps tendon posteriorly. Fat pads between the synovial lining and fibrous layer of the capsule are seen posteriorly in the olecranon fossa and anteriorly in the coronoid fossa of the humerus. These fossae render the trochlea waist-like on the sagittal section.

Bursae. These must be distinguished from cysts or other pathologic conditions. The superficial bursa at the olecranon is intratendinous or subtendinous underneath the subcutaneous tissue. The subtendinous bursae are best seen on transverse and sagittal sections and can be mistaken for a joint effusion if filled with fluid, but with no fluid seen anterior to the joint, a bursitis is more likely. The subcutaneous bursal involvement at the medial and lateral epicondyles must be distinguished from ligamentous lesions. Normally, these bursae are not identified unless they are altered by inflammation. If they are inflamed, they are well seen on the T_2-weighted images.

Arteries. These are hard to separate from the accompanying veins.

Nerves. The delineation of the nerves depends on the lipomatous content of the surrounding tissues. Median nerve and radial nerve are best identified on the proximal transverse sections. The ulnar nerve is well seen on transverse sections immediately dorsal to the medial epicondyle.

Radial annular ligament. This is of special importance clinically. MRI barely delineates its lesions directly, but can reveal any positional change of the radial head as an indirect sign of a ligamentous lesion (15).

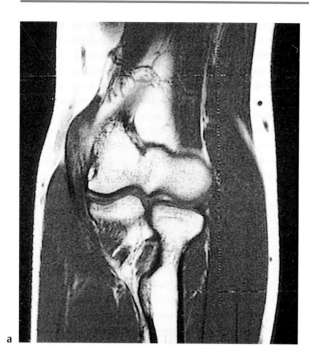

Figs. 4.1– 4.9   Sectional anatomy of the elbow:
4.1 a, b–**4.3 a, b**   Coronal plane
4.4 a, b– **4.6 a, b**   Sagittal plane
4.7 a, b– **4.9 a, b**   Transverse plane
a T₁-weighted SE images
b Annotated schematic drawings showing the level of each section

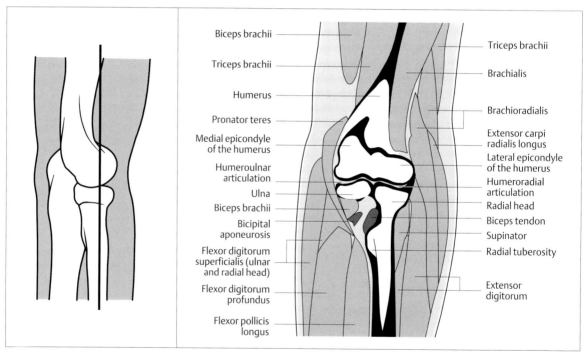

Biceps brachii

Triceps brachii

Humerus

Pronator teres

Medial epicondyle of the humerus

Humeroulnar articulation

Ulna

Biceps brachii

Bicipital aponeurosis

Flexor digitorum superficialis (ulnar and radial head)

Flexor digitorum profundus

Flexor pollicis longus

Triceps brachii

Brachialis

Brachioradialis

Extensor carpi radialis longus

Lateral epicondyle of the humerus

Humeroradial articulation

Radial head

Biceps tendon

Supinator

Radial tuberosity

Extensor digitorum

Figs. 4.**2 a, b**

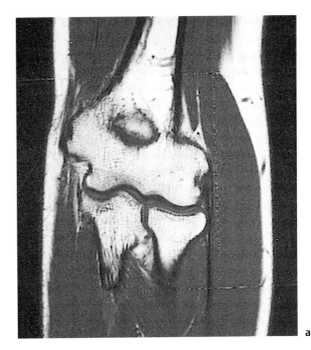

a

Triceps brachii

Humerus

Olecranon

Medial epicondyle
of the humerus

Humeroulnar
articulation

Brachialis tendon

Ulna

Flexor digitorum
superficialis (ulnar
and humeral head)

Flexor digitorum
profundus

Flexor pollicis
longus

Triceps brachii

Brachialis

Extensor carpi
radialis (longus)

Lateral epicondyle
of the humerus

Extensor digitorum
tendon

Humeroradial
articulation

Radial head

Supinator

Abductor
pollicis longus

Extensor carpi
radialis (brevis)

Extensor digitorum

Extensor pollicis
brevis et longus

b

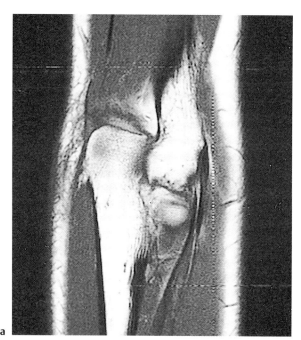

Figs. 4.**3 a, b**

a

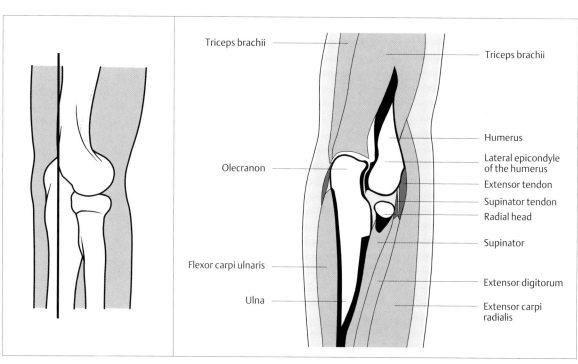

Triceps brachii

Triceps brachii

Olecranon

Humerus

Lateral epicondyle
of the humerus

Extensor tendon

Supinator tendon

Radial head

Supinator

Flexor carpi ulnaris

Extensor digitorum

Ulna

Extensor carpi
radialis

b

Figs. 4.**4 a, b**

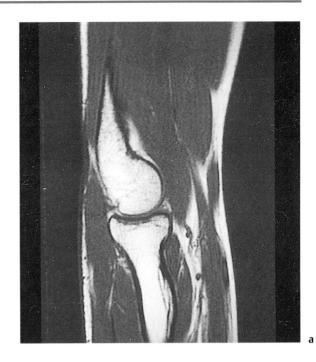

a

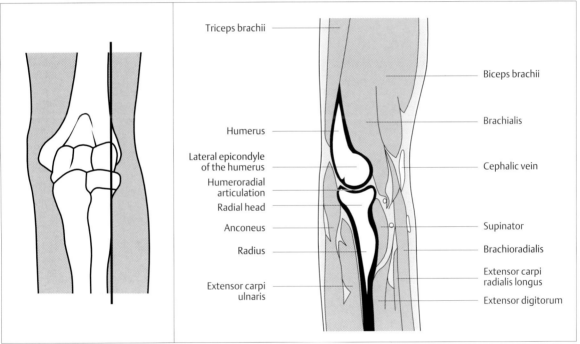

b

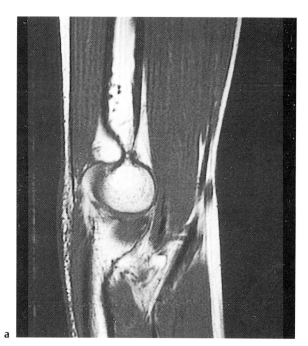

a

Figs. 4.**5 a, b**

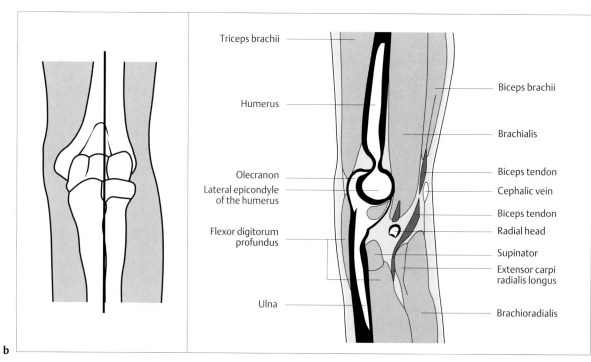

b

Figs. 4.**6 a, b**

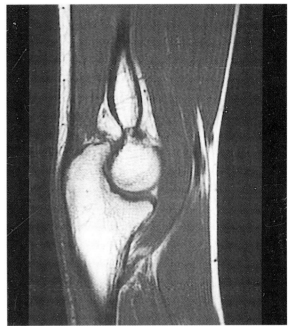

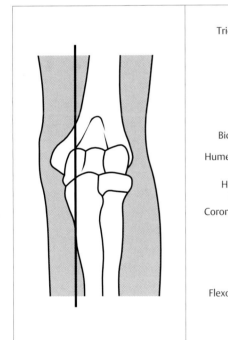

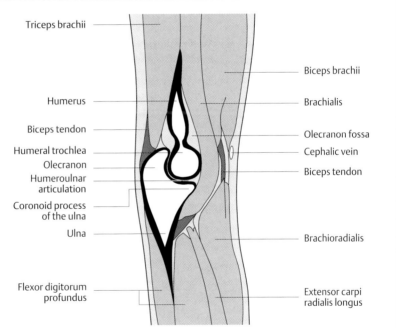

Triceps brachii

Biceps brachii

Humerus

Brachialis

Biceps tendon

Olecranon fossa

Humeral trochlea

Cephalic vein

Olecranon

Biceps tendon

Humeroulnar
articulation

Coronoid process
of the ulna

Ulna

Brachioradialis

Flexor digitorum
profundus

Extensor carpi
radialis longus

a

b

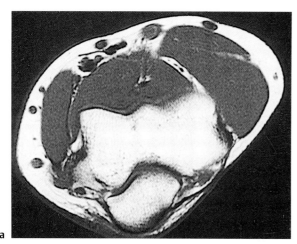

a

Figs. 4.**7 a, b**

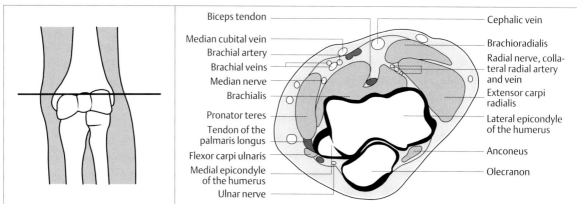

Biceps tendon	Cephalic vein
Median cubital vein	Brachioradialis
Brachial artery	Radial nerve, collateral radial artery and vein
Brachial veins	
Median nerve	Extensor carpi radialis
Brachialis	
Pronator teres	Lateral epicondyle of the humerus
Tendon of the palmaris longus	
Flexor carpi ulnaris	Anconeus
Medial epicondyle of the humerus	Olecranon
Ulnar nerve	

b

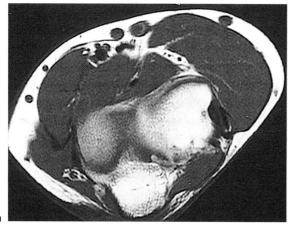

a

Figs. 4.**8 a, b**

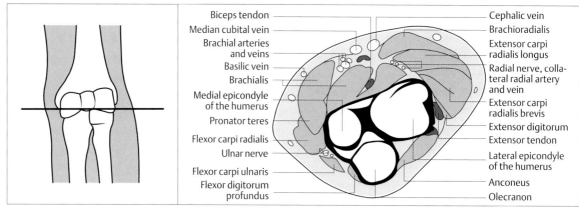

Biceps tendon	Cephalic vein
Median cubital vein	Brachioradialis
Brachial arteries and veins	Extensor carpi radialis longus
Basilic vein	Radial nerve, collateral radial artery and vein
Brachialis	
Medial epicondyle of the humerus	Extensor carpi radialis brevis
Pronator teres	Extensor digitorum
Flexor carpi radialis	Extensor tendon
Ulnar nerve	Lateral epicondyle of the humerus
Flexor carpi ulnaris	Anconeus
Flexor digitorum profundus	Olecranon

b

Figs. 4.**9 a, b**

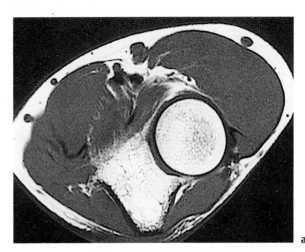

a

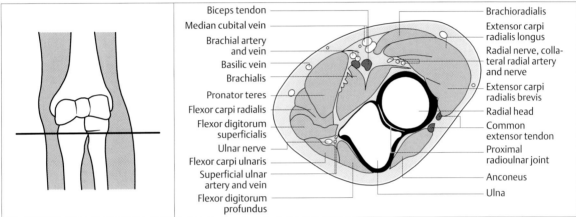

b

Table 4.**1**   Recommended sections for the examination of specific anatomic structures

	Anatomic structure	Recommended sections[1]	Remarks
Skeleton	Humerus, radius, ulna	Sagittal/coronal	
Articulations	Humeroulnar articulation	Sagittal/coronal	
	Humeroulnar articulation	Sagittal/coronal	
	Radioulnar articulation (proximal)	Transverse/coronal	
	Internal articular structures and articular surfaces	Sagittal/coronal	
	Hyaline cartilage	Sagittal/coronal	
	Joint capsule	Sagittal/coronal	
Bone	Humeral trochlea	Sagittal/coronal	
	Radial head	Coronal/transverse	
	Ulnar groove of the trochlea	Sagittal	
	Ulnar groove of the radius	Transverse	
	Coronoid process of the ulnar	Sagittal	
	Olecranon and ulnar fossa with fad pad	Sagittal	
Ligaments	Ulnar collateral ligament	Coronal/transverse	
	Radial collateral ligament	Coronal/transverse	
	Annular ligament of the radius	Transverse	Lesion only indirectly visible as displacement of the radial head
Bursae	Subtendinous bursa of the olecranon	Sagittal/transverse	DD[2]: Joint effusion
	Epicondylar bursa	Transverse/sagittal	DD: Ligamentous lesion
Muscles and tendon	Insertion of the biceps and triceps	Sagittal/transverse	
	Insertion of the anconeus	Sagittal	
	Entire elbow muscles in all four compartments	Transverse	
Vessels and Nerves	Arteries/veins	Transverse	
	Median nerve Radial nerve Ulnar nerve	Transverse	

[1] With free mobility of the elbow (especially full extension), otherwise oblique sections have to be considered
[2] DD = Differential diagnosis

Table 4.**2**   Signal intensity of different tissue in relation to the used sequence

Tissue	T_1	Proton density	T_2
Fat	+++	+++	+++
Musculature	+	+	+
Cortical bone	0	0	0
Tendons	0	0	0
Ligaments	0	0	0
Capsule	0	0	0
Fibrous cartilage (collagen type 2)	0	0	0
Hyaline cartilage (collagen type 1)	++	++	+
Inflammatory changes in soft tissue (fluid, edema)	+	+	+++

◄ Sequence
+++ = high signal intensity (white)
++ = medium signal intensity (various gray levels)
+ = low signal intensity (dark gray)
0 = no signal

Synovitis, Plicae, and Pannus Formation

The synovial membrane reacts to cartilaginous degeneration and lesions with inflammatory changes. Hypervascular membranous protrusions grow toward the site of the articular lesion and become arranged like folds or plicae through fibrous transformations. If these changes are extensive and cover a large area, they are referred to as pannus. Pannus formation has a predilection for the olecranon and the coronoid process, but a plica can arise wherever synovial lining changes to cartilaginous coating. Plicae can become trapped at the superior recess of the joint capsule as well as between the

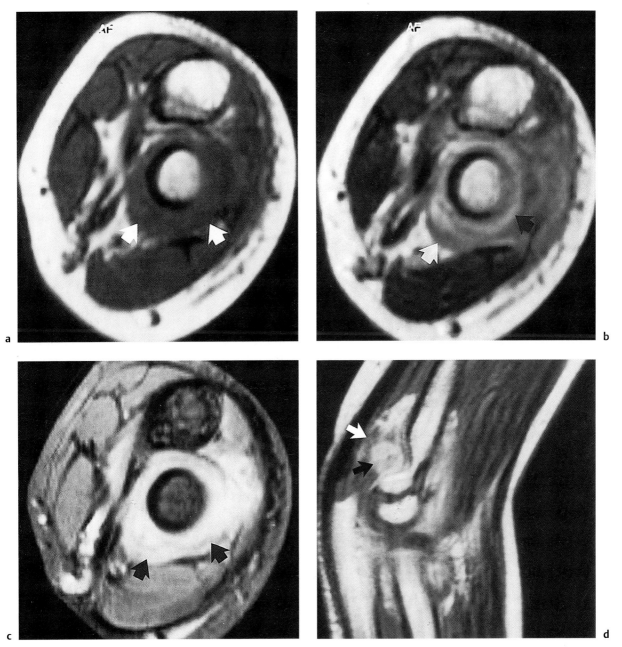

Figs. 4.**10 a–d** Juvenile rheumatoid arthritis. **a** T$_2$-weighted SE sequence, transverse plane. The lower aspect of the joint shows a low signal area around the radial head (arrows). **b** T$_1$-weighted SE sequence, transverse section after IV Gd-DTPA at 0.1 mmol/kg body weight. The joint effusion remains of low signal intensity (white arrow), while the synovial proliferations show definite enhancement (black arrow). **c** FLASH–2-D sequence, transverse section. Equal enhancement of tissue proliferation and joint effusion (arrows). **d** T$_1$-weighted SE sequences after IV Gd-DTPA at 0.1 mmol/kg body weight. The enhancement demarcates the extensive pannus formation (black arrow) from the non-enhancing joint effusion (white arrow).

capitellum of the humerus and radial head. The latter condition can be mistaken for a tennis elbow because of similar clinical presentation. MRI can resolve this problem.

One of the MRI finding of *arthritis* is effusion (Fig. 4.**10**). A few weeks after the onset of the disease, the joint space becomes narrowed due to cartilaginous damage and bone destruction (Fig. 4.**11**). In *hemophilia*, the elbow is the third most frequently involved joint, after knee and ankle. Extensive cartilaginous destructions are the result of hemorrhagic synovitis. MRI could increase the diagnosis of hemophilic arthritis by 40% in comparison with conventional imaging (14). The T_1-weighted sequences show the extent of the synovitis as well as subchondral cysts and erosions. GRE sequences can separate cartilage from joint effusion. Hemosiderin deposits in the joint capsule are detected as low signal intensities. The T_2-weighted sequences reveal multiloculated synovial cysts, especially in rheumatoid con-

ditions. All these findings, however, are only specific for inflammation and lack any differential diagnostic criteria. The joint effusion can be characterized further by the observation that the T_1 and T_2 relaxation times are longer for transudates than for exudates. Accordingly, a purulent and hemorrhagic joint effusion has medium signal intensities and can appear heterogeneous on the T_2-weighted images. Normal synovial fluid has a homogeneous, high signal intensity on T_2-weighted sequences. Early inflammatory changes involving the synovial membrane can be identified by their enhancement after IV contrast medium.

In *chronic polyarthritis*, the clinically painful synovitis is often visualized by MRI. While these changes are found in several joints in the early stage, its manifestation as monoarthritis of the elbow increases with progression of the disease process and ultimately affects about two-thirds of patients. MRI proves valuable for the indication of synovectomy since 15–20% of

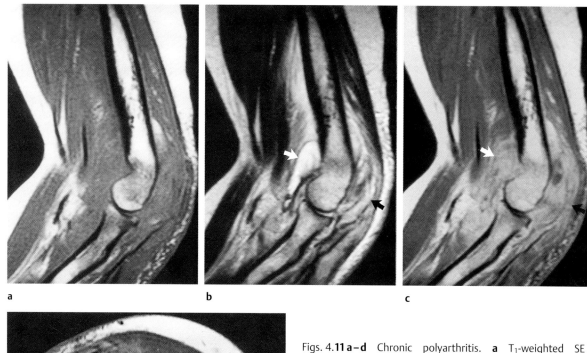

a   b   c

d

Figs. 4.**11 a–d** Chronic polyarthritis. **a** T_1-weighted SE sequence, sagittal plane. A low signal structure is just barely discernible in the anterior and posterior aspect of the joint. **b** T_2-weighted SE sequence, sagittal plane. The structure in the anterior joint capsule exhibits an increased signal intensity (white arrow). The dorsal joint capsule contains areas of increased and decreased signal intensity (black arrow). **c** T_1-weighted SE sequence, sagittal plane after IV Gd-DTPA at 0.1 mmol/kg body weight. The anterior structure enhances (white arrow). In addition an enhancing process is seen in the dorsal joint capsule at the level of the radial head and epicondyles (black arrow). This represents extensive callus formation. **d** T_1-weighted SE sequence, transverse section after IV Gd-DTPA at 0.1 mmol/kg body weight. Pannus permeates the entire joint and has destroyed the radial head and the epicondyles.

cases develop severe functional impairment, which can be approached with preventive measures on the basis of early MRI diagnosis. Cyst-like changes frequently affect the radial head. Coarse synovial protrusions are frequently seen by MRI.

Bursitis

Olecranon bursitis is most frequent (Fig. 4.**12**). Aside from mechanical irritation, other causes of bursitis must be considered, such as early manifestation of chronic polyarthritis or gout. The olecranon bursa is generally visualized on the sagittal section. Neighboring bursae are located at the insertion of the triceps tendon beneath the triceps muscle, while the olecranon bursa is subcutaneous. The signal intensity of the fluid-distended bursa is higher on T_2^*-weighted and STIR sequences than on regular T_2-weighted sequences. The signal intensity is low on the T_2-weighted sequences. The fluid is behind the lateral epicondyle and exhibits a tongue-like or concave-shaped extension toward it.

Osteomyelitis

Short TR-/TE-SE (T_1-weighted) sequences can be obtained quickly. They display the infection as decreased signal intensity relative to the high signal intensity of the normal bone marrow (Fig. 4.**13**). Changes of cortical bone, periosteum, and muscles are generally less apparent. T_2-weighted sequences show the infected area as high signal intensity. Furthermore, STIR sequences permit very good differentiation. By suppressing the fat signal, they bring out the infected areas as an easily distinguished increase in signal intensity. Similar findings are also observed in neoplasms and the specificity of MRI has to be further investigated. Increased signal intensity in the bone marrow surrounded by a low signal intensity is strong evidence of an infectious process. This finding has to be differentiated from a benign tumor.

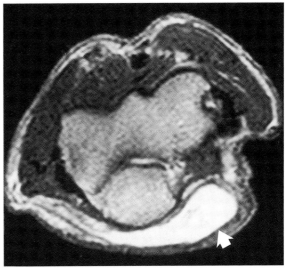

a

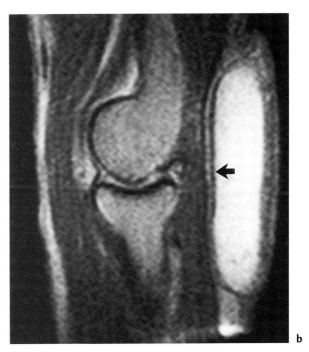

b

Figs. 4.**12a, b** Olecranon bursitis. **a** T_2-weighted SE sequence, transverse plane. The fluid in the olecranon bursa appears rather bright (arrow). **b** T_2-weighted SE sequence, sagittal plane. The fluid accumulation in the olecranon bursa extends from the humeral shaft distally to the radial head. The bursal capsule shows inflammatory thickening (arrow).

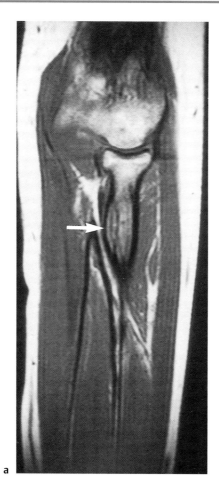

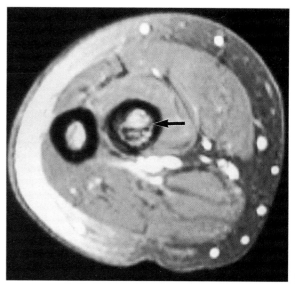

Figs. 4.**13 a, b**   Osteomyelitis. **a** T₁-weighted SE sequence, coronal plane. The radial shaft is thickened and shows decreased signal intensity. **b** T₁-weighted SE sequence, transverse plane, after IV Gd-DTPA at 0.1 mmol/kg body weight. Enhancement of the bone marrow (arrow).

Enthesopathy

Lateral (radial) humeral epicondylitis is well known as tennis elbow (Fig. 4. **14**) and *medial (ulnar) humeral epicondylitis* as golf elbow. These enthesopathies are characterized by lateral and medial pain syndromes due to overuse. In lateral epicondylitis, T₂-weighted and STIR sequences reveal an increased amount of water in the anconeus. This increased signal is absent in healthy subjects and is characteristic of lateral epicondylitis (5). In the differential diagnosis of tennis elbow, synovial plicae of the radiohumeral articulation should be looked for since they can develop on the basis of cartilaginous lesions and mimic epicondylitis refractory to therapy. MRI can also delineate the extent of the epicondylitis. *Degenerative changes* of the tendinous insertion present as increases in signal intensity on T₁-weighted images without further increase on T₂-weighted sequences. However, care must be taken when evaluating the T₁-weighted images as lack of complete signal void is not an uncommon finding in asymptomatic patients. Tendinosis may be associated with thickening of the tendon.

Partial tears are marked by tendinous thinning or defects and fluid accumulation on the T₂-weighted sequences. *Complete tears* are diagnosed by a fluid-filled gap between tendon and its osseous insertion. MRI is especially useful for high-degree partial tears and complete tears. At the same time, it can assess whether the radial collateral ligament, which can be injured together with traumatic tears of the extensor tendons, is intact. Pain in the presence of unremarkable capsuloligamentous structures raises the possibility of a nerve entrapment syndrome. Medial epicondylitis occurs in golf and baseball players as well as in those participating in sports with throwing activities. It is less frequent than lateral epicondylitis.

MRI can evaluate the ulnar collateral ligament, which is situated under the medial epicondyle and important for articular stability. Interpretation of the MRI findings must consider any preceding *therapeutic injections* since they can account for a signal increase on STIR and T₂-weighted sequences. Injection-induced MRI changes can be seen at the epicondyles for up to 4 weeks after the injection. In the growing skeleton, stress fractures and avulsions of the medial apophysis should be considered in the differential diagnosis.

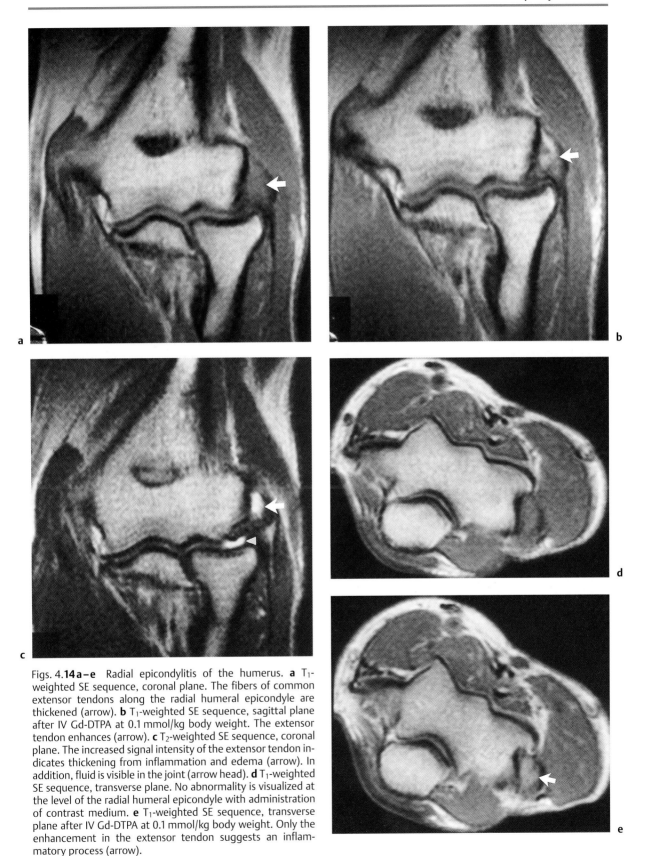

Figs. 4.**14 a–e** Radial epicondylitis of the humerus. **a** T_1-weighted SE sequence, coronal plane. The fibers of common extensor tendons along the radial humeral epicondyle are thickened (arrow). **b** T_1-weighted SE sequence, sagittal plane after IV Gd-DTPA at 0.1 mmol/kg body weight. The extensor tendon enhances (arrow). **c** T_2-weighted SE sequence, coronal plane. The increased signal intensity of the extensor tendon indicates thickening from inflammation and edema (arrow). In addition, fluid is visible in the joint (arrow head). **d** T_1-weighted SE sequence, transverse plane. No abnormality is visualized at the level of the radial humeral epicondyle with administration of contrast medium. **e** T_1-weighted SE sequence, transverse plane after IV Gd-DTPA at 0.1 mmol/kg body weight. Only the enhancement in the extensor tendon suggests an inflammatory process (arrow).

Ligamentous Injuries

MRI can detect medial and lateral ligamentous lesions, offer a differential diagnosis, and document their severity. The documentation of ligamentous lesions may be aided by the use of direct MR arthrography obtained with diluted gadolinium solution injected into the joint. Repetitive valgus stress, which occurs with javelin throwing but also with violin playing, causes a medial tensile stress, which can lead either to epicondylitis or, when the tensile stress increases further, to a stretched muscular insertion of the flexors and extensors as well as to a distorted ulnar collateral ligament. When the applied forces continue to increase, the resultant lateral compression produces characteristic intra-articular injuries, such as osteochondritis dissecans of the radial capitellum of the humerus or the radial head, with subsequent degenerative arthritis and synovitis. The functionally relevant anterior bundle of the ulnar collateral ligament can be examined on transverse and coronal sections. Chronic tensile stress causes ligamentous thickening that can be identified by MRI and occasionally can induce calcific deposits. In all cases, the ulnar coronoid process, which is the site of the origin of

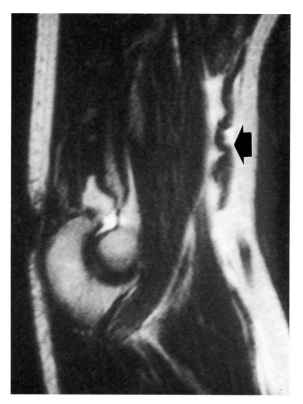

Fig. 4.**15** Tear of the biceps muscle. T$_2$-weighted SE sequence, sagittal plane. The tendon of the biceps muscle is torn above the attachment at the radial tuberosity. The proximal part of the fragment exhibits an undulated course (arrow) (with kind permission of Drs. Bültmann, Boye, Hermie and Grün, Aachen).

the collateral ligament, must be evaluated at the same time since the ligamentous attachment is crucial for articular stability. Partial and full-thickness tears of the ligament are associated with linear fluid accumulations, in particular, on the T$_2$-weighted sequences. This is in contrast to the diffuse soft tissue swelling of edema seen with distortion. At the same time, an edema or hematoma should be looked for in the surrounding soft tissues. Moreover, stretching and entrapment of the ulnar nerve, which can accompany a medial osseous or ligamentous lesions, can be diagnosed by MRI.

Tendon Tears

Tears of the triceps tendon are rare and comprise only 1% of all tendon tears. They are more common in patients with systemic diseases or on corticosteroid therapy. MRI can visualize the accompanying inflammatory reaction and the relationship to the ulnar nerve, which are best seen on the T$_2$-weighted images. The normal triceps tendon often displays an undulated course and contains regionally increased signals, which are less intense on T$_2$-weighted images. These findings are not pathologic and decrease with extension of the tendon during flexion of the elbow. Degenerative changes of the tendon are best seen on T$_2$*-weighted sequences. The same examination technique can be applied to tears of the distal biceps tendon, which are also rather rare (Fig. 4.**15**). Care should be taken not to mistake the anterior ulnar insertion of the brachial muscle for the intact biceps tendon. Sections proximal to the brachial insertion show absence of the biceps tendon. MRI can provide information useful for planning the surgical repair of the torn biceps tendon (6). Other tendon tears, such as avulsion of the common extensor tendon, are rare (Fig. 4.**16**).

Nerve Compression Syndromes

The course of the ulnar nerve is well delineated on transverse section in its groove on the dorsum of the humeral epicondyle, where it can be entrapped by inflammatory or degenerative changes as well as by post-traumatic changes (also secondary to chronic stress or growth disturbance) (Fig. 4.**17**). If the ulnar groove lacks a retinaculum, flexion of the elbow can cause subluxation of the nerve with corresponding paresthesia. However, subluxation of the ulnar nerve may be seen in around 15% of symptomatic individuals (18). In terms of a malformation, this band can also be replaced by a muscle (epitrochlear anconeous muscle) that might cause entrapment of the nerve. The anatomy of the radial nerve poses a more complex problem for the MRI examination. The radial nerve can be compressed at the lateral border of the triceps muscle, but also where it passes through the supinator muscle or after it has become the posterior interosseous branch. For adequate

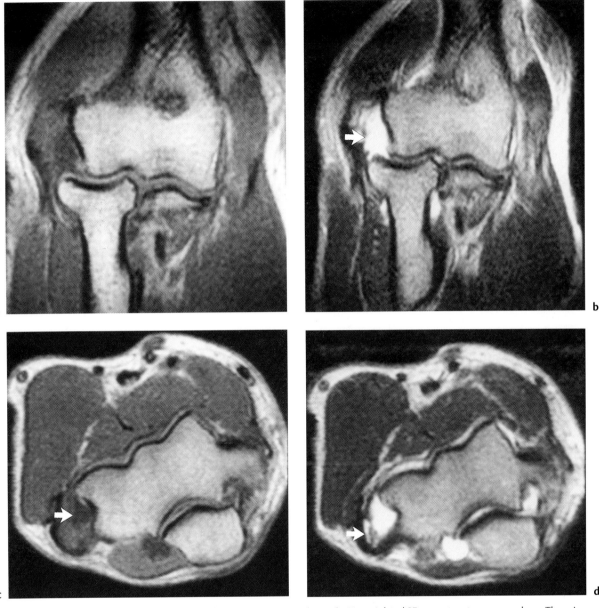

Figs. 4.**16 a–d**   Partial tear of the tendon of the extensor carpi radialis brevis and extensor digitorum muscles. **a** T_1-weighted SE sequence, coronal plane. The common extensor tendon is no longer demarcated as low signal structure. **b** T_2-weighted SE sequence, coronal plane. The extensor tendon together with the extensor carpi radialis muscle shows an increased signal (arrow) **c** T_1-weighted SE sequence, transverse plane. There is a decreased signal at the level of the extensor tendon (arrow). **d** T_2-weighted SE sequence, transverse plane. An increased signal intensity in the region of the extensor tendon without delineation of the extensor tendon suggest a torn tendon (arrow). Concomitant joint effusion.

evaluation, it is advisable to select thin sections. The most frequent compression occurs at the upper border of the supinator muscle. In addition, a motor paralysis of the extensor musculature can lead to a compression of the posterior interosseous branch. The ulnar nerve characteristically is compressed at the supracondylar process or near the pronator teres. These regions should be surveyed on coronal sections, to select the appropriate field of view. The subsequent transverse T_2- weighted images allow a better differentiation of anatomic detail.

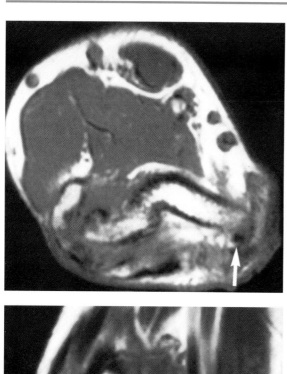

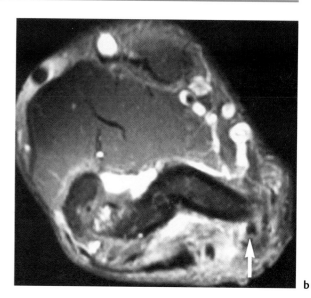

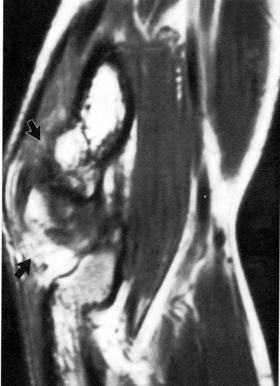

Figs. 4.**17 a–c** Ulnar nerve compression syndrome secondary to arthritis. **a** T$_1$-weighted SE sequence, transverse plane. Increased connective tissue is seen at the level of the epicondyles and olecranon. The connective tissue extends to the ulnar nerve (arrow). **b** T$_1$-weighted SE sequence, transverse plane after IV Gd-DTPA at 0.1 mmol/kg body weight. Strong enhancement of the pannus, which extends to the ulnar nerve (arrow). **c** T$_1$-weighted SE sequence, sagittal plane after IV Gd-DTPA at 0.1 mmol/kg body weight. The extensive pannus formation can be separated from the epicondyles to the olecranon (arrows).

Osteochondritis dissecans

Loose bodies (Fig. 4.**18**) in the joint are usually located anteriorly. They can be single or, as synovial chondromatosis, multiple. A loose body that arises from osteochondritis dissecans of the capitellum of the humerus does not differ from a detached cartilaginous fragment following acute trauma. The loose bodies can migrate posteriorly where they can cause a painfully impaired extension of the elbow because of the narrow joint space, and must then be searched for in the olecranon fossa. Loose bodies can also arise from primary or secondary osteoarthritis (Fig. 4.**19**). Osteochondritis dissecans has a predilection for the capitellum and the radial head. MRI is very sensitive at detecting loose bodies (17). If the elbow can be fully extended, transverse, coronal, and sagittal sections should be obtained. The section thickness generally is 3 mm. Loose bodies are frequently accompanied by a joint effusion.

As a non-invasive modality, MRI is indicated for planning the surgical therapy of loose bodies. It also visualizes the defect of the articular cartilage and possible other injuries. The articular defects contain granulation tissue, which can enhance after IV contrast medium. Osteochondritis dissecans should be distinguished from avascular osteonecrosis of the capitellum (Panner's disease, see below). While osteochondritis dissecans characteristically occurs between the ages of 13 and 16 years, Panner's disease is observed at an age (ages 5 to 10 years). Apart from a loose body, osteochondritis dissecans shows an articular defect of the capitellum, not usually seen with Panner's disease, which is characterized by fragmentation and a pathologic decrease in signal intensity of the ossifying capitellum on T_1-weighted images. Intra-articular gadolinium is also of value in the assessment of fragment stability when evaluating osteochondritis dissecans of the elbow (14 a).

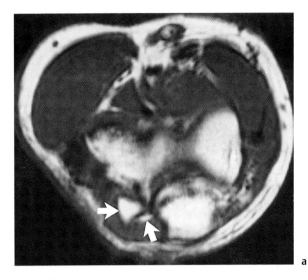

a

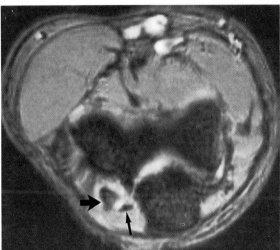

b

Figs. 4.**18a, b** Loose joint body. **a** T_1-weighted SE sequence, transverse plane. Two fragments of the lateral humeral epicondyle can be delineated at the level of the olecranon (arrows). **b** FLASH–2-D sequence, transverse plane. In addition to the loose bodies (arrows), a joint effusion is visualized.

Osteonecrosis

Osteochondrosis (avascular osteochondrosis) of the elbow occurs during the growth period or, in adults, as manifestation of a systemic disease or after corticosteroid therapy. In young adults, osteonecrosis occurs most frequently in the capitellum (capitulum humeri) (Panner's disease). In the growth period, it is observed between the ages of 7 and 12 years during the ossification of the capitellar epiphysis, affecting the anterior central region of the capitellum where it has the largest contact area with the radial head.

Since the imaging findings determine the indication for therapy, MRI staging of the lesion is important:

- Type 1 lesions are undisplaced fragments with intact cartilage.
- Type 2 lesions are articular cartilage defects, which may be partially detached.
- Type 3 lesions are completely detached.

Surgical treatment is indicated for lesions of type 1 and type 2. Sagittal and coronal T_2-weighted sequences are recommended. On T_1-weighted images, the area of necrosis is isointense with the bone marrow and surrounded by a rim of low signal intensity (Fig. 4.**20**). In the early phase of the disease, the low signal rim corresponds to hyperemia around the lesion. The T_2-weighted images show a high signal intensity in this hyperemic zone. New bone formation with encapsulation of the lesion decreases the signal intensity on the T_1-weighted and T_2-weighted sequences. Different signal intensities along the periphery of the necrosis corre-

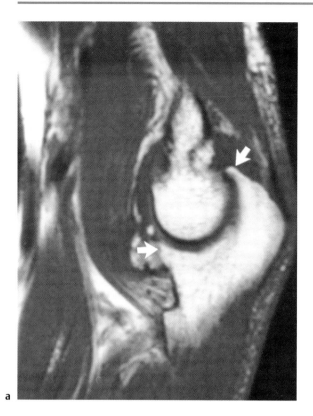

Figs. 4.**19a–c** Osteoarthritis. **a** T_1-weighted SE sequence, sagittal plane. In addition to joint space narrowing, osteophytes of the olecranon and the ulnar coronoid process are seen (arrows). **b** T_1-weighted SE sequence, transverse plane. An ulnar osteophyte is delineated (arrow). **c** FLASH–2-D sequence, transverse plane. In addition to osteophytes, fluid accumulation is visualized in the joint (arrow).

a

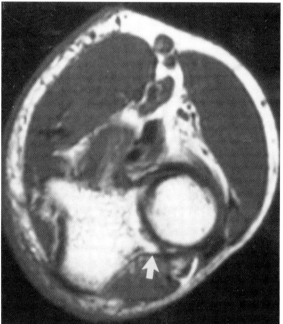

b

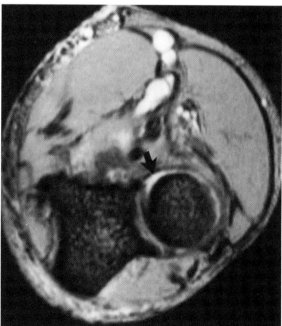

c

spond to the different rates of osseous resorption and apposition. Articular cartilage can be visualized both on T_1-weighted and T_2-weighted sequences because of its medium signal intensity. Delicate fissures or longitudinal defects are better detected on T_2-weighted images.

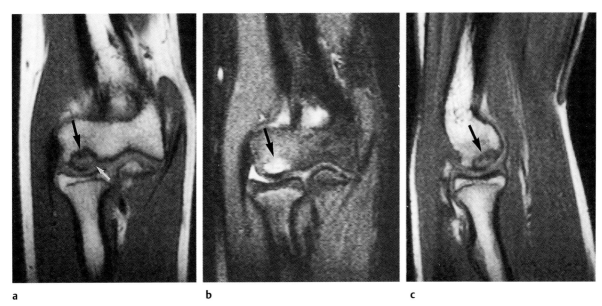

a   b   c

Figs. 4.**20a–c** Panner disease (type II). **a** T_1-weighted SE sequence, coronal plane. A low signal contour defect of the capitellum of the humerus is delineated. **b** STIR sequence, coronal plane. The defect exhibits an increased signal intensity (arrow). **c** T_1-weighted SE sequence, sagittal plane. The contour defect is also easily recognized on the sagittal plane (arrow).

Osseous Injuries

In addition to delineating the fracture line and bone marrow edema, MRI reveals the associated soft tissue changes. For the elbow, this is especially relevant in view of the destabilizing lesions of the ulnar collateral ligament and its insertion at the coronoid process since this affects the function of the elbow. MRI offers a multiplanar visualization of fractures and can delineate the fracture line better than conventional radiographs in two projections. Articular involvement of the fracture can be well determined by MRI (Fig. 4.21). In particular, microtraumas and contusions can be detected early on T_2-weighted images.

Epiphyseal injuries can be detected well by MRI. Depending on the age, the following ossifications should be identified:

- in the 1st year, the capitellum of the humerus,
- in the 2nd to 6th year, the radial head,
- in the 5th to 7th year, the medial epicondyle of the humerus,
- in the 9th to 10th year, the trochlea of the humerus,
- in the 9th to 13th year, the lateral epicondyle of the humerus (16).

Tumors

Osseous tumors of the elbow are rare (see Chapter 12). Benign soft tissue tumors, cysts or ganglions are usually smoothly outlined, of homogeneous signal intensity and without signs of infiltration (Fig. 4.22). Lipomas, which are frequently observed, have a homogeneous signal intensity on T_1-weighted and T_2-weighted images. They can contain fibrous septations. Most benign tumors differ from lipomas by showing a high signal intensity on T_2-weighted and a low signal intensity on T_1-weighted images. Only hemangiomas and desmoid tumors are an exception.

Soft Tissue and Muscle Injuries

Muscle injuries are among the most frequent sport injuries and consist of contusions with blunt separation of muscle fibers, edema, and hemorrhage. The exact site and the extent of these findings can be localized by MRI. Strains are probably more frequent than contusions. The severity of any possible tear of the musculotendinous transition can be visualized by MRI. This information determines the indication for surgical intervention by demonstrating a full-thickness tear, muscle herniation, or compartment syndrome. Edema and hemorrhage are visualized on standard sequences as abnormal signal intensity. The STIR sequence is especially sensitive for fluid or blood in the soft tissues. Moreover, sequelae of muscle strains, such as atrophy, fibrosis, or fatty infiltration, can be diagnosed by MRI.

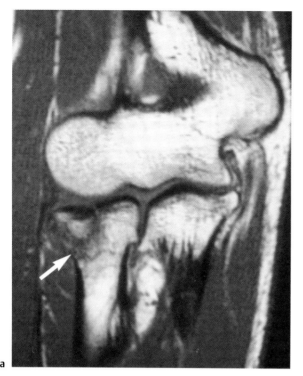

a

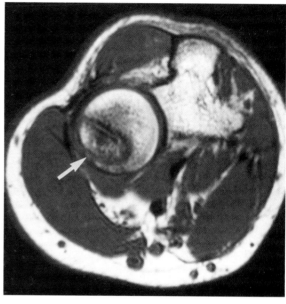

b

Figs. 4.**21 a, b** Radial head fracture. **a** T₁-weighted SE sequence, coronal plane. An undisplaced fracture of the radial head with intra-articular extension is visualized (arrow). **b** T₁-weighted SE sequence, transverse plane. The fracture line of the radial head is well delineated (arrow).

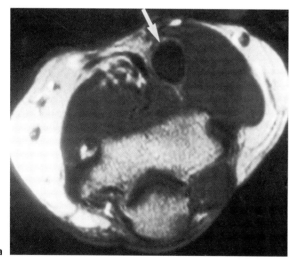

a

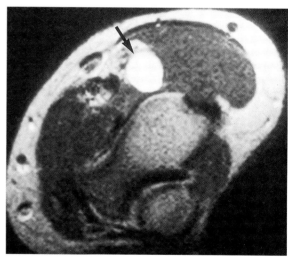

b

Figs. 4.**22 a, b** Ganglion cyst in the anterior cubital fossa. **a** T₁-weighted SE sequence, transverse plane. The ganglion (arrow) has a signal intensity that almost equals that of the surrounding musculature. **b** T₂-weighted SE sequence, transverse plane. The ganglion is demarcated from the surrounding tissue due to a very high signal intensity (arrow).

The high signal intensity seen with the compartment syndrome on T₂-weighted images and STIR sequences is pathognomonic for muscle edema (Chapter 10).

Post-Therapy Findings

Employing MRI for the evaluation of elbow lesions is relatively new and little is known about findings that appear after therapy. Most of the experience has been gathered with fractures, whereby MRI is compromised whenever metallic devices have been inserted. Its high resolution makes MRI especially suitable for traumatic changes of the elbow region. Osseous consolidation can be documented, particularly in contradistinction to fibrous incorporation of fragments and nonosseous fibrous bridging of fracture clefts. Fragments with fibrous connections between osseous fragments exhibit a decreased signal intensity on T_1- and T_2-weighted sequences. Without osseous bridging of the fracture cleft, the signal intensity increases on T_2-weighted sequences along the previous fracture line because of increased water content. What has been stated on page 97 also applies to avascular fracture fragments with impaired healing and clinical consequence.

In cases of prolonged post-therapeutic complaints, MRI can be useful for revealing complications of healing or concomitant lesions that were left untreated (e.g., missed tear of the ulnar collateral ligament associated with a surgically treated olecranon fracture or damage to the humeroradial cartilage with valgus injury associated with a tear of the ulnar collateral ligament). Furthermore, MRI can even be employed for postsurgical staging after tumor resection. It can also monitor inflammatory changes of the elbow joint needed for evaluating the therapeutic results of rheumatoid arthritis (20).

Pitfalls in Interpreting the Images

Misinterpretations of MRI findings of the elbow are usually attributable to anatomic variants or technical shortcomings, such as unsuitable coils as well as flow and motion artifacts.

The supracondylar process is a hook-shaped osseous prominence above the medial epicondyle and is asymptomatic in the majority of cases, but can occasionally compress the median nerve or the brachial artery. This process can be visualized radiographically, though its fibrous extension to the medial epicondyle, which can cause the entrapment syndrome mentioned previously, cannot (2). Coronal and transverse MRI images can delineate these soft tissue structures and establish the correct diagnosis.

The hyaline cartilage of the trochlear notch of the ulna only rarely forms a coherent articular surface in the adult. Instead, a partial or complete transverse groove devoid of cartilage is found, bisecting the articular surface. The subchondral bone can form a crest along the transverse groove that mimics a lesion but is actually a normal variant.

Most artifacts in the upper extremity are due to motion and blood flow. Flow artifacts can induce an in-creased vascular signal that can be mistaken for a cyst. To avoid interference from flow artifacts, it has been recommended that the direction of phase encoding is changed. Another asymptomatic normal variant that can be misinterpreted as pathologic is the spontaneously reducible subluxation of the ulnar nerve that creates a void in the ulnar groove of the humerus. This is positional and disappears when the forced position of the elbow is released at completion of the examination. Furthermore, accompanying vessels (a recurrent ulnar artery (18)) can be encountered in the ulnar groove. The accompanying veins can be distended. This finding is asymptomatic and represents a normal variant.

Clinical Relevance of MRI and Comparison with Other Imaging Modalities

The relative value of MRI for diagnosis in comparison with other imaging methods for a range of pathologic conditions is summarized in Table 4.**3**.

The diagnostic evaluation of the skeletal components of the elbow still includes conventional radiography. Radiographic views in two projections should precede the MRI examination to allow the osseous findings to be taken in to account when setting up the MRI protocol. Sonography is invaluable for the inexpensive diagnosis of soft tissue processes, in particular for tendon lesions. The choice between CT and MRI is less clear cut. Because of its multiplanar display and excellent contrast resolution of soft tissues, MRI achieves a high predictive value for evaluating tendon injuries, ligamentous lesions, cartilage defects, and loose intra-articular bodies. In one investigation, for instance, the detection of loose bodies had a sensitivity of 100% and a specificity of 67% (17). For the display of any complex anatomic relationship, MRI is the preferred modality. Furthermore, MRI is indicated for the traumatized pediatric elbow since it is noninvasive, does not involve ionizing radiation, and can even be performed with a plaster cast in place. Interpreting the findings, however, requires a profound anatomical knowledge in view of the complex anatomy of the ossification centers around the elbow joint. This is complicated further by the absence of radiographic visualization of the cartilaginous centers at the age of 11 to 12 years, but this is the very reason for MRI, especially in view of the fractures involving the cartilage and growth plates. For pediatric fractures of the epiphyseal region, MRI is suitable for determining adequate therapy, in particular for fractures that cannot be assessed adequately on the conventional radiograph and that involve the growth plate (1). Arthrography of the elbow for evaluating loose bodies is invasive, even if performed with CT, and because of its possible complications has been replaced by MRI.

The findings and management of hemophilic arthropathy were changed in 40% of the cases after a follow-up MRI (14). This indicates the sensitivity of MRI for

Table 4.**3** Diagnostic value of MRI in comparison with other imaging methods.

Lesionen/Diseases	Sequence of the Radiologic Examinations					
	Radiology	Sonography	Arthrography	CT	Arthro-CT	MRI
Capsule/ligament rupture	(3)	1				2
Tendon rupture		1				2
Fracture	1			2		2
Dislocation	1			2		2
Osteoarthritis	1					2
Osteochondritis dissecans	1		3		3	2
Osteonecrosis	1					2
Osteomyelitis	1			3		2
Arthritis	1	2				2
Synovitis		2				2
Bursitis/Tendinitis/Enthesopathy		1				2
Muscle lesions		1				2
Tumor	1	(3)				2
Nerve compression syndrome		1				2

1 = Modality should be used first
2, 3 = Modality should be used subsequently if findings inconclusive
(3) = Modality might provide additional information

soft tissue and cartilage lesions. Moreover, early stages of osteomyelitis can be assessed better because of the excellent tissue contrast and multiplanar display in comparison with conventional imaging modalities. As for other musculoskeletal lesions, the examination includes both T_1-weighted and T_2-weighted sequences as well as contrast enhancement.

MRI can render more specific indications for diagnostic arthrography. In particular, the therapeutic approach to loose intra-articular bodies can be planned more reliably with MRI. Radiographically occult fractures and fissures can be well visualized by MRI. An applied cast does not interfere with MRI. Even with a bulky cast in place, adequate image quality can be achieved by using a large surface coil, such as the head coil. In general, the findings of osseous trauma are clearly evident on T_1- and T_2-weighted sequences as well as on STIR sequences, but are often better delineated on T_2- and T_2^*weighted GRE sequences.

MRI has largely replaced CT of the elbow and can be expected to replace arthrography. The only advantage of CT over MRI is the better delineation of the osseous structures in cases of suspected trauma and its lower costs. MRI is superior for the evaluation of accompanying soft tissue changes. Cartilaginous fragments not visualized because of superimposition on CT or CT-arthrography can be delineated by MRI (22). Disadvantages of MRI are the long examination times, possible claustrophobia, the high costs and the exclusion of patients with pacemakers or other metallic foreign bodies (e.g., vascular clips, shrapnel).

Literatur

1 Beltran, J., Z. S. Rosenberg, M. Kawelblum, L. Montes, A. G. Bergman, A. Strongwater: Pediatric elbow fractures: MRI evaluation. Skelet. Radiol. 23 (1994) 277–281
2 Berquist, T. H.: The elbow. In Higgins, C. B., H. Hricak, C. A. Helms: Magnetic Resonance Imaging of the Body, 2nd ed. Raven, New York 1992 (p. 1163)
3 Bunnell, D. H., D. A. Fisher, L. W. Bassett, R. H. Gold, H. Ellman: Elbow joint: normal anatomy on MR images. Radiology 165 (1987) 527–531
4 Bunnell, D. H., L. W. Bassett: The elbow. In Bassett, L. W., R. H. Gold, L. L. Seeger: MRI Atlas of the Musculoskeletal System. Dunitz, London 1989 (p. 129)
5 Coel, M., C. Y. Yamada, J. Ko: MRImaging of patients with lateral epicondylitits of the elbow (tennis elbow): importance of increased signal of the anconeus muscle. Amer. J. Roentgenol. 161 (1993) 1019–1024
5a Cotten et al. Radiology 1997; 204: 806–812
6 Fitzgerald, S. W., D. R. Curry, S. J. Erickson, S. F. Quinn, H. Friedman: Distal biceps tendon injury: MR imaging diagnosis. Radiology 191 (1994) 203–206
7 Fritz, R. C., L. S. Steinbach: The elbow. In Chan, W. P., P. Lang, H. K. Genant: MRI of the Musculoskeletal System. Saunders, Philadelphia 1994 (p. 193)
8 Gires, F., A. Chevrot, A. Leroy-Willing, M. Wybier, C. Vallée, J. C. Roucayrol, G. Pallardy: Joints. In Vanel, D., M. T. McNamara: MRI of the Body. Springer, Berlin 1989 (p. 263)
9 Herzog, R. J.: Magnetic Resonance Imaging of the elbow. Magn. Reson. Quart. 9 (1993) 188–198
10 Herzog, R. J.: Efficacy of Magnetic Resonance Imaging of the elbow. Med. Sci. Sports Exerc. 26 (1994) 1193–1203
11 Ho, C. P., D. J. Sartoris: Magnetic Resonance Imaging of the elbow. Rheum. Dis. Clin. N. Amer. 17 (1991) 705–709
12 Ho, C. P.: Magnetic Resonance Imaging of the elbow. In Bloem, J. L., D. J. Sartoris: MRI and CT of the Musculoskeletal System. Williams and Wilkins, Baltimore 1992 (p. 294)

13 Middleton, W. D., S. Macrander, J. B. Kneeland, W. Froncisz, A. Jesmanowicz, J. S. Hyde: MR imaging of the normal elbow: anatomic correlation. Amer. J. Roentgenol. 149 (1987) 543–547

14 Nuss, R., R. F. Kilcoyne, S. Geraghty, J. Wiedel, M. Manco-Johnson: Utility of magnetic resonance imaging for management of hemophilic arthropathy in children. J. Pediat. 123 (1993) 388–395

14a Peiss et al. Skeletal Radiology 1995; 24: 17

15 Peters, P. E., G. Bongartz: MR-Anatomie des Ellenbogengelenkes. In Peters, P. E., H. H. Matthiaß, M. Reiser: Magnetresonanztomographie in der Orthopädie. Enke, Stuttgart 1990 (S. 39)

16 Pitt, M. J., D. P. Speer: Imaging of the elbow with an emphasis on trauma. Radiol. Clin. N. Amer. 28 (1990) 293–297

17 Quinn, S. F., J. J. Haberman, S. W. Fitzgerald, P. D. Traughber, R. J. Belkin, W. T. Murray: Evaluation of loose bodies in the elbow with MRImaging. Magn. Reson. Imag. 4 (1994) 169–175

18 Rosenberg, Z. S., J. Beltran, Y. Cheung, M. Broker: MR imaging of the elbow: normal variant and potential diagnostic pitfalls of the trochlear groove and cubital tunnel. Amer. J. Roentgenol. 164 (1995) 415–420

19 Schinz: Prinzipien der Beurteilung von Skeletterkrankungen. In Frommhold, W., W. Dihlmann, H.-St. Stender, P. Thurn: Radiologische Diagnostik in Klinik und Praxis, 7. Aufl. Thieme, Stuttgart 1991 (S. 276)

20 Schnarkowski, P., C. Bader, A. Goldman, J. M. Friedrich: Pannusdarstellung bei rheumatoider Arthritis mittels Kernspintomographie. Röntgenpraxis 45 (1992) 412–418

21 Stark, D. D., W. G. Bradley: Magnetic Resonance Imaging, 2nd ed. Mosby, St. Louis 1992 (p. 2493)

22 Stoller, D. W.: The elbow. In Stoller, D. W.: Magnetic Resonance Imaging in Orthopaedics and Sports Medicine. Lippincott, Philadelphia 1993 (p. 633)

23 Tehranzadeh, J., R. Kerr, J. Amster: Magnetic Resonance Imaging of tendon and ligament abnormalities: Part I. Spine and upper extremities. Skelet. Radiol. 21 (1992) 1–13

24 Treadwell, E. L.: Synovial cysts and ganglia: the value of magnetic resonance imaging. Semin. Arthr. Rheum. 24 (1994) 61–69

Wrist

A. Stäbler and M. Vahlensieck

Introduction

MRI is used less frequently for the wrist than for knee or shoulder since the wrist has fewer conditions with established MRI indications, such as ligamentous injuries, soft tissue and bone tumors, or inflammations. Furthermore, positioning in the MRI gantry is difficult and burdensome for the patient unless special coils are used. With the right auxiliary equipment, however, the ›small' wrist is suitable for imaging at a high resolution by using appropriate surface coils. The wrist is the most complex joint of the human body and poses high technical demands on diagnostic imaging, and it is here that MRI has opened new diagnostic avenues and will continue to forge the diagnostic and therapeutic approach in the future.

Examination Technique

■ Positioning

The position should be as comfortable as possible for the patient. The best results can be achieved by using small Helmholtz-type surface coils or flexible coils that keep the wrist next to the patient's body while the patient is placed in a comfortable supine position. An off-center field of view is a prerequisite for this examination technique.

For examinations performed in the center of the magnetic field, the patient has to be prone with the arm extended above the head. This position might be difficult for older patients and those with shoulder complaints.

Excellent images can be obtained by using a temporomandibular joint coil incorporated in a head coil, but the patient must be in the lateral decubitus or prone position with the arm extended above the head. This position again is uncomfortable and often the patient can hold still without moving the arm for a few image acquisitions only.

■ Coil

Examinations of the head require the highest spatial resolution and should be performed only with dedicated surface coils. Circular coils with a diameter of 8 – 15 cm are most frequently used. The wrist is placed on or into the coil. Usually a field of view of 6 – 8 cm is large enough, which can be achieved with a coil diameter of 5 – 6 cm. Such small surface coils must have strong gradient fields to achieve this field of view for the applied sequence parameters. Conventional coils have the disadvantage of a rapid signal loss with increasing distance from the center of the receiver coil. A homogeneous distribution can be achieved with Helmholtz-type coils or flexible coils.

■ Sequences and Parameters

Each examination of the wrist should include a coronal section. It provides a survey image of the bone marrow of all carpal bones and, at the same time, visualizes the distal forearm and the metacarpal bones. The sagittal plane is most suitable for visualizing the axial relationships of instabilities and for revealing any posterior or anterior subluxations. The transverse plane is primarily used for the evaluation of the carpal canal. Furthermore, it is the plane mandatory for delineating the extent of tumors and their pattern of infiltration. For the wrist proper, it can also assist evaluating the palmar or dorsal capsule and the synovial tendon sheaths.

Coronal T_1-weighted and T_2-weighted images as well as sagittal T_1-weighted images have been proven useful for finding the causes of unclear carpal pain. STIR sequences have been quite helpful for the sensitive detection of effusions and bone marrow edema.

■ Special Examination Techniques

Contrast Enhancement. This frequently provides additional information. IV contrast medium is indicated whenever the findings are unclear.

3D-GRE Sequences. These allow sections less than 1 mm in width, which are especially advantageous for evaluating the triangular cartilage complex, but are rarely obtained in routine imaging. Since GRE sequences are sensitive to different magnetic susceptibilities, they can display an increased sclerosis in osseous regions.

Rapid GRE Sequences Applying these sequences repetitively at short intervals (three sections within 10 sec.) can display enhancement dynamics in inflammatory and tumorous tissue. This technique can be used to monitor inflammatory conditions (rheumatoid arthritis) during therapy and, furthermore, might clarify the type of tumors (hemangioma) and reveal therapeutic responses (radiation therapy, chemotherapy).

MR Arthrography. The use of MR arthrography for the visualization and evaluation of the triangular fibrocartilage complex (TFCC) and interosseous ligaments is currently being assessed. Its fundamental disadvantage is the inability to visualize the flow of contrast medium from the mediocarpal joint into the radiocarpal joint and from the radiocarpal joint into the radioulnar joint as evidence of corresponding defects of the ligaments and triangular cartilage. Instilling contrast medium into several joint compartments is time consuming and currently its use is difficult to justify. However with more experience, use of the technique may increase.

Cinematic Examination of the Wrist. This can be achieved with rapid GRE sequences and in the future also with echo-planar sequences. An interesting approach is the realtime visualization of motion by recording the images during movement of the patient's hand. Whether this provides more information than conventional fluoroscopy remains to be seen and awaits the results of upcoming studies.

Anatomy

■ General Anatomy

The eight *carpal bones* can be divided functionally into a proximal row (scaphoid, lunate, triquetral, pisiform) and into a distal row (trapezium, trapezoid, capitate, hamate). The pisiform articulates with the triquetrum and can be considered to be a sesamoid in the flexor carpi ulnaris tendon. Functionally, it conforms neither to the proximal nor distal row.

The *articulation* between distal radial articulating surface, distal ulna, triangular articular disk and proximal carpal row forms the radiocarpal articulation. In about 15% of the cases, it communicates with the pisotriquetral articulation. The proximal and distal carpal rows form the midcarpal joint. The distal carpal row and metacarpal bases constitute the carpometacarpal articulation, which has no motion because of strong connecting ligaments (amphiarthrosis). The articulation between the metacarpal bases is also referred to as intermetacarpal articulation. Separate articulations are the first carpometacarpal articulation (the sellar joint of the thumb) and the distal radioulnar articulation. The articulating surface of the radius is concave and forms a sigmoid notch for the ulna.

The anatomic arrangement of the carpal *ligaments* is very complex. Interosseous (intercarpal) ligaments, which partially compartmentalize the internal joint capsule and as such are intrinsic, are distinguished from extracarpal ligaments, which reinforce the joint capsule and are extrinsic.

Intrinsic ligaments: The proximal carpal row is interconnected by the interosseous ligaments between scaphoid and lunate (SL ligament) and between lunate and triquetrum (LT ligament), (Fig. 5.1) and forms a functional unit. These ligaments prevent a communication between the radiocarpal and mediocarpal articulations. Like all fibrous and ligamentous structures of the body, they are subject to degeneration, and defects in the SL ligament and LT ligament are found in about 30% of asymptomatic older patients.

The distal carpal row is also interconnected by interosseous ligaments (Fig. 5.1).

The configuration of the interosseous ligaments and the ulnar disk creates different *joint compartments* (Fig. 5.1). Familiarity with these compartments is a prerequisite for the performance and interpretation of arthrography. In MRI, the distribution of fluid accumulation or effusion within the individual compartments can be used to localize the site of a pathologic process.

Extrinsic ligaments: The entire carpal region is enveloped by a firm fibrous capsule, partially reinforced by strong ligaments (Fig. 5.2). On the palmar side, the radiocapitate ligament, which is a part of the palmar radiocarpal ligament, extends from the radial styloid process across the waste of the scaphoid to the capitate. The radiotriquetral ligament, also part of the palmar radiocarpal ligament, arises from the ulnar aspect of the radial styloid process and follows a similar diagonal direction. It crosses the lunate and connects with fibrous extensions to it (part of the palmar radiocarpal ligament). On the ulnar aspect of the palmar carpal region, fibrous bands arise from the ulnar styloid process and fuse with the triangular fibrocartilage complex. Since these ligaments form a 'V' with the radial palmar ligaments, these structures are also referred to as proximal or distal V-ligaments.

There are two strong diagonal ligaments on the dorsal side. The proximal ligament extends from the radial styloid process over the lunate to the triquetrum, called the dorsal radiotriquetral ligament, and represents the dorsal component of the carpal sling. The triquetrum can be imagined as the stone placed in the sling. From the triquetrum, broadly fan-shaped fibers extend over the distal carpal row to the trapezium, constituting the dorsal carpal ligament. Radial and ulnar collateral ligaments are seen on the respective sides of the carpal region.

The triangular articular disk is composed of fibrocartilage and is positioned between the distal ulna proximally and the triquetrum and lunate distally. It has a flat triangular configuration, extends into the hyaline cartilage of the distal articulating surface of the radius and fuses imperceptibly with a complex structure of fibers and ligaments between the ulnar styloid process and proximal carpal rows.

Fig. 5.**1** Schematic drawing of a coronal section through the wrist to illustrate the compartmentalization of the carpal region into five articular compartments by the interosseous ligaments and triangular disk (after Greenspan).
1 = Compartment of the first carpometacarpal articulation
2 = Common carpometacarpal compartment
3 = Mediocarpal compartment
4 = Radiocarpal articulation
5 = Scapholunate ligament
6 = Distal radioulnar articulation
7 = Triangular disk
8 = Ligament between lunate and triquetrum
9 = Ligament between pisiform and triquetrum
10 = Intermetacarpal compartment

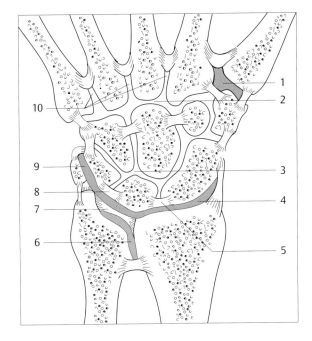

Fig. 5.**2a, b** **a** Posterior and **b** anterior view of the extrinsic ligaments (after Kahle and co-workers).
1 = Radius
Ligaments between distal forearm and carpal bones:
3 = Ulnar collateral ligament
4 = Radial collateral ligament
5 = Palmar radiocarpal ligament
6 = Posterior radiocarpal ligament
7 = Palmar ulnocarpal ligament
Ligaments between carpal bones:
8 = Radiate carpal ligament
9 = Pisohamate ligament
10 = Palmar intercarpal ligaments
11 = Posterior intercarpal ligaments
Ligaments between carpal and metacarpal bones:
12 = Pisometacarpal ligament
13 = Palmar carpometacarpal ligaments
14 = Posterior carpometacarpal ligaments
Ligaments between metacarpal bones:
15, 16 = Metacarpal ligaments

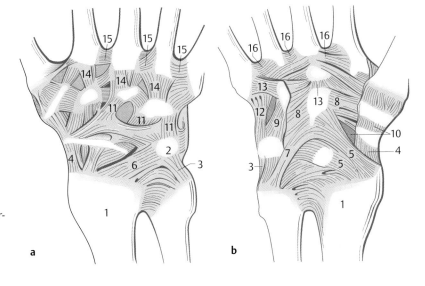

Two bands of fibers of the ulnar attachment are distinguished: one at the ulnar styloid process and one at the base of the distal ulna. Its undersurface glides over the head of the distal ulna covered with hyaline cartilage. The ulnar component of the radiocarpal articulation is distal to the triangular disk. The central and radial portions of the disk are not vascularized and, in contrast to the ulnar portion of the disc, show poor spontaneous healing after trauma. Because of its vascularization, the ulnar aspect of the disk has a higher signal intensity.

Since it is difficult to separate the multiple fibrous structures of the ulnar side of the carpal region by imaging, the triangular disk and its ligamentous complex are simply referred to as triangular fibrocartilage complex (TFCC). Apart from the disk, this complex includes the dorsal and palmar radioulnar ligaments, a variably manifested ligamentous structure between triquetrum and ulna (so-called ulnocarpal meniscus or meniscal homologue), the ulnar collateral ligament, two ulnocarpal ligaments, the ulnolunate ligament and the ulnotriquetral ligament. The ulnocarpal meniscus can occa-

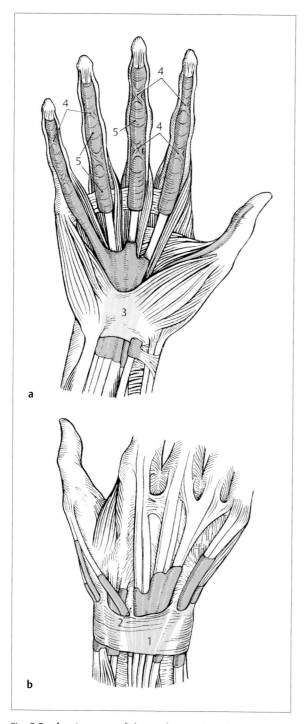

sionally contain an accessory ossicle, called the os triquetrum secundarium or os triangulare. The opening to the prestyloid recess, also referred to as the ulnar recess and representing an extension of the joint capsule, is between discus and meniscus.

Like the midcarpal articulation, the radiocarpal articulation contributes to flexion and extension as much as to radial and ulnar abduction. Flexion occurs to a greater degree in the radiocarpal articulation and extension is somewhat greater in the midcarpal articulation. The scaphoid undergoes the most conspicuous changes between radial and ulnar abduction of the wrist. Its normally 45 to 50 degree palmar inclination relative to the longitudinal axis of the radius rotates palmarly with radial abduction, while it extends upright and fills the space between distal radius, trapezium and trapezoideum with ulnar abduction.

After passing through the openings and channels of the wrist, the *muscle tendons* are surrounded by synovial sheaths, which are arranged in several tendon sheath compartments (Fig. 5.3 – 5.5).

Fig. 5.**3 a, b**   Anatomy of the tendons and tendon sheaths of the hand. **a** Anterior (palmar) view of the flexor tendons. **b** Posterior (dorsal) view of the extensor tendons (after Kahle and co-workers).
1 = Extensor retinaculum
2 = Septa of the retinaculum
3 = Flexor retinaculum
4 = Cruciate ligaments
5 = Annular ligaments

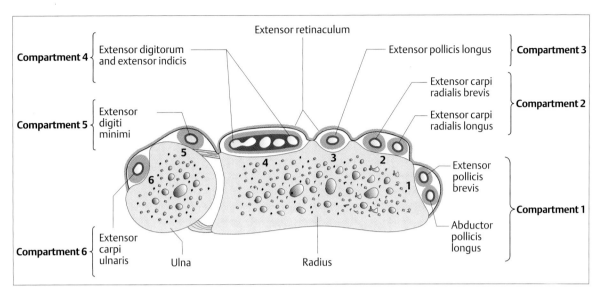

Fig. 5.**4** Anatomy of the tendons and tendon sheaths of the hand. Cross section at proximal wrist to illustrate the six extensor compartments (after Netter).

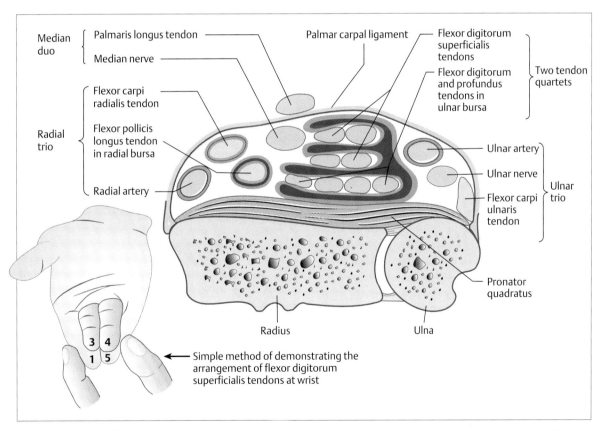

Fig. 5.**5** Anatomy of the tendons and tendon sheaths of the hand. Cross section proximal to the flexor retinaculum to illustrate the flexor tendons (after Netter).

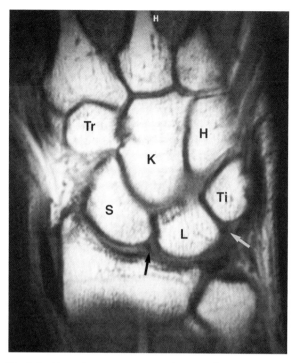

Fig. 5.**6** Normal anatomy. Coronal T$_1$-weighted SE image. The bone marrow spaces of the carpal bones exhibit a homogeneous signal. The interosseous ligaments (scapholunate ligament = SL, lunotriquetral ligament = LT) are identified as low signal structures (arrows).

S = Scaphoid	Ti = Triquetrum	C = Capitate
L = Lunate	Tr = Trapezoid	H = Hamate

■ Specific MRI Anatomy

Coronal Plane. This is the standard plane for visualizing the wrist. The bone marrow space of the carpal bones, especially lunate and scaphoid, can be easily evaluated, showing a homogeneous signal of high intensity on T$_1$-weighted sequences (Figs. 5.**6**– 5.**8**). Punctate decreases in signal intensity can correspond to bone islands, small cysts or nutrient vessels. The homogeneously high signal intensity reflects the absence of hematopoietic bone marrow in the distal extremities. The interosseous scapholunate and lunotriquetral ligaments are not definitively visualized in the coronal plane. Since the lunotriquetral ligament is slightly smaller, it can be evaluated less often than the scapholunate ligament. These ligamentous structures do not occupy the entire intercarpal spaces and are more arranged along the peripheral contact zone. Consequently, the coronal plane visualizes these ligaments at the radiocarpal articulation and not at the mediocarpal articulation (Fig. 5.**9**). As found at the remaining intercarpal articulations, the interspaces are filled with hyaline cartilage of the respective carpal bones. The somewhat stronger scapholunate ligament shows variations where it is attached at the hyaline cartilage of the scaphoid and lunate. A broad zone of attachment along the proximal articular surface of the lunate is the most frequently encountered finding. Like the capsular ligaments and fibrocartilaginous

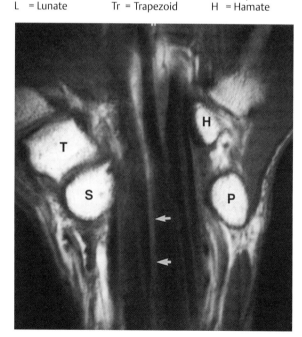

Fig. 5.**7** Normal anatomy. Coronal T$_1$-weighted SE image. The carpal canal with its low signal flexor tendon is visualized. The linear high signal structure seen centrally is a section of the median nerve (arrow). The Guyon canal is between the hamulus of the hamate and pisiform.

S = Distal pole of the scaphoid   P = Pisiform
T = Trapezium   H = Hamulus of the hamate

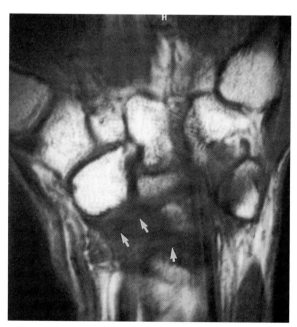

Fig. 5.**8** Normal anatomy. Coronal T$_1$-weighted SE image. The radial aspect of the proximal and distal V ligament (radiocapitate ligament, radiotriquetral ligament) is visualized.

disk complex, the interosseous ligaments exhibit a low signal intensity in all sequences.

These fibrocartilaginous structures can deviate by exhibiting an artificial increase in signal intensity on T_1- and T_2^*-weighted and protein density weighted images in certain joint positions, unrelated to and not to be mistaken for a pathologic process (see magic angle phenomenon, Appendix, p. 378). Furthermore, an increasing number of published articles have reported various patterns of increased signal intensities, particularly in thin sections, in the scapholunate and lunotriangular ligaments of asymptomatic pattern, attributed to degenerative changes (Fig. 5.**10**). These increases in signal intensity can be punctate or linear and can occur both along the course of the ligament or at the osseous attachment. Moreover, thin MRI sections can reveal morphologic variants that can be triangular, linear or amorphous.

The ulnar disk has degenerative changes beginning in the third decade, causing increased signal intensities not to be mistaken for acute ruptures or inflammations. Histologically, these areas show a decreased number of chondrocytes as well as an altered fibrous matrix. The T_1- and T_2-weighted images show focal and linear increases in signal intensity (Fig. 5.**10**). Linear signal intensities that extend to the surface generally correspond to a complete chronic rupture. These degenerative changes progress with age but are rarely symptomatic.

Fluid or effusion is not detectable in the capsule or recesses of the carpal joints of most healthy wrists, though it can be normal to observe a small amount of fluid on T_2-weighted, STIR and GRE sequences. An effusion exceeding 1–1.5 mm in width should be considered pathologic. The coronal plane also allows the evaluation of the triangular fibrocartilage disk. However, the disk is seen with 3 mm sections only on

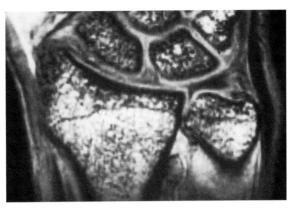

Fig. 5.**9**   Coronal 3D GRE image of a healthy subject. The scapholunate and lunotriquetral ligaments exhibit a triangular configuration and contain a somewhat heterogeneous signal increase centrally. High signal cartilage is seen at the base. The ulnar portion of the extrinsic ligaments is well delineated and consists of the triangular fibrocartilage complex with high signal radial attachment formed by the cartilaginous cover of the radius. The high signal on the ulnar site is caused by vascularized connective tissue. The so-called meniscus homologue (meniscus ulnocarpalis) is further distal with the ulnar collateral ligament along its ulnar side.

one or two sections. Thin sections of 1.5–2 mm are recommended for the region of the triangular fibrocartilage disk. The low-signal fibers of the triangular fibrocartilage disk radiate into the distal radial articular surface and exhibit a broad-based attachment along the radiocarpal articulation and more proximal along the radioulnar articulation.

Sagittal Plane. Images in the sagittal plane show the axial relationship of the carpal bones to each other. In particular, the axes of the radius, lunate, capitate and

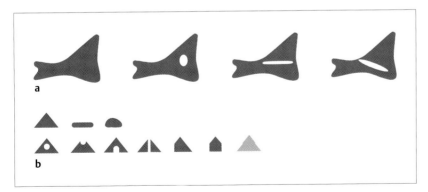

Fig. 5.**10a, b**   Variable visualization of the triangular disk and the intrinsic ligaments between the lunate and scaphoid and between the lunate and triquetrum. **a** The fibrocartilaginous triangular disk is usually seen as structure of low signal intensity or signal void (left). Age-related degeneration induces increases in signal intensity, which initially are focal and later appear linear with possible extension to the surface (from left to right). **b** The intrinsic ligaments of the proximal carpal row are

seen usually as low signal intensity to signal void and are triangular in shape (about 60%). Form variants can lead to a more linear (about 30%) or more amorphous (more than 10%) visualization. The signal changes consist of (from right to left) focal increase in intensity in the center, at the tip (about 5%) or base (about 3%), linear and still central increase (about 10%), and unilateral or bilateral increase at the attachment as well as a diffuse increase.

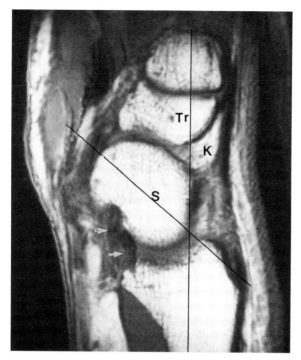

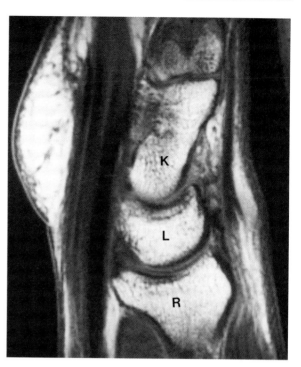

Fig. 5.**11** Normal anatomy. Sagittal T₁-weighted SE images. Scaphoid and its articulation with the trapezium and trapezoid are seen in part. On the palmar aspect, the radioulnar and radiotriquetral ligaments are diagonally transected (arrows). The longitudinal axis of the wrist (the vertical line along the radiolunate-capitate-metacarpal axis) and the 30 to 60 degree tilted scaphoid axis are superimposed.
S = Scaphoid
C = Capitate
T = Trapezoid

Fig. 5.**12** Normal anatomy. Sagittal T₁-weighted SE images. The normal alignment of radius, lunate and capitate is apparent. The flexor tendons are seen on the palmar aspect.
L = Lunate
C = Capitate
R = Radius

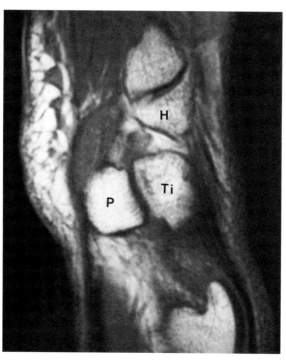

scaphoid can be measured as on a lateral radiographic view but without interfering superimpositions (Figs. 5.**11**–5.**13**). Palmar or dorsal subluxations are accurately visualized on the lateral plane only. Even minor subluxations as well as early localized cartilaginous degenerations can be detected. The sagittal plane is therefore mandatory for the evaluation of instabilities and degenerative changes. Furthermore, it discloses the structural changes of the lunate in patients with avascular necrosis of the lunate.

◄ Fig. 5.**13** Normal anatomy. Sagittal T₁-weighted SE images. The pisotriquetral articulation and the ulnar styloid process are visualized.
H = Hamate
Ti = Triquetrum
P = Pisiform

Transverse Plane. The axial or transverse plane displays the carpal tunnel with its contents.

The retinaculum, which extends between distal scaphoid, tubercle of the trapezium and hamulus of the hamate, is seen as structure of low signal intensity (Fig. 5.**14**). The median nerve is immediately beneath it and, because of its water and fat content, has a higher signal intensity than the flexor tendons in all sequences. Positional variants of the median nerve are well recognized on all transverse images and should not be mistaken for pathologic displacements. Moreover, the com-

partment for the ulnar nerve, the Guyon canal, can be adequately evaluated in this plane. The superficial and deep flexor tendons are also distinctly delineated (Fig. 5.**15**), and inflammatory changes or effusions of the tendon sheaths can be easily detected on T_2-weighted images. Furthermore, the palmar and dorsal capsular ligaments are displayed on the transverse images, especially if pathologic changes are present. Only the transverse images can adequately display the anatomic position of the radioulnar joint and can detect even minor palmar or dorsal subluxations (Fig. 5.**16**).

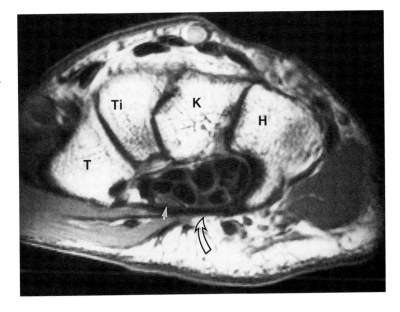

Fig. 5.**14**   Normal anatomy. Transverse T_1-weighted SE images. The flexor retinaculum is seen as structure of low signal intensity (open arrow). The flexor digitorum superficialis and profundus tendons also are seen as nearly signal void. The median nerve is relatively far on the radial aspect, appears transverse-ovoid and has an increased signal intensity relative to the flexor tendons (arrow).

T = Trapezium
Ti = Trapezoid
C = Capitate
H = Hamate with hamulus

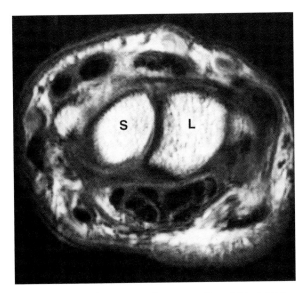

Fig. 5.**15**   Normal anatomy. Transverse T_1-weighted SE images at the level of the scapholunate joint space. The capsular ligaments are stronger on the palmar side than on the dorsal side.
S = Scaphoid
L = Lunate

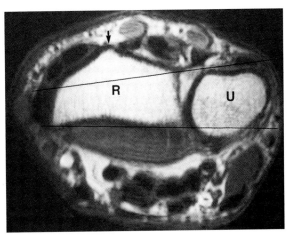

Fig. 5.**16**   Normal anatomy. Transverse T_1-weighted-weighted SE images at the level of the distal radioulnar articulation. Lister's tubercle is seen at the dorsal aspect of the radius (arrow). Lines are drawn between dorsal and palmar corners of the radius to determine any malposition of the ulna. The ulna should not project beyond these lines by more than half the shaft width.
R = Radius
U = Ulna

Spontaneous Avascular Necroses

MRI has been become established as a very sensitive method for the detection of avascular necroses due to the direct visualization of pathologic processes involving the internal osseous structures. Bone scintigraphy has an equally high sensitivity but a lower specificity. Conventional radiographs and CT are negative in the early stages of avascular necroses. The most common manifestations in the wrist are the spontaneous avascular necrosis of the lunate (Kienböck disease) and, somewhat less frequent, the spontaneous avascular necrosis of the scaphoid (Preiser disease). Only a few case reports describe spontaneous avascular necroses affecting other carpal bones: trapezoid (Agati disease), osteochondritis dissecans of the pisiform (Schmier disease) and triquetrum (Witt disease) as well as multiple avascular necroses involving capitate, trapezium, and hamate (Brainard disease).

■ Avascular Necrosis of the Lunate (Kienböck disease)

Lunate avascular necrosis represents the progressive necrotic collapse of the lunate. Men are affected three to four times more often than women. It is generally unilateral but can be bilateral, possibly affecting each wrist at a different stage.

Etiology. Various causative mechanisms are being discussed. Frequently, the patient remembers a trauma in the recent or remote past. Mechanical overuse of the wrist seems to play a role in some patients. For workers using a jackhammer, lunate avascular necrosis is a recognized occupational hazard. Incongruence of the radiocarpal articulation is considered a predisposing factor, most often manifested as relatively short ulna, less often as relatively long ulna (so-called ulna plus variant and ulna minus variant according to Hultén [Hultén 1928]).

Symptoms. The symptoms generally begin between the ages of 20 and 40 years, but can become manifest after the fifth decade. The complaints often begin insidiously. Radiating wrist pain can last for years, leading to progressing active and passive restriction of motion and declining strength of grip. A swelling is observed on the dorsum of the hand, associated with local tenderness. Characteristically, passive extension of the middle finger is painful.

Therapy. Depending on the stage of the disease, conservative therapy (immobilization for stage Decloux I and II) or surgically reconstructed articular congruence by means of ulnar extension or radial shortening (so-called leveling surgeries for stage Decloux II) should be considered. To avoid secondary degenerative changes and carpal collapse, a lunate resection is usually combined with plastic replacement using interposed tendons, silicon (Swanson prosthesis), Vitallium or even acrylic. Alternatively, an intercarpal fusion or extended resection with additional partial resection of adjacent carpal bones (e.g., Steinhäuser techniques) should be considered. Furthermore, transposing the pisiform into the lunate lodge is a surgical option. In stage IV disease, fusion or denervating surgeries as salvage procedures can provide symptomatic relief (Fig. 5.**17**). MRI is indicated if symptoms persist or worsen post-surgically and clinical and conventional radiologic findings are inconclusive. Familiarity with the surgical procedure is mandatory for interpreting postsurgical findings.

Diagnosis. Diagnosing avascular necrosis of the lunate can be difficult since its early stage is *radiographically* unremarkable. Bone scintigraphy is a sensitive method and already positive in the early stages. The first radiographic finding consists of a subtle increase in density in the lunate in comparison with the other carpal bones. Cysts can develop within the lunate. Later in the disease, the lunate becomes fragmented. The fragmentation generally begins in the proximal subchondral region that articulates with the distal radius. Already in this stage, a functional insufficiency of the scapholunate ligament can develop, leading to a moderate rotatory subluxation of the scaphoid (RSS). This instability can progress to degenerative changes of the styloid as the first manifestation of osteoarthritis of the carpal bones. This is followed by progressive collapse with loss of height and dorsovolar ribbon-like elongation of the lunate. The proximal migration of the capitate eventually leads to a carpal collapse followed by a generalized osteoarthritis of the radiocarpal and mediocarpal articulations. With the progression of the structural changes, grip strength and range of motion decline. The osseous changes can be visualized well by conventional and computed tomography.

Different staging classifications of lunate avascular necrosis on the basis of conventional radiographic findings have been advocated and described in publications by Stähl (1947, five stages), Decloux (1957, four stages) and Lichtman (1988, four stages). The staging proposed by Decloux is as follows:

- Stage I: Increased density of the lunate,
- Stage II: Geographic and/or linear radiolucencies,
- Stage III (end stage): Fragmentation and dorsal displacement of the posterior pole,
- Stage IV (late stage): Secondary osteoarthritis.

Fig. 5.**17 a–d**   Radiographic findings of four surgical treatments for avascular necrosis of the lunate. **a** Osteotomy for ulnar extension. **b** Tendon interposition arthroplasty. **c** Alloarthroplasty (Silicon implant). **d** Pisiform transposition arthroplasty.

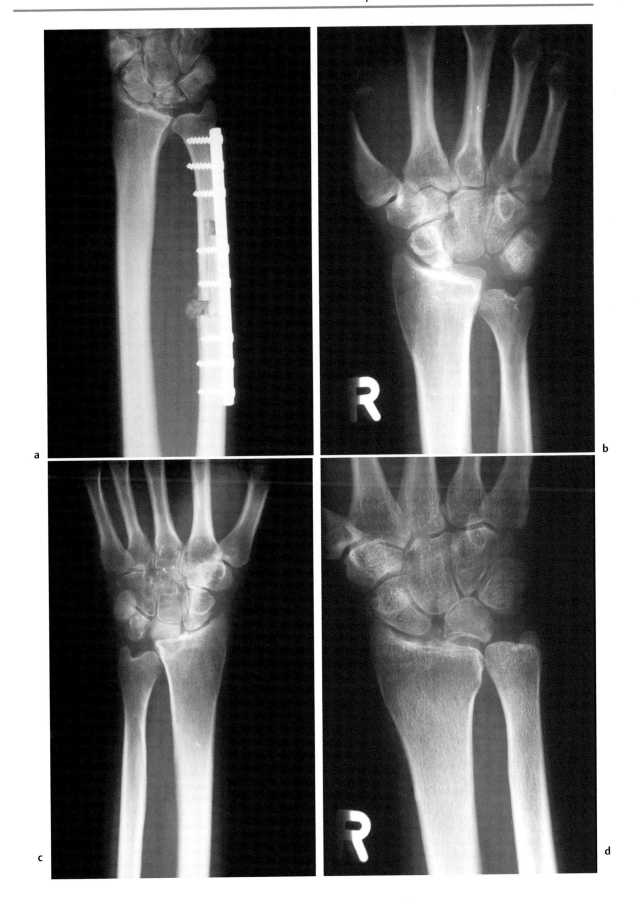

MRI. The use of MRI for diagnosing and staging avascular necrosis of the lunate as well as for following its course, especially after surgery, has led to fundamentally new criteria for interpreting its presentation and has enabled a new approach to the understanding of the underlying pathologic processes. The stages of the disease display different findings (Table 5.**1**):

- *Early stage (stage I):* Minimally decreased signal intensity affecting the entire lunate on the T_1-weighted image (Fig. 5.**18**). The T_2-weighted images show a slightly increased signal intensity. A homogeneous, moderate to intense enhancement can be observed after IV administration of Gd-DTPA. This enhancement is best appreciated on frequency selected fat suppression sequences. Radiographically, the lunate appears normal (stage Ia) or shows a homogeneous sclerosis (stage Ib).
- *Progression (stage II):* Localized punctate areas of more pronounced decreased signal intensity can appear on the T_1 sequences. These areas primarily affect the subchondral proximal trabeculae opposite the radius and show a progressive increase in signal intensity on the T_2-weighted images. They correspond to localized necrotic areas with beginning cystic transformation. In contrast to the remaining portion of the lunate, these areas fail to show contrast enhancement (Fig. 5.**19**). A progressing diffuse decrease in signal intensity can develop. Unlike the early stage, contrast enhancement is no longer detectable in the areas having decreased signal intensity on the T_1-weighted image. The T_2-weighted images no longer show an increased signal intensity.
- *Late stage (stage III):* The lunate undergoes structural changes with loss of height, fragmentation and extension in sagittal direction (Fig. 5.**20**). Between the necrotic osseous areas, localized or disseminated areas of increased or fluid-like signal intensity are detected on the T_2-weighted images. Contrast enhancement, if seen at all, is confined to the peripheral zones

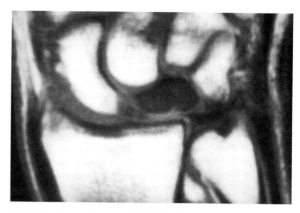

Fig. 5.**18** Avascular necrosis of the lunate, MRI stage Ia or Ib. Coronal T_1-weighted-weighted SE image. Homogeneously decreased signal intensity in the lunate, without deformity. Mild minus variant of the ulna. The radiographic examination was unremarkable (stage Ia).

or to punctate areas in the reparative granulation tissue. Contrast enhancement is no longer homogeneous.

- *Chronic avascular necrosis of the lunate (stage IV):* The instability caused by the fragmented lunate is, in part, that of a scapholunar instability. This can lead to degenerative changes at the radial styloid process and later even at the mediocarpal articulation (Fig. 5.**21**). It is of great clinical importance to recognize these degenerative changes since they markedly worsen the prognosis of revascularizing or reconstructive surgeries. Consequently, local fusion should be carried out if secondary degenerative changes are present.

Pathophysiology. The signal patterns described for the different stages suggest that idiopathic lunate avascular necrosis represents a particular manifestation of an avascular necrosis. A single trauma causing an abrupt disruption of the vascular supply is rare and can be

Tabelle 5.**1**   MRI stages of avascular necrosis of the lunate. In stage I and II, configuration and architecture of the lunate are preserved. In stage III, the lunate is fragmented. Stage IV is characterized be secondary degenerative changes, in particular at the styloid process of the radius. Aside from the usual criteria, these changes are recognized by synovial proliferations and vascularized granulation tissue that shows marked enhancement.

MRI Stage	T_1	MR Morphology	Enhancement	T_2	Radiology
Ia	↓	homogeneous, diffuse signal change	yes	↑	unremarkable
Ib	↓	homogeneous, diffuse signal change	yes	↑	sclerosis
II	↓	heterogeneous, geographic signal change	focally no	↓	sclerosis, possible cysts
III	↓	loss of height, fragmentation	no	↓	cysts, loss of height, fragmentation
IV	↓	secondary degenerative arthritis	in lunate: no, synovial proliferationen: yes	↓	as stage III and degenerative changes

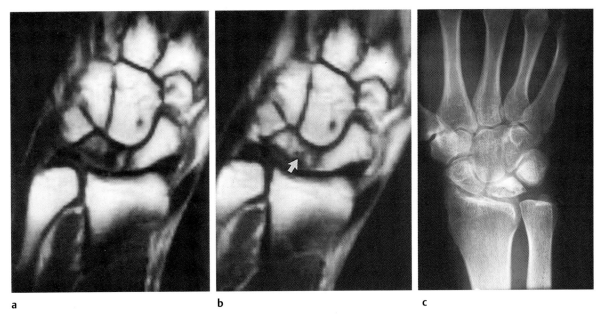

a   b   c

Fig. 5.**19a–c**   Avascular necrosis of the lunate, stage II. **a** T$_1$-weighted SE sequence before IV administration of Gd-DTPA. **b** T$_1$-weighted SE sequence after IV administration of Gd-DTPA. Decreased signal intensity in the lunate with preserved contour. A band-like zone near the radius remains a signal void even after administration of contrast medium (arrow), while portions near the midcarpal articulation enhance. **c** Radiographic view of another patient with avascular necrosis of the lunate. A heterogeneous increase in density with geographic and linear radiolucencies and with preserved size and shape of the lunate. Mild plus variant of the ulna.

found with complete separation of the lunate from its nourishing capsule and ligaments, as occurs with perilunate injuries and palmar displacement of the lunate. Even multiple traumas might not disrupt the blood supply.

The early stage probably does not represent an avascular necrosis in the majority of cases, but a bone marrow edema as stress reaction to a permanently increased pressure on the lunate. This is induced by the exposed anatomic position of the lunate and the unfavorable load transmission from the capitate through the lunate to the radius, and can be accentuated by a coexisting ulnar minus variant. Over months and years, the chronic bone marrow edema causes the marrow to become fibrotic and sclerotic. During this period, the vascular flow to the lunate is augmented, accounting for the increased uptake seen on the bone scan. Only the progression of the sclerosis and fibrosis in the bone marrow impairs the blood supply. If areas of increased pressure cause microfractures, particularly on the radial side of the subchondral trabecular bone, localized avascular necroses can develop on the basis of mechanical bone destruction. It is conceivable that the decreased elasticity of the sclerotic lunate predisposes to subchondral trabecular infractions. Only then can osteonecroses be detected histopathologically. These are only depicted as localized findings in the fractured regions of the lunate, while the remaining regions of the bone marrow are vital despite a decreased signal intensity on T$_1$-weighted images.

■ Spontaneous Avascular Necrosis of the Scaphoid (Preiser disease, Köhler-Mochet disease)

In 1910, Preiser described a disease of the scaphoid that causes spontaneous osseous collapse similar to that found in the lunate. This condition affects adults and leads to progressive painful carpal weakness and point tenderness of the anatomical snuff-box. The dominant hand is more often affected. Like Kienböck disease, its etiology is not known definitively. It could represent a type of stress reaction of bone associated with ischemia. Many patients recall an acute or remote trauma. Discrete sclerotic and cystic changes are observed radiographically early in the disease. With progression, the scaphoid undergoes deformation and loss of height, eventually leading to its complete fragmentation. MRI initially shows a predominately local decrease in signal intensity on the T$_1$-weighted image, later extending to the entire bone. Late in the disease, fragmentations become apparent interrupted osseous lines.

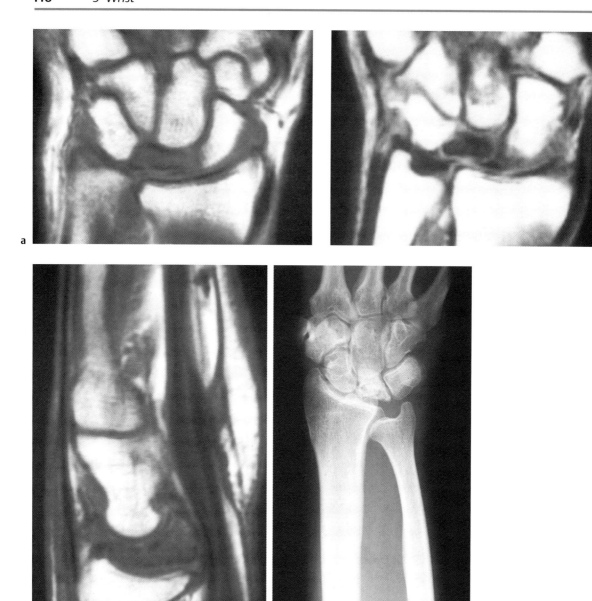

Fig. 5.**20a–d** Avascular necrosis of the lunate, MRI stage III. **a** The coronal T_1-weighted SE sequence shows a heterogeneous decrease in signal intensity as well as a loss of height of the lunate. **b** On the coronal contrast-enhanced image of another patient, the lunate mostly lacks any enhancement. **c** On the sagittal T_1-weighted SE image, the lunate shows a heterogeneous decrease in signal intensity and fragmentation, with carpal collapse and proximal dislocation of the capitate beginning. **d** The radiograph of another patient with an avascular necrosis of the lunate at the same stage. The lunate is fragmented and a ulnar minus variant is apparent.

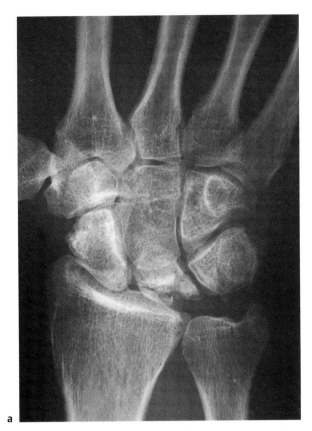

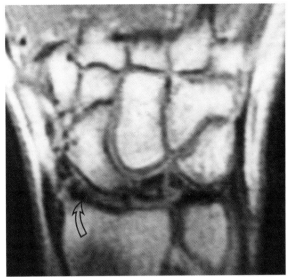

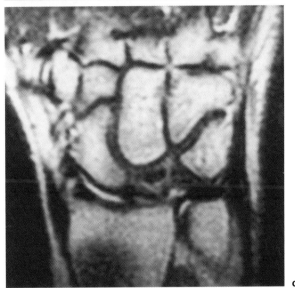

Figs. 5.**21 a–c**   Avascular necrosis of the lunate, stage IV. **a** Radiograph with fragmented, collapsed lunate, with sclerosis of the fragments. **b** T$_1$-weighted SE image with a lunate showing a decreased signal intensity and loss of height. Secondary osteoarthritis of the radiocarpal articulation with subchondral sclerosis of the radial styloid process and osteophytes (arrow) are almost better appreciated than on the conventional radiograph. **c** T$_2$-weighted SE image with effusion at the radial styloid process and increased signal intensity between the fragments of the lunate, properly corresponding to reparative fibrovascular granulation tissue.

Ulnar Compression Syndrome of the Lunate

After non-reduced compression fractures of the distal radial metaphysis or with congenital ulnar variance with relative shortening of the radius (Hultén's ulnar plus variant), the articulating surface of the radiocarpal articulation has a step deformity. The resultant unfavorable load distribution on the joint can damage the cartilage, lunate, ulnar disk and ulna. MRI can reveal the asymmetric osseous changes of the lunate or ulna manifested as cyst formation, sclerosis and edema.

Traumatic Lesions of the Carpal Bone

■ Contusion, Occult Fractures

MRI generally is not indicated for detecting or excluding wrist fractures. Conventional radiography and CT are the primary imaging methods.

Bone bruises. MRI can detect these reliably, even in the wrist, because of its high sensitivity for post-traumatic diffuse bone marrow edema.

Occult fractures. This term describes fractures seen by MRI but not detected by radiography. In the pre-MRI era, such fractures could be established by serial radiographic examinations since resorption processes widen the fracture line within 2 to 5 days and render it radio-

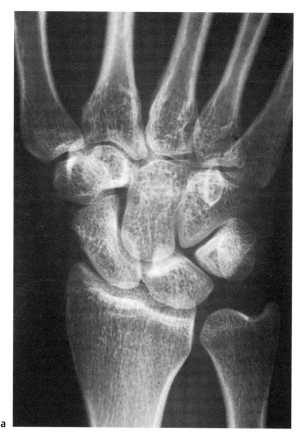

a

graphically visible. An alternative approach to detecting an occult fracture is the follow-up by bone scintigraphy, which also becomes positive after trauma with some temporal delay. MRI allows the diagnosis of radiographically occult fractures immediate after the trauma (2 a). The characteristic signs are the same as found with radiographically visible fractures, such as linear bone marrow edema (with decreased signal intensity on T_1-weighted and increased signal intensity on T_2-weighted images) as well as a central zone of decreased to absent activity (Fig. 5.**22**).

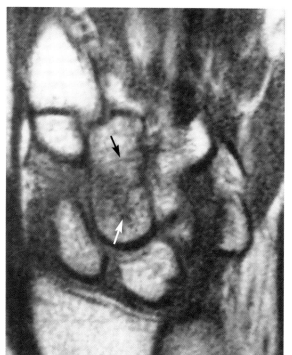

b

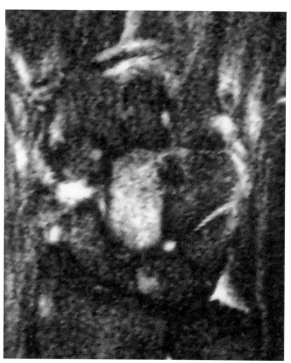

c

Figs. 5.**22a–c**   Occult fracture of the capitate. **a** Unremarkable radiograph. **b** Coronal T_1-weighted SE image with decreased signal intensity of the capitate, especially in the central region (arrows). **c** The STIR image displays the high signal intensity of the bone marrow edema.

■ Traumatic Lesions and Postsurgical Findings of the Scaphoid

Because of its high incidence and the possible clinically relevant complications, such as pseudarthrosis and necrotic fragmentation, the post-traumatic and post-surgical changes are presented separately.

Scaphoid Fractures

About 70–80% of the fractures involve the waist of the scaphoid. Less frequently involved are the tubercle (5–10%), the distal pole (5–10%) and the proximal pole (15–20%). In most cases, conventional radiographic examinations, including special views and conventional tomography, are adequate for fracture detection. The MRI findings are bone marrow edema and decreased to absent signal along the fracture line as well as edema of the surrounding soft tissues with edematous infiltration of the fat around the scaphoid (Fig. 5.**23**).

Pseudarthrosis, Fibrous and Partial Osseous Union

Pseudarthrosis. Non-union of a fracture three months after the trauma is referred to as delayed osseous healing and persistent non-union for more than six months as pseudarthrosis. The more proximal a fracture is located, the more likely is delayed healing. Other factors favoring a pseudarthrosis are initially overlooked and inadequately immobilized scaphoid fractures. The incidence of pseudarthrosis is stated to be 5–10%.

Radiographically, the pseudarthrosis is seen as persistent fracture line and increased density as well as cystic changes in the adjacent osseous fragments. Based on the radiographic findings, three stages with different therapeutic implications can be distinguished:

- Stage I: Resorption with widening of the fracture line (immobilization)
- Stage II: Cyst formation (surgery)
- Stage III: Sclerosis of the fragments (surgery)

On MRI, the pseudarthrosis appears heterogeneous. The pseudoarthrotic separation is typically seen as increased signal intensity on T_2-weighted images. The bone marrow edema in the adjacent fragments is shown as decreased signal intensity, of variable extent, on T_1 weighting and increased signal intensity on T_2 and STIR images. The evolving cysts exhibit a round signal with low intensity on T_1-weighted images and high intensity on T_2-weighted images. The sclerotic transformation gradually reduces the signal intensity in all sequences. IV contrast medium can disclose useful information as to the viability of the osseous fragments.

Fibrous Union. The pseudarthrosis must be distinguished from fibrous union of the fracture, constituting the restoration of load bearing through union and stabilization of the fracture by means of non-ossified fibrous tissue. This fibrous callus is not reliably detected radiographically. At the most, it represents tissue of slightly increased density relative to the surrounding soft tissues. Remaining instability observed on fluoroscopically guided stress views speaks for a pseudarthrosis.

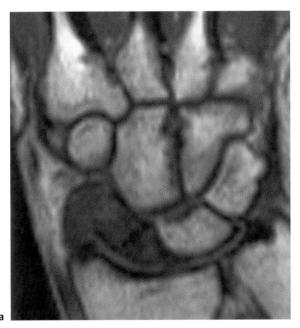
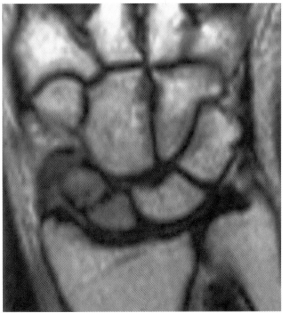

a   b

Figs. 5.23 a, b Old fracture through the waste of the scaphoid. **a** Coronal T_1-weighted SE image. **b** T_2-weighted image. Fracture line with decreased to no signal intensity, step deformity and extensive bone marrow edema in both fragments. Surrounding soft tissue edema, especially also in the periscaphoid fat.

MRI makes the documentation of a pseudarthrosis easier. The intervening fibrous tissue shows a low signal intensity and the adjacent bone fragments fatty bone marrow without evidence of edema.

Partial osseous union. Since the scaphoid fracture also can be bridged by partial ossification, a pseudarthrosis should diagnosed only if the fracture line remains visible across the entire width of the affected bone.

Post-traumatic Avascular Necrosis

The nutrient vessels of the scaphoid enter the bone through the waist primarily in the region of the lateral tubercle. The proximal scaphoid pole, which is essentially covered completely by hyaline cartilage, predominantly receives its supply from the distal pole. Fractures through the middle third of the scaphoid and, particularly, fractures through the junction of the middle and proximal thirds sever the blood supply to the proximal fragment of the scaphoid, frequently leading to a necrosis of the proximal fragment. Depending on the type of trauma, a necrosis of the distal fragment can occur but is uncommon. Necroses can occur late, especially in conjunction with delayed healing and pseudarthrosis. On conventional radiographs, the post-traumatic avascular necrosis is seen as relative increase in density since the absent or impaired perfusion results in no or delayed demineralization relative to the surrounding osseous structures during the course of post-traumatic immobilization. Later, the trabecular space shows an increased sclerosis.

MRI reveals various findings. The signal intensity of a necrotic fragment is low on the T_1-weighted image and initially high on the T_2-weighted image, and cannot reliably differentiated from an edema secondary to fracture or pseudarthrosis. Persistence of these signal changes in one of the fragments for more than six weeks after the trauma with normalization of the signal in the other fragment strongly suggests an avascular necrosis or impaired viability (Fig. 5.**24**). Another relatively reliable finding indicative of a necrosis is the lack of contrast enhancement in the presence of enhancement in the other fragment, as well as unchanged evidence of edema in both fragments (Fig. 5.**25**).

Determining the viability of the fragments of a scaphoid fracture has prognostic and therapeutic relevance. Impaired viability increases the probability for the development of a pseudarthrosis and decreases the success of conservative therapy.

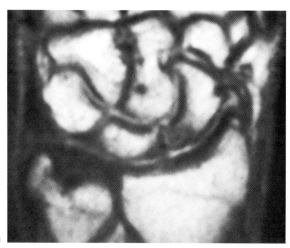
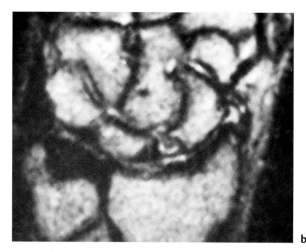

a   b

Figs. 5.**24a, b** Post-traumatic avascular necrosis of the proximal scaphoid fragment. Persistent edema-equivalent signal changes in the proximal fragment of a three-month-old fracture, with return to a normal signal in the distal fragment. **a** Coronal T_1-weighted SE image. **b** T_2-weighted image. Both sequences show low-signal bone islands in the capitate.

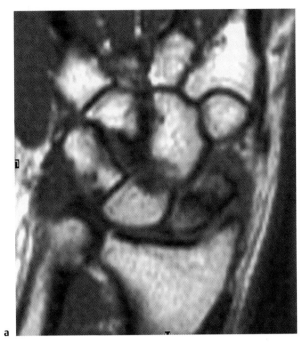

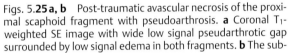

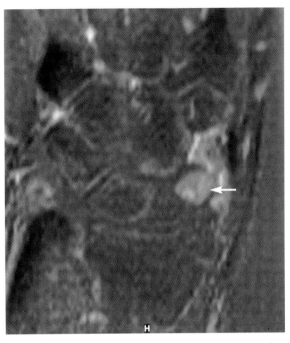

a   b

Figs. 5.25 a, b   Post-traumatic avascular necrosis of the proximal scaphoid fragment with pseudoarthrosis. **a** Coronal T_1-weighted SE image with wide low signal pseudarthrotic gap surrounded by low signal edema in both fragments. **b** The sub-traction image after IV administration of contrast medium fails to show enhancement in the proximal fragment in the presence of definite edema-induced enhancement in the distal fragment.

Postsurgical Findings of the Scaphoid

When interpreting MRI examinations performed after surgical repair of a pseudarthrosis, it should be kept in mind that the bone marrow edema can persist for several months to up to one year after the surgery, in particular on STIR images. Moreover, the type of surgery must be known when evaluating the osseous or fibrous union (Fig. 5.26). The success rate of the Matti-Russe graft is 87 – 95%. Modern materials for internal fixation (e.g., Herbert screw made of titanium) cause less interfering susceptibility artifacts and permit a limited evaluation of the viability of the proximal fragment and of the former pseudarthrotic gap (Fig. 5.27) (34 a).

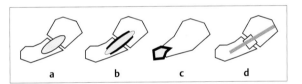

a   b   c   d

Fig. 5.**26 a–d**   Schematic drawing of the surgical treatment for scaphoid pseudarthrosis. **a** Inlay cancellous bone graft (Russe). **b** Inlay cancellous bone graft with added cortical chips (Matti-Russe). **c** For a small proximal fragment: replacement of the proximal fragment by a corticocancellous graft (Russe II), with sacrifice of the attached intercarpal ligaments. **d** Internal fixation with Ender plate or Herbert screw combined with cancellous bone graft.

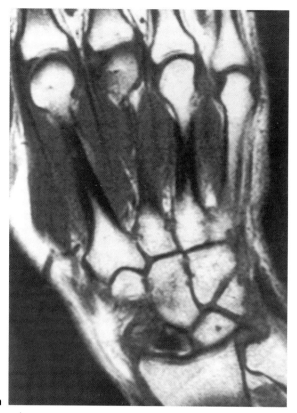
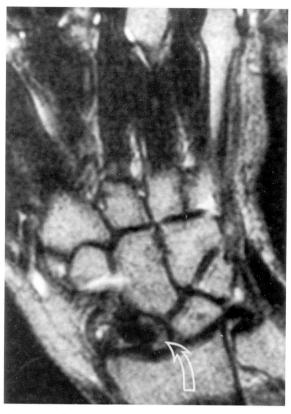

a   b

Figs. 5.**27 a, b**   Surgical repair of a pseudoarthrosis of the scaphoid by means of a Herbert screw. **a** Coronal T₁-weighted SE image. **b** Coronal T₂-weighted image. Being made of titanium, the screw only induces minor artifacts and the proximal fragment can still be evaluated. As seen, the proximal fragment shows a normal signal intensity.

Diseases of the Interosseous (Intrinsic) Ligaments

Three-compartment arthrography with the mediocarpal articulation injected first is the gold standard for the detection of a rupture of the ligament between the scaphoid and lunate (scapholunate or SL ligament) and of the ligament between lunate and triquetrum (lunotriquetral or LT ligament). The visualization of the ligaments by MRI is between 70% and 90% and is rather variable. Consequently, the diagnostic accuracy of MRI is low for these ligaments and is about 70% for the SL ligament and 50% for the LT ligament. The *direct signs* of a rupture comprise a break in continuity and an increased signal intensity. The *indirect signs* include local fluid accumulation and an increased distance between the affected carpals at rest or with the joint in a particular position, possibly with subluxation (Fig. 5.**28**).

In a complete or partial tear of an interosseous ligament, vascularized granulation fibrous tissue is formed and extends into the residual ligamentous structures. IV administration of Gd-DTPA shows enhancement (Fig. 5.**29**). Even this technique, however, fails to allow a complete tear, a partial tear or a severe degenerative process to be distinguished definitively.

Diseases of the Capsular Ligaments (Extrinsic Ligaments)

Multiple ligamentous structures are incorporated as reinforcement into the palmar and posterior joint capsule of the wrist. Even on the anatomic specimen, these ligamentous structures are difficult to visualize as separate ligaments. With MRI, the delineation of these ligamentous structures as separate entities is only successful in about 50–70% of cases. The likelihood of a reliable diagnostic statement is even lower and it can be concluded that non-enhanced MRI is not suitable for a diagnostic visualization of the extrinsic ligaments.

Laxity and rupture of the capsular ligaments can lead to instability, which usually is well visualized on conventional radiographs, but is also recognizable on MRI. The zigzag deformities with dorsal rotation of the lunate and dorsal displacement of the axis of the capitate, referred to as dorsal intercalated segment instability (DISI), and the variation with palmar rotation of the lunate and palmar displacement of the capitate, referred to as palmar intercalated segment instability (PISI), are easily recognized on sagittal MR images.

Table 5.**2** summarizes the malpositions found after ligamentous injuries.

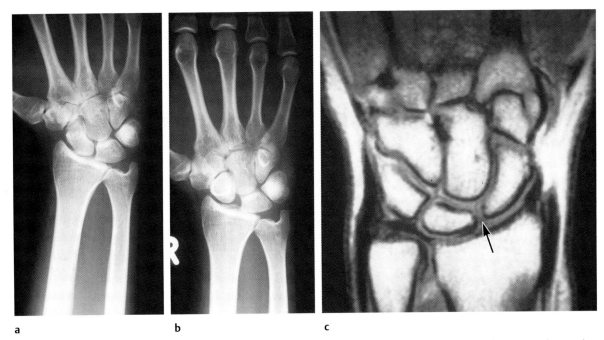

a   b   c

Fig. 5.**28 a–c** Scapholunate diastasis (rotatory subluxation of the scaphoid) owing to rupture of the scapholunate ligament. **a** The conventional radiograph is unremarkable. **b** The radiograph obtained with ulnar stress applied and after a 'click' was felt shows the distance between scaphoid and lunate to be increased to more than 2 mm (Terry-Thomas sign) as well as a ring-like structure in the distal scaphoid corresponding to the waist projected over the tilted and foreshortened scaphoid ('signet ring'). **c** The coronal T_1-weighted SE image of another patient shows an increased distance between scaphoid and lunate as well as an increased signal intensity and a questionable break in the scapholunate ligament (lunate).

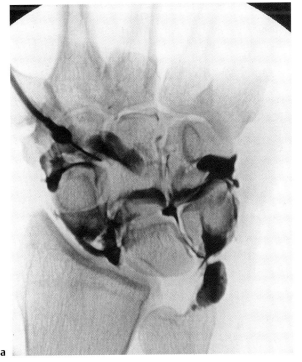

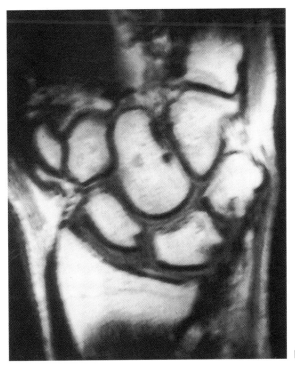

a   b

Fig. 5.**29 a–c** Lesion of the scapholunate ligament. **a** Arthrography following mediocarpal injection of contrast medium shows extension of the contrast medium into the radiocarpal joint through the interosseous scapholunate and lunotriquetral ligaments. **b** The unenhanced T_1-weighted image shows slight widening of the scapholunate joint space.

Fig. 5.**29 c** ▶

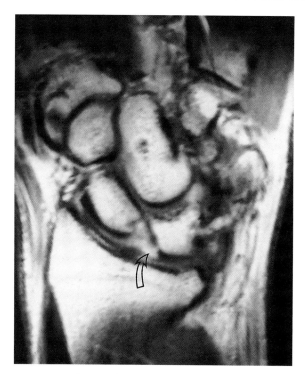

Fig. 5.**29c**   After IV administration of Gd-based contrast medium, marked enhancement of the scapholunate ligament. Furthermore, the lunotriquetral ligament shows contrast enhancement.

Ulnar Fibrocartilage Complex

Pain in the ulnar aspect of the proximal wrist can be caused by pathologic changes of the triangular disk and the surrounding capsulofibrous structures. Based on the clinical complaint, the differential diagnosis of a disk rupture includes lesions of the lunotriquetral ligament, extensor carpi ulnaris tendon, pisotriquetral joint and distal radioulnar joint. The triangular disk can be completely ruptured, creating a communication between radiocarpal joint and distal radioulnar joint. Furthermore, incomplete tears can occur distally (radiocarpal), but also proximally (undersurface of the disc). Chronic irritation and rupture are associated with vascularized granulation tissue as manifestation of an attempted repair. Moreover, synovial irritation with synovial proliferation can induce secondary vascularization of the fibrocartilage complex.

Negative ulnar variance is rarely associated with tears of the TFCC. However positive ulnar variance predisposes to tears of the developmentally thin TFCC. In this situation, an ulna impingement syndrome affecting the lunate can arise with increasing age due to a relative extension of the lunar length.

Arthrography used to be the only method for detecting pathologic changes and ruptures of the triangular disc. Following injection into the radiocarpal joint,

contrast medium extends into the distal radioulnar joint if the disk is ruptured. In some disk ruptures, contrast medium only extends in one direction. Consequently, following a negative finding after radiocarpal injection, an additional injection into the distal radioulnar joint is indicated to exclude a ruptured disk with certainty.

MRI shows the triangular disk as low signal intensity structure in all sequences. Toward the ulnar side with its transition to the adjacent fibrous complex, the signal increases in intensity. The ruptured disk causes localized areas with increased signal intensity on the T_2-weighted or STIR images. The distal radioulnar articulation usually contains a small effusion, which has a high positive correlation with the presence of a ruptured disc. Secondary vascularization manifested as synovial pannus or vascularized granulation tissue due to stress-induced damage or a chronic degenerative processes in the triangular fibrocartilage complex can be sensitively detected on T_1-weighted images after IV administration of Gd-DTPA. Imaging with frequency-selected fat suppression is useful in this situation. Coronal unenhanced T_2-weighted GRE sequences have also proved helpful in detecting disk ruptures.

Most disks rupture on the basis of degenerative changes. A defect or rupture of the triangular disk is already found in 8% of patients aged between 30 and 40 years and in 50% of patients older than 60 years. Since ruptures of the triangular disk increase with advancing age and most ruptured disks are clinically asymptomatic, corresponding MRI findings must be assessed cautiously and only in close correlation with the clinical complaints. Most degenerative ruptures affect the central region of the disk and usually exhibit a round configuration (Fig. 5.**30**). The extent of the secondary vascularization found with chronic degenerative changes

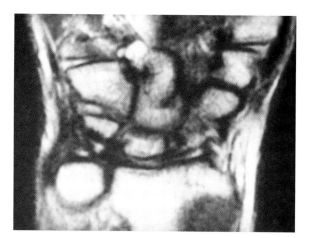

Fig. 5.**30**   Degenerative tear of the ulnar disk. Coronal T_2-weighted SE image. Essentially spherical foci of contrast enhancement are seen in the center of the disk (IIc after Palmer). Only a small amount of fluid is noted in the radiocarpal articulation and no fluid in the distal radioulnar articulation. Symptoms were present for many years without any known trauma.

Table 5.**2**   Relatively frequent dislocations and instabilities of the wrist. Dislocations can be associated with fractures, resulting in numerous combinations. A fracture together with a dislocation is given a term with the prefix ›trans,‹ followed by the name of the fractured bone and then followed by the type of dislocation: e.g., transscaphoid-perilunar dislocation. In addition, there are rare types of dislocation related to the mechanism of trauma. These findings are based on the radiographic findings, but can be applied to the corresponding MRI plane. On the lateral view, the lunate is normally angled 0 – 30 degrees relative to the longitudinal axis (radius-lunate-capitate-metacarpals). The normal angulation of the scaphoid relative to the longitudinal axis is 30 – 60 degrees (Fig. 5.**11**).

It can generally be assumed that palmar or posterior perilunar dislocations, palmar or posterior midcarpal dislocations, and palmar and posterior dislocations of the lunate represent perilunar injuries. To determine the malposition of the ulna using known CT criteria, the axial section with the apparently smallest radioulnar articulation is selected. The measuring lines are the lines between the palmar corner of the radial articulating surface and the outer corner of the radius as well as the lines between the posterior and corners of the radial articulating surface. The ulna normally should not project beyond these lines by more than half a shaft width (Fig. 5.**16**). Other measuring methods have been described by Wechsler and co-workers (36).

	Injury	Findings
Dislocationen:		
• I scapholunate dissociation or posterior rotatory subluxation of the scaphoid	Scapholunate ligament, radioscaphoid ligament, palmar radiocapitate ligament	Scapholunate distance > 2 mm, provoked by ulnar deviation (Terry Thomas sign), ring structure in the scaphoid (signal ring sign), palmar tilting of the scaphoid
• II perilunate dislocation	Radiocapitate ligament	Posterior and proximal displacement of the capitate relative to the lunate
• III midcarpal dislocation	Lunotriquetral ligament, radiotriquetral ligament, ulnotriquetral ligament	As in II and subluxation of the lunate with slight palmar tilting of the lunate axis
• IV lunate dislocation (lunatotriquetral dissociation)	All lunate ligaments	Palmar tilting of the lunate, triangular appearance of the lunate and interrupted lunatotriquetral (second carpal) arc Deviation from the radioulnar tangent by half a shaft width (subluxation) and one shaft width (dislocation) (Fig. 5.10)
ulnar subluxation and dislocation	TFCC (triangular fibrocartilaginous complex radioulnar ligaments	
Instabilities:		
• Dorsal intercalated segmental instability (DISI)	Scapholunate ligament, volar radiocarpal ligament, scaphoid pseudoarthrosis	Posterior tilting of the lunate by more than 30 degrees and palmar tilting of the scaphoid by more than 60 degrees
• Palmar intercalated segmental instability (PISI)	Triquetrohamate ligament	Palmar tilting of the lunate by more than 30 degrees, often also posterior tilting of the capitate by more than 30 degrees

seems to correlate with the clinical complaints (Fig. 5.**31**).

Acute traumatic ruptures of the disk usually are on the radial side where the disk is thin and close to where hyaline articular cartilage extends from the distal radius (Fig. 5.**32**). Typically, they extend vertically from surface to surface. Traumatic lesions also occur in the region of the ulnar attachment. Aside from an increased signal intensity on the T_1-weighted and T_2-weighted images, particularly on the fat suppression images, a lesion is suggested by localized fluid accumulation, especially if found in the distal radioulnar articulation, caused by a communication between the radiocarpal recess and the distal radioulnar compartment.

A classification of triangular fibrocartilage complex lesions suggested by Palmer is increasingly gaining acceptance. It is based on differentiating between degenerative and traumatic changes as well as on considering associated and evolving findings, and distinguishes nine types, in part with therapeutic implications (Tab. 5.**3**) (23, 24).

Incorporating all diagnostic criteria, MRI should be effective in evaluating triangular fibrocartilage tears with a sensitivity of more than 90% (45). These good results, however, have not been achieved by other authors and are influenced by the choice of sequences and hardware, especially adequate magnet homogeneity.

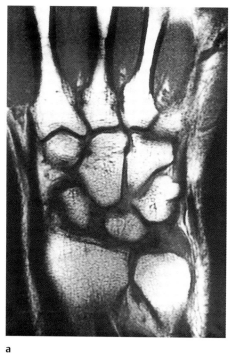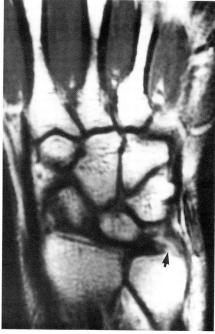

a   b

Figs. 5.**31 a, b**   Lesion of the ulnar triangular disk. Chronic pain on the ulnar side after a twisting injury. **a** T_1-weighted unenhanced SE image showing a normal bone marrow signal without convincing pathologic finding. **b** After IV administration of Gd-based contrast medium, definite enhancement of the fibrovascular tissue in the region of the TFCC (arrow).

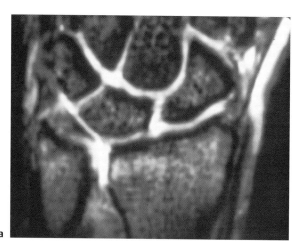
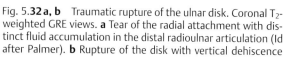

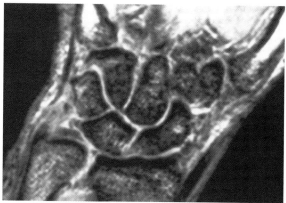

a   b

Fig. 5.**32 a, b**   Traumatic rupture of the ulnar disk. Coronal T_2-weighted GRE views. **a** Tear of the radial attachment with distinct fluid accumulation in the distal radioulnar articulation (Id after Palmer). **b** Rupture of the disk with vertical dehiscence and some fluid in the distal radioulnar articulation (Ia after Palmer). Both patients had persistent complaints after an adequate trauma.

Nerve Compression Syndromes

■ Carpal Tunnel

Median nerve and the flexor tendons (flexor digitorum profundus, flexor digitorum superficialis, flexor pollicis longus) pass from the distal forearm to the palm of the hand through an anatomical tunnel, which is bordered dorsally by the carpal bones and palmarly by the flexor retinaculum, a fibrous band. The median nerve normally is palmar to the flexor tendons. As a developmental variant, however, the nerve can be in the dorsal aspect of the tunnel. With flexion of the wrist, slight displacements and deformities of the median nerve occur, in particular, flattening of its diameter. Compression of the median nerve in the carpal tunnel produces the carpal tunnel syndrome, constituting a neuropathy with pain, paresthesias of the radial $2^1/_2$ fingers and weakness or atrophy of the thenar muscles, usually with nocturnal worsening. This condition characteristically effects patients between the age of 30 and 60 years and is bilateral in up to 50% of the cases.

Table 5.**3**   Classification of the injuries of the triangular fibrocartilage complex lesions according to Palmar

Stage	Lesion	Therapy
I Traumatic:		
• Ia	Vertical tear on radial side	Poor spontaneous healing; debridement
• Ib	Tear on the ulnar side, often with avulsion of the ulnar styloid process and radioulnar stability because of torn radioulnar ligaments	Spontaneous healing, immobilization
• Ic	Torn ulnocarpal ligaments with ulnocarpal instability	Ligamentous repair
• Id	Avulsion of the disk from the radius, possibly with osseous avulsion	Debridement
II Degenerative:		
• IIa	Thin disk without tear	Possible shortening of the ulna, debridement
• IIb	IIa plus chondromalacia	As in IIa
• IIc	Central, usually oval tear	As in IIa
• IId	IIc and torn LT ligament with resultant instability	Debridement, lunatotriquetral fusion
• IIe	Large central tears (often completely absent visualization of the disk), osteoarthritis, synovitis, torn LT ligament	As in IId

Space-occupying lesions within the carpal tunnel can cause the carpal tunnel syndrome. Recognized specific lesions include tumors, ganglion cysts, muscular hypertrophy, rheumatoid arthritis, excessive fat deposits, tendonitis, tendosynovitis, amyloid deposits, and edema (pregnancy), in addition to extrinsic processes that narrow the carpal tunnel, such as fractures with exuberant callus formation. Furthermore, congenital anomalies such as a persistent medial artery or dystrophic lumbrical muscles can produce a carpal tunnel syndrome.

The diagnosis of carpal tunnel syndrome is normally based on clinical findings, supported by nerve conduction studies and electromyography. Conventional radiographs and CT might detect osseous causes.

MRI can clearly delineate numerous causative soft tissue and osseous lesions. An increased volume of the carpal tunnel, for instance, bulges the flexor retinaculum. This can be quantified by measuring the distance between the flexor retinaculum and an imaginary line between the hamate of the hamulus and trapezium. Furthermore, the nerve itself can become altered, revealed as increased signal intensity on the T_2-weighted images (Fig. 5.**33**) and thickening. The increased signal intensity probably reflects an edema. The neural swelling is usually most pronounced at the level of the pisiform. Occasionally, a flattening of the nerve is observed, particularly at the level of the hamate of the hamulus. In late stages of a chronic course, atrophy of the thenar muscles becomes apparent, manifested as increased signal intensity on T_1-weighted and T_2-weighted sequences and occasionally as decreased signal intensity on T_1-weighted and T_2-weighted images, probably caused by fibrosis.

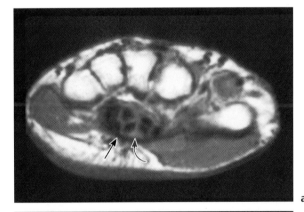

a

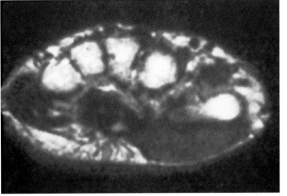

b

Fig. 5.**33 a, b**   Carpal tunnel compression syndrome. **a** Axial proton density SE image. **b** T_2-weighted SE image. The images show the bulging flexor retinaculum (arrow) as well as the increased signal intensity of the median nerve in both sequences.

In persistent or recurrent complaints of carpal tunnel syndrome after surgical therapy, MRI can directly detect possible causes, such as inadequate surgical division of the flexor retinaculum and scar tissue or neurinomas.

■ Guyon Canal

Together with the ulnar artery, the ulnar nerve passes through a physiologic narrowing, the Guyon canal, from the distal forearm to the palm of the hand. This canal extends from the pisiform to the hamate of the hamulus and is bordered by the flexor retinaculum, abductor digiti minimi (hypothenar), pisiform and hamate of the hamulus. The palmar border is the palmar aponeurosis strengthened proximally by the palmar carpal ligament (proximal hiatus) and distally by the palmar brevis tendon as well as by the fibrous attachment of the flexor digiti minimi brevis (distal hiatus) (Fig. 5.**34**).

Narrowing of this canal can cause neuropathy of the ulnar nerve, analogous to the carpal tunnel syndrome of the median nerve. Numerous conditions can narrow the canal and often are detected by MRI. These conditions include:

- Ganglion cysts (Fig. 5.**35**)
- Tumors
- Extrinsic pressure, e.g., bicycle riding
- Aneurysm of the ulnar artery
- Muscular anomalies
- Thickening of the flexor carpi ulnaris tendon
- Dupuytren disease
- Osteoarthritis of the pisotriquetral joint

- Fractures of the hamate of the hamulus or pisiform
- Fractures of the metacarpal bases.

Tumors

Tumors of the osseous structures and soft tissues are discussed in a separate chapter (Chapter 12: Bone and Soft Tissue Tumors). Only the spectrum of tumor types that can be encountered in the wrist and hand is listed here (Tab. 5.**4** and 5.**5**). Tumors of the hand are rare.

Ganglion Cysts, Other Cysts

Ganglion cysts. These are periarticular gelatinous space-occupying lesions that arise from ligamentous, osseous, or tendinous structures. They can be intraosseous (Fig. 5.**36**). The most frequent intraosseous location of a ganglion is in the lunate near the scapholunate joint space, with the scapholunate ligament or radioscapholunate ligament the most frequent site of origin. Ganglion cysts are a common disorder of the wrist and often become symptomatic by their mass effect.

Ganglions have a typical signal intensity on MRI. They have of low signal intensity on T_1-weighted images and an extremely high signal intensity on T_2-weighted images. Septations seen as linear signal voids often appear within the ganglion (Fig. 5.**37**). In addition, funnel-shaped tapering of the lesion is often identified, probably representing the neck of the site of origin (Fig. 5.**38**).

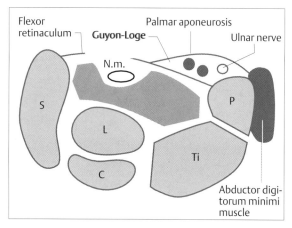

Fig. 5.**34** Schematic drawing of an axial section of the hand at the level of the pisotriquetral articulation to illustrate the location of the Guyon canal.
N. m. = Median nerve in the carpal tunnel
S   = Scaphoid
L   = Lunate
C   = Capitate
Ti   = Triquetrum
P   = Pisiform

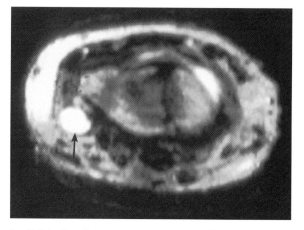

Fig. 5.**35** Ganglion cyst in Guyon canal. Transverse T_2-weighted TSE image at the level of the lunate. Partially transected scaphoid and triquetrum (palmar = inferior). On the left (ulnar) side, a very high-signal space-occupying lesion with displacement of the ulnar neurovascular bundle (arrow) is visualized.

Table 5.**4**   Bone tumors of the hand and wrist, listed in order of dignity and incidence (for instance, 37% of all observed enchondromas [90 of 245] are in the hand and wrist). The total group comprised more than 8000 tumors (1 a)

Dignity	Entity	Totel number	Number and percentage in the hand and wrist
Benign	Enchondroma	245	90 (37%)
	Giant cell tumor	425	63 (15%)
	Osteoid osteoma	245	18 (7%)
	Osteochondroma	727	28 (4%)
	Aneurysmal bone cysts	134	6 (4%)
	Osteoblastoma	63	2 (3%)
	Chondromyxoid fibroma	39	1 (2,6%)
	Hemangioma/lymphangioma	80	0
	Chondroblastoma	79	0
Malignant	Hemangioendothelioma	60	6 (10%)
	Chondrosarcoma	634	14 (2,2%)
	Parosteal osteosarcoma	56	1 (2%)
	Osteosarcoma	1274	13 (1%)
	Ewing sarcoma	402	5 (1%)
	Lymphoma	469	4 (0,9%)
	Fibrosarcoma	207	1 (0,5%)
	Metastases	3000	2 (0,1%)
	Myeloma	556	0

Cysts. Pure cysts that contain serous fluid can be distinguished from ganglion cysts. They also can be intraosseous or extraosseous. They probably differ pathogenetically from ganglion cysts and most likely represent synovial inclusions or proliferations.

Clinically, their differentiation from ganglion cysts is usually not possible. Even differentiation by MRI is problematic since the signal intensities of both entities are identical. Septations and a visualized neck speak against pure cysts. On magnetization transfer contrast images, ganglions show a distinctly lower signal intensity than pure cysts. In general, a differentiation between ganglions and pure cysts is clinically irrelevant since the therapy is the same for symptomatic cases.

Table 5.**5**   Frequent soft tissue tumors of the hand and wrist and their peculiarities

Epidermoids	Often post-traumatic subcutaneous implantation of dermal tissues at the distal phalanx; causes painful swelling
Glomus tumors	Subungual, very painful mass lesion of the neuromyoarterial glomus < 1 cm
Giant cell tumors of the tendons	Relatively frequent; often involving the extensors; owing to hemosiderin deposits, often has low signal intensities on T_1- and T_2-weighted sequences
Lipoma	Often large lobulated mass lesion; usually in the thenar
Hemangioma, lymphangioma	Often diffuse spread; very high signal intensities on T_2-weighted sequences
Ganglion cyst	See Page 130

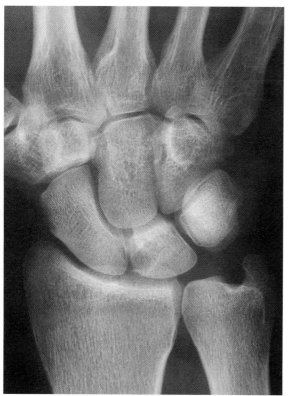

Fig. 5.**36a–d**   Intraosseous ganglion cyst of the lunate. **a** Cystic defect with sclerotic rim in the radial aspect of the lunate. **b** The unenhanced T_1-weighted image shows a low signal defect, which arises from the interosseous scapholunate ligament. **c** Definite enhancement after IV administration of Gd-based contrast medium. **d** The ganglion cysts characteristically show a high signal intensity on the T_2-weighted image.

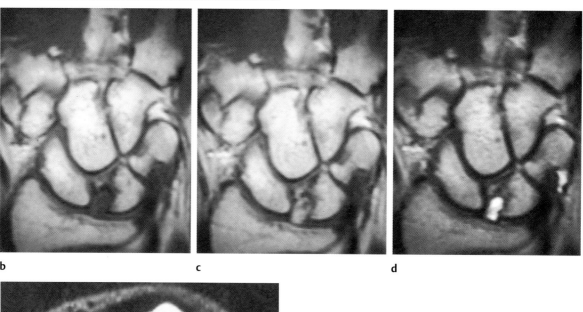

b   c   d

◀ Fig. 5.**37**   Ganglion cyst of the wrist. Transverse T_2-weighted SE image. Good demarcation of the septa as lines of low signal intensity.

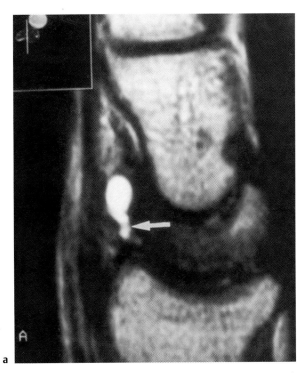
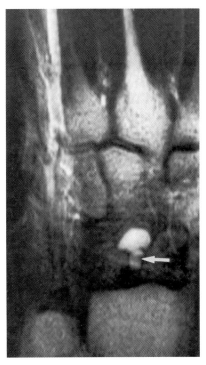

Fig. 5.**38 a, b**   Ganglion cyst of the wrist. T_2-weighted TSE sequences. **a** Sagittal section. **b** Coronal section. Visualization of the neck (arrows).

Disorders of the Synovial Membrane

As with other joints, MRI can delineate a synovial proliferation as synovial thickening, with the thickening showing increased signal intensity on T_2-weighted images and strong enhancement. The unenhanced image often cannot distinguish between an effusion and active pannus, which is easily resolved after IV contrast medium. Chronic pannus with fibrotic changes has slightly decreased signal intensity on T_2-weighted images. Furthermore, early osseous erosions have been detected by MRI (Fig. 5.**39**).

Disorders of the Tendons

Tendinitis causes the tendon to thicken and to become isointense with muscle on T_1-weighted and hyperintense on T_2-weighted images. In addition, fluid can accumulate within the synovial tendon sheath (tenosynovitis), which distends and exhibits a definite increase in signal intensity on the T_2-weighted images.

The most frequent tenosynovitis of the wrists is the inflammation of the tendon sheath of the abductor pollicis longus and extensor pollicis brevis (the so-called first extensor compartment, see page 109) at the level of the radial styloid process (de Quervain's tenosynovitis) (Fig. 5.**40**). Furthermore, inflammations of the tendon of the flexor or extensor carpi ulnaris are common (Fig. 5.**41**).

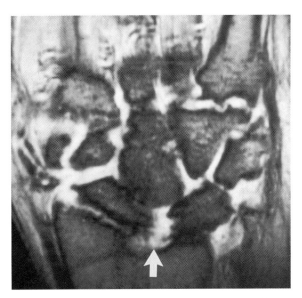

Fig. 5.**39**   Rheumatoid arthritis. Coronal T_2-weighted GRE image. Erosions with bone destruction. Large erosions at the radius (so-called radial crypt) (arrow).

Tendon ruptures cause a visible gap in the continuity as well as increased signal intensity on the T_2-weighted image. Incomplete and chronic ruptures lead to irregular thickening or thinning of the tendon with or without increased signal intensity or contrast enhancement.

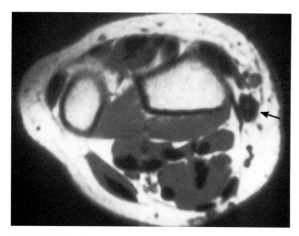

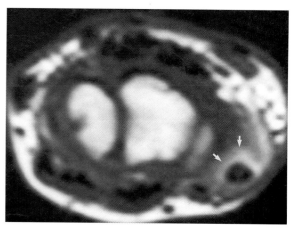

Fig. 5.**40** De Quervain's tenosynovitis pollicis. Axial T_1-weighted SE image. Low-signal expansion of the tendons and their sheaths in the extensor compartment (tendons of the abductor pollicis longus and extensor pollicis brevis) (arrow). The T_2-image (not shown) exhibits a corresponding increase in signal intensity.

Fig. 5.**41** Tenosynovitis. Contrast-enhancement in the thickened tendon sheath of the flexor carpi ulnaris (arrows).

Tendinitis and ruptured tendons frequently accompany chronic polyarthritis, infections and trauma.

Pitfalls in Interpreting the Images

Incorrect positioning of the wrist. This can mimic subluxations or instability. Radial abduction or palmar flexion can mimic a palmar rotation of the scaphoid. With the hands in pronounced flexion, the lumbricals can project over the carpal tunnel and appear as a space-occupying lesion. Ulnar adduction of the wrist causes a dorsal tilt of the lunate axis that should not be mistaken for a dorsal instability. A distinction between instability and malposition should be possible on the basis of the position of the lunate relative to the capitate. Ulnar malposition, but not instability, causes a palmar displacement of the lunate. Pronation causes a slight dorsal displacement of the ulna relative to the radius and supination a slight palmar displacement. These normal positional changes should not be mistaken for an ulnar subluxation.

Variations in the development and insertion of the lumbricals. These variations should not be mistaken for tumors. Vascular variants, such as a persistent median artery, can also cause diagnostic problems.

Chemical shift artifact. This causes a variable visualization of the thickness of the hyaline articular cartilage related to the direction of the frequency encoding. In particular, this affects the interosseous spaces of the scapholunate, lunotriquetral, radiocarpal, and mediocarpal articulations. It might be necessary to change the frequency encoding and to use sequences with broader band widths.

Magnetic angle phenomenon. This refers to the known artificial increase in signal intensity in tendons related to their orientation to the magnetic field, observed with sequences of short echo times (T_1-weighted and proton density-weighted sequences) (see Appendix, page 378).

Osseous variants. Coalitions (frequently lunotriquetral), accessory ossicles, absent or incomplete fusion of the ossification centers (especially scaphoid, capitate and hamate of the hamulus), dysplasias, aplasias, or bone islands (9a) can also cause diagnostic problems with MRI. Absent fusion of ossification centers can be problematic in differentiating from fractures. Generally, fractures can be recognized by associated edema and incomplete fusion by intact cartilage cover or synchondrosis between the ossification centers. Fusions are characterized by a bridge of fat-containing bone marrow.

Openings for nutrient vessels in the carpal bones dorsally and palmarly. They are rather variable and are seen on conventional radiographs as radiolucencies of different sizes and surrounded by sclerosis (9a, 29). They are seen as small foci of a few millimeters in diameter and in variable locations, with low signal intensity on T_1-weighted images and high signal intensity on T_2-weighted images, in particular with GRE sequences and fat suppression (35a). Such nutrient channels should not be mistaken for bone cysts as manifestation of early avascular necrosis of the lunate (Fig. 5.**42**).

Flexor tendon sheaths of the wrist and hand. Their development is rather variable (Fig. 5.**43**). Consequently, in patients with tenosynovitis or peritendinitis, the distribution of the increase in signal intensity on T_2-weighted image has a rather variable interindividual pattern.

Figs. 5.**42a–d** **a** Schematic drawing of the frequent locations of 'cystoid' lesions representing nutrient canals (after Köhler and Zimmer). **b** Coronal T₁-weighted SE image. Several nutrient canals are seen as spots of low signal intensity. **c** They exhibit a high signal intensity on the T₂-weighted image (coronal GRE image). **d** In another patient, the coronal 3D GRE image shows a relatively large area of high signal, compatible with a nutrient canal.

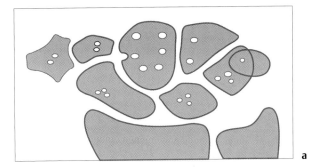

a

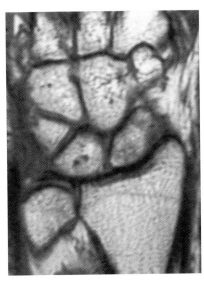

b

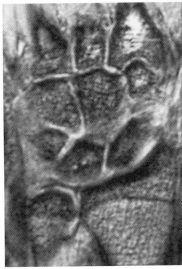

c

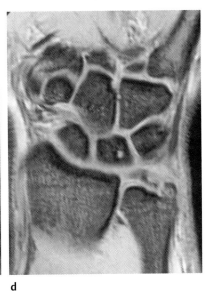

d

Fig. 5.**43a–c** Three examples of the most common manifestations of the extent and communications of the flexor tendons of the hand. Corresponding interindividual variations of fluid accumulations are seen with tenosynovitis on the T₂-weighted MRI image (after Kahle *et al.*).

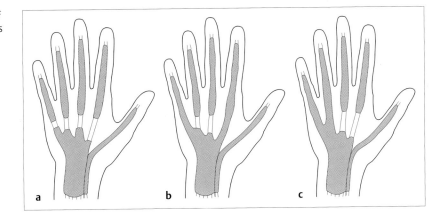

a   b   c

Literatur

1 Berger, R. A., R. L. Linscheid, T. H. Berquist: Magnetic Resonance Imaging of the anterior radiocarpal ligaments. J. Hand Surg. 19 A (1994) 295–303

1a Berquist, T. H.: MRI of the Musculoskeletal System. Raven, Lippincolt, Philadelphia, 1996 (pp. 673–734)

2 Brahme, S. K., D. Resnick: Magnetic Resonance Imaging of the wrist. Rheum. Dis. Clin. Amer. 17 (1991) 721–739

2a Breitenseher, M., V. Metz, L. Guilula, C. Gaebler, C. Kukla, D. Fleischmann, H. Imhof, S. Trattnig: Radiographically occult scaphoid fractures: value of MR imaging in detection. Radiology 203 (1997) 245–250

3 Bruhn, H., M. L. Gyngell, W. Hänicke, K.-D. Merboldt, J. Frahm: High-resolution fast low-angle shot Magnetic Resonance Imaging of the normal hand. Skelet. Radiol. 20 (1991) 259–265

4 Cardinal, E., K. A. Buckwalter, E. M. Braunstein, A. D. Mih: Occult dorsal carpal ganglion: comparison of US and MR Imaging. Radiology 193 (1994) 259–262

5 Desser, T. S., S. McCarthy, T. Trumble: Scaphoid fractures and Kienböck's disease of the lunate: MR Imaging with his-

topathologic correlation. Magn. Reson. Imag. 8 (1990) 357 – 361

6 Dion, E., C. Oberlin, R. Codanda, I. Idy-Peretti, O. Jolivet, M. C. Dauge, J. J. Sarcy, J. Grellet: High-resolution MRI of the carpal tunnel. Anatomical correlations. J. Radiol. 73 (1992) 293 – 301

7 Hofmann-Preiß, K., J. Grebmeier, B. Reichler, M. Flügel, G. Lenz: Vergleich Arthrographie – Kernspintomographie bei schmerzhaften Bewegungseinschränkungen der Hand. Radiologe 30 (1990) 380 – 384

8 Hooper, G.: Kienböck's disease. J. Hand Surg. 17 B (1992) 3 – 4

9 Imaeda, T., R. Nakamura, T. Miura, N. Makino: Magnetic Resonance Imaging in Kienböck's disease. J. Hand Surg. 17 B (1992) 12 – 19

09 a Köhler/Zimmer: Grenzen des Normalen und Anfänge des Pathologischen im Röntgenbild des Skeletts, 13. Aufl. Thieme, Stuttgart 1989

10 Koenig, H., D. Lucas, R. Meissner: The wrist: a preliminary report on high-resolution MR Imaging. Radiology 160 (1986) 463 – 467

11 Koman, L. A., J. F. Mooney, G. C. Poeling: Fractures and ligamentous injuries of the wrist. Hand Clin. 6 (1990) 477 – 491

12 Krahe, T., W. Dölken, R. Schindler: Hochauflösende MRT der Hand: Normalanatomie. Fortschr. Röntgenstr. 150 (1989) 417 – 420

13 Lichtman, D. M., G. R. Mack, R. I. MacDonald, S. F. Gunther, J. N. Wilson: Kienböck's disease: the role of silicone replacement arthroplasty. J. Bone Surg. 59-A (1977) 899 – 908

14 Lener, M., W. Judmaier, M. Gabl, S. Pechlaner, A. Dessl, M. Hackl: Diagnostik des ulnokarpalen Komplexes im MR-Movie. Handchir. Mikrochir. plast. Chir. 26 (1994) 115 – 119

15 Mesgarzadeh, M., C. D. Schneck, A. Bonakdarpour: Carpal tunnel MR Imaging part I: normal anatomy. Radiology 171 (1989) 743 – 748

16 Mesgarazadeh, M., C. D. Schneck, A. Bonakdarpour: Carpal tunnel MR Imaging part II: Carpaltunnel syndrome. Radiology 171 (1989) 749 – 754

17 Meske, S., H. Friedburg, J. Henning, W. Reinbold, K. Stappert, C. Scgumichen: Rheumatoid arthritis lesions of the wrist examined by rapid gradient-echo Magnetic Resonance Imaging. Scand. J. Rheumatol. 19 (1990) 235 – 238

18 Metz, V. M., M. Schratter, W. Dock, F. Grabenwöger, R. Kuzbari, S. Lang, A. H. Wanivenhaus, S. Puigg, H. Imhof: Age-associated changes of the triangular fibrocartilage of the wrist: evaluation of the diagnostic performance of MR Imaging. Radiology 184 (1992) 217 – 220

19 Munk, P. L., A. D. Vellet, M. F. Levin, L. S. Steinbach, C. A. Helms: Current status of Magnetic Resonance-Imaging of the wrist. Canad. Ass. Radiol. J. 43 (1992) 8 – 18

20 Nägele, M., W. Kuglstatter, D. Hahn, K. Wilhelm: Kernspintomographie der Lunatummalazie. Fortschr. Röntgenstr. 148 (1988) 652 – 658

21 Nägele, M., K. Wilhelm, W. Kuglstatter, D. Hahn: Kienböck'sche Erkrankung: Kernspintomographische und röntgenologische Vergleichsstudie. Handchir. Mikrochir. plast. Chir. 22 (1990) 23 – 27

22 Neidl, K., K. D. Hagspiel, G. K. Schulthess: Orthopäde 22 (1993) 13 – 18

23 Oneson, S. R., L. M. Scales, M. E. Timis, S. J. Erickson, L. Chamony: MR Imaging interpretation of the palmer classification of triangular fibrocartilage complex lesions. Radiographics 16 (1996) 97 – 106

24 Palmer, A. K.: Triangular fibrocartilage complex lesions: a classification. J. Hand Surg. 14 (1989) 594 – 605

25 Peterfy, C. G., R. Linares, L. S. Steinbach: Recent advances in Magnetic Resonance Imaging of the musculoskeletal system. Radiol. Clin. N. Amer. 32 (1994) 291 – 311

26 Reinus, W. R., W. F. Conway, W. G. Totty, L. A. Gilula, W. A. Murphy, B. A. Siegel, P. M. Weeks, V. L. Young, P. R. Manske: Carpal

avascular necrosis: MR Imaging. Radiology 160 (1986) 689 – 693

27 Reuther, G., R. Erlemann, J. Grunert, P. E. Peters: Untersuchungstechnik und ligamentäre Binnenmorphologie in der MRT des Handgelenkes. Radiologe 30 (1990) 373 – 379

28 Rominger, M. B., W. K. Bernreuter, P. J. Kenney, D. H. Lee: MR Imaging of anatomy and tears of wrist ligaments. Radiographics 13 (1993) 1233 – 1246

29 Schmidt, H., M., U. Lanz: Guonsche Loge. In Schmidt, H. M., U. Lanz: Chirurgische Anatomie der Hand. Hippokrates, Stuttgart 1992

30 Schweitzer, M. E., S. K. Brahme, J. Hodler, G. J. Hanker, T. P. Lynch, B. D. Flannigan, C. A. Godzik, D. Resnick: Chronic wrist pain: spin-echo and short tau inversion recovery MR Imaging and conventional and MR arthrography. Radiology 182 (1992) 205 – 211

31 Shahabpour, M., B. Lacotte, P. David, D. Roth, M. Osteaux: MRI des poignets. Ann. Radiol. 35 (1992) 341 – 348

32 Sowa, D. T., L. E. Holder, P. G. Patt, A. J. Weiland: Application of Magnetic Resonance Imaging to ischemic necrosis of the lunate. J. Hand Surg. 14-A (1989) 1008 – 1016

33 Sullivan, P. P., T. H. Berquist: Magnetic Resonance Imaging of the hand, wrist and forearm: utility in patients with pain and dysfunctionas a result of trauma. Mayo Clin. Proc. 66 (1991) 1217 – 1221

34 Szeglowski, S. D., J. P. Hornak: Asymmetric single-turn solenoid for MRI of the wrist. Magn. Reson. Med. 30 (1993) 750 – 753

34 a Tomczak, R., P. Mergo, A. J. Aschof, A. Rieber, E. Merkle, H.-J. Brambs: MRI follow-up of pisiform bone transposition for treatment of lunatomalacia. Skeletal Radiol. 27 (1998) 26 – 29

35 Trumble, T. E., J. Irving: Histologic and Magnetic Resonance Imaging correlations in Kienböck's disease. J. Hand Surg. 15-A (1990) 879 – 884

35 a Vahlensieck, M., P. Brüser, H. Schild: Differentialdiagnose zystischer Läsionen im und um das Os lunatum. Fortschr. Röntgenstr. 166 (s) (1997) s 142

36 Wechsler, R. J., M. A. Wehbe, M. D. Rifkin: Computed tomography diagnosis of distal radioulnar subluxation. Skelet. Radiol. 16 (1987) 1 – 5

37 Weiss, K. L., J. Beltran, O. M. Shamam, R. F. Stilla, M. Levey: High field MR surface-coil imaging of the hand and wrist: normal anatomy and pathologic correlations. Radiology 160 (1986) 143 – 152

38 Williams, C. S., J. B. Jupiter: Orthopäde 22 (1993) 36 – 45

39 Wright, T. W., M. Del Charco, D. Wheeler: Incidence of ligament lesions and associated degenerative changes in the elderly wrist. J. Hand Surg. 19-A (1994) 313 – 318

40 Yanagawa, A., Y. Takano, K. Nishioka, J. Shimada, Y. Mizushima, H. Ashida: Clinical staging and Gadolinium-DTPA enhanced images of the wrist in rheumatoid arthritis. J. Rheumatol. 20 (1993) 781 – 784

41 Yoshida, T., K. Yamamoto, T. Shibata, K. Shimada, H. Kawai: Aged-onset Kienböck's disease. Arch. Orthop. traum. Surg. 109 (1990) 241 – 246

42 Yoshioka, S., Y. Okuda, K. Tamai, Y. Hirasawa, Y. Koda: Changes in carpal tunnel shape during wrist joint motion. MRI evaluation of normal volunteers. J. Hand Surg. 18 B (1993) 620 – 623

43 Zeiss, J., M. Skie, N. Ebraheim, W. T. Jackson: Anatomic relations between the median nerve and flexor tendons in the carpal tunnel: MR evaluation in normal volunteers. Amer. J. Roentgenol. 153 (1989) 533 – 536

44 Zeiss, J., E. Jakab, T. Khimji, J. Imbriglia: The ulnar tunnel at the wrist (Guyon's canal): normal MR anatomy and variants. Amer. J. Roentgenol. 158 (1992) 1081 – 1085

45 Zlatkin, M. B., P. C. Chao, A. L. Osterman, M. D. Schnall, M. K. Da Linka, H. Y. Kressel: Chronic wrist pain: Evaluation with high-resolution MR Imaging. Radiology 173 (1989) 723 – 729

6 Hip and Pelvis

M. Reiser and A. Heuck

Introduction

Soon after its clinical introduction, MRI was used to examine the pelvis and, especially, the hips. It became apparent that the avascular necrosis of the femoral head could be detected early, before any visible radiographic findings (48). Furthermore, the sensitive visualization of inflammatory changes of the bone marrow, such as those seen with septic arthritis, proved diagnostically useful. The technical advances of MRI, above all the markedly improved spatial resolution and shorter time for examination of the musculoskeletal system, allowed a more refined visualization of even small anatomic structures.

New entities, such as bone marrow contusions, were discovered by MRI and different patterns of edema were recognized which advanced the understanding of several diseases.

The general availability of MRI today makes it feasible to utilize it early in evaluating cases with radiographic findings that are inconclusive or do not explain the patient's complaints. The goal of reaching a definitive diagnosis quickly and cost effectively has led to MRI as the initial 'problem solving' technique, bypassing conventional tomography, bone scintigraphy and CT. As is true when MRI is applied in other areas, the prerequisite for its appropriate use in disorders of the osseous pelvis and hips is a meticulous examination technique and an understanding of the clinical conditions and their correlation with imaging findings (19).

Examination Technique

As in other anatomic regions, the examination technique for examining the pelvis is determined by the clinical question. The patient should be positioned with both hips in a neutral position. Analogous to the radiographic examination, both patellae should be anterior, ensuring that the hip is not rotated externally, which would otherwise occur spontaneously since this is the more comfortable position for the patient. To make it easier for the patient to maintain this position, pillows can be placed under the legs.

Pelvis and hip are generally examined with the *body coil* or a suitable *phased-array coil*. If an especially high spatial resolution is desired, for instance for a detailed visualization of the cartilage, surface coils can

be used. The section thickness should be 3–5 mm. To select the sections, fast axial T_1-weighted sections with a coarser matrix are recommended.

For most clinical questions, T_1-weighted and T_2-weighted SE sequences are appropriate (35, 36). For inflammations, tumors and bone marrow edema, STIR sequences or T_2-weighted sequences with spectral fat suppression can improve sensitivity and image contrast. GRE sequences are advantageous for a detailed visualization of the articular cartilage (47).

In general, the combination of axial, coronal and sagittal sections achieves an adequate visualization of the anatomic structures. For particular questions, it might be worthwhile to orient the sections parallel or perpendicular to the axis of the femoral neck or sacrum (Fig. 6.1).

For a differentiated and detailed delineation of the articular cartilage of the acetabulum and femoral head, Rosenberg and co-workers (47) recommend T_1-weighted 3D GRE pulse sequences (TR = 26–35 ms, TE = 8–14, flip angle = 45 degrees, FFE of 0.5 T). Fat saturated sequences, which have been found advantageous for the knee, were not applied by these authors, but it can be assumed that GRE sequences with fat saturation are also suitable for examining the hip. It is noteworthy that no chemical shift artifacts appear along the interface of the fat containing bone marrow and hyaline articular cartilage. When T_1-weighted and T_2-weighted SE and 3D GRE sequences are compared, the cartilage thickness measured on the frozen anatomic specimen agrees best with the T_1-weighted 3D GRE technique.

By applying *traction* with a weight of 15 kg, Rosenberg *et al.* (47) could visualize the articular car-

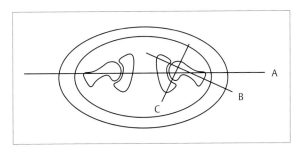

Fig. 6.**1** Schematic drawing of the imaging plane of the hip.
A = Coronal plane
B = Oblique coronal plane parallel to the axis of femoral neck
C = Oblique sagittal plane, perpendicular to B

tilage of the acetabulum and femoral head separately. Using T_1-weighted 3D GRE sequences, the relative high signal of the hyaline cartilage could be distinguished from the synovial fluid, which extends into the joint space during traction. By contrast, SE and T_2-weighted 3 D GRE sequences could not visualize the articular surfaces separately.

MR arthrography can improve the imaging of the acetabular labrum and joint capsule (24). Following intra-articular instillation of a 1 : 100 diluted solution of gadopenetate dimeglumine, the acetabular labrum can be delineated readily from the joint capsule. These structures could not be distinguished from each other without intra-articular contrast medium.

Nishi and co-workers (44) used contrast-enhanced MRI (IV injection of contrast medium) under continuous leg traction to improve the visualization of the acetabular labrum. Analogous to other joints, the hip shows an increased signal intensity in the synovial fluid after IV injection of Gd-based contrast medium. With motion of the hip, the diffusion of the contrast medium into the synovial fluid increases, rendering a clear distinction between acetabular labrum and surface of the articular cartilage, while this is not possible without traction and contrast enhancement.

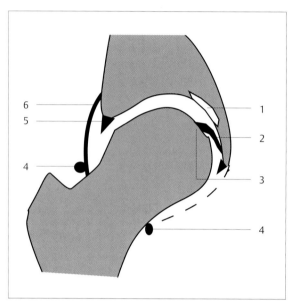

Fig. 6.**2** Schematic drawing of the anatomic structures of the hip in the adult.
1 = Fat in the acetabular fossa
2 = Ligament of the femoral head
3 = Fovea of the femoral head
4 = Zona orbicularis
5 = Acetabular labrum
6 = Iliofemoral ligament

Anatomy (Figs. 6.**2**–6.**5**)

The pelvis has to transmit the weight of the body to both feet and at the same time allow extensive movements of the hips. The sacroiliac joint and symphysis pubis only permit little movement. The hip bone is formed by the ilium, ischium, and pubis, and encloses the acetabulum. In infants, the acetabulum is united by a Y-shaped cartilage.

The hip is a *ball-and-socket joint*, formed by the articulation of the spherical femoral head with the acetabulum. The hyaline cartilage covering the semilunar surface of the acetabulum is shaped like an inverted horseshoe. It contains a non-articulating central depression, the acetabular fossa. Within the acetabular fossa, MRI visualizes fat and the round ligament of the femoral head, which is delineated by lower signal intensity (Figs. 6.**2** and 6.**5**).

The *femoral head* is almost completely coated by hyaline cartilage, sparing only the depression of the

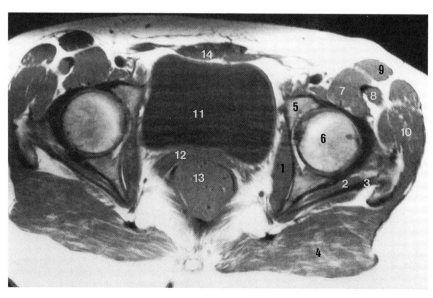

Fig. 6.**3** Axial T_1-weighted SE image at the level of the femoral head.
1 = Obturator internus
2 = Gemellus inferior
3 = Obturator internus tendon
4 = Gluteus maximus
5 = Acetabulum
6 = Femoral head
7 = Iliopsoas
8 = Rectus femoris with tendon
9 = Sartorius
10 = Gluteus medius
11 = Urinary bladder
12 = Vagina
13 = Rectum
14 = Rectus abdominalis

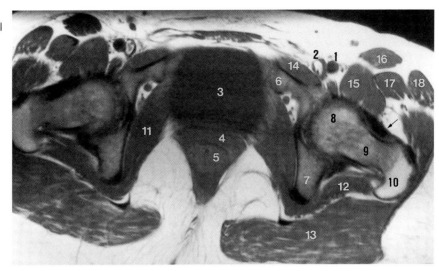

Fig. 6.**4**   Axial T$_1$-weighted SE image at the level of the femoral neck.
1 = Femoral artery
2 = Femoral vein
3 = Urinary bladder
4 = Vagina
5 = Rectum
6 = Pubic bone
7 = Ischial bone
8 = Femoral head
9 = Femoral neck
10 = Greater trochanter
11 = Obturator internus
12 = Gemellus inferior
13 = Gluteus maximus
14 = Pectineus
15 = Iliopsoas
16 = Sartorius
17 = Rectus femoris
18 = Tensor fasciae latae
Arrow = Iliofemoral ligament

acetabular fovea, where the round ligament of the femoral head inserts.

The *femoral neck* separates the femoral shaft from the pelvis, allowing a wide range of motion of the leg. It is anteriorly angulated in relation to the femoral shaft (antetorsion). The *joint capsule* arises from the osseous rim of the acetabulum. Anteriorly, it covers the entire femoral neck and attaches along the intertrochanteric line. Posteriorly, it covers two thirds of the femoral neck. The joint capsule is reinforced by various ligaments. The iliofemoral ligament arises from the anterior inferior iliac spine and broadens posteriorly in a fan shape to attach the greater trochanter and along the intertrochanteric line. The pubofemoral ligament arises from the superior pubic ramus, blends laterally and anteriorly with the joint capsule and continues to the inferior aspect of the intertrochanteric line. The ischiofemoral ligament is located dorsally. It arises from the ischial tuberosity, extends nearly horizontally and attaches at the upper aspect of the intertrochanteric line.

The *sacroiliac joints* have restricted movements. The articulating surfaces of the sacral alar and ilium serve to transmit weight. The articular surfaces are covered by hyaline cartilage and bound together by strong ligaments: the anterior, interosseous, and posterior sacroiliac ligaments.

Avascular Necrosis of the Femoral Head

Avascular necrosis (AVN) of the femoral head can occur with numerous diseases and after trauma. Ischemia or anoxia of the bone marrow of the femoral head is considered to be the common underlying mechanism. Since large areas of the femoral head are covered by hyaline articular cartilage with no vessels entering the bone marrow through it, the vascular supply of the

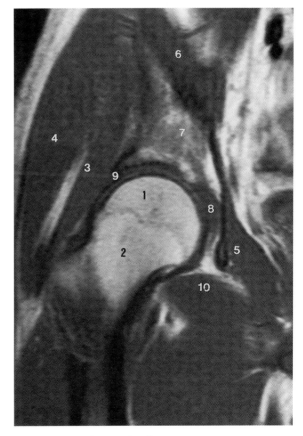

Fig. 6.**5**   Coronal T$_1$-weighted SE image.
1 = Femoral head
2 = Femoral neck
3 = Gluteus minimus
4 = Gluteus medius
5 = Obturator internus
6 = Iliacus
7 = Acetabulum
8 = Acetabular fossa
9 = Acetabular labrum
10 = Obturator externus

femoral head is rather fragile, relying almost exclusively on the deep branch of the medial circumflex artery of the femoral head and the artery of the teres ligament of the femoral head. Furthermore, no pressure can be released from the femoral head in the case of an intracapital space-occupying process. This can greatly hinder the venous drainage.

Subcapital fractures of the femoral neck, acetabular fractures, and hip dislocations can interrupt the arterial supply of the femoral head. In addition, a hemarthrosis of the hip can increase intra-articular pressure and impair venous drainage. (In the newborn and infants, the purulent joint effusion of septic arthritis can also cause avascular necrosis of the femoral head epiphysis.)

Non-traumatic avascular necrosis of the femoral head can be caused by vascular obstruction at the arterial, capillary, or venous level. The following diseases or pathologic conditions are frequently associated with avascular necrosis of the femoral head:

- Corticosteroid therapy
- Cushing's disease
- Collagen vascular disorders
- Barotrauma (Caisson disease)
- Pancreatitis
- Hyperlipidemia
- Sickle cell anemia
- Diabetes mellitus
- Alcohol abuse
- Gaucher's disease
- Hyperuremia
- Polycythemia vera

Not infrequently, neither an adequate trauma nor a predisposing condition can be elicited, and these cases are referred to as idiopathic avascular necrosis. Males are affected more often than females with a ratio of 4 : 1. Avascular necrosis most often occurs in the third to fifth decade of life. Both hips are involved in 40% of the cases. The contralateral involvement can be synchronous or metachronous.

Early detection of avascular necrosis is important. It provides a diagnostically correct explanation of the hip pain and, above all, allows commencement of adequate therapy, which is largely determined by the stage of the disease. It is of great importance to prevent collapse of the femoral head since this invariably progresses to severe degenerative joint changes.

Classification. Different classifications have been proposed for staging avascular necrosis of the hip joint. The most commonly used is the classification of Ficat (18) (Tab. 6.1).

This classification is based primarily on clinical symptoms and the radiographic changes. In *stage 0 and 1*, the necrosis is already histologically detectable. The radiographic findings are unremarkable and the patient is asymptomatic (stage 0) but might complain of pain of sudden onset and restricted motion. Especially in this early stage, MRI is of great value since it is frequently already diagnostic at this time.

In *stage 2* of avascular necrosis, MRI has also proven extremely valuable. The radiographic changes are often non-specific precluding a definitive diagnosis. MRI can invariably diagnose an avascular necrosis at this stage (11).

Bone scintigraphy can detect avascular necrosis with greater sensitivity than radiography, but it is less sensitive than MRI. The specificity of bone scintigraphy and its morphologic detail is inferior to MRI (1, 37, 38).

CT only plays a secondary role in the diagnosis of avascular necrosis today (15). Several studies show that CT is superior to conventional radiography but less accurate than MRI. Only the subchondral fracture in avascular necrosis is detected better by CT than by MRI.

As mentioned above, MRI is especially suited to detect and characterize stages 0 and 1 of avascular necrosis (36, 58). In asymptomatic patients with renal transplants and on corticosteroid therapy, an avascular necrosis could be detected in 6–7.6% of the cases (20, 40, 55), confirming the known associated high risk of avascular necrosis. In patients examined for 24 months at various intervals following a renal transplant, 14 of 104 patients were found to have an avascular necrosis, with spontaneous resolution in some.

The various cellular components of the bone marrow have a different sensitivity to anoxia and ischemia. Hematopoietic cells become necrotic after 6–12 hours and osteoblasts and osteoclasts after 12 to 48 hours. Fat

Table 6.**1** Staging of avascular necrosis of the femoral head according to Ficat

Stage	Clinical Findings	Radiographic findings	Morphologic changes
0	None	Normal	histologic necrosis in the bone marrow
1	Pain, restricted motion	Normal	Necrosis
2	Pain, restricted motion	Sclerosis, radiolucency	Necrosis
3	Increasing complaints	Flattening of the femoral head, crescent sign as evidence of subchondral fracture	Necrosis and subchondral fracture
4	Inceasing complaints	Degenerative arthritis, joint destruction	Necrosis, degenerative arthritis

cells die after 2 to 5 days. The MRI signal of the bone marrow depends on its microscopic composition, in particular on the proportion of fat cells (34, 57).

Edema or biochemical changes of the fatty tissue in bone marrow cause the most significant alterations of MR signals. It is, therefore, not surprising that anoxic necrosis of osteocytes and osteoclasts are not detected by MRI as long as other changes are absent.

Nadel and co-workers (41) conducted investigations in dogs after complete devascularization of the entire femoral head. During the first hours after the total anoxia, no signal changes were detected on SE or STIR sequences. Dynamic imaging with injection of contrast medium (GD-DTPA), however, revealed neither perfusion nor enhancement.

The necrotic area predominately involves the cranial aspect of the femoral head, usually the anterosuperior aspect, and usually has a biconcave or planoconcave configuration (Fig. 6.**6**). The necrosis is separated from the normal bone marrow by a low signal line.

The central areas of necrosis can exhibit different signal patterns, which have been classified by Mitchell and co-workers (39) in four different stages (Tab. 6.**2**).

The different necrotic patterns have no prognostic relevance, however. The prognosis is determined exclusively by the size of the necrotic area. In addition, a heterogeneous signal pattern not found in the stages listed in Tab. 6.**2** can be encountered.

In T_2-weighted images, the highly specific double line sign can be detected in about 80% of the cases (39, 54). A high signal line along the necrotic side and an adjacent low signal line along the healthy bone marrow characterize this sign (Fig. 6.**6**). This double line sign reflects the hypervascular peripheral region of the necrotic area surrounded by fibrosed and sclerotic zone. The hypervascular peripheral zone of the avascular necrosis can show marked enhancement following the administration of gadolinium-based contrast medium.

Unless prosthetic joint replacement is considered regardless of the outcome of the imaging study, MRI is excellently suited for planning any surgical interventions. Sagittal and coronal images can determine exactly the location and extent of the necrosis (Fig. 6.**7**). Beltran and co-workers (2) and Lafforgue and co-workers (31) found that core decompression of the femoral head is especially promising if the necrosis involves less than 25% of the femoral head.

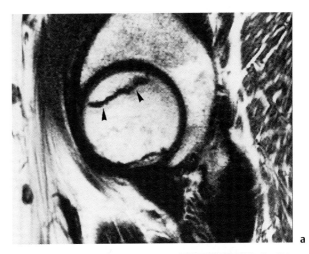

a

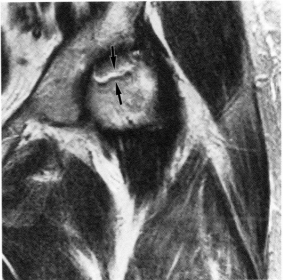

b

Fig. 6.**6 a, b**   Avascular necrosis of the left hip. **a** Sagittal, T_1-weighted SE image. **b** Coronal T_2-weighted image.
On the T_1-weighted image, the necrotic zone has the same signal intensity as the normal bone marrow. In the anterosuperior segment, the necrotic zone is demarcated by a line of low signal intensity (arrowhead). On the T_2-weighted image, the typical double line sign (arrow), considered pathognomonic for avascular necrosis of the femoral head, is seen.

▪ Indication of MRI in Femoral Head Avascular Necrosis

- Suspected AVN in cases of negative or inconclusive radiographic findings
- Exclusion or detection of contralateral involvement in cases of unilaterally established AVN
- Determining the location and extent of the necrotic zone
- Inconclusive differential diagnosis of a hip disorder

Table 6.**2**   Signal pattern of the central regions of the necrosis according to Mitchell

Class	T_1-weighted	T_2-weighted	
A	↑	–	Fat
B	↑	↑	Subacute hemorrhage
C	↓	↑	Fluid
D	↓	↓	Fibrosis

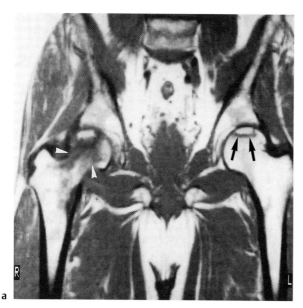

a

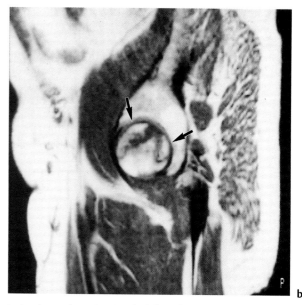

b

Fig. 6.**7 a, b** Avascular necrosis of both femoral heads.
a Coronal T₁-weighted SE image. **b** Sagittal T₁-weighted SE
image of the right hip.
An extensive necrosis with definitely altered signal intensity
(arrowhead) is present on the right, with extension to the remaining femoral head and the femoral neck as well as to the in-

tertrochanteric region. On the left, only a small necrotic area is
seen in the cranial segment of the femoral head demarcated by
a band of low signal intensity (arrow). The sagittal image of the
right hip shows involvement of an extensive area of the femoral
head, with two demarcated necrotic zones anterosuperiorly
and dorsally (arrows).

Transient Osteoporosis

Transient osteoporosis is a relatively rare condition that
is not entirely understood etiologically. In general,
young and middle aged adults are affected, frequently
following an infection or trauma.

The conventional radiograph reveals demineralization of the femoral head and neck. The bone scan reveals
increased uptake. Histologically, increased bone turnover as well as inflammatory changes are seen in transient osteoporosis. Signs of a low grade chronic inflammation can be found in the synovial membrane.

In general, clinical symptoms and radiologic findings resolve spontaneously within 6–12 months.

Distinguishing transient osteoporosis from other
disorders, in particular from bacterial and tuberculous
arthritis as well as from inflammatory rheumatoid arthritis, is of great importance, since therapeutic measures are rather different. Transient osteoporosis displays a characteristic pattern of involvement on MRI.
Diffuse signal changes are found in the femoral head
and neck, possibly extending into the femoral neck
(Fig. 6.**8**). The T₁-weighted image shows a definite
decrease in signal intensity of the bone marrow, while
the T₂-weighted SE images and particularly the STIR images show a definite increase in signal intensity (Figs.
6.**9** and 6.**10**). The Turbo (Fast) SE sequences show less
contrast relative to the normal bone marrow in comparison with conventional SE sequences. The signal

changes of transient osteoporosis are attributed to bone
marrow edema (60). Serial examinations have shown
resolution of edematous pattern within 6–10 months
(3).

Several authors have discussed the etiologic relationship between transient osteoporosis and femoral
head avascular necrosis (23, 42, 43, 59). An MRI controlled study of treatment by core decompression found
changes suggesting an early avascular necrosis of the
femoral head when bone marrow edema was found in
femoral head and neck (25). From these findings it has
been concluded that bone marrow edema is a reversible
intermediate stage in the development of femoral head
avascular necrosis and that the different repair mechanisms determine whether the process heals by resolution of the bone marrow edema or progresses to avascular necrosis of the femoral head (Fig. 6.**11**).

Kramer and co-workers (30) report nine patients
who had severe therapy-resistant pain in one or both
hips in the last trimester of pregnancy. Of 11 diseased
hips, bone marrow edema was found in eight and
avascular necrosis of the femoral head in three. The core
decompression performed in patients with bone marrow edema resulted in rapid pain relief and resolution
of the signal alterations on MRI. Conservative therapy
had a definitely protracted course of healing, lasting 4 to
6 months. All cases with bone marrow edema were
found to have increased intramedullary pressure.

Fig. 6.**8 a, b**   **a** Axial and **b** coronal STIR image. Transient osteoporosis of the left hip. Bone marrow edema (triangles) with high signal intensity in the femoral head, femoral neck, and portions of the intertrochanteric region.

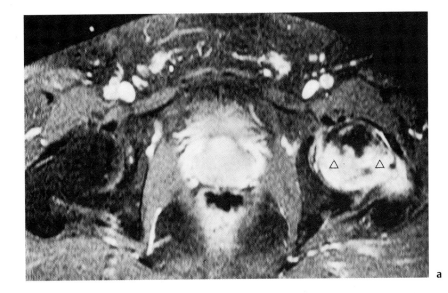

a

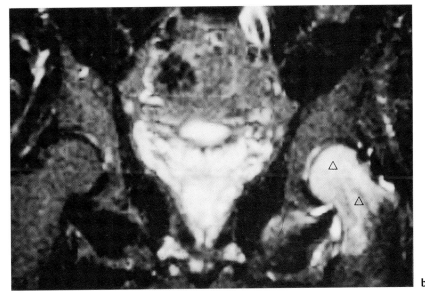

b

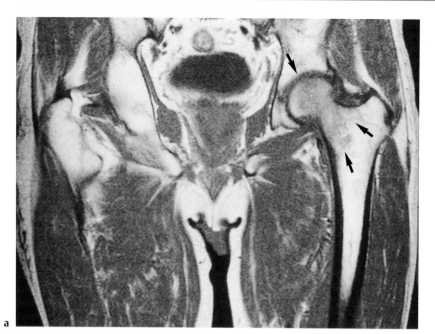

a

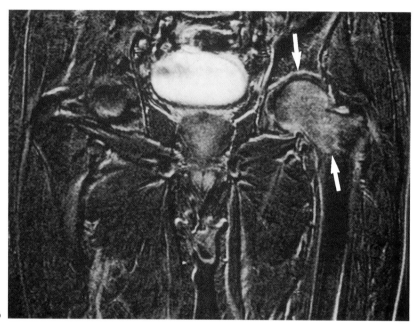

b

Fig. 6.**9 a, b**   Transient osteoporosis of the left hip. **a** Coronal
T$_1$-weighted SE sequence.
b Coronal STIR image. Femoral
head and neck show large ill-
defined areas of decreased signal
intensity (arrows) on the T$_2$-
weighted image and of increased
signal intensity on the STIR
image.

Fig. 6.**10 a–c** Transient osteoporosis of the left femur and avascular necrosis of the right femoral head. **a** Coronal T_1-weighted SE image. The subchondral region of the right hip exhibits a smoothly outlined decrease in signal intensity (arrows), corresponding to early avascular necrosis. The left proximal femur shows an extensive and indistinctly outlined decrease in signal intensity within the bone marrow (arrowhead). **b** Coronal T_1-weighted SE image of the left hip. Clearly visualized decreased signal intensity in the femoral head, femoral neck and intertrochanteric region. **c** Axial T_2-weighted SE image with fat saturation. Clearly increased signal intensity (arrowhead) in the dorsal aspect of the femoral head as well as in the femoral neck. Effusion in the anterior aspect of the joint capsule of the left hip (arrow).

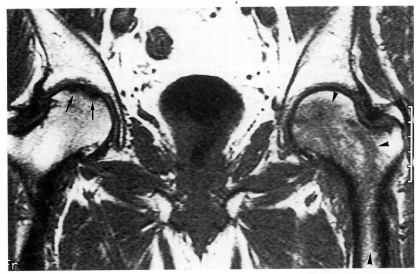

a

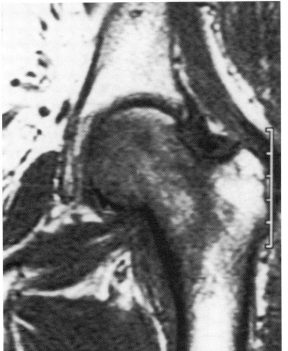

b

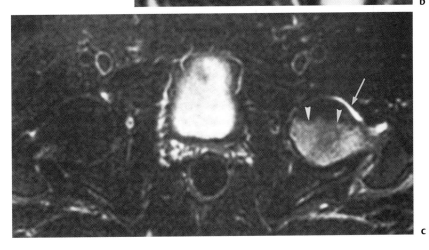

c

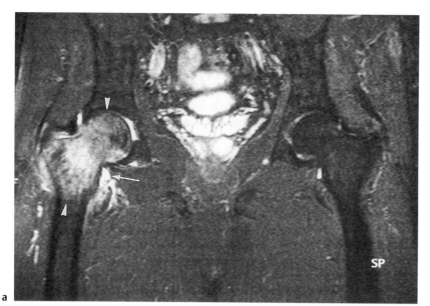

a

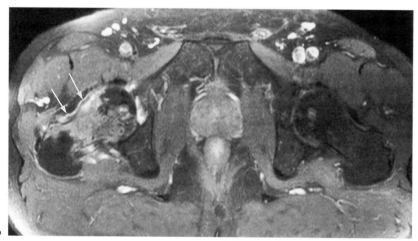

b

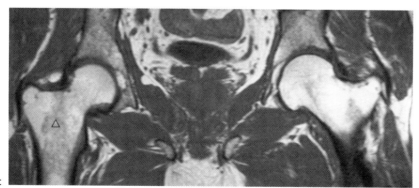

c

Fig. 6.**11 a–c**   Transient osteoporosis of the left proximal femur.
a Coronal STIR image. Extensive increase in signal intensity in the femoral head, femoral neck and intertrochanteric region (arrowhead) on the left. The joint effusion shows a high signal intensity (arrow). **b** Axial T_1-weighted SE image with fat saturation after intravenous administration of contrast medium. Definite contrast enhancement in large areas of the femoral head and neck. Intense enhancement of anterior synovial membrane (arrow).
c Coronal T_1-weighted SE image. Only a discrete decrease in signal intensity (triangle) is seen in the right proximal femur.

Legg-Perthes Disease

Legg-Perthes disease primarily occurs between the age of 4 and 8 years. Boys are more often affected than girls. Its etiology is not clearly known. It is believed to be an idiopathic form of avascular necrosis of the femoral head in the pediatric age group.

Legg-Perthes disease is staged on the basis of clinical and radiologic findings:

- *Initial stage* with definite complaints but without radiographic findings,
- *Fragmentation stage* with sclerosis, patchy radiolucencies, and flattening of the epiphysis of the femoral head,
- *Repair stage* with restoration of the epiphysis.

Depending on the severity of the disease and the response to therapy, a more or less complete restoration can occur or a residual deformity remains, with coxa vara and an enlarged, mushroom-shaped femoral head. This can lead to early degenerative osteoarthritis of the hip (pre-osteoarthritic deformity).

As in the femoral head avascular necrosis in adults, bilateral involvement is observed in one-third of the cases, which can be synchronous or metachronous.

MRI is suitable for the early detection of Legg-Perthes disease (Fig. 6.**12**) before radiographic or scintigraphic findings are apparent (5, 10, 50). Contradicting this favorable assessment of MRI for the early diagnosis of Legg-Perthes disease, Rix and co-workers (46) found a sensitivity of 58%, specificity of 85% and accuracy of 74% for MRI (radiography: sensitivity = 50%, specificity = 83%, accuracy = 71%). MRI could establish the diagnose of Legg-Perthes disease earlier than radiography only in selected cases.

The bone marrow of the epiphysis of the femoral head normally has a high signal intensity on T_2-weighted images. In Legg-Perthes disease, the epiphysis of the femoral head has a low signal intensity on T_1-weighted and T_2-weighted images (16). In the early stages of Legg-Perthes disease, a patchy or segmental decrease in signal is observed in the epiphysis of the femoral head. Eventually, the signal intensity is decreased in the entire epiphysis of the femoral head (Fig. 6.**13**), occasionally also in portions of the metaphysis (Fig. 6.**14**). During the repair phase, fat-containing bone marrow returns to the epiphysis and a high signal reappears.

Thickening of the hyaline articular cartilage has been described in Legg-Perthes disease, leading to a lateral displacement of the femoral head and resultant loss of the congruence of the articular surfaces (Fig. 6.**15**). Thickening of the synovial membrane, which is observed within the entire capsule of the hip joint (49), contributes to the displacement. Rix and co-workers (46) could not confirm the thickening of the hyaline

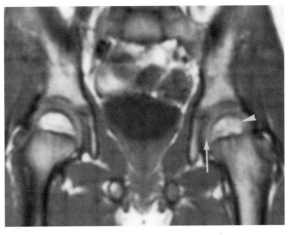

Fig. 6.**12**   Early manifestation of Legg-Perthes disease of the left hip. The configuration of the epiphysis of the left femoral head has not yet changed. A discrete decrease in signal intensity (arrowhead) is seen on the T_1-weighted SE image. The articular cartilage (arrow) is thickened with slight lateral displacement of the left femoral head.

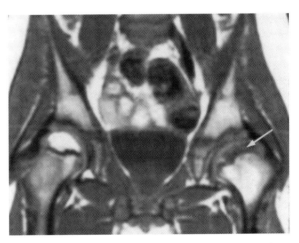

Fig. 6.**13**   Legg-Perthes disease of the left hip. Coronal T_1-weighted SE sequence. Definitely decreased signal intensity in the left femoral head epiphysis, which is flattened and deformed (arrow). Normal bone marrow signal in the right femoral head epiphysis.

articular cartilage. Loss of joint stability was only observed in cases with flattening of the epiphysis of the femoral head.

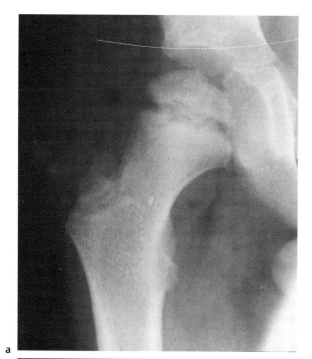

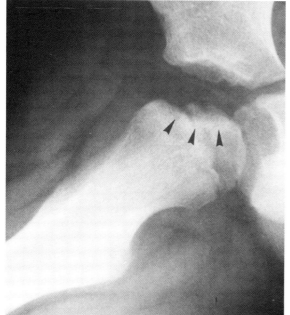

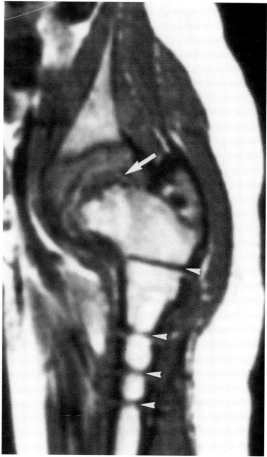

Fig. 6.**15** Legg-Perthes disease of the left hip, post osteotomy. Coronal T₁-weighted SE sequence. Flattening and deformity as well as extensive decrease in signal intensity involving the entire epiphysis of the left femoral head (arrow). The burr holes for the screws of the osteotomy fixation device are seen as bands of decreased signal intensity (arrowheads) in the bone marrow of the proximal femur.

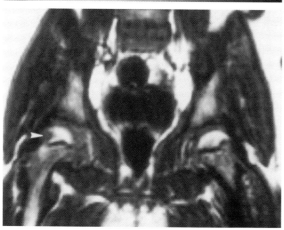

◀ Fig. 6.**14 a–c   a, b** Radiographs of the right hip in AP and lateral projection. The AP projection shows an irregular density distribution in the lateral aspect of the epiphysis of the femoral head. The axial projection demonstrates a defect and collapse involving the lateral aspect of the femoral head (arrowheads). **c** Coronal T₂-weighted SE sequence. Large areas of the femoral epiphyseal head still have a normal fat signal. A wedge-shaped decrease in signal intensity is apparent laterally (arrowhead).

Trauma, Stress and Fatigue Fractures

In most cases, fractures of the femoral neck, femoral head, and acetabulum can be definitively evaluated by conventional radiography, possibly supplemented by CT. For complex pelvic fractures, which frequently involve the sacroiliac joints, CT is advantageous since it allows detailed analysis of the fracture lines and position of the osseous fragment.

MRI is indicated for the evaluation of suspected *occult* fractures as well as stress and fatigue fractures (21). Occult fractures refer to traumatic fractures that cannot be detected on adequately performed radiographic examinations and generally represent undisplaced fractures with subtle or no morphologic changes. It has been proven that such occult fractures of the proximal femoral shafts can be reliably detected or excluded by MRI (14, 33).

The T_1-weighted image shows occult fractures as low signal intensity in the bone marrow, extending as indistinct bands or lines to the cortex (Fig. 6.**16**). This finding corresponds to the fracture line and its surrounding bone marrow edema or hematoma. A band-like zone of increased signal intensity is seen on the T_2-weighted images, in particular with fat saturation, and most conspicuous on STIR images (Fig. 6.**17**). The fracture line itself can appear as an even more intense signal or as linear decrease in signal intensity. Such a decreased signal intensity is believed to represent trabecular compression. The susceptibility sensitive T_2-weighted GRE sequences can show extensive areas of decreased signal intensity.

Quinn and McCarthy (45) examined 20 patients with clinically suspected hip fractures and indeterminate radiographs. Only coronal T_1-weighted sequences were used. A femoral neck fracture could be established in 13 patients and excluded in seven. In comparison to serial radiographs, bone scintigraphy, conventional tomography and CT, this shortened MRI protocol was less expensive.

Haramati and co-workers (22) examined 15 elderly patients with osteoporosis and clinically suspected fracture of the proximal femur and an unremarkable or indeterminate radiographic finding. In seven patients, MRI detected an occult fracture of the femoral neck. To find an occult fracture of the femoral neck, the authors recommend MRI as the only examination to be added to conventional radiography in old patients with osteoporosis.

Bone scintigraphy is extremely sensitive for the detection of occult fracture, though not very specific. False positive findings can be caused by degenerative joint changes and ligamentous avulsions. False negative findings can be found primarily in old age, chronic renal insufficiency, corticosteroid therapy, and local synovitis. False negative findings can also be encountered in the immediate post-traumatic phase (24 hours).

Feldman and co-workers (17) examined 30 patients with discrepancy of the clinical and imaging findings (radiography, bone scintigraphy, CT). Twenty-two patients had a preceding acute trauma and eight patients a trauma or unusual stress with worsening of pain over a period of 1 – 4 weeks. An occult fracture was found in the sacrum in 10 patients, in the proximal femur in eight and in the acetabulum in two. Bone scintigraphy showed a slight or diffuse uptake, precluding a correct anatomic assignment. Feldman and co-workers (17) conclude from their results that MRI is the modality to be selected after an inconclusive radiographic examination whenever the clinical findings suggest a fracture.

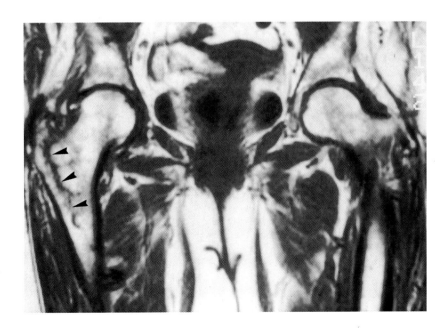

Fig. 6.**16** Occult fracture of the right proximal femur. Conventional radiographs and AP tomography fail to detect a fracture. The coronal T_1-weighted SE image shows an irregularly outlined band-like decrease in signal intensity (arrowheads) extending from the base of the femoral neck and the intertrochanteric region to the proximal femoral shaft. (By kind permission of Dr P. Lang, San Francisco.)

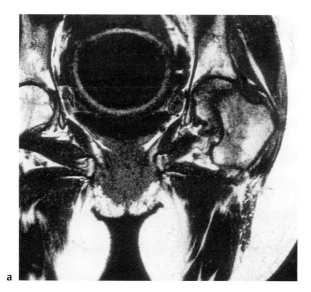

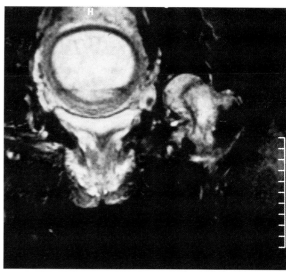

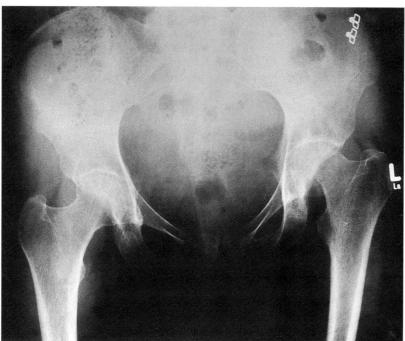

Fig. 6.**17 a – c**   Subcapital fracture of the femoral neck with a varus position of the fracture fragments. The patient complained of severe pain in the left hip during her pregnancy. To avoid radiation to the fetus, an MRI was performed. **a** Coronal T_1-weighted SE image. **b** Coronal T_1-weighted STIR image. An extensive bone marrow edema is seen in the proximal femur and a line of low signal intensity in the medial femoral shaft corresponding to the fracture line. The femoral head is medially angulated. **c** Radiographs obtained after delivery confirm the diagnosis of a subcapital fracture of the femoral neck and show definite demineralization of the proximal femur. It is conceivable that in this case a transient osteoporosis predisposed the femoral neck to fracture without adequate trauma.

Bogost and co-workers (6) examined 70 patients with suspected occult fracture of the femoral neck. Coronal T_1-weighted, SE and STIR images were used. A femoral neck fracture was found in 37% of the patients and a pelvic fracture in 23%. In addition, soft tissue injuries were found in 74% of the cases, primarily represented as tears, hematomas, and contusions of the muscles, most frequently involving the adductors, quadratus femoris and pectineus. The authors conclude that in a relatively high proportion of examinations performed because of suspected occult pelvic fracture MRI reveals previously unsuspected pelvic fracture and, also, soft tissue injuries that can explain the patient's complaints. They advise against a shortened examina-

tion protocol designed exclusively for the detection of occult fractures of the femoral neck.

Several authors question whether MRI can predict the *development of avascular necrosis* following a femoral neck fracture. Speer and co-workers (52) found no signal changes in the femoral head in 15 patients 48 hours after intracapsular fracture of the femoral neck. In view of the known high incidence of avascular necrosis in these injuries, these results suggest that unenhanced MRI is not suitable to detect early signs of post-traumatic avascular necrosis.

Lang and co-workers (32) performed contrast-enhanced MRI on 10 patients with acute femoral neck fracture and compared the results with those of selective angiography of the femoral head. Whenever the vessels were angiographically patent, contrast enhancement was found on MRI and this corresponded to the non-affected hip. However, if angiography revealed interrupted vessels of the femoral head, MRI failed to show any enhancement. These results could have therapeutic implications as to whether internal fixation or primary hip replacement should be performed.

Furthermore, MRI can contribute to the clarification of suspected *stress fractures*. Stress fractures can be further divided into fatigue and insufficiency fractures (13). Insufficiency fractures are caused by normal strain acting on weakened bone (osteoporosis, osteomalacia, post radiation state, rheumatoid arthritis, steroid therapy), while fatigue fractures occur in normal bone subjected to increased strain (such as a march fracture).

Radiographically, the stress fracture is seen as a fracture line perpendicular or oblique to the longitudinal axis of the affected bone, often surrounded by perifocal sclerosis and periosteal new bone formation. In the absence of such typical signs, the diagnosis of a stress fracture can be difficult. In particular, during the initial 10–14 days before visible endosteal and periosteal callus formation, definitive radiographic findings are usually absent. In these cases, MRI can be helpful and contribute to the differential diagnostic evaluation.

On the T_1-weighted image, the stress fracture presents as a band-like zone of decreased signal intensity in the bone marrow with extension to the cortex. On the T_2-weighted image, primarily with added fat saturation, and on the STIR image, extensive zones of increased signal intensity are detected, caused by edema and possible hemorrhage into the bone marrow.

In the pelvis, fatigue fractures are seen in the sacrum (frequently bilateral) and in the supra-acetabular region of the ilium. In the ilium, fatigue fractures are usually parallel to the acetabulum and horizontally oriented and, in the sacrum, they are usually parallel to the SI joint and vertically oriented (Fig. 6.**18**).

Blomlie and co-workers (4) examined 18 patients who had radiotherapy for malignant tumors of the pelvis and developed radiation-induced insufficiency fracture of the sacrum. They mentioned the risks of misinterpreting the corresponding MR findings as metastases. In the region of the insufficiency fractures, extensive zones of decreased signal intensity were seen on the T_1-weighted image and increased signal intensity on the STIR image. In 16 patients, both sacral ala were involved. In some patients, fatigue fractures were also found in the medial and supra-acetabula ilium, pubic bone and lumbar vertebrae, which were also within the radiation field.

Bone scintigraphy is also extremely sensitive for stress fractures, but not very specific. In elderly patients and in patients with known tumor, the combination of the clinical presentation of pain and the scintigraphic finding of focally increased uptake is often attributed to osseous metastases. In these cases, MRI is well suited to

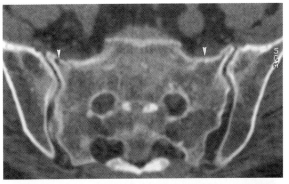

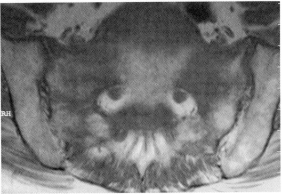

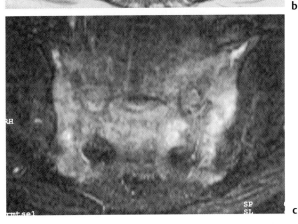

Fig. 6.**18 a – c** Insufficiency fracture of the sacrum bilaterally. **a** The CT shows a break in the anterior cortex of the sacrum and subtle sclerosis (arrowheads). **b** Axial T_1-weighted SE image. Extensive decrease in signal intensity in both sacral ala. **c** Axial STIR image. Diffuse increase in signal intensity throughout the sacrum.

establish the correct diagnosis. CT can also be helpful for insufficiency fractures of the sacrum.

MR arthrography, e.g., MRI after intra-articular injection of diluted contrast medium, can detect injuries and degenerative changes of the acetabular roof that are invisible on other non-invasive diagnostic imaging methods.

Hip Dysplasia

Sonography has been proven extremely useful in the early diagnosis of hip dysplasia and represents the method of choice during the first year of life. It can dis-

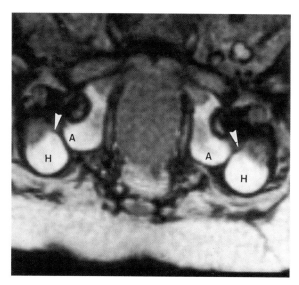

Fig. 6.**19** Bilateral hip dislocation with posterior displacement of the femoral heads (arrowheads). Six-month-old male patient. Axial GRE sequence. Examination performed with 0.5 Tesla. High signal intensity of the cartilaginous components of the acetabulum and femoral heads.
A = acetabulum
H = femoral head

play the anatomic relationship between femoral head and acetabulum. Since avoiding ionizing radiation is particularly important in the newborn and infants, sonography has replaced radiography as a screening method.

After the age of one year, radiography of the hips is needed. It can reveal the relationship of the femoral head to the acetabulum, particularly excluding any cranial or lateral displacement of the femoral heads. The radiographic image does not display the complex anatomic relationship found in hip dysplasia, especially any ventral and dorsal position of the femoral head relative to the acetabular roof. Furthermore, joint capsule, ligament and vasculature cannot be directly visualized (Figs. 6.**19** and 6.**20**).

MRI can display the non-osseous components of the femoral head and acetabulum, the joint capsule and the labrum. The three-dimensional display of the MRI finding can illustrate the anatomic relationships superbly.

On T_1-weighted and T_2-weighted SE images, the fibrocartilage acetabular labrum is seen as a triangular signal void at the edge of the acetabular roof (28). In a congenitally dislocated hip, displacement, infolding or hypertrophy of the acetabular labrum or joint capsule can prevent reduction by conservative measures (9). Furthermore, the ligamentum teres of the femoral head, which is seen as a band-like signal void structure on MRI, can interfere with reduction of the femoral head.

MRI can also display the cartilaginous components of the acetabulum and femoral head, including acetabular labrum. Nishii and co-workers (44) examined patients with hip dysplasia and secondary degenerative

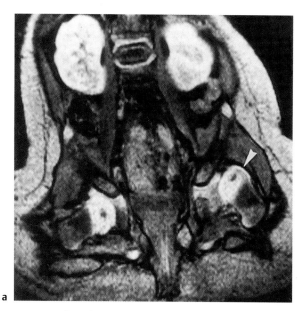

a

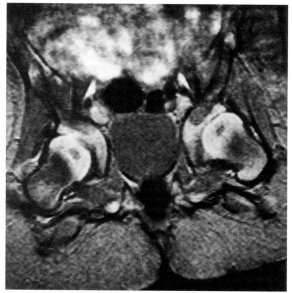

b

Fig. 6.**20a, b**   Bilateral hip dysplasia with dislocation on the left (arrowhead). **a** Before reduction. **b** After reduction. Restoration of the normal position of the femoral heads to the acetabulum. The ossification centers of the femoral heads are

demarcated as oval structures of low signal intensity. The cartilaginous components of both hips show a high signal intensity.

osteoarthritis and could identify tears of the acetabular labrum on contrast enhanced MR images obtained during continuous leg traction, which were not apparent on unenhanced MR images.

Degenerative and Rheumatoid Joint Changes and Other Conditions Arising from the Synovial Membranes

In chronic degenerative and inflammatory rheumatoid joint diseases, MRI is not used for the initial diagnosis. Instead, it is employed to address a difficult differential diagnosis, in addition to answering scientific questions.

Using standard examination protocols, especially T_1-weighted and T_2-weighted SE sequences, advanced stages of degenerative osteoarthritis of the hip can be definitively identified. Joint space narrowing, subchondral sclerosis, osteophytes, and cysts are clearly identifiable (Figs. 6.**21**–6.**23**). The sectional visualization without superimposition and the free selection of the imaging plane, with the coronal plane preferred for the hip, allows MRI to reveal morphologic details that are radiographically invisible.

Rosenberg and co-workers (47) examined patients who underwent total hip replacement following MRI. This allowed them to investigate correlation between the MRI findings and the microscopic and histologic examination of the removed femoral head. Using 3-D-GRE images with T_1-weighted sequences, they found good agreement with microscopic and histologic findings (Tab. 6.**3**).

In active osteoarthritis of the hip, signs of bone marrow edema occasionally can be observed in the femoral head and acetabulum (Fig. 6.**24**). Such cases can also have detectable joint effusion and synovial thickening. These synovial proliferations are not synonymous with chronic rheumatoid joint changes.

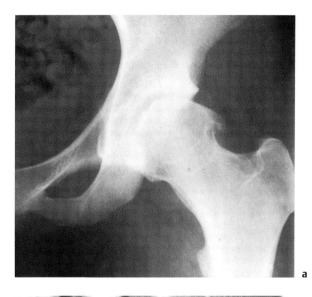

a

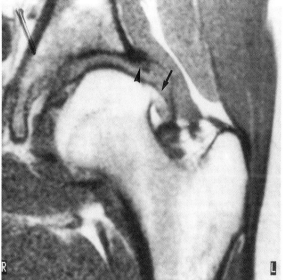

b

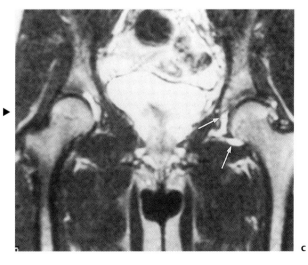

c

Fig. 6.**21 a–c** Osteoarthritis of the left hip in a 19-year-old female patient. **a** The conventional radiograph of the left hip shows a large marginal osteophyte of the femoral head and periosteal bone apposition along the medial cortex of the femoral neck as a manifestation of the Wiberg sign. **b** Coronal T_1-weighted image of the left hip. A bone marrow signal of high intensity is seen in the osteophyte of the femoral head (arrow). A small area of increased signal intensity (arrowhead) is seen in the lateral aspect of the acetabular labrum, suggesting a tear. **c** Coronal T_2-weighted SE sequence. Increased fluid accumulation (arrows) around the left hip joint. The left femoral head has less acetabular coverage than the right femoral head. An underlying hip dysplasia is the presumptive cause of the osteoarthritis.

Table 6.**3**   Staging of osteoarthritis by MRI

Stage	MRI	Macroscopic findings	Histologic findings
Normal	Normal cartilage width, homogeneous signal, smooth surface	→	No surface fibrillations, tangential arrangement of the cartilage cells in the lamina splendens, vertical arrangement of the chondrocytes in the zone III, no cluster formation or ballooning
1	Normal cartilage width, heterogeneous signal (decreased signal intensity)	→ Smooth surface	Decrease and swelling of the chondrocytes in the tangential zone, in the middle zone cartilaginous clusters, ballooning; decreased staining of the matrix
2	Thinning and irregular surface of the cartilage	→	Marked surface fibrillations, loss of the tangential cells, moderate hypocellularity of the middle and basal zones, cluster in the middle zone
3	Loss of cartilage cover	→	→

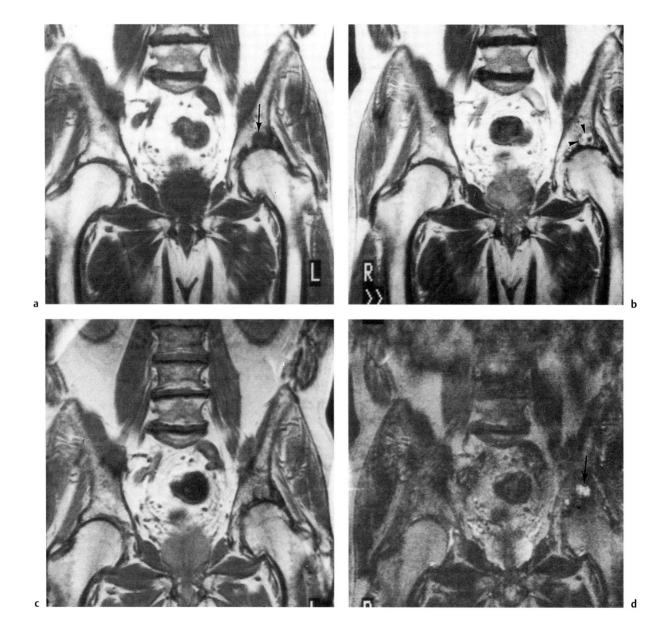

a   b   c   d

Fig. 6.**23 a, b**   Dislocated left hip with secondary osteoarthritis.
a Coronal T$_1$-weighted SE image after IV contrast medium.
b Coronal T$_2$-weighted SE sequence.
There is marked deformity and flattening of the left femoral head, with lateral and upward displacement. A large subchondral cyst is present in the acetabulum (arrow). This cyst exhibits a low signal intensity on the T$_1$-weighted image and a high signal intensity on the T$_2$-weighted image.

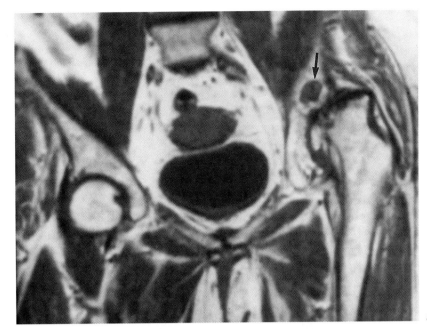

a

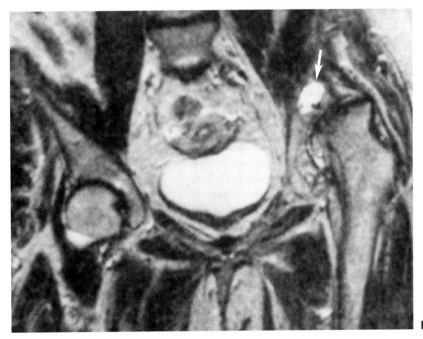

b

◀ Fig. 6.**22 a–d**   Severe osteoarthritis of the left hip. Early osteoarthritis of the right hip. Coronal MR images. **a** T$_1$-weighted SE image. **b** T$_1$-weighted SE image after IV administration of Gd-based contrast medium. **c** Proton density-weighted image. **d** T$_2$-weighted SE image.
There is definite joint space narrowing bilaterally. On the left, subchondral cysts (arrows) are seen in the acetabulum, with the cysts showing a low signal intensity on the T$_1$-weighted image, an intermediate intensity on the proton density-weighted image and a high signal intensity on the T$_2$-weighted image. After injection of Gd-based contrast medium, the cysts show definite peripheral enhancement (arrowheads). Synovial contrast enhancement is also seen in the inferior aspect of the left hip, indicative of reactive synovitis.

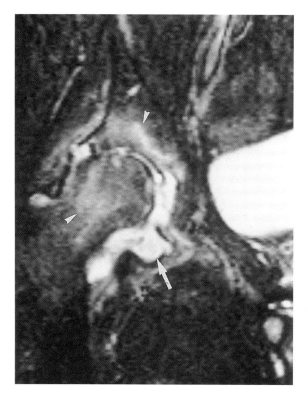

Fig. 6.24 Active osteoarthritis of the right hip. Coronal STIR image. Edema (arrowhead) in the femoral head, femoral neck, and juxta-articular portions of the acetabulum. Extensive joint effusion (arrow).

■ Inflammatory Rheumatoid Diseases

In rheumatoid arthritis and rheumatoid variant diseases of the hips, MRI can reveal several morphologic changes shown only poorly or not at all by other imaging methods (51). The T_2-weighted images have an 'arthrographic effect,' displaying joint effusion as high signal intensity and clearly visualizing even small joint effusions and fluid in bursae and synovial extensions (53). TSE sequences, however, have relatively little contrast relative to the surrounding fat-containing structures. The fat saturated T_2-weighted SE and STIR sequences achieve high contrast relative to the adjacent fat-containing structures.

Synovial proliferations of inflammatory rheumatoid conditions show a marked and rapid enhancement following IV administration of contrast medium, clearly separating them from joint effusion and surrounding soft tissue structures. The T_2-weighted fat saturated sequences are particularly useful.

Dynamic contrast enhanced examinations can quantitatively determine the speed and extent of the enhancement in the synovial proliferations. Several authors have pointed out that the rate of enhancement and the intensity achieved correlates with the activity of the inflammatory rheumatoid processes and can be used to evaluate therapeutic methods. It should be

mentioned that synovial enhancement does not prove that the process represents an inflammatory rheumatoid arthritis. Similar enhancement can be observed in severe osteoarthritis, post-traumatic changes, bacterial arthritis and tumorous changes. In particular, this applies to the intracapsular osteoid osteoma of the femoral neck and head. Periosteal and endosteal new bone formation are not very marked or are even absent in these cases. An extensive joint effusion and synovial proliferations are often detectable, mimicking the picture of an inflammatory rheumatoid condition.

■ Pigmented Villonodular Synovitis

Pigmented villonodular synovitis (PVNS) most frequently involves the knee, but can also occur in the hip. Though the etiology of PVNS is not completely known, it is generally agreed that it is a condition with benign tumor-like lesions of the synovial membrane.

The radiographic examination is characterized by periarticular osseous destruction caused by tumor-like intra-articular synovial proliferations. These destructions are round and surrounded by sclerotic margins. For the localization of these destructions, it must be kept in mind that the joint capsule inserts distally at the femoral neck and that, consequently, PVNS-related destructions can extend along the femoral neck. Characteristically, the periarticular osseous structures of the acetabulum and proximal femora are equally involved.

These findings, which are seen radiographically as well as by MRI, are not invariably present. Instead, intra-articular manifestation of PVNS can occur before causing any osseous destruction. In most of these cases, MRI can already establish a specific diagnosis.

PVNS characteristically has a low signal intensity on T_1-weighted and T_2-weighted images, distinguishing it from almost all tumorous and inflammatory conditions, which have a high signal intensity on the T_2-weighted image. The low signal intensity on the T_2-weighted images is caused by the variable degree of hemosiderin deposits (26, 29). The hemosiderin content can be detected especially well on T_2-weighted GRE sequences. In addition to low signal areas, PVNS frequently has cystic components and an accompanying joint effusion. After IV administration of contrast medium, a definite synovial enhancement is apparent. In contrast to osteoarthritis and rheumatoid arthritis, articular cartilage and widths of the joint space remain characteristically preserved in PVNS.

■ Synovial Osteochondromatosis

Synovial osteochondromatosis is characterized by loose intra-articular bodies that arise from the synovial membrane following cartilaginous metaplasia. It is found most frequently in the knee and hip. Primary idiopathic osteochondromatosis has to be distinguished from secondary osteochondromatosis, which primarily arises on the basis of severe osteoarthritis. As long as the loose intra-articular bodies contain calcium, the condition can be diagnosed on conventional radiographs.

MRI also visualizes the cartilaginous intra-articular bodies, seen as defects in the high signal intensity joint effusion on the T_2-weighted image. The signal intensity of the intra-articular body depends on its composition. If they are completely calcified, they appear as signal void. Purely cartilaginous intra-articular bodies have an intermediary signal intensity on the T_1-weighted and T_2 weighted image. Ossified intra-articular bodies with bone marrow display a fat equivalent signal intensity centrally.

Osteomyelitis and Septic Arthritis

MRI is extremely sensitive for the diagnosis of bacterial and tuberculous infections. The morphologic changes seen on MRI are only diagnostic in the context of the clinical and laboratory findings. An arthritis originating from the surrounding bone is generally marked by an extensive bone marrow edema and joint effusion in its early stage (Fig. 6.**25**). This allows differentiation from inflammatory rheumatoid diseases, which characteristically do not alter the bone marrow signal. Joint space narrowing and extensive osteoporosis are frequently seen radiographically, both with rheumatoid arthritis and tuberculosis arthritis. Though MRI misses the osteoporosis, it makes an important contribution by detecting or excluding any bone marrow changes.

Infections confined to the joint cavity and not arising from a hematogenous focus in the adjacent bone marrow can pose a differential diagnostic problem. In these cases, a septic joint effusion is detected that does not differ in its signal pattern from serous effusion (arthrographic effect on T_2-weighted sequences). For clarification, the joint effusion has to be aspirated for staining and bacterial cultures.

Furthermore, the sacroiliac joint and adjacent osseous sections of the sacrum and ilium are often affected by tuberculous and bacterial infections. Detecting a focal osseous abscess or an extraosseous extension of an abscess can be an important sign for bacterial infection and excludes spondyloarthropathy.

MRI can display severe cartilaginous and subchondral erosions caused by arthritis. Discrete osseous erosions are only seen with high resolution techniques, possibly with the examination performed during continuous leg traction.

For treatment planning, especially when surgical intervention is considered, MRI can disclose the extent of the infection (Fig. 6.**26**). In particular, it should be determined whether and how far osseous structures, soft tissues, and joints are involved (12). Fat-saturated T_2-weighted SE sequences and contrast-enhanced T_1-weighted sequences with fat saturation are particularly informative in this regard.

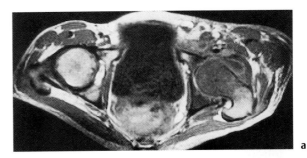

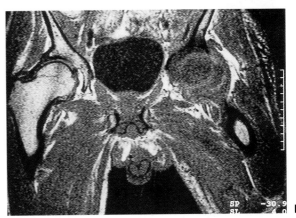

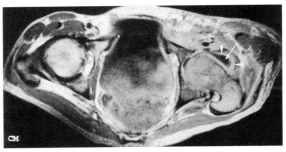

Fig. 6.**25 a–c** Non-specific arthritis of the left hip. **a** Axial and T_1-weighted SE image. **b** Coronal T_1-weighted SE image. Decreased signal intensity is seen in the left femoral head and femoral neck as well as in the acetabulum. Because of severe pain, the left hip is fixed in external rotation and abduction and obliquely sectioned on the coronal image. Joint effusion is present anterior to the femoral head and neck. **c** Axial contrast-enhanced T_1-weighted SE image. There is marked enhancement in those parts of the acetabulum, femoral heads and femoral neck altered by inflammation, as well as in the surrounding soft tissues. The contrast of normal bone marrow, compared to the unenhanced examination, is markedly decreased. The joint effusion shows a low signal intensity (arrow) and is clearly distinguishable from the intensely enhancing thickened synovial membrane (arrowhead).

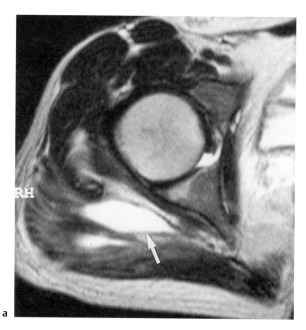

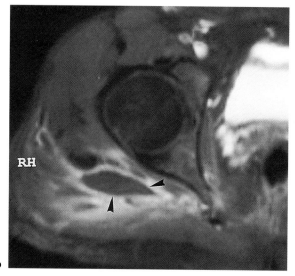

Fig. 6.**26 a, b** Abscess in the gluteal region. **a** Axial T$_2$-weighted SE image. Lentiform fluid accumulation (arrow) is seen between gluteus medius and maximus. Extensive edema is present in the surrounding muscular sections. **b** Axial T$_1$-weighted SE image with fat suppression after IV injection of contrast medium. There is definite enhancement of the capsule (arrowheads) encompassing the abscess and in the inflammatory changes involving the adjacent muscle.

Pitfalls in Interpreting the Images

As in the proximal humerus, the spatial distribution of epiphyseal and metaphyseal remnants in the hematopoietic bone marrow of the metaphysis can be mistaken for infiltrative processes, particularly on the axial sections. The details of the age-related distribution of hematopoietic and fatty bone marrow will be discussed in Chapter 11. Remnants of the epiphyseal plate appear as linear low signal zones and should not be mistaken for linear signal changes secondary to avascular necrosis of the femoral head.

■ Transcortical Synovial Herniation

In up to 5% of radiographs, the femoral neck shows osteolytic lesions that are variable in size, characteristically measuring up to 10 mm in diameter, and are surrounded by a sclerotic rim. These lesions are attributed to a transcortical synovial herniation of the joint capsule with erosions of the anterior femoral neck, in particular affecting the zona orbicularis. They are characteristically observed in the upper outer quadrant of the proximal femoral neck, but are also encountered, though less frequently, mediocaudally (Fig. 6.**27**). MRI shows corresponding defects in the typical location (12 a). If they are predominately fluid-filled, they are of low signal intensity on the T$_1$-weighted image and of high signal intensity on the T$_2$-weighted image. They display a low signal intensity if they are predominately fibrous. A signal void halo encircles these lesions. They are also referred to as herniation pits and should not be mistaken for erosions due to inflammatory synovial proliferations or tumors.

■ Bursitis

Inflammation of the bursae can be isolated or concomitant with an inflammatory joint condition. The inflammation leads to swelling, which can be mistaken for a tumor if it is an isolated finding (Fig. 6.**28**). The location of the bursae should be known when cross-sectional images are interpreted (Fig. 6.**29**). The iliopsoas bursa is the largest bursa of the hip region (3 – 7 × 2 – 4 cm) and is absent in only 2% of cases. In 15% of cases, it communicates with the joint.

MRI displays the inflamed bursa with low signal intensity on T$_1$-weighted images and high signal intensity on T$_2$-weighted images, with the latter occasionally showing low signal inclusions if it is a long-standing inflammation. The bursal lining can be of variable thickness and enhances. Interpreting the bursae is further complicated by their multifarious manifestations and possible communications with the joint cavity, which cannot always be identified on the MRI image.

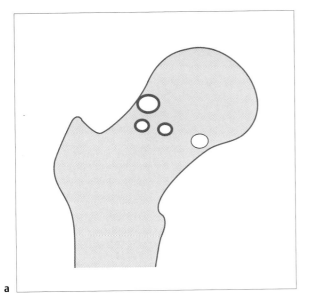

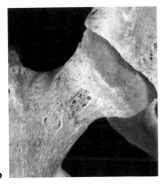

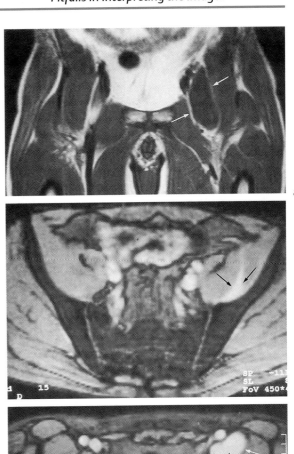

Fig. 6.**27 a, b**   **a** Schematic drawing of the coronal section. Typical location of the defects caused by transcortical synovial herniation in the upper outer quadrant of the femoral neck are shown (bold circles). These defects occur less frequently in the medial inferior aspect (thin circle). It is conceivable that pressure and erosions along the zona orbicularis of the joint capsule perforate the cortex and lead to synovial herniation. **b** The anterior view of an anatomic specimen of the hip. Several round cortical defects are seen in the cranial third of the femoral neck, compatible with openings of transcortical synovial herniations. (By kind permission of Professor Dr H. M. Schmidt, Anatomic Institute of the University of Bonn.)

Fig. 6.**28 a–c**   Rheumatoid arthritis of the hip and visualization of the iliopsoas bursa. **a** Coronal T_1-weighted SE image. **b** and **c** Axial T_2-weighted GRE image. The iliopsoas bursa (arrow) has a low signal intensity on the T_1-weighted SE image, barely demarcating it from the musculature. The vessels are displaced medially by the bursa. The T_2-weighted GRE image shows a high signal in the bursa that is equal to the intensity of the effusion in the hip joint. The axial sections at the level of the hip show the communication (arrowhead) between bursa and hip joint. The bursa extends upward under the iliopsoas and is visualized anterior to the ilium.

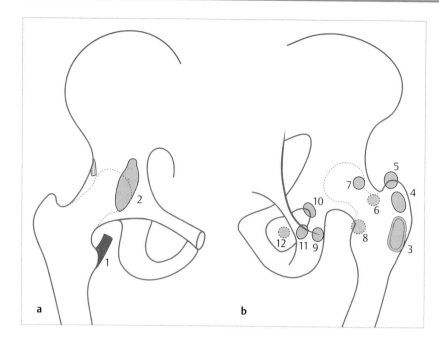

Fig. 6.**29 a, b**   Schematic drawing of the hip, seen from the front (**a**) and from the back (**b**), to illustrate the position of the constant bursae (semicircle) and the facultative bursae (dotted circle) (after 32 and 51).

1 = Attachment of the iliopsoas
2 = Iliopsoas bursa
3 = Subcutaneous and subfascial trochanteric bursae of the gluteus maximus
4 = Trochanteric bursa of the gluteus medius
5 = Trochanteric bursa of the gluteus minimus
6 = Bursa of the obturator internus (attachment) (variable)
7 = Bursa of the piriform muscle
8 = Bursa of the quadratus femoris (variable)
9 = Bursa of the biceps femoris
10 = Bursa of the obturator internus
11 = Ischial bursa of the gluteus maximus
12 = Subcutaneous ischial bursa

References

1 Beltran, J., L. J. Herman, J. M. Burk et al.: Femoral head avascular necrosis: MR Imaging with clinical-pathologic and radionuclide correlations. Radiology 166 (1988) 215–220

2 Beltran, J., C. T. Knight, W. A. Zuelzer et al.: Core decompression for avascular necrosis of the femoral head: correlation between long-term results and preoperative MR staging. Radiology 175 (1990) 533–536

3 Bloem, J. L.: Transient osteoporosis of the hip: MR Imaging. Radiology 167 (1988) 753–755

4 Blomlie, V., H. H. Lien, T. Iversen et al.: Radiation-induced insufficiency fractures of the sacrum: evaluation with MR Imaging. Radiology 188 (1993) 241–244

5 Blümm, R. G., T. H. M. Falke, B. G. Z. des Plantes et al.: Early Legg-Perthes disease (ischemic necrosis of the femoral head) demonstrated by magnetic resonance imaging. Skelet. Radiol. 14 (1985) 95–98

6 Bogost, G. A., E. K. Lizerbram, J. V. Crues: MR Imaging in evaluation of suspected hip fracture: frequency of unsuspected bone and soft-tissue injury. Radiology 197 (1995) 263–267

7 Bongartz, G. E., E. Bock, T. Horbach et al.: Degnerative cartilage lesions of the hip – magnetic resonance evaluation. Magn. Reson. Imag. 7 (1989) 179–187

8 Boos, S., G. Sigmund, P. Huhle: Magnetresonanztomographie der sogenannten transitorischen Osteoporose. Fortschr. Röntgenstr. 158 (1993) 201–206

9 Bos, C. F. A., J. L. Bloem, W. R. Obermann et al.: Magnetic Resonance Imaging in congenital dislocation of the hip. J. Bone Jt Surg. 70-B (1988) 174–178

10 Bos, C. F. A., J. L. Bloem, R. M. Bloem: Sequential Magnetic Resonance Imaging in Perthes' disease. J. Bone Jt Surg. 73-B (1991) 219–224

11 Coleman, B. G., H. Y. Kressel, M. K. Dalinka et al.: Radiographically negative avascular necrosis: detection with MR Imaging. Radiology 168 (1988) 525–528

12 Conway, W. F., W. G. Totty, K. W. McEnery: CT and MR Imaging of the hip. Radiology 198 (1996) 297–307

12a Daenen, B., K. W. Preidler, S. P. Paadmanabhan, J. Bossmann, R. Tyson, D. W. Goodwin, G. Bergmann, D. Resnick: Symptomatic herniation pits of the femoral neck. AJR 168 (1997) 149–153

13 Daffner, R. H., H. Pavlov: Stress fractures: current concepts. Amer. J. Roentgenol. 159 (1992) 245–252

14 Deutsch, A. L., J. H. Mink, A. D. Waxman: Occult fractures of the proximal femur: MR Imaging. Radiology 170 (1989) 113–116

15 Dihlmann, W.: CT analysis of the upper end of the femur: the asterisk sign and ischemic bone necrosis of the femoral head. Skelet. Radiol. 8 (1982) 251–258

16 Egund, N., H. Wingstrand: Legg-Calvé-Perthes disease: imaging with MR. Radiology 179 (1991) 89–92

17 Feldman, F., R. Staron, A. Zwass et al.: MR Imaging: its role in detecting occult fractures. Skelet. Radiol. 23 (1994) 439–444

18 Ficat, R. P.: Treatment of avascular necrosis of the femoral head. Hip 2 (1983) 279–295

19 Gabriel, H., S. W. Fitzgerald, M. T. Myers et al.: MR Imaging of hip disorders. Radiographics 14 (1994) 763–781

20 Genez, B. M., M. R. Wilson, R. W. Houk et al.: Early osteonecrosis of the femoral head: detection in high-risk patients with MR Imaging. Radiology 168 (1988) 521–524

21 Gregg, A., M. D. Bogost, E. K. Lizerbram et al.: MR Imaging in evaluation of suspected hip fracture: frequency of unsuspected bone and soft-tissue injury. Radiology 197 (1995) 263–267

22 Haramati, N., R. B. Staron, C. Barax et al.: Magnetic Resonance Imaging of occult fractures of the proximal femur. Skelet. Radiol. 23 (1994) 19–22

23 Hayes, C. S., W. F. Conway, W. W. Daniel: MR Imaging of bone marrow edema pattern: transient osteoporosis, transient bone marrow edema syndrome, or osteonecrosis. Radiographics 13 (1993) 1001–1011

24 Hodler, J., J. S. Yu, D. Goodwin: MR arthrography of the hip: improved imaging of the acetabular labrum with histologic correlation in cadavers. Amer. J. Roentgenol. 165 (1995) 887–891

25 Hofmann, S., A. Engel, A. Neuhold: Bone-marrow oedema syndrome and transient osteoporosis of the hip. An MRI-controlled study of treatment by core decompression. J. Bone Jt Surg. 75-B (1993) 210–216

26 Jelinek, J., M. Kransdorf, J. Utz et al.: Imaging of pigmented villonodular synovitis with emphasis on MR Imaging. Amer. J. Roentgenol. 152 (1989) 337 – 342

27 Jiang, C. C., T. T. F. Shih: Epiphyseal scar of the femoral head: risk factor of osteonecrosis. Radiology 191 (1994) 409 – 412

28 Johnson, N. D., B. P. Wood, K. V. Jackman: Complex infantile and congenital hip dislocation: assessment with MR Imaging. Radiology 168 (1988) 151 – 156

29 Kottal, R., J. Vogler, A. Matamoros et al.: Pigmented villonodular synovitis: a report of MR Imaging in two cases. Radiology 163 (1987) 551 – 553

30 Kramer, J., S. Hofmann, A. Engel: Hüftkopfnekrose und Knochenmarksödemsyndrom in der Schwangerschaft. Fortschr. Röntgenstr. 159 (1993) 126 – 131

31 Lafforgue, P., E. Dahan, C. Chagnaud et al.: Early-stage avascular necrosis of the femoral head: MR Imaging for prognosis in 31 cases with at least 2 years of follow-up. Radiology 187 (1993) 199 – 204

32 Lang, P., M. Mauz, W. Schörner et al.: Acute fracture of the femoral neck: assessment of femoral head perfusion with gadopentetate dimeglumine-enhanced MR Imaging. Amer. J. Roentgenol. 160 (1993) 335 – 341

32a Lanz, T., W. Wachsmuth: Praktische Anatomie I, 4, 2. Aufl. Springer, Berlin 1959

33 Lee, J. K., L. Yao: Stress fractures: MR Imaging. Radiology 169 (1988) 217 – 220

34 Li, K. C. P., P. Hiette: Contrast-enhanced fat saturation magnetic resonance imaging for studying the pathophysiology of osteonecrosis of the hips. Skelet. Radiol. 21 (1992) 375 – 379

35 Littrup, P., A. Aisen, E. Bruanstein et al.: Magnetic Resonance Imaging of femoral head development in roentgenographically normal patients. Skelet. Radiol. 14 (1985) 159 – 163

36 Markisz, J. A., J. R. Knowles, D. W. Altchek et al.: Segmental patterns of avascular necrosis of the femoral heads: early detection with MR Imaging. Radiology 162 (1987) 717 – 720

37 Miller, I. L., C. G. Savory, D. W. Polly et al.: Femoral head osteonecrosis. Detection by Magnetic Resonance Imaging versus single-photon emission computed tomography. Clin. Orthop. 247 (1989) 152 – 162

38 Mitchell, D. G., H. L. Kundell, M. E. Steinberg et al.: Avascular necrosis of the hip: comparison of MR, CT and scintigraphy. Amer. J. Roentgenol. 147 (1986) 67 – 71

39 Mitchell, D. G., V. M. Rao, M. K. Dalinka et al.: Femoral head avascular necrosis: correlation of MR Imaging, radiographic staging, radionuclide imaging, and clinical findings. Radiology 162 (1987) 709 – 715

40 Mulliken, B. D., D. L. Renfrew, R. A. Brand et al.: Prevalence of previously undetected osteonecrosis of the femoral head in renal transplant recipients. Radiology 192 (1994) 831 – 834

41 Nadel, S. N., J. F. Debatin, W. J. Richardson et al.: Detection of acute avascular necrosis in the femoral head in dogs: Dynamic contrast-enhanced MR Imaging vs spin-echo and STIR sequences. Amer. J. Roentgenol. 159 (1992) 1255 – 1261

42 Neuhold, A., S. Hofmann, A. Engel et al.: Bone marrow edema of the hip: MR findings after core decompression. J. Comput. assist. Tomogr. 16 (1992) 951 – 955

43 Neuhold, A., S. Hofmann, A. Engel: Knochenmarködem – Frühform der Hüftkopfnekrose. Fortschr. Röntgenstr. 159 (1993) 120 – 125

44 Nishii, T., K. Nakanishi, N. Sugano et al.: Acetabular labral tears: contrast-enhanced MR Imaging under continuous leg traction. Skelet. Radiol 25 (1996) 349 – 356

45 Quinn, S. F., J. L. Mc Carthy: Prospective evaluation of patients with suspected hip fracture and indeterminate radiographs: use of T_1-weighted MR Images. Radiology 187 (1993) 469 – 471

46 Rix, J., R. Maas, G. M. Eggers-Stroeder: Legg-Calvé-Perthes. Wertigkeit der MRT in der Frühdiagnostik und Verlaufsbeurteilung. Fortschr. Röntgenstr. 156 (1992) 77 – 82

47 Rosenberg, R., L. Bernd, W. Wrazidlo: Magnetresonanztomographische Optimierung der Hüftknorpeldarstellung durch die Wahl einer T_1-Volumen-Gradienten-Echo-Sequenz und die Anwendung einer Hüftgelenktraktion. Fortschr. Röntgenstr. 163 (1995) 321 – 329

48 Rupp, N., M. Reiser, E. Hipp et al.: Diagnostik und Knochennekrose durch magnetische Resonanz-(MR-)Tomographie. Fortschr. Röntgenstr. 142 (1985) 131 – 137

49 Rush, B. H., R. T. Bramson, J. A. Ogden: Legg-Calvé-Perthes disease: detection of cartilaginous and synovial changes with MR Imaging. Radiology 167 (1988) 473 – 476

50 Scoles, P. V., Y. S. Yoon, J. T. Makley et al.: Nuclear Magnetic Resonance Imaging in Legg-Calvé-Perthes disease. J. Bone Jt Surg. 66-A (1984) 1357 – 1363

51 Senac, M. O., D. Deutsch, B. H. Bernstein et al.: Mr Imaging in juvenile rheumatoid arthritis. Amer. J. Roentgenol. 150 (1988) 873 – 878

51a Sobotta, J.: Atlas der Anatomie des Menschen, Band 2, 20. Aufl. Urban & Schwarzenberg, München 1993

52 Speer, K. P., C. E. Spritzer, J. M. Harrelson et al.: Magnetic Resonance Imaging of the femoral head after acute intracapsular fracture of the femoral neck. J. Bone Jt Surg. 72-A (1990) 98 – 103

53 Steinbach, L. S., R. Schneider, A. B. Goldman et al.: Bursae and cavities communicating with the hip. Radiology 156 (1985) 303 – 307

54 Sugimoto, H., R. S. Okubo, T. Ohsawa: Chemical shift and the double-line sign in MRI of early femoral avascular necrosis. J. Comput. assist. Tomogr. 16 (1992) 727 – 730

55 Tervonen, O., D. M. Mueller, E. L. Matteson et al.: Clinically occult avascular necrosis of the hip: prevalence in an asymptomatic population at risk. Radiology 182 (1992) 845 – 847

56 Totty, W. G., W. A. Murphy, W. I. Ganz et al.: Magnetic Resonance Imaging of the normal and ischemic femoral head. Amer. J. Roentgenol. 143 (1984) 1273 – 1281

57 Turner, D. A., A. C. Templeton, B. Selzer et al.: Femoral capital osteonecrosis: MR findings of diffuse marrow abnormalities without focal lesions. Radiology 171 (1989) 135 – 140

58 Van de Berg, B. E., J. Malghem, M. A. Labaisse et al.: Avascular necrosis of the hip: comparison of contrast-enhanced and nonenhanced MR Imaging with histologic correlation. Radiology 182 (1992) 445 – 450

59 Van de Berg, B. E., J. J. Malghem, M. A. Labaisse et al.: MR Imaging of avascular necrosis and transient marrow edema of the femoral head. Radiographics 13 (1993) 501 – 520

60 Wilson, A. J., W. A. Murphy, D. C. Hardy et al.: Transient osteoporosis: Transient bone marrow edema? Radiology 167 (1988) 757 – 760

Knee

M. Reiser and M. Vahlensieck

Introduction

The knee joint is one of the weight-bearing joints of the human body. The joint-moving levers of the tibia and femur are longer than for any other joint. Furthermore, complex and extensive movements are possible, involving numerous active and passive mechanisms. It is therefore not surprising that the knee is frequently affected by traumatic and degenerative conditions.

Controlled investigations have revealed that the value of clinical examinations was overrated in the past (68), in particular, for the detection of meniscal tears. MRI has been found to be an informative and safe imaging method for the joints, especially for the knee. Today, MRI of the knee is the second most frequently performed MRI after spinal and cerebral MRI. It is often performed to support or reject the indication for arthroscopy. If applied in a meaningful way, it should reduce the number of diagnostic arthroscopies and, at the same time, pave the way for a targeted, therapy-oriented arthroscopy.

Examination Technique

■ Patient Positioning and Coil Selection

The patient is examined supine in the foot first position. The knee is lightly flexed and the leg minimally externally rotated. As for all MRI examinations, the patient should be comfortable and in a position that he or she can maintain without motion for an extended period of time. Even small bumps or a hard surface can cause pain within minutes, invariably leading to undesirable movements by the patient. To avoid vibrations or movements when examining the extremities, small sandbags have been used with success. All manufacturers offer a high-resolution cylindrical coil for the knee. For very obese patients, it may be necessary to use a surface coil, such as the ring coil or the flexible rectangular coil. The joint space should be in the center of the coil. Often, the patella is incorrectly placed in the center, causing an undesirable loss of signal from the distal structures of the knee that are already outside the optimal field of the receiver coil. Points of tenderness or palpable lesions can be marked by taping a vitamin E capsule to the skin.

■ Sequences

Injuries and diseases of the knee usually involve several anatomic structures. The examination strategy should follow both a standard protocol that addresses most clinical questions and specific protocols used selectively for any specific question. The numerous recommendations that have been made are only partially based on empirical data and therefore should not be considered binding.

Most authors recommend coronal and sagittal T_1-weighted and T_2-weighted SE sequences. For the sagittal sections, the leg should be externally rotated 15 to 20 degrees to encompass the anterior cruciate ligament in its entire length and along the axis of its course. As a double echo sequence, the T_2-weighted pulse sequence can also generate proton density images. In one investigation, discrete meniscal tears that were undetectable on T_1-weighted and T_2-weighted images could be depicted only on the proton density weighted images (23). When interpreting the proton density images it must be kept in mind that they are susceptible to the magic angle effect and that not every increase in signal intensity corresponds to a pathologic lesion.

Fast (turbo) SE sequences have no intrinsic disadvantage in comparison to conventional SE sequences as long as it is taken into consideration that they display fat at a higher signal intensity. All things considered, the fast SE technique is superior (120). However, when using sequences with long echo trains and short TEs, as used to image to image the menisci, loss of accuracy due to blurring effects is of concern. As result, short TE FSE sequences for the echo train length should probably not exceed four. Especially for acute injuries, the fat saturated T_2-weighted SE and STIR sequences are superior since they visualize the edematous zones in the bone marrow and soft tissue at high contrast.

The section thickness should not exceed 3–4 mm for SE sequences. The sequential sections should encompass the entire knee, including the peripheral meniscal regions.

For the evaluation of the hyaline articular cartilage, numerous pulse sequences have been recommended. Fat saturated 3-D-GRE techniques give a high contrast between hyaline articular cartilage, intra-articular fluid and fatty tissue. Recht and co-workers (88) achieved the best results with a spoiled GRASS sequence with a TE of 10 msec and a flip angle of 60 degrees.

Eckstein and co-workers (32) found the best signal-to-noise and contrast-to-noise ratios in comparison with other pulse sequences (T1-weighted and T$_2$-weighted sequences, MTC-FISP, DESS) by using a 3-D-FLASH sequence with fat saturation. This also had the highest correlation with the anatomically measured thickness and volume of the cartilage (32, 33, 41). Using the MTC technique, Vahlensieck and co-workers could detect cartilage defects with an exquisite sensitivity (123).

Anatomy

■ General Anatomy

Menisci of the human knee. These are crescentic fibrocartilage laminae (Fig. 7.**1**) that largely compensate for the incongruity between femoral and tibial articular surfaces and protect against points of excessive pressure by distributing the weight uniformly over a wider area. The standing adult transmits 40–60% of the weight through the menisci, reducincing compression of the articular cartilage.

The menisci are 3–5 mm in height peripherally, decreasing to 0.5 mm at the inner free border. Both menisci have an anterior horn and a posterior horn, as well as a pars intermedia constituting the central two-thirds of the meniscus.

Seen from above, the *lateral meniscus* exhibits a largely round configuration. It is attached anteriorly and posteriorly to the anterior and posterior tibial intercondylar area, respectively, and is only loosely fixed to the joint capsule elsewhere. The tendon of the popliteus passes freely through the joint capsule. The posterior horn of the lateral meniscus is unattached where it is passed by the popliteal tendon. The posterior horn of the lateral meniscus can send two ligaments to the medial femoral condyle, which pass posteriorly (posterior meniscofemoral ligament of Wrisberg) or anteriorly (anterior meniscofemoral ligament of Humphrey) to the posterior ligament. Either ligament is found in about 30–40% of cases and both together in about 10%.

The *medial meniscus* has a slightly larger radius and is ovoid or comma-shaped (Fig. 7.**2**). Its width is larger in the region of the posterior horn than in the pars intermedia or anterior horn. The anterior horn is fixed to the anterior intercondylar area of the tibia (Fig. 7.**3**). The pars intermedia is attached to the deep layers of the medial collateral ligament. The anterior horns of both menisci are connected by the meniscofemoral ligament, which forms several components in about 10% of cases.

The menisci consist of fibrocartilage with a large proportion of collagenous fibers containing individual cartilage cells. The stronger collagenous fibers are predominantly peripherally and longitudinally oriented. They are crossed by thinner, radially oriented fibers.

In adulthood, the menisci are poorly vascularized. The capillary loops of the vascularized peripheral zone provide nourishment for the inner avascular meniscal regions.

Anterior cruciate ligament. Its role is the prevention of anterior subluxation of the tibia. It arises from the posterior aspect of the inner surface of lateral femoral condyle and inserts in the anterior intercondylar area, anterolaterally to the anterior intercondylar eminence (Fig. 7.**3**). It is about 35 mm long and about 11 mm thick (57). The anterior ligament consists of three components: the anteromedial, intermediate, and posterolateral bundles. With the knee in extension, the entire ligament is uniformly taut; in flexion, the anteromedial bundle remains taut with the remaining bundles relaxed.

Posterior cruciate ligament. This arises from the inner surface of the medial femoral condyle and inserts at the posterior aspect of the tibia in the posterior intercondylar area. It is considerably stronger than the anterior cruciate ligament. It is about 38 mm long and about 13 mm thick. When the knee is extended, the posterior cruciate ligament is relaxed and exhibits a superoposte-

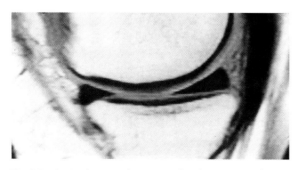

Fig. 7.**1**   Sagittal proton density weighted SE image with visualization of the medial meniscus. Anterior and posterior horns of the meniscus are delineated as signal void triangles.

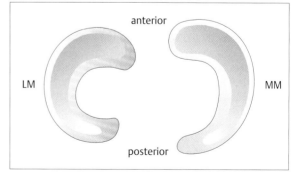

Fig. 7.**2**   Surface view of lateral (LM) and medial meniscus (MM).

Fig. 7.**3** Schematic drawing of the attachment of the menisci and cruciate ligaments to the tibial plateau.

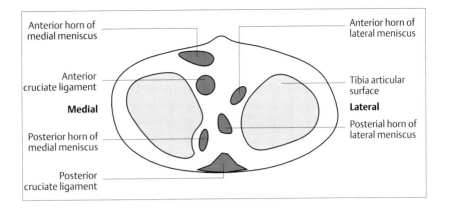

Anterior horn of medial meniscus

Anterior cruciate ligament

Medial

Posterior horn of medial meniscus

Posterior cruciate ligament

Anterior horn of lateral meniscus

Tibia articular surface

Lateral

Posterial horn of lateral meniscus

rior convexity (›boomerang' configuration). In flexion, the posterior cruciate ligament is taut and exhibits a straight course. The anterior (Wrisberg) and posterior (Humphrey) meniscofemoral ligaments respectively pass in front and behind the posterior cruciate ligament.

Medial collateral ligament. This is especially important for the stability of the knee joint. It constitutes a superficial and deep layer (Fig. 7.**4**). It arises from the medial femoral epicondyle and extends to the medial surface of the tibia, about 7.5 – 10 cm distal to the joint space. The deep layer is firmly attached to the pars intermedia of the medial meniscus. Deep and superficial layers are separated by fatty tissue and a bursa.

Lateral collateral ligament. This extends obliquely from the lateral femoral epicondyle posteroinferiorly to the fibular head. The popliteal tendon passes between the lateral meniscus and lateral collateral ligament and inserts at the distal femur laterally.

Extensor mechanism. This comprises the quadriceps muscle and tendon, the patella and the patellar tendon. The quadriceps tendon inserts into the upper pole of the patella. Some fibers continue over the patella and insert as the patellar tendon at the tibial tuberosity. The majority of the fibers of the patellar tendon originate from the rectus femoris.

■ Specific MR Anatomy

The fibrocartilage of the *menisci* contains only a small proportion of free protons and, consequently, is displayed as signal void, regardless of the pulse sequences selected. It should be kept in mind that the somewhat higher signal intensity seen on GRE images should not inevitably be attributed to a pathologic process.

T_1-weighted and proton density-weighted sequences can show artificially increased signal intensities because of the magnetic angle phenomenon (40). Globular and linear meniscal increases in signal intensity can be caused by mucoid degeneration or a tear. The

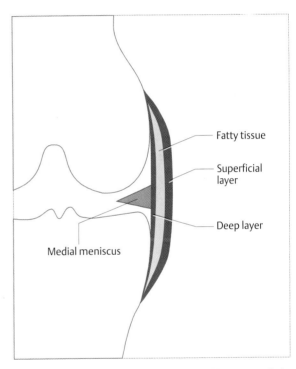

Fatty tissue

Superficial layer

Deep layer

Medial meniscus

Fig. 7.**4** Structure of the medial collateral ligament of the knee.

differentiation and prosposed classifications will be discussed later. Coronal and sagittal sections display the menisci as having a 'bow tie' configuration on the peripheral sections and as signal void triangles on the more central sections (Fig. 7.**5**).

Familiarity with a few anatomic peculiarities is required to avoid misidentifying them as pathologic findings. The transverse ligament connects the anterior horns of both menisci. It is located posterior to Hoffa's fat pad and anterior to the joint capsule. In 22 – 38% of the sagittal sections, a high signal line (Fig. 7.**6**) is seen where the transverse ligament joins the anterior horn of the lateral meniscus (48, 129). This high signal line should not be misinterpreted as a tear in the anterior

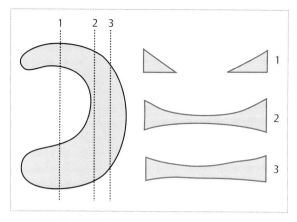

Fig. 7.**5** Schematic drawing showing the sagittal MR visualization of the meniscus in relationship to the sagittal plane.

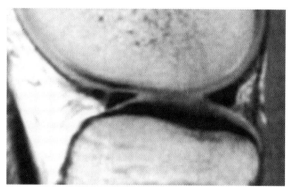

Fig. 7.**6** High signal zone at the junction of the transverse ligament with the anterior horn of the lateral meniscus.

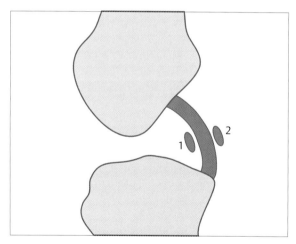

Fig. 7.**7** Sagittal topography of the anterior (1) and posterior (2) meniscofemoral ligaments relative to the posterior cruciate ligaments visualized in cross section.

horn of the lateral meniscus. Review of sequential sagittal sections allows the distinction since the transverse ligament is identified passing medially to its insertion on the medial meniscus. Likewise, the anterior meniscofemoral ligament can mimic a tear where it inserts at the posterior horn of the lateral meniscus (118). In particular, it may be mistaken for a 'bucket handle' tear with a fragment dislodged into the intercondylar space (Fig. 7.**7**).

The tendon sheath of the popliteus tendon is seen as a vertically or slightly obliquely oriented zone of high signal intensity, posteriorly bordering the posterior horn of the lateral meniscus. Unfamiliarity with this situation can lead to the misinterpretation of a vertical tear of the posterior horn of the lateral meniscus or a meniscocapsular separation. Finally, it should be remembered that the pars intermedia of the lateral meniscus is not attached to the lateral collateral ligament to avoid interpreting a signal void zone between the lateral meniscus and ligament as a meniscocapsular separation.

The sagittal sections delineate the *anterior cruciate ligament* in its entire length as long as the knee is 15 – 20 degrees externally rotated. Paracoronal sections angled on the basis of the course of the ligament identified on the sagittal sections are often a useful addition since they can demonstrate the femoral origin of the ligament. The anterior cruciate ligament is depicted as signal-void band, which can exhibit signal intensity, especially in the tibial region because of fatty tissue interposed between individual fiber fascicles. The magic angle phenomenon can also be responsible for higher signal intensities.

The *posterior cruciate ligament* has a homogeneously low signal intensity and is easily identified on sagittal sections. It displays a superoposterior convexity.

The *medial collateral ligament* is seen in its entirety on the midcoronal sections. It exhibits a low signal intensity on all pulse sequences, distinguishing a superficial and deep ligamentous layer. The superficial layer extends from the medial femoral epicondyle to the inner aspect of the tibial metaphysis, 7.5 – 10 cm distal to the joint space. The deep layer of the medial collateral ligament represents an enforcement of the joint capsule and is separated anteriorly from the superficial layer. It is clearly shorter than the superficial layer and extends from the distal aspect of the medial femoral epicondyle to the proximal tibia. It sends fibrous connections to the medial collateral ligament. The deep layer of the medial collateral ligament is not discernible in normal cases. Fatty tissue is usually deposited between superficial and deep layers of the medial collateral ligament.

MRI shows the normal patellar tendon as a straight structure that exhibits a signal void on all sequences (24). Its average AP diameter is 5 mm. With advancing age and increased body weight the patellar tendon may develop an undulating appearance. This has been

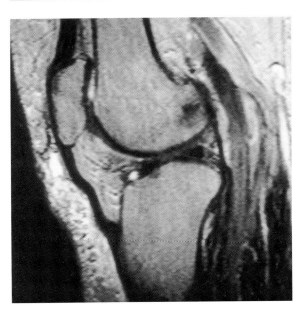

Fig. 7.**8** Marked undulation of the patellar tendon in an asymptomatic female patient without any history of trauma to the knee.

found to be the case in 71% of asymptomatic patients (Fig. 7.**8**).

Schweitzer and co-workers (102) found discrete, V-shaped foci of increased signal intensity in the patellar tendon, located in the proximal end of the tendon in 82% of the cases and in the distal end in 32%. These foci show no further signal increase on the T_2-weighted image in comparison with the proton density-weighted images. It is undetermined whether these high signal foci reflect a clinically undetectable tendon degeneration or the complex internal structure of the patellar tendon.

A variety of pulse sequences have been recommended for visualizing the hyaline articular cartilage (69, 92, 116). Exact anatomic correlations have revealed that fat-suppressed T_1-weighted 3-D-GRE sequences can determine cartilage thickness and volume reliably and reproducibly (31, 33, 34). Using this technique in patients, loss of cartilage and surface alterations can be reliably detected (108). In contrast, heavily T_2-weighted TSE sequences are better able to diagnose structural changes in the hyaline cartilage. Furthermore, magnetization transfer contrast (MTC) and MTC subtraction have been shown to be useful for depicting superficial cartilage defects and intracartilaginous lesions (123).

The hyaline articular cartilage has an intermediate signal intensity on the T_1-weighted SE images. The basal calcified cartilage layers cannot be distinguished from the subchondral bone. On the T_2-weighted images, the hyaline articular cartilage has low signal intensity. The display of the image contrast is variable on the GRE sequences and depends on the examination parameters. Intermediate flip angles (20–40 degrees) are usually recommended for visualization of the hyaline artic-

ular cartilage. In the presence of a joint effusion, heavily T_2-weighted sequences create an 'arthrographic effect,' which can be used diagnostically to demonstrate superficial lesions of the articular cartilage.

The amount of *joint fluid* within the knee is variable and can increase after physiologic stress or athletic activities. A joint effusion should be diagnosed only when visible fluid accumulation in the suprapatellar recess or posterior to the cruciate ligaments (posterior recess) exceeds 10 mm in width on sagittal MR images (42).

Meniscal Lesions

■ Degenerative Changes and Tears

Acute traumatic changes of the menisci result from forced rotation applied to the flexed knee, with resultant longitudinal (bucket handle) or transverse (radial) tears (Fig. 7.**9**). Longitudinal tears follow the dominating

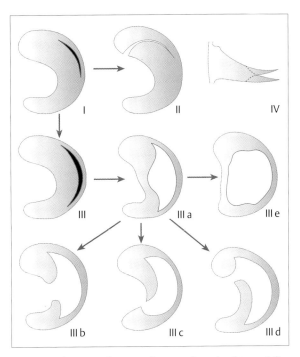

Fig. 7.**9** Schematic drawing of types of meniscal tears (after Jäger and Wirth):

I: Small longitudinal tear
II: Vertical tear
III: Large longitudinal tear and large longitudinal tear with partial (IIIa) and total (IIIe) displacement of the medial fragment (bucket-handle tear)
IIIb-IIId: Complex tears with displaced fragments
IV: Horizontal tear at the superior and inferior surface (fish-mouth tear)

Fish-mouth tears are usually degenerative in nature and only detectable arthroscopically by probing the meniscal surface. Individual tears can be the beginning of other types of tears (arrows).

Table 7.**1**   Classification of increased signal intensities in the menisci (after 72)

Grade	MRI	Histology
0	Triangular signal void, possible increased signal	Normal meniscus
I	One or several punctate or globular increased signals not extending to the articular surface	Mucinous degeneration, magic angle artifact
II	Linear increased signal not extending to the articular surface	Extensive mucinous degeneration or intrameniscal tear
III	Linear increased signal extending to one or both articular surfaces	Tear
IV	Several areas of increased signal as well as deformity and fragmentation	Complex Tear

longitudinal arrangement of the peripheral fibers. Transverse and small tears (fibrillations) occur more frequently centrally or at the inner free edge since here the transverse fibers dominate. Degenerative changes of the meniscus cause loss of elasticity of the collagenous fibers, predisposing them to tears when subjected to trauma. Characteristically, these tears are horizontal or oblique and arise from the inferior meniscal surface.

Several studies comparing the increased signal intensity within the menisci with the pathologic specimen (112) have revealed a correlation between signal pattern and histologic findings (Fig. 7.**10**). Classification of the meniscal signal pattern is based on the findings seen on the T_1-weighted and proton density weighted sequences (Tab. 7.**1**)

In children and adolescents, the central meniscal regions are markedly more vascularized than in adults. Increased signal intensities in these age groups do not have the same meaning as in adults.

Serial examinations have shown that grade II lesions remain stable in the majority of cases and rarely progress to tears or regress (29).

From the visualization of the meniscal tears in the sagittal and coronal planes, the extent and configuration of the tear can be deduced. The pattern of the tear should be described as accurately as possible since this information might be relevant to the therapeutic approach (Tab. 7.**2**). Very thin transverse sections depict the extent of the tears well (Fig. 7.**11**). However, ultrathin sections are not generally required for diagnostic evaluation of the menisci.

Bucket-handle tears result from a vertical or oblique tear that extends along the entire length of the

Table 7.**2**   Morphologic classification of the meniscus tears

Vertical tears	Horizontal tears	Complex tears
Vertical tear	Horizontal cleft	Combination of variable tears (Figs. 7.**16** and 7.**18**)
Peripheral tear	Radial tear	Rounded fragments
Capsulomeniscal separation	Oblique tear (Figs. 7.**14** and 7.**15**)	
Bucket handle tear	Parrot beak tear (Fig. 7.**17**)	

meniscus. The medial segment becomes displaced into the intercondylar space. This medial fragment can be identified in the region of the intercondylar space on contiguous coronal sections.

Bucket-handle tears (Fig. 7.**12**) can display the following signs on MRI:

- double posterior cruciate ligament sign (Fig. 7.**13**),
- flipped meniscus sign,
- detection of a fragment in the intercondylar space (130, 132)

The 'double posterior cruciate ligament' sign refers to the visualization of the medially displaced meniscus segment as a low signal band parallel to and under the posterior cruciate ligament on the sagittal sections. The flipped meniscal sign describes the visualization of the fragment immediately posterior to the anterior

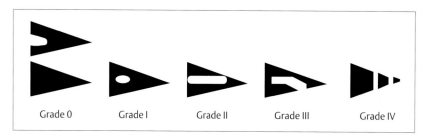

Fig. 7.**10**   Classification of signal alterations in the meniscus (modified after 72).

| Grade 0 | Grade I | Grade II | Grade III | Grade IV |

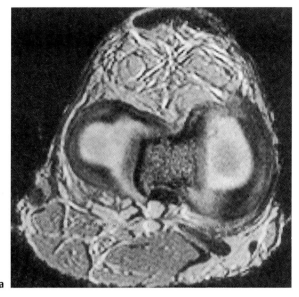
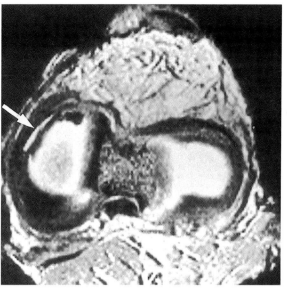

Fig. 7.**11 a, b**   Axial visualization of the meniscus of an anatomic specimen using GRE sequence (TR = 30 msec, TE = 9
msec, flip angle 25 degrees, section thickness 0.7 mm, resolution 0.5 mm). **a** Normal finding. **b** Athrotomically created
longitudinal tear (arrow).

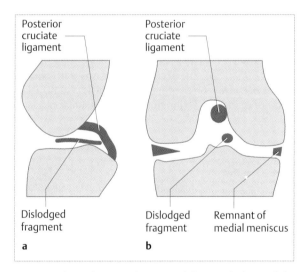
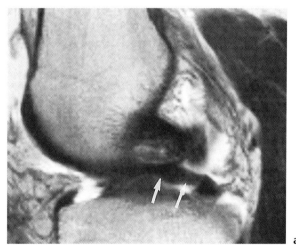

Fig. 7.**12 a, b**   Schematic drawings of the MRI findings of the
bucket-handle tear of the medial meniscus. **a** Sagittal plane.
b Coronal plane.

Fig. 7.**13 a, b**   Sagittal T$_1$-weighted and T$_2$-weighted SE ▶
sequence, showing the 'double posterior cruciate ligament
sign' of a bucket-handle tear of the medial meniscus. A band-
like structure is seen parallel to and beneath the course of the
posterior cruciate ligaments (arrow) corresponding to the medially displaced bucket-handle fragment of the meniscus.

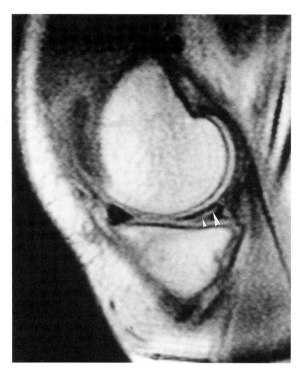

Fig. 7.**14**   Oblique tear in the posterior horn of the medial meniscus. Sagittal T₁-weighted SE sequence. Examination performed with an 0.2 Tesla MR system. The obliquely oriented linear zone of increased signal intensity (arrowhead) extends to the undersurface of the meniscus.

horn, resulting in an apparent magnification of the anterior horn. Bucket-handle tears involve the medial meniscus considerably more frequently than the lateral meniscus. Of course, small fragments of a bucket-handle tear are more difficult to identify than larger fragments.

Peripheral vertical tears can be sutured since this region of the meniscus is vascularized ('red zone'), while this approach has little success if applied to the inner avascular ('white') zone.

Normally, no fluid is detectable between the medial meniscus and the joint capsule. In cases of meniscal capsular separation, the meniscus itself is unremarkably visualized, though fluid is seen between meniscus and joint capsule.

Aside from direct evidence of a tear as linear increase in signal intensity with extension to the meniscal surface, the interpretation of the MRI examination must also consider morphologic changes without associated signal alterations, such as shortening and rounding of the triangular cross section or failed visualization in the normal anatomic position. On sagittal sections, the normal posterior horn of the medial meniscus is clearly larger than the anterior horn. Loss of this difference suggests a bucket-handle tear. The coronal sections show the body of both menisci to be about equal in size. A high diagnostic accuracy can be achieved by using signal alterations of Type III as well as the morphologic changes mentioned previously as criteria for diagnosing meniscal tears (Tab. 7.**3**). The accuracy increases with confirmation of the tear on a second plane and its visualization on more than one section of the same imaging plane.

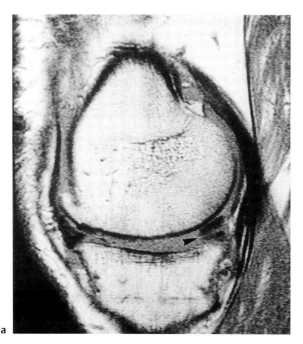

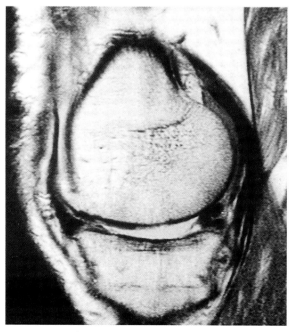

a   b

Fig. 7.**15 a, b**   Posterior horn of the medial meniscus with horizontal tear (arrowhead) and shortening. **a** Sagittal T₁-weighted SE image. **b** Sagittal T₂-weighted SE image.

Table 7.**3** Results of diagnosis of meniscal tears using MRI

Author	Sensitivity		Specifity		Accuracy	
	MM	LM	MM	LM	MM	LM
Jackson *et al.*	98	85	89	99	93	97
Mink *et al.*	97	92	89	91	94	92
Boeree *et al.*	97	96	91	98	94	98
Fisher *et al.*	93	69	84	94	89	88
De Smet *et al.*	93	80	87	93	90	89
Justice and Quinn	96	82	91	98	95	93

MM = medial meniscus LM = lateral meniscus

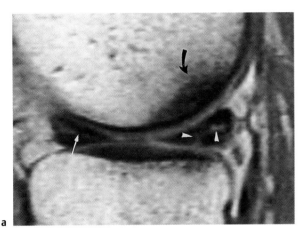

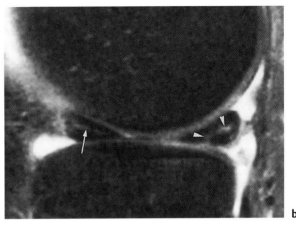

a

b

Fig. 7.**16 a, b**   Grade III lesion of the posterior horn of the medial meniscus and grade II lesion of the anterior horn. **a** Sagittal
T_1-weighted SE sequence. **b** Sagittal T_2-weighted SE sequence
with fat saturation.

Branching increased signal intensity with extension to the surface in the posterior horn of the medial meniscus (arrowheads). Linear increase in signal intensity with extension to the
surface in the anterior horn (arrow). Subchondral decrease in
signal intensity in medial femoral condyle due to osteoarthritis.

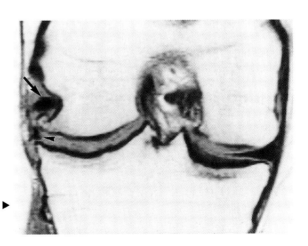

Fig. 7.**17**   Osteoarthritis of the lateral femorotibial compart- ▶
ment with tear near the base of the lateral meniscus (arrowhead) and displaced fragment in the superior recess (arrow).

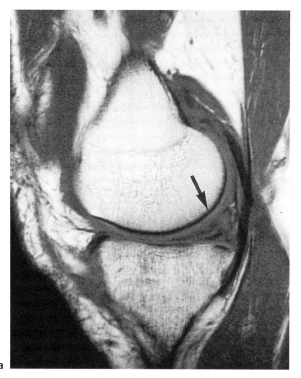 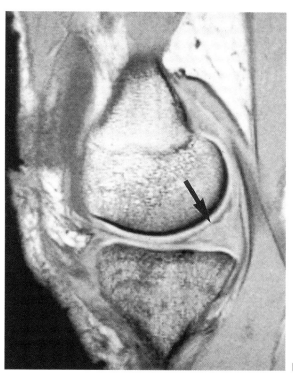

Fig. 7.**18a, b** Complex tear of the medial meniscus following severe trauma to the knee. **a** Sagittal T₁-weighted SE sequence. **b** Sagittal 2-D FLASH sequence. Fragmentation and complete destruction with hemorrhage of the posterior horn of the medial meniscus (arrow).

Conventionally, arthroscopy is used as the standard reference for assessing the precision of MRI, but arthroscopy is an imperfect 'gold standard' with its stated accuracy of 70–98%. In particular, tears of the peripheral meniscus and tears under the surface of the posterior horn of the medial meniscus can escape detection (86). Tolin and Sapega (113) point out that the complete arthroscopy of the posterior horn of the medial meniscus should include a posterior portal in addition to the arthroscopic standard anterior portal.

Possible semantic differences between the descriptive terminology of MRI and arthroscopy may also add to the discrepancies between the technologies. For instance, a free edge abnormality may be described as fraying by the arthroscopist and as small tear by the radiologist (55).

Other causes of false positive MRI interpretations are:

- Vacuum phenomenon,
- Magic angle phenomenon in the lateral meniscus,
- Anatomic variants.

For tears of the lateral meniscus, false negative interpretations outnumber false positive ones, while errors of interpretation are evenly divided between false negatives and false positives for the medial meniscus.

To improve the results of MRI even further, several refinements and improvements of the examination technique have been recommended, such as the in-travenous (124, 131) and intra-articular (4) application of paramagnetic contrast medium or three-dimensional reconstruction of 2-D MR data (30). In particular, axial 3-D GRASS T₂*-weighted images showed a high sensitivity in the diagnosis of radial meniscal tears (5, 70). Radial MRI imaging (87) was found to be statistically equal to sagittal spin-echo imaging in the evaluation of meniscal abnormalities.

■ Postsurgical Changes

Meniscal operations include meniscal suture, partial resection and meniscectomy. In general, solely peripheral tears are *sutured* since healing with ingrowth of granulation tissue can be expected in this location. Long-term grade III signal changes can persist, following conservative therapy and meniscal suture, even in asymptomatic patients. Only if additional changes suspicious for a tear are identified on follow-up examination, a recurrent tear should be considered. Signal changes in terms of a grade III tear are indistinguishable from a healing process with granulation and scar tissue and a renewed tear. New complaints also raise the possibility of a fresh tear at a different site.

Following *partial resection of the meniscus*, an area of central increase in signal intensity without extenion to the surface (type II signal) might be noted at the resection margin. Following surgery it will appear as type III signal change extending to the meniscal surface.

However, it should not be interpreted as a new tear since it represents meniscal degeneration that was present preoperatively.

Frequently, the MR image only reveals a discrete deformity along the meniscal margin following partial resection (Fig. 7.**19**). Without knowledge of any previous surgery, these postsurgical findings are easily overlooked. Intra-articular administration of contrast medium can be useful in diagnosing a new meniscal tear after partial resection or meniscal suture (4). Whether indirect MR arthrography is clinically useful in diagnosing recurrent tears remains to be investigated further.

Following *total meniscectomy*, the meniscus is no longer visualized at its typical location. Cartilaginous calcifications or the vacuum phenomenon, whether as part of pre-existing osteoarthritis or a gradually progressing post-operative osteoarthritis, can be visualized as signal void and as such might be mistaken for meniscal remnants or post-operatively developing free intra-articular bodies. The post-operative development of osteoarthritis is characterized by progression of osteoarthritic signs, such as cartilaginous lesions, osteophytes, subchondral cysts, and sclerosis.

As with all surgical interventions, open meniscectomies have corresponding skin changes and can have susceptibility artifacts caused by metallic and osseous chips left behind.

■ Discoid and Ring Meniscus

Discoid menisci are morphologic variants caused by the persistence of central portions of the meniscal disks after the fetal period. Complete and incomplete forms as well as a rare ring form can be distinguished. The prevalence is about 3% for the lateral meniscus and 0.1–0.3% for the medial meniscus.

A discoid meniscus may lead to a loud snapping sound heard with flexion or extension of the knee. Otherwise, the discoid meniscus is asymptomatic. Discoid menisci, however, are susceptible to premature degeneration and tears and become symptomatic at that point.

MRI generally can diagnose a discoid meniscus unequivocally, when the characteristic deviations from the normal morphologic findings are displayed. A height differential of 2 mm is evident also between discoid menisci and normal menisci of the same knee (106).

■ Meniscal Cysts and Parameniscal Cysts

Parameniscal cysts are fluid accumulations in the region of the meniscal capsular interface. They are generally associated with horizontal or complex meniscal tears (Fig. 7.**20**). In contrast, meniscal ganglion cysts are not necessarily associated with a damaged meniscus. Medial meniscal cysts are frequently eccentric, because of the meniscal attachment along the medial collateral ligaments, and larger than lateral cysts. This means that

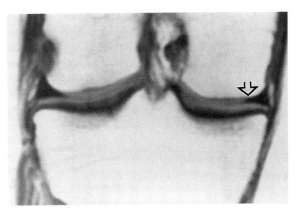

Fig. 7.**19** S/P partial resection of the medial meniscus. Coronal T_1-weighted SE image. The medial meniscus border is blunted (arrow).

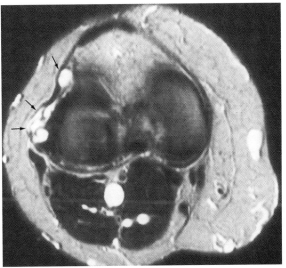

a

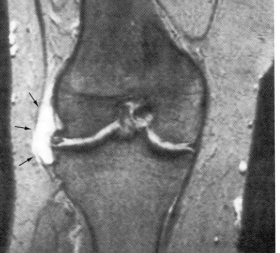

b

Fig. 7.**20a, b** Parameniscal cysts, arising from a markedly deformed and hyperintense lateral meniscus and protruding in a lobular fashion beneath the collateral ligament and the patellar retinaculum. High signal intensity of the parameniscal cyst (arrow) on **a** axial and **b** coronal T_2-weighted SE images.

they are not at the immediate level of the underlying tear. Meniscal cysts have a high recurrence rate following resection. MRI shows meniscal cysts and ganglion cysts with fluid-equivalent signal intensities. Parameniscal cysts often display a stalk toward the meniscus. Meniscal ganglion cysts, in contrast, are not connected with the articular cavity.

Injuries of the Cruciate Ligaments

Anterior cruciate ligament. Tears of the anterior cruciate ligament (ACL) are frequently accompanied by tears of the medial collateral ligament and injuries to the joint capsule. Isolated tears of the ACL are rare. The

accuracy of clinical diagnosis is stated to be relatively high (sensitivity: 75–95%, specificity 95–100%). Lee and Yao (68) reported a sensitivity of 87% and a specificity of 89% for clinical tests. In acute injuries, the clinical examination can be markedly compromised (51).

MRI can diagnose tears of the ACL by applying direct and indirect criteria. The constellation of findings depends on the nature of the tear, whether it is acute or chronic, partial or complete (Fig. 7.**21**).

The *direct signs* of a tear of the ACL are discontinuity or absence of the ligament in its anatomic position in the lateral intercondylar space (Fig. 7.**22** and 7.**23**), wavy or irregular contour of the ligament, and displacement of the tibial and femoral ligamentous components. Frequently, the tibial remnant of the ligament assumes

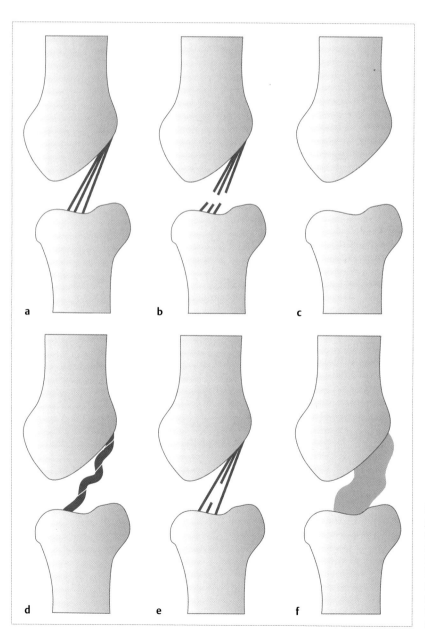

Fig. 7.**21 a–f**   Schematic drawing of abnormalities of the anterior cruciate ligament. **a** Normal. **b** Gap in the ligament. **c** Absent delineation in expected anatomic position. **d** Tortuous course with focally increased signal intensity. **e** Focally increased signal intensity. **f** Thickening and diffuse increase in signal intensity.

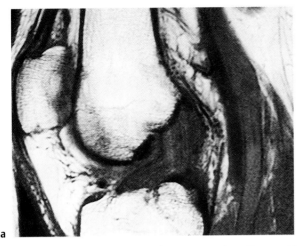
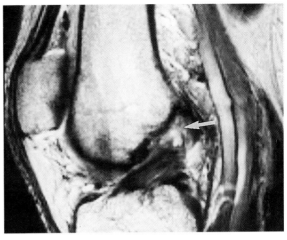

Fig. 7.**22 a, b**   Anterior cruciate ligament tear in a 49-year-old female patient. **a** Sagittal T$_1$-weighted SE sequence. **b** Sagittal T$_2$-weighted SE sequence.
Tear of the anterior cruciate ligament close to the femoral attachment. The tibial remnant has assumed a flattened course.

In particular, a definite increase in signal intensity (arrow) is seen in the tear adjacent to the femur on the T$_2$-weighted image. The T$_1$-weighted image shows a low signal structure throughout the intercondylar space and posterior joint capsule, barely discernible from ligamentous remnants.

an almost horizontal position. In acute injuries, the T$_2$-weighted image shows a diffuse or focal increase in signal intensity within and around the ligament, as well as an indistinct outline and thickening of the ligament (Fig. 7.**24**) (119). The direct signs of the tear have a stated sensitivity of 93% and specificity of 97% (3, 68, 91, 94, 126). Fat saturated T$_2$-weighted and STIR sequences show these changes with an exquisite contrast. As manifestation of an associated capsular injury, increased signal intensity might be observed in the soft tissues posterior to the articular cavity.

The *indirect signs* of a tear of the ACL include the increased angulation or buckling of the posterior cruciate ligament (Figs. 7.**25**– 7.**27**) and the 'uncovered lateral meniscus' sign due to the posterior displacement of the lateral meniscus relative to the posterior cortical margin of the tibial plateau. These changes reflect anterior instability and essentially are based on the anterior displacement of the tibial plateau compared with the femoral condyles (114). A distance of more than 5 mm between the vertical lines drawn tangentially to the posterior cortical margins of the lateral femoral condyle and tibial plateau suggests a complete tear of the ACL (Figs. 7.**28** and 7.**29**).

In acute injuries of the ACL, subchondral bone bruises are frequently observed in the mid portion of the lateral femoral condyle and in the posterolateral portion of the tibial plateau (Fig. 7.**30**) (56 a, 20 a). They are caused by transient subluxation and impaction of the medial portion of the lateral femoral condyle on the posterolateral tibial plateau. Aside from subchondral bone bruises, osteochondral and chondral compression fractures can occur in the lateral femoral condyle. Subchondral bone bruises are exquisitely displayed on fat saturated T$_2$-weighted SE images and on STIR images (98). Occasionally, a focal bone bruise can also be de-

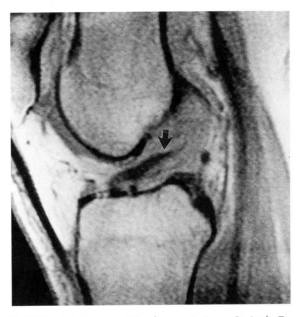

Fig. 7.**23**   Anterior cruciate ligament tear. Sagittal T$_1$-weighted SE sequence obtained with a 0.2 Tesla MRI system dedicated for imaging extremities. The tibial remnant of the anterior cruciate ligament is displaced inferiorly (arrow). Relatively low signal intensity next to the femoral attachment of ligaments in the posterior aspects of the joint capsule of the knee.

tected next to the attachment of the anterior cruciate ligament (Tab. 7.**4**).

With tears of the ACL, the patellar tendon may exhibit focal areas of increased signal intensity, more frequently localized in its tibial than patellar aspect.

In the majority of cases, direct signs can establish the diagnosis of a tear of the anterior cruciate ligament.

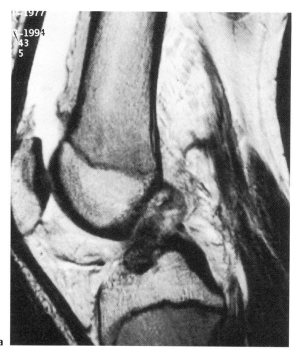
a

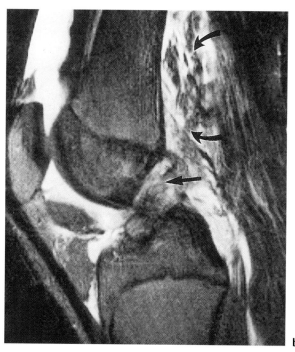
b

Fig. 7.**24 a, b** Severe knee trauma in a 17-year-old patient with complex internal derangement of the knee. **a** T₂-weighted TSE sequence. **b** T₂-weighted TSE sequence with fat saturation. Extensive effusion in the knee joint and suprapatellar recess. Fluid accumulation in the soft tissues posterior to the popliteal fossa and the distal femora (curved arrows) as evidence of a capsular lesion. Acute tear of the anterior cruciate ligament with swelling, irregular outline, and heterogeneous signal. In particular, the femoral aspect of the ligament shows a definite increase in signal intensity and a gap in the ligamentous structures (arrow). The heterogeneity of the signal distribution in the anterior cruciate ligaments is most conspicuous on the fat saturated image.

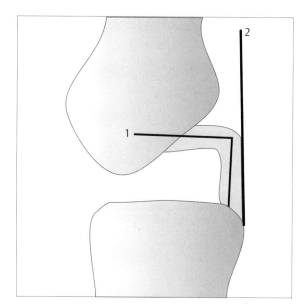

Fig. 7.**25** Changes in the posterior cruciate ligament as indirect sign of a tear of the anterior cruciate ligament.
1 = Reduced angle of the posterior cruciate ligament (normal: about 123 degrees; with a tear of the anterior cruciate ligament: about 106 degrees).
2 = The posterior cruciate ligament line does not transect the distal femur (within the distal 5 cm).

Indirect signs are rarely taken as exclusive evidence of a torn anterior cruciate ligament, but are valuable confirmation of the diagnosis and increase the level of confidence. Robertson and co-workers (98) analyzed a total of 22 different MRI signs of tear of the anterior cruciate ligament and gave the following signs the highest predictive value (in decreasing order):

- Disruption of the anterior cruciate ligament,
- Disruption of individual fascicles,
- Bone bruise in the posterolateral tibial plateau,
- Buckled posterior cruciate ligament,
- Failure of the posterior cruciate ligament line to intersect the distal femur within 5 mm

Aside from sagittal sections with external rotation of the leg, oblique coronal sections parallel to the ACL are helpful, in particular if other findings are inconclusive and a partial tear is suspected (Fig. 7.**32**) (49). Close to the femoral origin of the ACL, a partial volume effect can cause false positive or false negative findings on the sagittal sections, requiring further evaluation with oblique coronal sections. Axial sections may also be useful in the evaluation of the ACL particularly at its insertion into the lateral femoral condyle. Here it is normally well seen on axial sections and its absence (the so-called 'empty notch sign') is suggestive of an ACL tear.

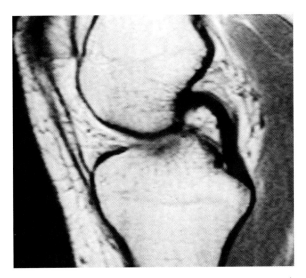

Fig. 7.**26** Rupture of the anterior cruciate ligament. Moderately increased angulation of the posterior cruciate ligament.

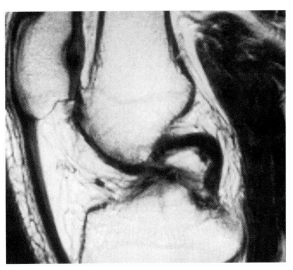

Fig. 7.**27** Rupture of the anterior cruciate ligament. Marked angulation of the posterior cruciate ligament.

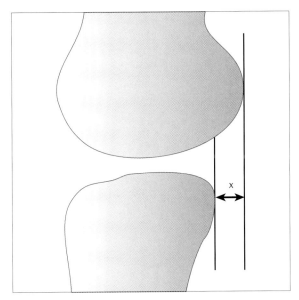

Fig. 7.**28** Interior displacement of the tibial plateau as indirect sign of a rupture of the anterior cruciate ligament (x < 5 mm favors a tear).

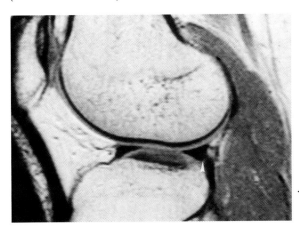

Fig. 7.**30** Patient with a tear of the anterior cruciate ligament. Sagittal T$_2$-weighted SE sequence with fat saturation. The section through the lateral femoral condyle shows bone bruises in the medial aspect of the femoral condyle (arrowhead), as well as in the dorsal aspect of the tibial plateau (arrow), considered an indirect sign of a tear of the anterior cruciate ligament.

◀ Fig. 7.**29** Tear of the anterior cruciate ligament. Posterior displacement of the posterior horn of the lateral meniscus (arrowhead).

Table 7.**4**   Sensitivity of indirect signs (Fig. 7.**31**) of the anterior cruciate tear (42)

	Normal	Acute	Chronic	Sensitivity	
				Acute	Chronic
ACL angle	55 degrees	30.7 degrees	27.2 degrees	87	100
Angle between ACL and Blumensaat line	– 1.6 degrees	26.6 degrees	27 degrees	87	100
Bone bruise	NA	NA	NA	76	100
Posterior PCL line	NA	NA	NA	45	76
PCL angle	123 degrees	109 degrees	95 degrees	42	84
Posterior displacement of the lateral meniscus	0.5	2.1	5.1	30	76
Anterior translocation of the tibia (anterior drawer sign)	2.2	5.4	8.7	27	61

ACL angle =	Angle between tangent to the anterior ACL and the tibial plateau
Angle between ACL and Blumensaat line =	Angle between tangent to the anterior ACL and the Blumensaat line
Posterior PCL line =	Line drawn along the posterior PCL to intersect the medullary cavity within 5 cm of the distal femur
PCL angle =	Angle between lines through the center of the proximal and distal portion of the PCL
Posterior diaplacement of the lateral meniscus =	Posterior displacement of the posterior cortex of the tibial plateau
Anterior translocation of the tibia (anterior drawer sign) =	Distance between tangent to the posterior cortex of the lateral femoral condyle and tangent to the posterior cortex of the tibial plateau

NA = not applicable
ACL = anterior cruciate ligament
PCL = posterior cruciate ligament

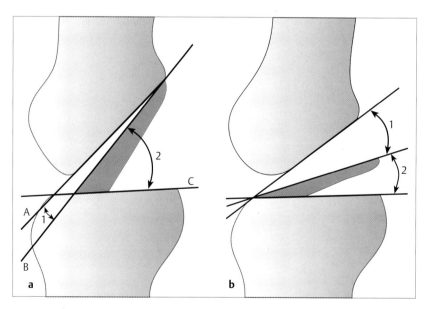

Fig. 7.**31 a, b**   Indirect signs of a tear of the anterior cruciate ligament. **a**
A = Tangent to the Blumensaat line
B = Tangent to the anterior contour of the anterior cruciate ligament
C = Tangent to the contour of the tibial plateau
1 = Angle between anterior cruciate ligament and Blumensaat line
2 = Anterior cruciate ligament

b Tear of the anterior cruciate ligament
1 = The angle between the anterior cruciate ligament and the Blumensaat line normally measures about 1.6 degrees; with an anterior ligament tear it is positive and measures > 26 degrees.
2 = The anterior cruciate ligament angle, which normally measures about 55 degrees, is markedly reduced to about 30 degrees.

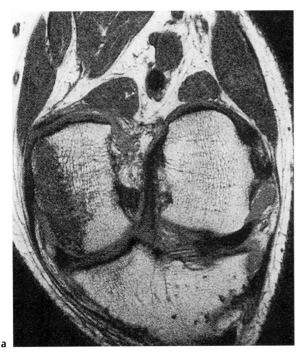

a

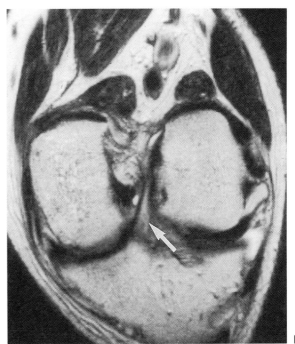

b

Fig. 7.**32a, b**   Partial tear of the anterior cruciate ligament. Oblique coronal sections parallel to the course of the anterior cruciate ligament. **a** T$_1$-weighted SE sequence. **b** T$_2$-weighted SE sequence.
The T$_1$-weighted image shows an extensive bone contusion with decreased signal intensity in the region of the medial femoral condyle. This bone marrow contusion is not seen on the T$_2$-weighted image. Increased signal intensity, especially in the tibial aspect of the anterior cruciate ligament, is best appreciated on the T$_2$-weighted sequence (arrow). The continuity of the ligament is preserved.

Detecting a partial tear of the ACL is clinically relevant since partial tears can progress to a complete tear and predispose to subsequent knee instability. These severe sequelae can be avoided through early surgical intervention (101).

On MRI, partial tears of the ACL are characterized by the following findings (117):

- Increased intrasubstance signal intensity with definable intact ligamentous fibers in continuity between femoral and tibial attachments,
- Bowing and undulating contour of the otherwise intact anterior cruciate ligament,
- Nonvisualization of the anterior cruciate ligament on the T$_1$-weighted image with concomitant discernible intact fibers seen on either STIR or GRE image,
- Absence of secondary signs of a complete anterior cruciate ligament tear.

In particular, no anterior subluxation of the tibia greater than 5 mm is a reliable additional sign for excluding a complete tear of the ACL (20).

The MRI diagnosis of a partial ACL tear has been found to be difficult. The reported sensitivity of 40–75% and specificity of 62–89% are not sufficient to establish the diagnosis and to direct treatment (117).

Posterior Cruciate Ligament. Tears of the posterior cruciate ligament (PCL) are considerably less frequent than tears of the anterior cruciate ligament. The following trauma mechanisms (Fig. 7.**33**) are common:

- Direct force on the proximal and anterior portion of the tibia while the knee is bent, displacing the tibia posteriorly; this injury usually causes a tear in the mid portion of the ligament and a tear of the posterior joint capsule,
- Hyperextension; this is frequently accompanied by an osseous avulsion of the tibial insertion of the posterior cruciate ligament,
- Severe abduction and adduction with rotatory component.

Using an anterior portal, arthroscopic detection of injuries of the PCL can be difficult when the anterior ligament is intact (74). Frequently, these injuries are combined with complex damage to the remaining internal structure, particularly to the posterolateral capsular complex and the collateral ligaments, resulting in a marked instability.

In general, MRI can unequivocally diagnose PCL tears, and the criteria applied are essentially the same as those used for diagnosing anterior cruciate ligament tears (Figs. 7.**34** and 7.**35**) (43, 110). Bone contusions in the anterior tibial plateau are frequent indirect evidence of acute tears of the posterior cruciate ligament (Fig. 7.**36** and Tab. 7.**5**) (56).

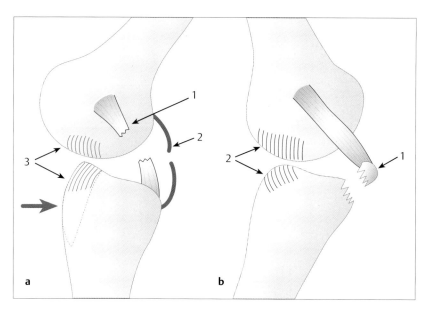

Fig. 7.**33 a, b** Trauma mechanisms and pattern of findings seen with a posterior cruciate ligament tear.
a Force acting on the proximal tibia with the knee flexed.
1 = Tear of the posterior cruciate ligament at its mid portion.
2 = Tear of the posterior joint capsule.
3 = Bone marrow contusion in the anterior aspect of the tibial plateau and (lateral) femoral condyle.
b Hyperextension injury
1 = Osseous avulsion of the tibial attachment of the posterior cruciate ligament.
2 = Bone marrow contusions in the anterior aspect of the tibial plateau and femoral condyles.

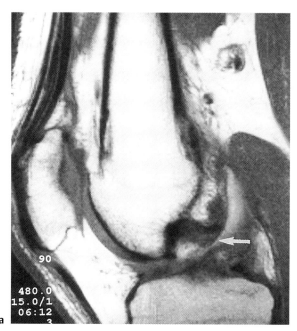

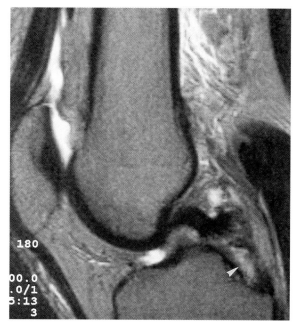

Fig. 7.**34 a, b** Tear of the posterior cruciate ligament. **a** Sagittal T₁-weighted SE sequence. **b** Sagittal T₂-weighted SE sequence.

Gap in the posterior cruciate ligament near its tibial attachment (arrow). Definite increased signal intensity in the region of the attachment of the posterior cruciate ligaments, especially on the T₂-weighted image (arrowhead).

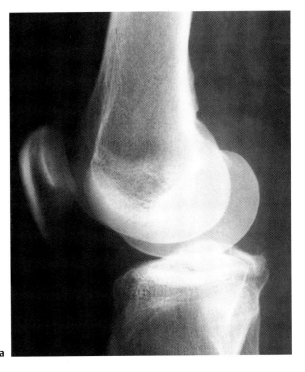

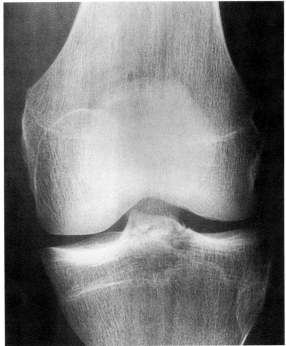

a

b

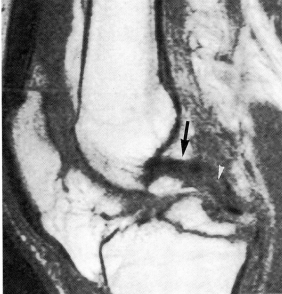

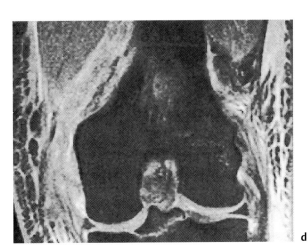

c

d

Fig. 7.**35a–d**   Osseous avulsion of the posterior cruciate ligament involving both intercondylar spines. **a**, **b** AP and lateral radiographs. **c** Sagittal T₁-weighted image. **d** Coronal GRE image.

The course of the posterior cruciate ligament (arrow) approaches the horizontal plane. The tibial aspect of the posterior cruciate ligament is thickened and irregular in outline and shows a definite increase in signal intensity (arrowhead). Extensive edema and hemorrhage in the periarticular soft tissues.

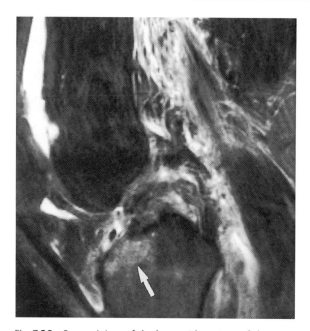

Fig. 7.**36** Severe injury of the knee with rupture of the anterior and posterior cruciate ligaments. Sagittal T_2-weighted SE sequence with fat saturation. Irregularly oriented ligamentous remnants are seen in the intercondylar space. Extensive fluid accumulation in the popliteal fossa and posterior to the distal femur as evidence of an injury of the posterior joint capsule. Bone bruise in the anterior aspect of the tibia (arrow).

Table 7.**5**   Injuries associated with the posterior cruciate ligament (n = 47) (after 110)

Associated injury	Incidence (%)
Joint effusion	64
Bone contusion	36
Medial meniscus	32
Lateral meniscus	30
Medial collateral ligament	23
Anterior cruciate ligament	17
Lateral collateral ligament	6

■ Postsurgical Changes of the Cruciate Ligament

Torn cruciate ligament can be repaired by ligament reconstruction or by autoplastic or alloplastic grafts. A potential donor site is the patellar tendon. The most common technique of ACL reconstruction involves drilling tunnels into the femoral condyle and tibial plateau. Bone plugs attached to each end of the graft are then inserted into these tunnels and secured with interference screws. MRI occasionally displays multiple focal signal voids caused by osseous or metallic chips, as well as by the metallic screws. The tunnels are seen as signal voids and can be assessed for orientation and angulation with the same approach used for radiographic views. The reconstructed ligament is visualized as a low

signal intensity structure on all sequences. In addition, focal or linear areas of increased signal intensity are observed, attributed to fibrous or, at least in part, fatty tissue and should not be mistaken for a new tear (21, 100). A wavy contour to the ligament reconstruction may be a normal postsurgical finding. The detection of a ligamentous gap is a definite sign of renewed tear.

Injuries of the Collateral Ligaments

Complex injuries of the knee frequently involve the collateral ligaments as well as the posterior joint capsule (50, 54). The clinical examination cannot reliably distinguish between a tear of the medial meniscus and an isolated injury of the medial collateral ligament. The injuries of the collateral ligaments (Fig. 7.**37**) can be graded on the basis of severity:

- Grade 1: sprain with local tenderness, no instability,
- Grade 2: partial tear of the ligament; local tenderness, opening of the medial joint space with valgus stress,
- Grade 3: complete tear of the ligament, definite instability.

The medial collateral ligament is considerably more frequently injured than the lateral ligamentous structures. The injuries are caused by excessive valgus stress during flexion. In general, the deep structures of the medial collateral ligament tear first, accompanied by a meniscocapsular separation of the medial meniscus. Tears are far more frequent in the femoral portion of the medial collateral ligament, occasionally extending to the level of the joint space. They are rarely found in the tibial aspect.

Coronal T_2-weighted images are best suited for the MRI evaluation of tears of the collateral ligament (134). Depending on the severity of the injury, the following findings (Figs. 7.**38**– 7.**41**) can be encountered (103):

- Indistinctly outlined local increase in signal intensity in the medial collateral ligaments (edema, hemorrhage),
- Discontinuity of the ligament, wavy ligamentous contour, avulsion of the osseous attachments,
- Lost demarcation between collateral ligament and subcutaneous fatty tissue,
- Bone bruise in the medial femoral condyle (Fig. 7.**42**) or in the tibial tableau.

It is important that associated injuries, such as a tear of the anterior cruciate ligament, meniscocapsular separation and bone bruises in the lateral aspect of the tibia and femur, are searched for. Tears of the anterior cruciate ligaments are frequently accompanied by torn medial collateral ligaments.

In about one-quarter of patients, bone bruises were observed in the medial aspect of the tibia and femur adjacent to the collateral ligament attachments. These are best recognized on fat saturated T_2-weighted SE and STIR images.

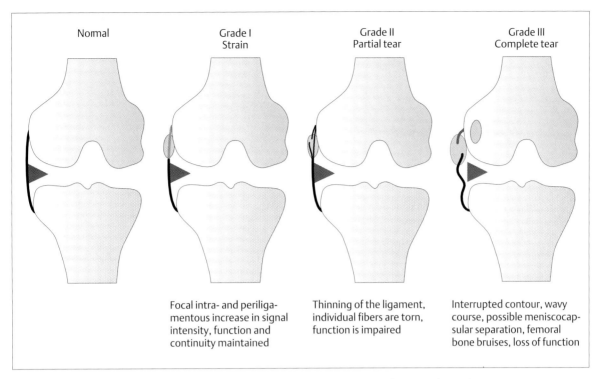

Fig. 7.**37**   Schematic drawing of the injuries of the collateral ligaments as seen on the coronal MRI plane.

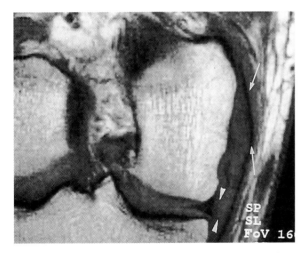

Fig. 7.**38**   Coronal T_1-weighted SE sequence. Damaged deep layer of the medial collateral ligament. Low signal zone (arrowheads) between meniscal base and medial collateral ligament, as well as low signal zone around the ligament.

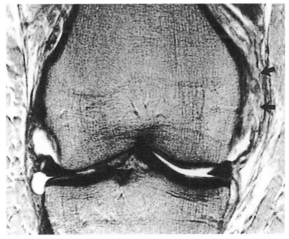

Fig. 7.**39**   Coronal T_2-weighted SE sequence. The medial collateral ligament is complete, frayed, and thickened with irregularly increased signal intensity (arrow).

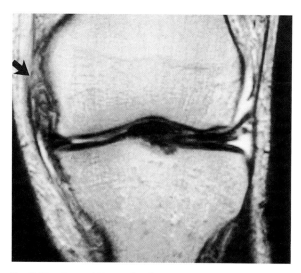

Fig. 7.**40**   Coronal T$_2$-weighted SE sequence. Tear of the medial collateral ligament, which is thickened, with its femoral aspect no longer discernible (arrow). Increased signal intensity in the region of the course of the medial collateral ligament.

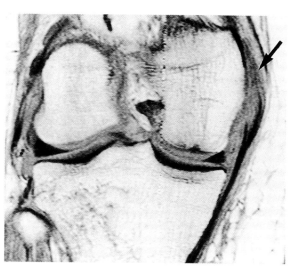

Fig. 7.**41**   Coronal proton density-weighted SE image. Complete tear of the medial ligament with avulsion of the ligament from its femoral origin (arrow).

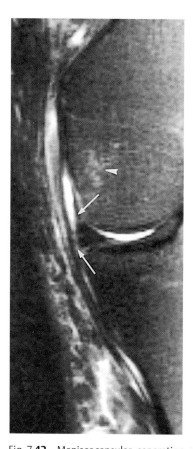

Fig. 7.**42**   Meniscocapsular separation with damage of the deep layers of the medial collateral ligament. Zone of increased signal intensity (arrows) between the base of the medial meniscus and the collateral ligament, which itself is surrounded by increased signal intensity. Subtle bone marrow edema in the medial aspect of the femoral condyle (arrowhead).

Comparing clinical findings and MRI grading of medial collateral ligament (MCL) injuries, Schweitzer and co-workers (103) reported that grading of MR appearances was not accurate for the classification of MCL injury. They found that the most sensitive signs of medial collateral ligament tears included fascial edema and loss of sharp demarcation of the ligament from adjacent fat. The authors discovered a frequent association with bone bruises and hypothesize that the medial bone bruises may be a manifestation of microavulsions. Yao and co-workers (134) could correctly classify the grade of severity in 87% of cases of medial collateral ligament injuries (Tab. 7.**6**).

Injuries of the lateral collateral ligament are considerably less frequent than those of the medial collateral ligaments and are caused by excessive varus stress. The MRI findings correspond to those of the medial collateral ligament injuries.

Table 7.**6**   Signs of injuries of the medial meniscus at MRI (103)

	Sensitivity (%)	Specificity (%)
Proximal discontinuity	7	98
Distal discontinuity	12	100
Internal signal intensity	31	98
Adjacent subcutaneous edema	57	96
Adjacent fascial edema	76	96
Bone bruise (medial)	53	95

Dyskinesias of the Femoropatellar Articulation and Patellar Dislocations

As a sesamoid bone, the patella glides over the trochlear groove of the femur. Disturbances of these gliding motions may lead to retropatellar pain, chondromalacia and, after several years, osteoarthritis. Numerous morphologic and functional conditions leading to these disturbances are known. The morphologic causes, such as incongruence of the cartilaginous joint facets, which normally consist of a small medial facet and a large lateral facet, are manifestations of patellar dysplasia, horizontal and vertical dystrophia and trochlear dysplasia. They are not further discussed here since they are adequately visualized on radiographic views. MRI, however, can visualize the resultant cartilaginous damage.

Functional disturbances of tracking (dyskinesia). To some extent, the underlying abnormalities can be detected on tangential radiographs obtained at 30, 60, and 90 degrees flexion. However, subluxation or excessive pressure frequently occur between 0 and 30 degrees of flexion, precluding radiographic detection. Cinematographic MRI examinations have become increasingly important in these situations. The following syndromes are distinguished:

- *Lateral subluxation syndrome*: with minimal flexion, the lateral facet of the patella overlaps the lateral aspect of the femoral trochlea (Figs. 7.**43** and 7.**44**).
- *Excessive lateral pressure syndrome*: the lateral facet of the patella moves toward the femoral condyle without evidence of subluxation.
- *Medial subluxation syndrome*: the patella is medially displaced and overlaps the medial femoral trochlea.
- *Lateral-to-medial subluxation syndrome*: with increasing flexion of the knee, the patella starts in a laterally displaced position and moves medially, subluxing over the medial trochlea.

Patellar misalignment can be classified by tracking abnormalities of the patella, such as the position of the patella relative to the femoral trochlear groove (105), and by static quantitative criteria (patellar tilt angle, bisect offset, extent of lateral displacement) (15, 81).

Dyskinesias can be treated conservatively (strengthening training of the vastus lateralis and medialis) or surgically (retinaculum incision).

Patellar Dislocation. Following a traumatic patella dislocation, which usually reduces spontaneously, MRI can demonstrate typical constellations of findings (58, 127): tear of the opposite retinaculum, serous or hemorrhagic joint effusion, subchondral contusion, focus of the contusion on the contralateral patella facet (for instance, medial patellar contusion found after lateral dislocation) and bone contusion of variable size in the ipsilateral femoral condyle.

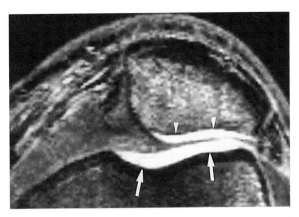

Fig. 7.**43** Fat saturated 3-D FLASH sequence. Hypoplasia of the medial patellar facet and lateral subluxation of the patella. High signal intensity of the retropatellar (arrowhead) and femoral (arrows) articular cartilage.

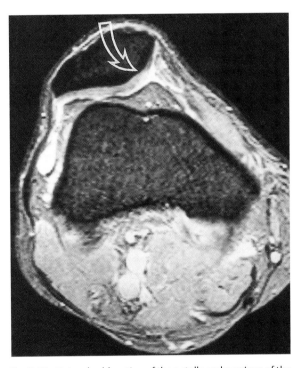

Fig. 7.**44** Lateral subluxation of the patella and erosions of the cartilage (curved arrow) in the region of the medial patellar facet. Axial T$_2$-weighted GRE image. Examination performed with the knee in 5 degree flexion.

Lesions of the Patellar Tendon

The patellar tendon represents the ligamentous connection between patella and tibial tuberosity and is the continuation of the quadriceps tendon. Some anterior fibers extend over the patellar surface and are firmly attached to it. A posterior group of the fibers insert directly at the patellar apex.

Patellar tendinitis (jumper's knee) usually develops at the patellar insertion of the tendon. The tendinitis is thought to result from chronic overuse and typically occurs in track and field athletes and in joggers. The clinical findings of this overuse damage include localized pain at the inferior patellar apex during as well as after athletic activities, point tenderness on palpation, quadriceps atrophy, partial or complete tear of the patellar tendon with a palpable tendon gap, impaired function of the quadriceps muscles, and high position of the patella. The diagnosis is generally made clinically and may be confirmed sonographically. However, MRI is also a useful investigation for this condition, and is particularly helpful at distinguishing patellar tendinitis from other causes of anterior knee pain such as patellofemoral osteoarthritis, chondromalacia or plica syndrome resulting from an infrapatellar plica. MRI visualizes the normal patellar tendon on midsagittal sections as a low signal structure that usually decreases somewhat in signal in a caudal direction. The thickness of the normal tendon should not exceed 7 mm.

Patellar tendinitis may produce the following findings:

- Increased thickness exceeding 7 mm immediately inferior to the patellar apex,
- Increased signal intensity on all sequences, most often located at the posterior aspect of the proximal tendon,
- Indistinct margin, especially posterior to the thickened area,
- Decreased signal intensity in Hoffa's fat pad on the T_1-weighted image,
- Equal signal intensity on T_2-weighted and contrast-enhanced images (associated Hoffa's disease) (Fig. 7.**45**).

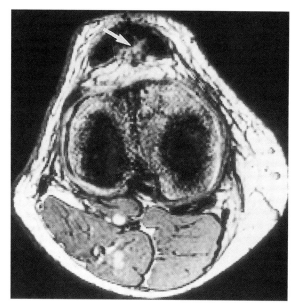

Fig. 7.**45**   Tendinitis of the patellar tendon, which is thickened and displays areas of increased signal intensity centrally and posteriorly (arrow).

Complete tear of the tendon is shown as a discontinuity of the tendon, a tortuous course of the residual distal fibers and high position of the patella (13, 35, 76).

If a joint effusion is present, the normal patellar tendon exhibits a wavy course. This is even more pronounced in patients with a torn anterior cruciate ligament since the tibia is frequently displaced anteriorly. This changes the angle of the patellar tendon insertion at the tibial tuberosity and the distance between the patella and the tibial tuberosity (102).

The painful avascular necrosis of the apophysis of the tibial tuberosity in childhood (Osgood-Schlatter disease) can be associated with a distal patellar tendinitis. This presents as indistinct swollen distal tendon with increased signal intensity, particularly on the T_2-weighted and fat suppression image.

Cartilaginous Lesions

Damage to the hyaline articular cartilage occurs with osteoarthritis, chondromalacia, inflammatory joint diseases and osteochondral injuries.

Chondromalacia Patellae. Chondromalacia patellae is a degenerative condition of the articular cartilage of the patella, characteristically occurring in adolescents and young adults. In this age group it is the most frequent cause of knee pain. Shahriaree (104) identifies four stages of chondromalacia patellae on the basis of arthroscopic findings:

- Stage I: softening of the articular cartilage due to broken vertical collagenous fibers,
- Stage II: blister formation in the articular cartilage due to the separation of the superficial from the deep cartilaginous layers,
- Stage III: ulceration and fragmentation of the surface of the articular cartilage,
- Stage IV: crater formation and eburnation of the exposed subchondral bone.

T_1-weighted fat saturated 3-D GRE (SPGR) sequences are especially suitable for evaluating the altered surface of the patellar cartilage (Fig 7.**46**). Furthermore, this technique can accurately measure cartilage thickness. Direct MR arthrography using intra-articular gadolinium has also proved useful in evaluating the surface of the cartilage.

T_2-weighted FSE sequences with fat saturation are also useful in the diagnosis of chondromalacia patellae. They reveal changes to the internal structure of the cartilage as focally globular or linearly increased signal intensity (Figs. 7.**47** and 7.**48**). In comparison with arthroscopy, MRI can detect chondromalacia patellae with a sensitivity of 86%, a specificity of 74%, and an accuracy of 81% (75).

Chondral and Osteochondral Injuries. These occur when the cartilage is subjected to strong shearing, rotatory or tangential forces, whereby the injury can be confined to the hyaline articular cartilage (chondral lesions) or extend through the cartilage to the underlying subchondral bone (osteochondral trauma). The subchondral bone can be impacted or fragmented with partial or complete detachment of the fragment (Fig. 7.**49**). The chondral and osteochondral injuries are often associated with changes of the subchondral bone marrow, referred to as bone bruises and characterized by an 'edema pattern' (see Chapter 7, bone marrow contusion of the knee).

Degenerative Osteoarthritis. This is characterized by asymmetric thinning of the hyaline articular cartilage. In advanced osteoarthritis, all compartments of the knee (medial and lateral femorotibial articulation, patellofemoral articulation) may be involved, with the severity of the changes being variable. As a weight bearing joint, the knee is frequently affected by osteoarthritic changes.

Conventional radiography is usually adequate to establish the diagnosis. Characteristic changes are joint space narrowing, subchondral sclerosis, osteophytes, and subchondral cysts. In preparation for prosthetic knee replacement, some orthopedic surgeons perform pre-operative arthroscopy to obtain detailed information about the status of the knee joint. For this indication, MRI can be considered a non-invasive alternative.

MRI allows reproducible assessment of the cartilaginous thickness and the detection of focal cartilaginous erosions (Figs. 7.**50**– 7.**52**). Where radiography shows involvement of only one or two joint com-

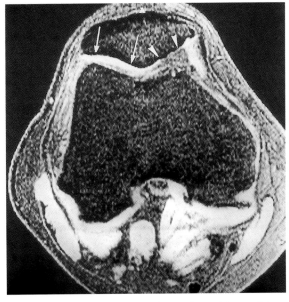

Fig. 7.**46**   Ulceration of the articular cartilage of the medial patellar facet. Axial fat saturated FLASH sequence. High signal intensity of the hyaline articular cartilage (arrows). Broad-based ulcerations involving the medial patellar facet (arrowhead).

partments, MRI frequently reveals bicompartmental or tricompartmental disease (Figs. 7.**53**– 7.**54**) (19). Thin MRI sections also demonstrate more osteophytes and subchondral cysts than conventional radiographs. The osteophytes often exhibit a normal bone marrow signal. The subchondral sclerosis that extends from the joint margin into the bone marrow is characterized by low

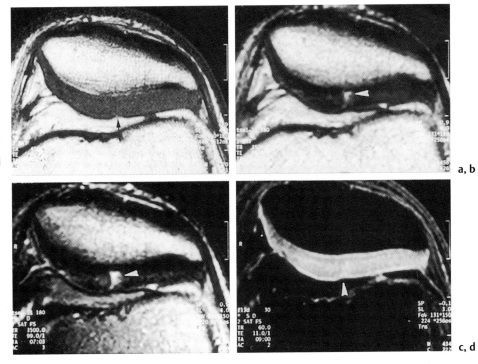

Fig. 7.**47 a – d**   Deep fissures of the articular cartilage of the lateral patellar facet. **a** The T$_1$-weighted SE sequence only shows a subtile irregularity along the surface of the cartilage (arrow). **b** The heavily T$_2$-weighted SE sequence delineates a zone of increased signal intensity that extends to the subchondral bone (arrowhead). **c** Fat saturated T$_2$-weighted SE sequence. Heterogeneous and incomplete fat saturation. The increase in signal intensity in the region of the lateral patellar facet (arrowhead) is better visualized due to improve contrast. **d** 3-D FLASH sequence with fat saturation (TR = 60 msec, TE = 11 msec, flip angle 30 degrees). The fissure in the region of the lateral patellar facet (arrowhead) is barely discernible.

a, b

c, d

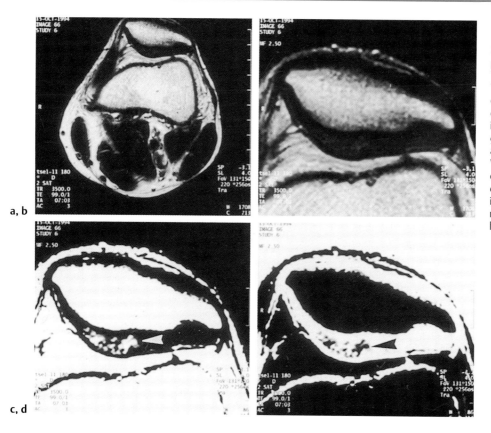

Fig. 7.**48 a–d** Structural changes in the articular hyaline cartilage. Retropatellar articular cartilage. T_2-weighted SE sequence. With the standard setting of the CRT display, only a discrete increase in signal intensity is noted in the region of the patellar crest and lateral patellar facet. With the CRT display changed to a narrow window setting, the increase in signal intensity becomes more conspicuous (arrowhead).

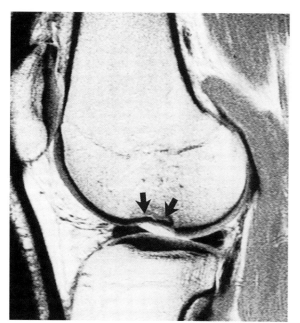

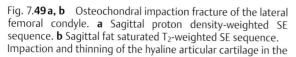

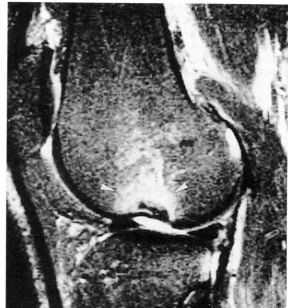

Fig. 7.**49 a, b** Osteochondral impaction fracture of the lateral femoral condyle. **a** Sagittal proton density-weighted SE sequence. **b** Sagittal fat saturated T_2-weighted SE sequence. Impaction and thinning of the hyaline articular cartilage in the region of the lateral femoral condyle (arrows). Subchondral bone marrow edema with low signal intensity on the proton density image and high signal intensity on the fat saturated T_2-weighted image (arrowheads).

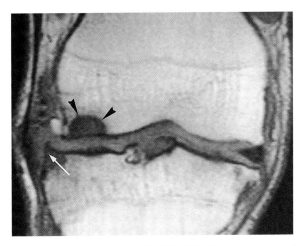

Fig. 7.**50** Severe osteoarthritis of the lateral compartment of the knee joint. Coronal proton density-weighted SE image. Marginal osteophytes (arrows). Joint space narrowing and subchondral cysts (arrowheads).

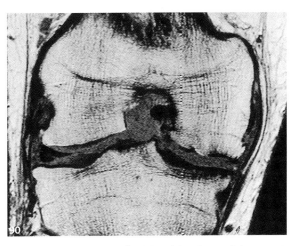

Fig. 7.**51** Severe osteoarthritis involving the medial compartment of the knee. Coronal T_1-weighted SE sequence. The medial meniscus is no longer identifiable. An oblique tear is identified laterally, extending to the undersurface of the meniscus. The hyaline articular cartilage, especially of the medial femoral condyle, is completely destroyed.

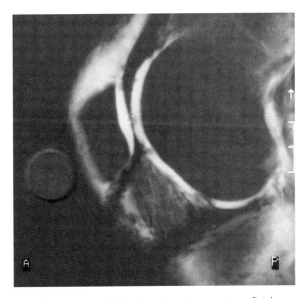

Fig. 7.**52** Sagittal MTC subtraction image. Superficial cartilaginous erosions in the region of the femoral articular cartilage.

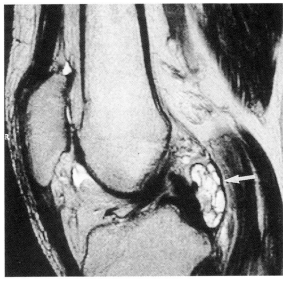

Fig. 7.**53** Sagittal T_2-weighted SE sequence. Severe thinning of the retropatellar articular cartilage. Minimal retropatellar effusion. With this examination technique, the hyaline cartilage has low signal intensity, rendering it indistinguishable from subchondral bone. In addition, a posterior intra-articular ganglion (arrow) is visualized.

signal intensity within the high signal intensity bone marrow, best seen on the T_2^*-weighted GRE sequences, which are especially sensitive to altered susceptibility. In patients with osteoarthritis, Bergmann and co-workers (9) found low to intermediate signal intensity in the subchondral bone on T_1-weighted and T_2-weighted images, displaying a hemispheric configuration and corresponding to bone marrow replacing fibrous tissue. In addition, trabecular thickening was detected.

Patients with severe osteoarthritis of the knee are often found to have associated internal joint derangements involving the menisci, primarily the posterior horn of the medial meniscus, and the ACL.

Hemophiliac Arthropathy. MRI can detect damage to the cartilage manifest as focal cartilaginous erosions, diffuse thinning, or complete loss of cartilage (Fig. 7.**55**). Furthermore, MRI can detect synovial proliferations

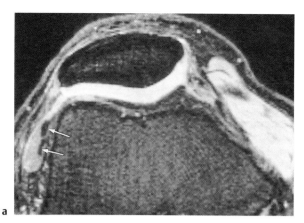

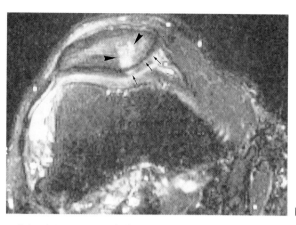

Fig. 7.54 a, b   Severe chondromalacia patellae. **a** Axial fat saturated 3-D FLASH image. High signal intensity of the retropatellar articular cartilage, which is of normal thickness. Two low signal areas are seen in the lateral articular cavity (arrows), corresponding to loose intra-articular bodies. **b** Axial T$_2$-weighted SE image with fat saturation. The medial patellar facet shows definite cartilaginous damage (arrow) and the patellar bone marrow an extensive edematous zone (arrowhead).

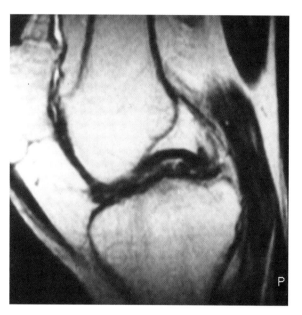

Fig. 7.55   Sagittal T$_2$-weighted SE image of hemophiliac osteoarthropathy of the knee. Severe damage of the retropatellar cartilage and evidence of impaired osseous growth.

found in hemophilic arthropathy secondary to recurrent intra-articular hemorrhage. Because of hemosiderin deposition, these synovial proliferations are of low signal intensity on T$_1$-weighted and T$_2$-weighted SE images. On the T$_2^*$-weighted GRE image, the hemosiderin-induced susceptibility artifact can cause excessive loss of signal (Fig. 7.56).

Cartilaginous and Osseous Erosions in Rheumatoid Arthritis. These are better visualized on MRI than by conventional radiography (8). This is attributed to the tomographic nature and the inherent high contrast resolution of MRI.

Bone Marrow Edema

Only after the introduction of MRI, *bone contusions* have been identified and this has offered new insights into understanding osseous pathology. On the one hand, bone contusions frequently explain otherwise unclear post-traumatic changes; on the other, they can support an otherwise suspected internal joint derangement.

Bone contusions (bone bruising) represent trabecular microfractures with edema and hemorrhage into the bone marrow. The histologic confirmation is rarely obtained. In one case of bone marrow biopsy during surgical cruciate ligament reconstruction, the bone marrow was found to contain edema with hemorrhage. MRI shows a characteristic 'edema pattern': decreased signal intensity on the T$_1$-weighted and increased signal intensity on the T$_2$-weighted image (Fig. 7.57). T$_2$-weighted fast spin-echo sequences with fat saturation and fast spin-echo STIR sequences are superior to conventional sequences for the diagnosis of bone marrow contusion (Fig. 7.58) (6, 121, 122). The fat saturated T$_1$-weighted sequences also show a pronounced contrast enhancement.

Osseous contusions can occur after direct blunt trauma or after a complex trauma that might include capsular and ligamentous derangement (Fig. 7.59). Following blunt trauma, bone marrow edema develops at the site of the impact. Capsular and ligamentous injuries produce a typical distribution pattern of bone marrow edema. In about half of the cases of acute anterior cruciate ligament tears, an edematous zone is detected in the lateral femoral condyle and in the posterior lateral aspect of the tibial plateau (73, 79, 133). In acute injuries of the posterior cruciate ligament, bone marrow edema is seen in the anterior aspect of the tibial plateau and in the femoral condyles.

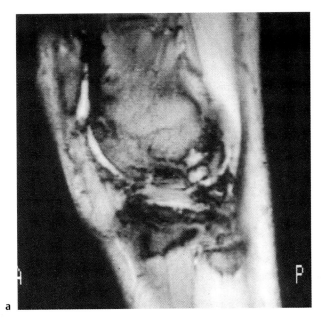

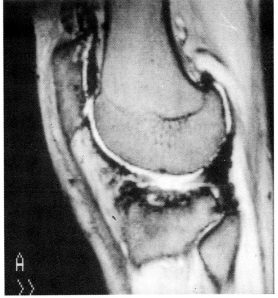

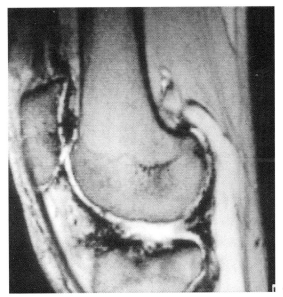

Fig. 7.**56 a–c** Hemophiliac arthropathy of the knee. T_2^*-weighted GRE images. The iron deposits in the synovial membrane induce extensive susceptibility changes with signal voids.

When Virolainen and co-workers performed MRI on 25 patients with acute dislocation of the patella, they found bone bruises in the lateral femoral condyles in all patients, in the medial aspect of the patella in eight and in the lateral aspect of the tibial plateau in two patients (127). In all cases, the medial retinaculum was injured with disruption of the fibers at or near the site of patellar attachment. All patients had a hemarthrosis. Osteochondral and chondral lesions could not be reliably detected at MRI.

Subchondral bone marrow edema is also observed in chondral and osteochondral injuries. While geographic distributions frequently lead to early osteoarthritis (125), changes confined to a reticular pattern can be expected to heal completely without sequelae (Fig. 7.**60**).

Occult fractures, i.e., fractures that are not recognized on technically adequate radiographs, can be reliably recognized on MRI. Aside from the fracture lines, the diagnosis is suggested by the edema pattern.

Recognizing bone marrow contusions has important therapeutic ramifications. Adequate immobilization can prevent permanent osteochondral damage or progression to overt fractures. Osseous contusion usually resolves within 6 to 8 weeks.

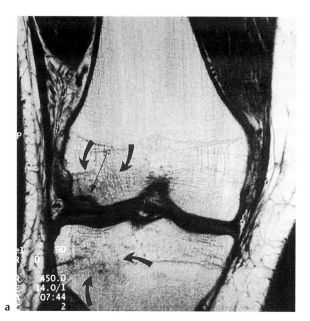
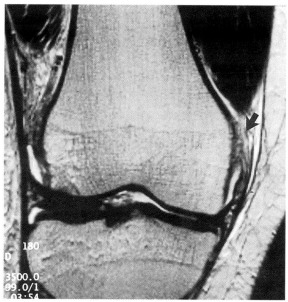

Fig. 7.**57 a, b**   Lesion of the medial collateral ligament and bone contusion in the region of the lateral femoral condyle and tibia. **a** Coronal T$_1$-weighted SE sequence. **b** Coronal T$_2$-weighted SE sequence.

On the T$_2$-weighted image, the femoral aspect of the medial collateral ligament shows increased signal intensity and a ligamentous gap (thick arrow). On the T$_1$-weighted image, the

lateral femoral condyle exhibits a subchondral area of decreased signal intensity (long arrow) as well as a reticular pattern of decreased signal intensity in the adjacent areas of the tibial plateau and femoral condyles (curved arrow). The T$_2$-weighted image shows the subchondral osseous changes as barely discernible subtle increases in signal intensity.

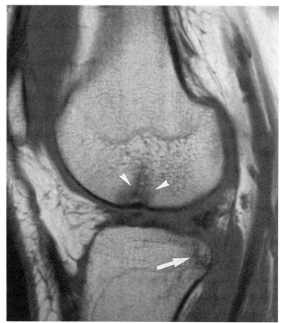
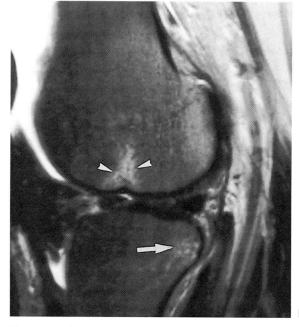

Fig. 7.**58 a, b**   Patient with an anterior cruciate ligament tear and areas of contusion in the lateral femoral condyle (arrowhead) and lateral aspect of the tibial plateau (arrow). **a** Sagittal T$_1$-weighted SE sequence. **b** Sagittal T$_2$-weighted SE sequence with fat saturation.

These sagittal sections through the lateral aspect of the knee show the signal intensity of the contusions to be low on the T$_1$-weighted image and high on the fat saturated T$_2$-weighted SE image.

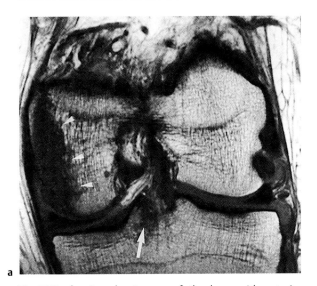
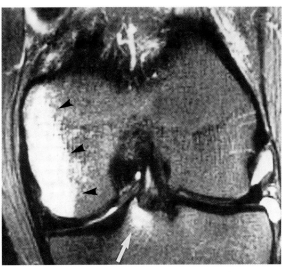

a b

Fig. 7.**59 a, b** Complex trauma of the knee with anterior cruciate ligament tear and areas of contusion in the medial femoral condyle (arrowhead) in the region of the medial inter-condylar spine (arrow). **a** Low signal intensity of the contusions on the coronal T_1-weighted SE image and **b** high signal intensity on the T_2-weighted fat saturated image.

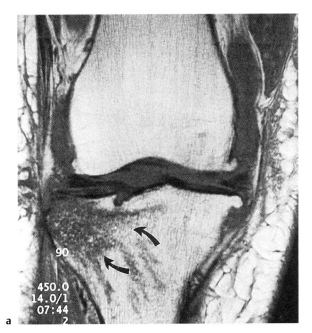
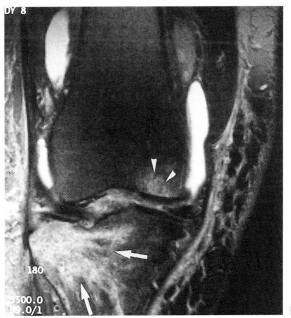

a b

Fig. 7.**60 a, b** Contusion in the region of the lateral tibial condyle. Large joint effusion. Low signal intensity in the region of the massive osseous contusion (arrows and curved arrows) on the **a** T_1-weighted SE image and **b** high signal intensity on the fat saturated T_2-weighted image. The T_2-weighted image also shows an additional subchondral contusion in the lateral femoral condyle (arrowhead).

Osteochondritis Dissecans and Avascular Necroses

Osteochondritis Dissecans. The etiology of osteochondritis dissecans is not definitely established. Etiologies that are considered include recurrent trauma, focal ischemia, and impaired normal ossification. Early detection and treatment of osteochondritis dissecans is prognostically relevant since otherwise this condition can lead to early osteoarthritis. Adolescents constitute by far the largest patient group affected by osteochondritis dissecans. In the knee, osteochondritis dissecans has a predilection for the intercondylar aspect of the medial femoral condyle (71).

The therapeutic approach is determined by the condition of the hyaline articular cartilage and the stability of the osteochondral fragment (77). The *staging* proposed by Clanton and DeLee (22) has been modified by Kramer and co-workers to incorporate the characteristic MRI findings (64) (Fig. 7.**61** and Tab. 7.**7**).

The type I lesion of osteochondritis dissecans is characterized by a lentiform or oval subchondral decrease in signal intensity on the T_1-weighted image. Since the covering articular cartilage is intact, no changes can be detected arthroscopically. The conventional radiograph is also normal. The type II lesion has an area of subchondral bone demarcated by a signal void line (Fig. 7.**62**). The type III lesion can be demonstrated arthroscopically and is seen on MRI as a circumscribed disruption of the cartilaginous layer and partial separation of the fragment. This can be accompanied by small cysts in the underlying subchondral bone. Synovial fluid and contrast medium, at MR arthrography, can penetrate into the space between the necrotic fragment and the osseous crater (Fig. 7.**63**).

The type IV lesion is completely separated from the osseous crater and encircled by fluid (25). Finally, the type V lesion has left the crater and is seen as loose body in distant regions within the articular cavity. Unenhanced MRI achieves a sensitivity of 92% and a specificity of 90% in differentiating between stable and unstable necrotic fragments.

The signal intensity of the necrotic fragment varies relative to the signal in the normal bone marrow, primarily depending on its content of fatty tissue, sclerosis and edema (Fig. 7.**64**). In general, higher stages have a proportionate decrease in signal intensity, correlating to the increasing density observed radiographically. The fat saturated T_2-weighted SE and STIR images occasionally show extensive bone marrow edema around the donor site (Fig. 7.**65**).

Some authors recommend the examination with intravenous or intra-articular contrast enhancement.

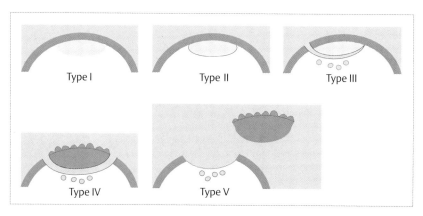

Type I   Type II   Type III

Type IV   Type V

Fig. 7.**61**   Types of osteochondritis dissecans (modified after 64).

Table 7.**7**   Staging of osteochondritis dissecans (after 22, 64)

Type	MRI	Arthroscopy/arthrotomy	Therapy
I	Subchondral area of decreased signal intensity	Unremarkable	Immobilization
II	Demarcation	Unremarkable	Drilling
III	Cartilaginous defect, partial separation, cysts	Cartilaginous defect, partial separation	Drilling, curettage, internal fixation (pins)
IV	Cartilaginous defect, complete separation, cysts	Cartilaginous defect, complete separation	Curettage, drilling, resection, transplantation
V	Loose intra-articular body	Loose intra-articular body	Removal of the loose body, transplantation

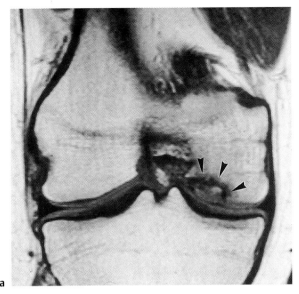

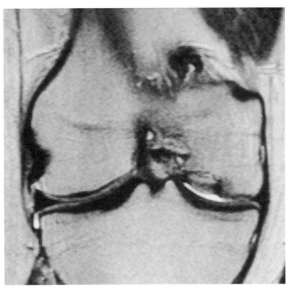

a

b

Fig. 7.**62 a, b** Osteochondritis dissecans of the medial femoral condyle. **a** Coronal T$_1$-weighted SE image. The necrotic fragment shows a decreased signal intensity and is demarcated from the bone marrow by a sclerotic rim (arrowhead).

b Coronal T$_2$-weighted SE image. The signal intensity of the fragment corresponds to the bone marrow. The high signal joint effusion does not extend between the fragment and the osseous crater. Irregular outline of the cartilage surface.

Enhancement of the zone along the junction between the necrotic fragment and osseous crater suggests fibrous bridging with fixation of the fragment (1). MR arthrography can assess the cartilage overlying the osteochondritis dissecans exactly and differentiate between partial and complete separation of the osteocartilaginous fragment, improving the staging accuracy in comparison to unenhanced MRI (62).

Spontaneous Osteonecrosis of the Femoral Condyle (Ahlbäck Disease). This condition affects the medial femoral condyle predominately and occurs in middle aged and older patients (2). Characteristically, and in contrast to osteochondritis dissecans, the weight-bearing aspects of the femoral condyles are affected. The patients complain of sudden onset of severe pain, often long before radiographic changes are detectable.

With progression of the disease, a subchondral radiolucent line appears in the affected femoral condyle, which becomes increasingly flattened and osteoarthritically deformed. Associated tears of the medial meniscus are often observed.

MRI can establish the diagnosis early and can also estimate the size of the necrotic area (66). The prognosis is poor if the width of the lesion multiplied by its length is over 5 cm^2 or if the ratio between the transverse width of the lesion and the width of the affected condyle is over 0.4 (11).

The T$_2$-weighted image shows a band-like or lentiform subchondral area of decreased signal intensity. The T$_2$-weighted images, particularly when used with fat saturating pulse sequences, and the STIR images frequently display an extensive indistinctly demarcated

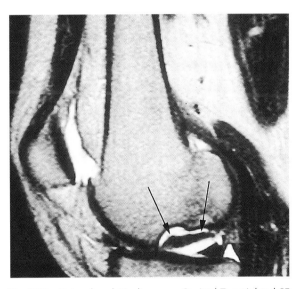

Fig. 7.**63** Osteochondritis dissecans. Sagittal T$_2$-weighted SE image. The fragment has left the crater. Its signal intensity is decreased. Fluid is seen between osseous crater and fragment (arrows).

increase in signal intensity in the adjacent bone marrow. Even the soft tissues can show extensive edematous zones.

Additional Osteonecroses in the Region of the Knee. These conditions are summarized in Table 7.**8**. The changes in signal intensity found in these relatively rare conditions correspond to the changes described earlier.

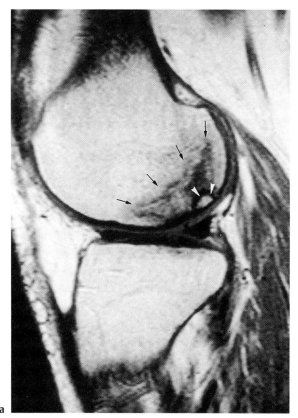

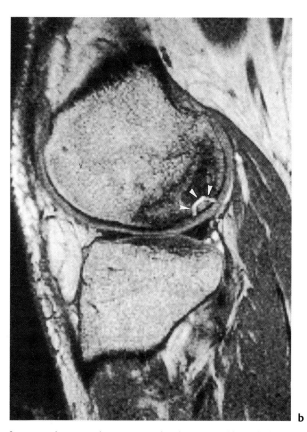

Fig. 7.**64a, b**   Corticosteroid-induced necrosis of the femoral condyles with the development of an osteochondritis dissecans. **a** Sagittal T_1-weighted SE image. The necrosis of the femoral condyle is visualized as an irregularly outlined area of decreased signal intensity (arrows). The osseous fragment has fat-equivalent signal intensity and is demarcated by a dark rim (arrowhead). **b** Sagittal T_2-weighted SE image. The necrosis of the femoral condyle continues to show a low signal intensity. The fragment is surrounded by a rim of high signal fluid (arrowhead).

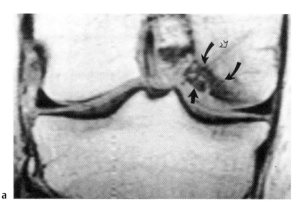

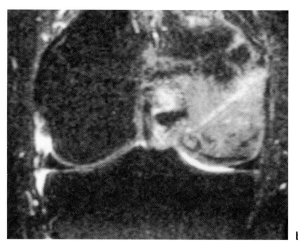

Fig. 7.**65a, b**   Osteochondritis dissecans following drilling. **a** Coronal T_1-weighted SE image. The fragment (arrow) and the adjacent bone marrow of the femoral condyles (curved arrow) show a decreased signal intensity, as well as the drill hole (open arrow). **b** Coronal STIR image. Clearly increased signal intensity in the fragment and femoral condyle.

Table 7.**8**   Osteonecroses of the knee

Name	Location	Predilection age
Sinding-Larsen disease	Secondary patellar ossification center	Adolescence
Caffey disease	Tibial spine	Adolescence
Blount disease	Medial tibial condyle	Infancy
Osgood-Schlatter disease	Tibial tuberosity	Infancy, adolescence

Changes of the Synovial Membrane and Joint Capsule

MRI does not identify the normal synovial membrane, but the joint capsule is demonstrated as a linear structure of decreased signal intensity.

In numerous joint conditions, the synovial membrane is thickened and shows contrast enhancement, frequently accompanied by a joint effusion. These changes are especially conspicuous in rheumatoid arthritis, hemophiliac arthropathy and PVNS.

Rheumatoid Arthritis. This induces hypertrophy and villous thickening of the synovial membrane. These synovial proliferations are considered to be the determining pathogenetic factor for the progressive joint destruction ('synovial arthropathies'). The synovial proliferations are hypervascular during the active phase of rheumatoid arthritis and become fibrous with loss of vascularization in the chronic inactive phase.

On the unenhanced T_1-weighted image, the synovial proliferations exhibit a low signal intensity and are barely distinguishable from a joint effusion. The synovial proliferations can have a low, high or mixed signal intensity on the T_2-weighted image. Active hypervascular synovial proliferations can be expected to have a high signal intensity on the T_2-weighted image.

After IV injection of Gd-based contrast medium, the synovial proliferations show a definite enhancement, resulting in a clear contrast in comparison to the joint effusion (Fig. 7.**66**). This enhancement is best appreciated on fat saturated images (Fig. 7.**67**).

Dynamic MRI with application of contrast medium shows rapid enhancement in the synovial proliferations (Figs. 7.**68** and 7.**69**). Hypervascular active pannus has a more rapid enhancement with maximum intensity reached at about 60 seconds, while the fibrous pannus reaches a maximum only after 120 seconds (59). The enhancement factor was 145% for hypervascular pannus and 25% for fibrous pannus.

Several studies have shown that dynamic contrast-enhanced MRI can document the results of anti-rheumatic therapy. It is still undetermined whether this technique might be helpful for following patients undergoing therapy. Furthermore, it is unclear whether any prognostic information can be derived from dynamic contrast-enhanced MRI. It is already established that MRI can be useful for planning synovectomy and for evaluating diagnostic problem cases. MRI can clearly document popliteal cysts, which are frequently filled with synovial proliferations, as well as involvement of tendon sheaths and tears or destruction of ligaments.

Pigmented Villonodular Synovitis (PVNS). This condition is characterized by frondose or nodular synovial proliferations, which can be found in the larger joints, bursae and tendon sheaths. With an incidence of 60–80%, mono-articular involvement of the knee is frequent. The etiology of PVNS is unclear. The synovial proliferations of PVNS are heavily vascularized and have a tendency to bleed. PVNS infiltrates the hyaline articular cartilage and the subchondral bone, producing lobulated destructions with sclerotic borders.

PVNS has characteristic MRI findings: the joint cavity is distended by a synovial mass, which shows a low signal intensity on all pulse sequences due to its high hemosiderin content. (53, 61). The severe susceptibility effect of hemosiderin produces conspicuous signal voids, especially on T_2^*-weighted GRE sequences (Fig. 7.**70**) (111).

Hemophiliac Arthropathy. This condition also produces synovial proliferation with hemosiderin deposition. The remaining morphologic changes and the history allow its diagnosis.

Sarcoidosis. Aside from osseous involvement, synovial changes have also been described in sarcoidosis. MRI shows uniform synovial thickening with contrast enhancement (85).

Lipoma Arborescens. This is a rare disease of the synovial membrane consisting of villous lipomatous proliferation. The condition tends to be associated with post-traumatic osteoarthritis and can cause joint locking, weakness, and, if the knee is affected, atrophy of the quadriceps. MRI findings are almost pathognomonic and include frond-like distention of the joint capsule with fat signal intensity on the T_1-weighted image and a signal void after fat suppression. The frond-like mass predominantly occupies the suprapatellar recess. The therapy consists of a total synovectomy (38).

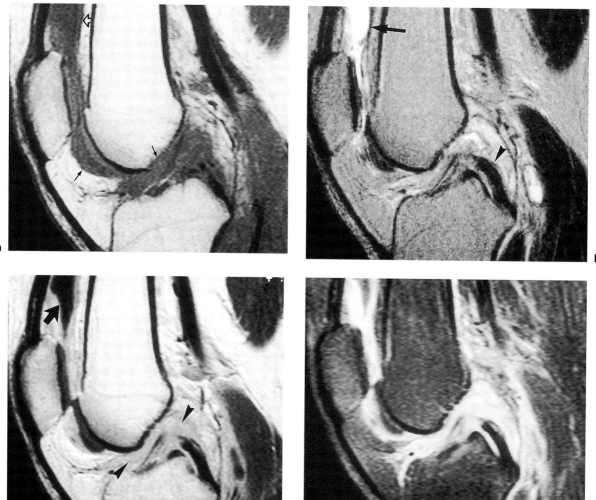

Fig. 7.**66 a – d**   Rheumatoid arthritis of the knee. **a** Sagittal T₁-weighted SE image. Synovial proliferations (arrows) and the effusion (open arrow) in the suprapatellar recess show an intermediate signal intensity, in marked contrast to the fat-containing surrounding structures, such as Hoffa's fat pad. **b** Sagittal T₂-weighted SE image. High signal intensity of the joint effusion in the suprapatellar recess (arrow). The synovial proliferations exhibit a heterogeneous, relatively high signal intensity. Faint contrast in comparison with the fatty tissue. The ligamentous structures are better delineated (arrowhead = posterior cruciate ligament). **c** Contrast-enhanced T₁-weighted sagittal SE image. Strong enhancement of the synovial proliferations (arrowhead). Marked contrast relative to the effusion in the suprapatellar recess (dark, arrow). The synovial proliferations are not discernible from the fatty tissue. **d** Sagittal contrast enhanced T₁-weighted SE image with fat saturation. The signal intensity of the synovial proliferations is high while it is low for the remaining structures.

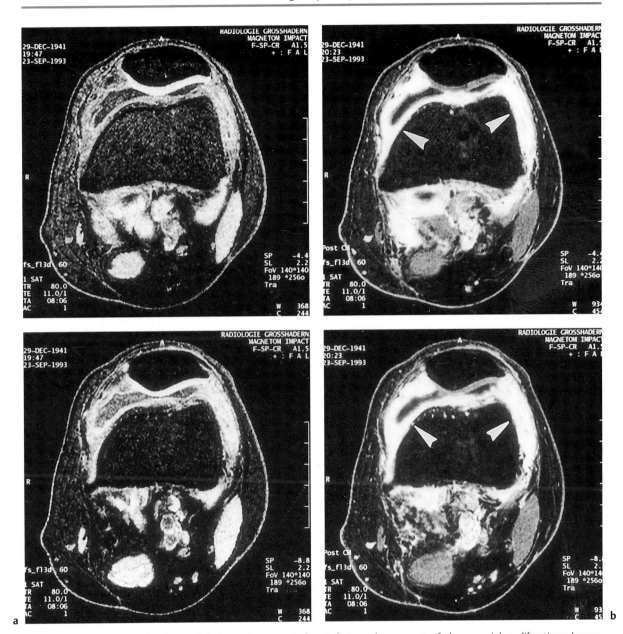

Fig. 7.**67 a, b**　Rheumatoid arthritis of the knee. Fat saturated 3-D FLASH sequence (**a** without, **b** with IV contrast medium).

Definite enhancement of the synovial proliferations (arrowhead).

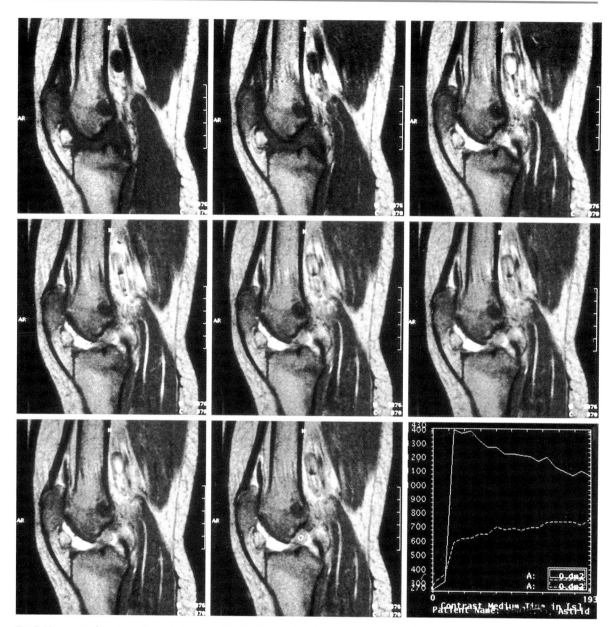

Fig. 7.**68**   Sagittal sections through the knee joint before and after IV contrast medium in rheumatoid arthritis. Definite enhancement in the synovial proliferation within the knee. The time–activity curve of the signal intensity (right lower corner) shows a contrasting enhancement pattern. The rapid enhancement corresponds to hypervascular active pannus and the slow enhancement to fibrous pannus.

Fig. 7.**69** Contrast-enhanced FLASH image in rheumatoid arthritis of the knee. The synovial proliferations in the articular cavity and the tibial infiltrations (arrowhead) exhibit a high signal intensity.

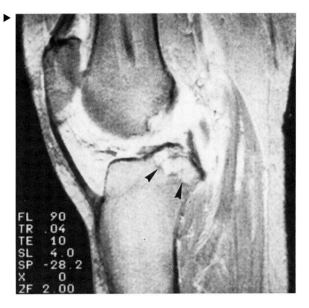

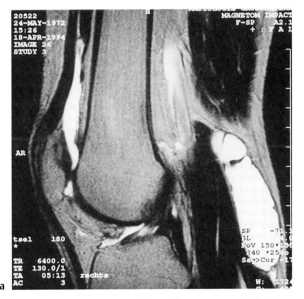

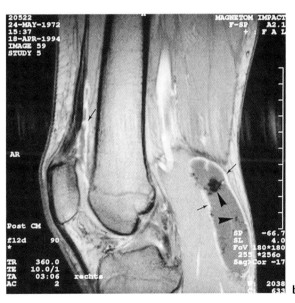

Fig. 7.**70 a, b** Pigmented villonodular synovitis of the knee with development of a Baker's cyst. **a** Sagittal T$_2$-weighted TSE image. Effusion in the joint capsule, suprapatellar recess and Baker's cyst, with the latter showing nodular changes. The sagittal FLASH image after IV contrast medium. Strong enhancement of the thickened synovial membrane (arrow). Due to iron deposits, susceptibility-induced signal voids in the Baker's cyst (arrowhead).

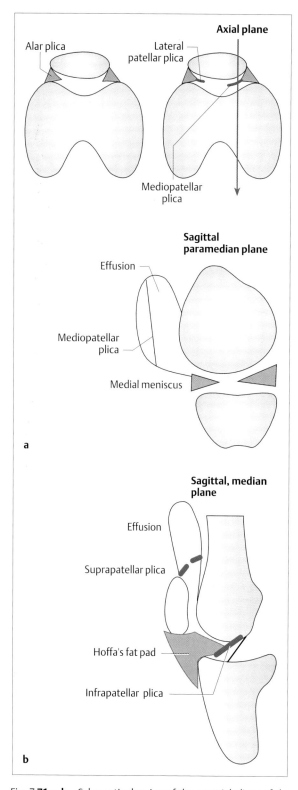

Fig. 7.**71 a, b**   Schematic drawing of the synovial plicae of the knee. **a** Normal visualization of the alar plicae on the axial image (left). Persistently thickened lateral patellar plica and mediopatellar plicae on the axial image (top right) and mediopatellar plicae on the sagittal image (right lower quadrant). **b** Suprapatellar plicae with small residual opening (porta) and infrapatellar plica on the sagittal image.

Synovial Plicae

During the embryonal phase, the knee consists of three separate synovial compartments: one suprapatellar compartment and two infrapatellar (lateral and medial) compartments. The dividing septa regress during normal embryonal development, creating a large single synovial cavity. The synovial plicae found in adults represent remnants of these embryonal membranes. They may be seen bilaterally, adjacent to the patellar and extending to Hoffa's fat pad (alar plicae) (Fig 7.**71**) and between the intracondylar fossa and the tip of Hoffa's fat pad, anterior and parallel to the ACL (infrapatellar plica). MRI shows the alar plicae on axial and coronal images as linear signal void, in particular, if an effusion is present. The infrapatellar plicae are normally invisible on MRI.

Through variations in normal development, the embryonal septa can partially persist as diversely formed remnants that appear as additional synovial plicae on MRI. They present as signal void structures, especially in the presence of an effusion. Persistence of the septum between infrapatellar and suprapatellar compartments constitutes the suprapatellar plica (Figs. 7.**72** and 7.**73**). If it remains completely intact, the adult knee is divided into two separate compartments. More frequently, however, it is partially resolved with a central opening (porta) of variable size and peripheral residues. The suprapatellar plica is usually asymptomatic. It is best visualized on sagittal MRI sections.

If the infrapatellar septum of the knee does not resolve, two infrapatellar compartments persist in adults. It is more common to encounter partial resolution with infrapatellar plicae of variable size (also referred to as ligamentum mucosum). The incompletely resolved infrapatellar plica is usually asymptomatic and generally not discernible on MRI. A thickened infrapatellar plica can be mistaken for an anterior cruciate ligament, making the diagnostic evaluation for ligamentous tears more difficult.

The complete persistence of embryonal knee joint compartments alters the spread of infections, affects the planning of surgical intervention and can account for asymmetric joint effusions. This condition is best proven by arthrography. Complete persistence of the suprapatellar plicae creates a suprapatellar bursa, which can present as a palpable suprapatellar mass in bursitis.

Thickened plicae can also occur in the medial and lateral knee joint with normal alar plicae. The mediopatellar plica is considerably more frequent than the lateral patellar plica. These plicae are especially well visualized on axial and paramedian sagittal sections in the presence of an effusion. The medial patellar plicae can become symptomatic (plica syndrome). In these cases, medially located pain and locking can develop after trauma. Later in the disease process, cartilaginous ulcerations can occur at the medial femoral condyle. The plicae can be arthroscopically resected if conservative therapy fails.

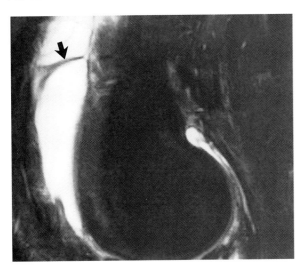

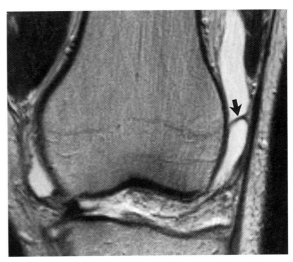

Fig. 7.**72** Suprapatellar synovial plica. T$_2$-weighted SE sequence with fat saturation. High signal intensity of the synovial fluid with clear demarcation of the plica (arrow). Gross fragmentation is seen in the region of the incidentally visualized posterior horn of the medial meniscus.

Fig. 7.**73** Coronal T$_2$-weighted SE image. The synovial suprapatellar plica (arrow) is outlined by the high signal intensity joint effusion.

The incidence of persistent synovial plicae is stated to be between 20 and 60%.

Synovial Popliteal Cysts and Bursitis

Synovial Popliteal Cysts. These are cystic lesions in the popliteal fossa, outlined by a synovial membrane and characteristically communicating with the joint cavity.

Though their exact pathogenesis is unclear, it is presumed that they represent localized perforations of the joint capsule in the region of the neighboring bursa with subsequent communication between bursa and joint cavity (Fig. 7.**74** and Tab. 7.**9**). The resultant increased pressure in the bursa leads to its cystic distention. This mechanism would explain the high incidence of popliteal cysts with increasing age as well as its frequent association with preceding injuries (characteristically constituting tears of the meniscus and ante-

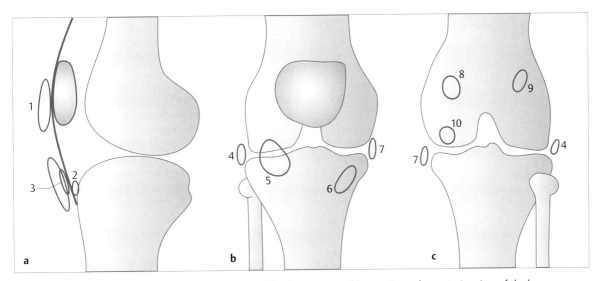

Fig. 7.**74a–c** Schematic drawing of the bursae around the knee. **a** Lateral **b** anterior and **c** posterior view of the knee.

1 = Prepatellar bursa and posterior component. Low signal debris within the Baker's cyst.
2 = Deep infrapatellar bursa
3 = Subcutaneous infrapatellar bursa
4 = Bursa of the lateral collateral ligaments
5 = Iliotibial bursa
6 = Pes anserine bursa
7 = Bursa of the medial collateral ligament
8 = Medial gastrocnemius bursa
9 = Lateral gastrocnemius bursa
10 = Semimembranous bursa

Table 7.**9**   Summary of the bursae of the knee and their inflammations

Bursa	Location	Cause of inflammation	Differential diagnosis
Prepatellar bursa	Between patella and subcutis	Kneeling occupation	Patellar tendinitis
Deep infrapatellar bursa and subcutaneous infra-patellar bursa	Around the tibial insertion of the patellar ligament	Jogging, jumping	Osgood-Schlatter disease
Medial and lateral gastrocnemius bursae and semimembranosus bursa	See section on popliteal synovial cysts		
Pes anserine bursa	Between pes anserinus and medio-anterior tibia	Jogging	Ganglion cysts
Bursae of the lateral and medial collateral ligament	Beneath the collateral ligaments		Meniscus lesion, injuries of the collateral ligaments
Iliotibial bursa	Beneath the insertion of the iliotibial tract at the latero-anterior tibia	Jogging, varus stress	

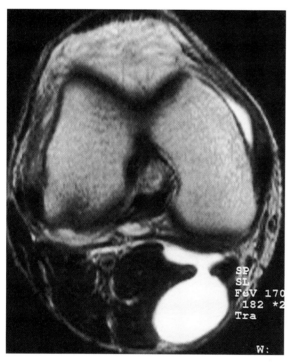

Fig. 7.**75**   Baker's cyst with high signal intensity on the T$_2$-weighted SE sequence. Communication of the Baker's cyst with the joint cavity.

rior cruciate ligament). Furthermore, the increased incidence of large Baker cysts in patients with rheumatoid arthritis can be attributed to increased intra-articular pressure caused by joint effusion.

The most frequently affected bursa is the gastrocnemius-semimembranosus bursa at the medial femoral condyle (Figs. 7.**75**– 7.**77**). The membrane-like tissue between bursa and joint is very thin, possibly predisposing this area to tears. The incidence of a communication between bursa and joint has been stated to be 35 – 55%. In the presence of a communication, the incidence of a bursa presenting as symptomatic mass effect (the so-called Baker's cyst) is 5%. Due to persistent pressure increase in the bursa or cyst caused by a check-valve mechanism or chronic arthritis, the bursa can extend deep into the soft tissues of the lower leg (so-called dissection). A sudden pressure increase can result in rupture.

The differential diagnosis for gastrocnemius-semimembranosus bursitis should include aneurysm of the popliteal artery, varicose veins, hematoma and tumors of the soft tissues or bones.

Bursitis. The inflammation of a bursa (*bursitis*) is usually caused by chronic overuse of the corresponding tendon or myotendinous transition in conjunction with athletic activities or by mechanical encroachment, for instance, by osteophytes. The clinical findings are characterized by pain during activity or at rest and by point tenderness (Tab. 7.**9**). Symptomatic relief after corticosteroid injections into the affected bursa is diagnostic of bursitis. Infectious bursae are diagnosed by aspiration. If the clinical symptoms are inconclusive, further evaluation by MRI is indicated (52, 67).

The bursae are not normally visible on MRI. A bursitis is seen as fluid-distended bursa with the signal intensity of the fluid decreased on the T$_1$-weighted image and increased on the T$_2$-weighted image. In chronic

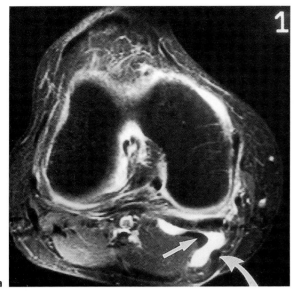

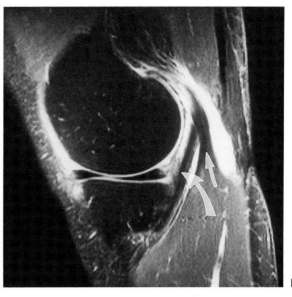

a   b

Fig. 7.**76** Indirect MR arthrography of a 30-year-old female patient with pain in the popliteal fossa. **a** Axial section. **b** Sagittal section.
A relatively small Baker's cyst is filled with contrast medium and displays a high signal intensity. It extends posteriorly between the medial head of the gastrocnemius (straight arrow) and the tendon of semimembranosus (curved arrow). Suggestive finding if a medial communication with the joint space.

bursitis, the T_1-weighted image can occasionally show a thickened wall of somewhat increased signal intensity as well as signal-void defects in the effusion caused by debris. Increased protein content in chronic bursitis can slightly increase the signal intensity on the T_1-weighted image. Contrary to a bursitis at other sites, prepatellar bursitis is characteristically accompanied by indistinct subcutaneous signal change as a manifestation of inflammatory reaction of the surrounding soft tissue structures (Fig. 7.**78**).

Ganglion Cysts (Excluding So-Called Meniscal Cysts)

Ganglion cysts contain a gelatinous material and can arise from tendons, ligaments, tendon sheaths, the joint capsule, bursae, subchondral bone, menisci or disks. They can become symptomatic due to pressure on neighboring structures. Furthermore, a ganglion cyst can present with nerve palsy and atrophy of the innervated muscle.

On MRI, ganglion cysts are of low signal intensity on the T_1-weighted image and of homogeneously increased signal intensity on the T_2-weighted image. Frequently, a neck to the anatomic structures, from where the ganglion arises, as well as linear signal void septations are seen. These criteria permit reliable differentiation of ganglion cysts from other space-occupying lesions (18, 52).

Intra-articular ganglion cysts of the knee arising from the cruciate ligaments can be anterior or posterior

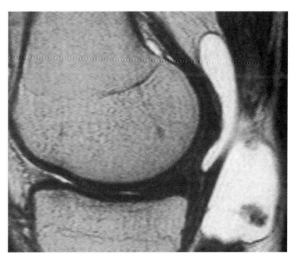

Fig. 7.**77** Sagittal T_2-weighted SE sequence Baker's cyst with high signal intensity of the synovial fluid and showing an upward and posterior component. Low signal debris within the Baker's cyst.

to the cruciate ligament or even within it. If they are symptomatic, they can be removed arthroscopically or through arthrotomy (Fig. 7.**79**). They are most frequently anterior to the tibial aspect of the anterior cruciate ligament.

A tibiofibular ganglion cyst can present with peroneal nerve palsy. In contrast to meniscal cysts, ganglion cysts are not associated with meniscal tears (see above).

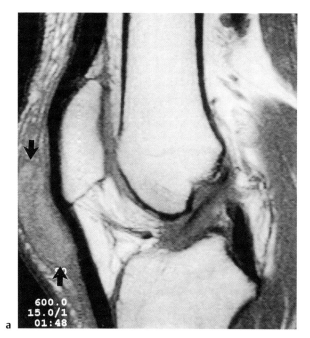

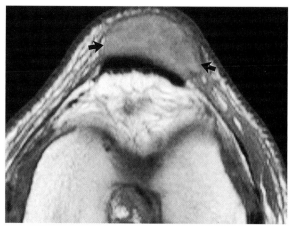

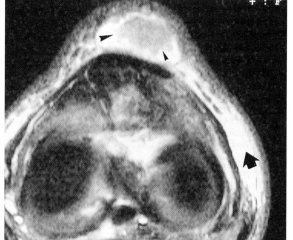

Fig. 7.**78 a–c** Chronic bursitis of the subcutaneous infra-patellar bursa. **a** Sagittal T₁-weighted SE image. **b** Axial T₁-weighted SE image. Ovoid structure of intermediate signal intensity, located subcutaneously and anterior to the patellar tendon (arrow). Reticular decrease in signal intensity in the adjacent subcutaneous tissue. **c** Axial STIR image. High signal intensity in the subcutaneous infrapatellar bursa and in the subcutaneous fatty tissue (arrow) as manifestation of inflammatory reaction. Intermediate signal intensity within the bursa (arrowhead).

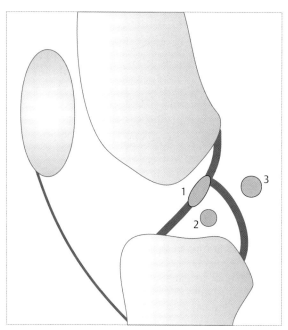

◄ Fig. 7.**79** Schematic drawing of the intra-articular ganglion cyst of the cruciate ligament. The topography is relevant for planning arthroscopic or open resection.
1 = Ganglion cyst of the cruciate ligament
2 = Ganglion cyst between the cruciate ligament
3 = Ganglion cysts behind the cruciate ligament

Pitfalls in Interpreting the Images

Intrameniscal increases in signal intensities are to be differentiated from *increased signal intensity* in the periphery of the meniscus, caused by fibrovascular fascicles. These areas of increased signal intensity are uniformly shaped and symmetric and radiate from the meniscal border. In one-third of cases, the sagittal images show a linear increase in signal intensity where the transverse ligament inserts at the anterior horn of the lateral meniscus, not to be mistaken for a meniscal tear. An increase in signal intensity is seen less frequently where the transverse ligament inserts at the anterior horn of the medial meniscus. It is conceivable that this change is related to branches of the accompanying lateral inferior geniculate artery or to fat surrounding the ligament (Fig. 7.**80**). Chondrocalcinosis may mimic tears as well (18 a).

In the superior aspect of the posterior horn of the lateral meniscus, the insertion of the meniscal femoral ligaments can mimic a tear on the sagittal images in one-third of cases.

The mid portion of the lateral meniscus is not attached to the lateral collateral ligament. The tendon and the tendon sheath of the popliteus pass between meniscus and joint capsule, which also might mimic a vertical tear of the posterior horn of the lateral meniscus or a meniscal capsular separation, especially on coronal images.

Pulsatile flow artifacts of the popliteal artery can mimic a fragmentation of the posterior horn of the lateral meniscus. In questionable cases, the pulsatile flow artifacts can be recognized as a ghost-like band across the anterior image in the direction of the phase decoding by changing the window of the CRT display. Furthermore, changing the direction of the phase decoding immediately reveals the nature of such an artifact.

Truncation artifacts, which are known from other body regions, can occur with a 128×256 matrix. They can mimic longitudinal meniscal tears (115). This is no longer a problem with the use of higher resolution matrix.

As is known from conventional radiography, a *bipartite or multipartite patella* can be mistaken for a fractured patella. In contrast to fractures, the anatomic fragmentation of the patella shows no bone marrow edema and the fragments are connected with cartilaginous material that is delineated as high signal intensity on the T_2-weighted image. The cartilaginous coverage is intact. The distinction between fracture and bipartite patella can usually be made by the typical location of the small fragment of the bipartite patella at the superolateral border of the patella. The bipartite patella is found in 1% of the population and usually is bilateral. The fragment can be absent, causing an indentation of the patella (patella emarginata). Such a morphologic variant should not be mistaken for an avulsion fracture.

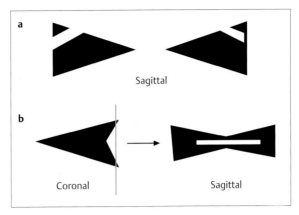

Fig. 7.**80 a, b** MRI artifacts of the knee: possible causes of misinterpretation of the menisci. **a** Increased signal intensity at the superior surface caused by the transverse ligament of the knee at the anterior meniscal horns and by the posterior meniscofemoral ligament at the posterior horn. **b** Linear increase in signal intensity of the menisci as seen on the sagittal section due the partial volume effect.

Accessory posterior sesamoids (fabellae) should not be mistaken for loose articular bodies or fracture fragments. Based on their typical location and size of 5–20 mm, they are readily recognized on conventional radiographs. A lateral fabella is observed in 10–20% of the population. It is imbedded in the lateral half of the gastrocnemius and articulates with the lateral femoral condyle. It is bilateral in 75% of cases. A medial fabella in the medial half of the gastrocnemius or a distal fabella in the popliteal tendon posterior and medial to the fibular head is rare. In contrast to loose intra-articular bodies, fabellae show hyaline articular cartilage where they articulate with the femora or fibula, which is easily recognized on MRI.

Clinical Relevance of MRI and Comparison with Other Imaging Modalities

Apart from conventional radiographs, a multitude of radiologic modalities were and some are still used for the diagnostic evaluation of the knee:

- Single or double contrast arthrography,
- CT and CT arthrography,
- Sonography,
- Stress views.

All of these methods are unsuitable or too cumbersome for a discerning and precise evaluation of the internal structures of the knee. Though MRI is subject to several constraints, it has become the method of choice for non-invasive or minimally invasive (MR arthrography, 36, 44 to 46) diagnostic evaluation of possible internal derangement of the knee. It is generally advisable to obtain conventional radiographs before the MRI examination. Juxta-articular osseous tumors or a stress fracture, which might be clinically attributed to internal derangement, can often be easily identified on conventional radiographs. Furthermore, conventional radiography is indicated to detect or exclude fractures of the juxta-articular bones.

A thorough clinical evaluation should precede any imaging evaluation!

Not infrequently, pathologic changes of the hip present with referred pain in the knee. It is not only embarrassing to the radiologist but also detrimental to the patient's health to perform the MRI examination on the wrong joint because of an inadequate preceding clinical evaluation. Arthroscopy, which has witnessed a dramatic increase over recent years, represents a major competitor to MRI.

Several investigations have shown that MRI can yield therapeutically relevant findings in acute injuries or chronic changes of the knee, clearly outperforming the clinical assessment. The MRI evaluation of chronic inflammatory joint diseases is less convincing. In particular, its therapeutic relevance has not been established. The use of MRI in diagnostic problem cases is essentially uncontested.

Several cost-benefit studies have confirmed the cost-effectiveness of MRI. Ruwe and co-workers (99) performed MRI on 103 consecutive patients with knee injuries that justified arthroscopy. Based on the MRI findings, 44 patients underwent immediate arthroscopy. The remaining 59 patients did not undergo arthroscopy, except for six patients who were later sent to arthroscopy on the basis of their clinical course. Without MRI, all patients enrolled in this study would have undergone arthroscopy. Because of the MRI diagnosis, arthroscopy was avoided in 51.4% patients, resulting in net savings of $103 700.

The results of this study might not be reproducible in other centers with different equipment and other patient populations. In addition, costs associated with lost work and arthroscopic complications are not included in this calculation. Nevertheless, the MRI-guided management of knee injuries can be expected to result in cost savings since diagnostic arthrography is more expensive than MRI and can be avoided if the MRI is normal.

References

1 Adam, G., J. Neuerburg, J. Peiß, K. Bohndorf, R. W. Günther: Magnetresonanztomographie der Osteochondrosis dissecans des Kniegelenkes nach intravenöser Gadolinium-DTPA-Gabe. Fortschr. Röntgenstr. 160 (1994) 459–464

2 Ahlbäck, S., G. C. H. Bauer, W. H. Bohne: Spontaneous osteonecrosis of the knee. Arthr. u. Rheum. 11 (1968) 705–733

3 Allgayer, B., Y. Gewalt, K. Flock, A. I. Henze, K. Lehner, R. Gradinger, G. Luttke: Diagnostische Treffsicherheit der KST bei Kreuzbandverletzungen. Fortschr. Röntgenstr. 155 (1991) 159–164

4 Applegate, G. R., B. D. Flannigan, B. S. Tolin, J. M. Fox, W. Del Pizzo: MR diagnosis of recurrent tears in the knee: value of intraarticular contrast material. Amer. J. Roentgenol. 161 (1993) 821–825

5 Araki, Y., F. Ootani, I. Tsukaguchi, M. Ootani, T. Furukawa, T. Yamaoto, K. Tomoda, M. Mitomo: MR diagnosis of meniscal tears of the knee: Value of axial three-dimensional Fourier transformation GRASS images. Amer. J. Roentgenol. 158 (1991) 587–590

6 Arndt, W. F., A. L. Truax, F. M. Barnett, G. E. Simmons, D. C. Brown: MR diagnosis of bone contusions of the knee: comparison of coronal T2-weighted fast spin-echo with fat saturation and fast spin-echo STIR images with conventional STIR images. Amer. J. Roentgenol. 166 (1996) 119–124

7 Bassett, L. W., J. S. Grover, L. L. Seeger: Magnetic Resonance Imaging of the knee trauma. Skelet. Radiol. 19 (1990) 401–405

8 Beltran, J., J. L. Caudill, L. A. Herman, S. M. Kaontor, P. N. Hudson, A. M. Noto, A. S. Baran: Rheumatoid arthritis: MR Imaging manifestations. Radiology 165 (1987) 153–157

9 Bergmann, A. G., H. K. Willén, L. Lindstrand, H. T. A. Pettersson: Osteoarthritis of the knee: Correlation of subchondral MR signal abnormalities with histopathologic and radiographic features. Skelet. Radiol. 23 (1994) 445–448

10 Berlin, R. C., E. M. Levinsohn, H. Chrisman: The wrinkled patellar tendon: an indication of abnormality in the extensor mechanism of the knee. Skelet. Radiol. 20 (1991) 181–185

11 Björkengren, A. G., A. Al Rowaik, A. Lindstrand, H. Wingstrand, K.-G. Thorngren, H. Petterson: Spontaneous osteonecrosis of the knee: value of MR Imaging in determining prognosis. Amer. J. Roentgenol. 154 (1990) 331–336

12 Bloem, J. L., M. F. Reiser, D. Vanel: Magnetic Resonance contrast agents in the evaluation of the musculoskeletal system. Magn. Reson. Q 6 (1990) 136–163

13 Bodne, D., S. F. Quinn, W. T. Murray: Magnetic Resonance Images of chronic patellar tendonitis. Skelet. Radiol. 17 (1988) 24–28

14 Boeree, N. R., A. F. Watkinson, C. E. Ackroyd, C. Johnson: Magnetic Resonance Imaging of meniscal and cruciate injuries of the knee. J. Bone Jt Surg. 73-B (1991) 452–457

15 Brossmann, J., C. Muhle, C. Schröder, U. H. Melchert, C. C. Büll, R. P. Spielmann, M. Heller: Patellar tracking patterns during active and passive knee extension: evaluation with motion-triggered cine MR Imaging. Radiology 187 (1993) 205–212

16 Buckwalter, K. A., E. M. Braunstein, D. B. Janizek, T. N. Vahey: MR Imaging of meniscal tears: narrow versus conventional window with photography. Radiology 187 (1993) 827–830

17 Buirski, J. P. P.: MR Imaging of the knee: a prospective trial using a low field strength magnet. Aust. Radiol. 34 (1990) 59–63

18 Burk, B. L., M. K. Dalinka, E. Kanal, M. L. Schiebler, E. K. Cohen, R. J. Prorok, W. B. Gefter, H. Y. Kressel: Meniscal and ganglion cysts of the knee: MR evaluation. Amer. J. Roentgenol. 150 (1987) 331–336

18a Burke, B. J., E. M. Escobedo, A. J. Wilson, J. C. Humter: Chondrocalcinosis mimicking a meniscal tear on MRI. AJR 170 (1998) 69–70

19 Chan, W. P., P. Lang, M. P. Stevens, K. Sack, S. Majambar, D. W. Stoller, G. Brasch, H. D. Genant: Osteoarthritis of the knee: comparison of radiography, CT, and MR Imaging to assess extent and severity. Amer. J. Roentgenol. 157 (1991) 799–806

20 Chan, W. P., C. Peterfy, R. C. Fritz, H. K. Genant: MR diagnosis of complete tears of the anterior cruciate ligament of the knee: importance of anterior subluxation of the tibia. Amer. J. Roentgenol. 162 (1994) 355–360

20a Chan, K. K., D. Resnick, D. Godwin, L. L. Seeger: Posteromedial Tibial Plateau Injury including Avulsion Fracture of the Semimembranous Tendon Insertion Site: Ancillary Sign of Anterior Cruciate Ligament Tear at MRI. Radiology 211 (1999) 754–758

21 Cheung, Y., T. H. Magee, S. Z. Rosenberg, D. J. Rose: MRI of anterior cruciate ligament reconstruction. J. Comput. assist. Tomogr. 16 (1992) 134–137

22 Clanton, T. O., C. DeLee: Osteochondritis dissecans: history, pathophysiology and current treatment concepts. Clin. Orthop. 167 (1982) 50–64

23 Crues, J. V., J. Mink, T. Levy, M. Lotysch, D. W. Stoller: Meniscal tears of the knee: accuracy of MR Imaging. Radiology 164 (1987) 445–448

24 Davies, S. G., C. J. Boudonin, J. B. King, J. D. Perry: Ultrasound, Computed Tomography and Magnetic Resonance Imaging in patellar tendonitis. Clin. Radiol. 43 (1991) 52–56

25 De Smet, A. A., D. R. Fisher, B. K. Graf, R. H. Lange: Osteochondritis dissecans of the knee: value of MR Imaging in determining lesions stability and the presence of articular defects. Amer. J. Roentgenol. 155 (1990) 549–553

26 DeSmet, A. A., M. A. Norris, D. R. Yandows, F. A. Quintana, B. K. Graf, J. S. Keene: MR diagnosis of meniscal tears of the knee: importance of high signal in the meniscus that extends to the surface. Amer. J. Roentgenol. 161 (1993) 101–107

27 De Smet, A. A., M. J. Tuite, M. A. Norris, J. S. Swan: MR diagnosis of meniscal tears: analysis of causes of errors. Amer. J. Roentgenol. 163 (1994) 1419–1423

28 Deutsch, A. L., J. H. Mink, J. M. Fox, S. P. Arnoczky, B. J. Rothmann, D. W. Stoller, W. D. Cannon: Peripheral meniscal tears: MR findings after conservative treatment and arthroscopic repair. Radiology 176 (1990) 485–488

29 Dillon, E. H., C. F. Pope, P. Jokl, K. Lynch: The clinical significance of stage 2 meniscal abnormalities on Magnetic Resonance knee images. Magn. Reson. Imag. 8 (1990) 411–415

30 Disler, D. G., S. V. Kattapuram, F. S. Chews, D. I. Rosenthal, D. Patel: Meniscal tears of the knee: preliminary comparison of three dimensional MR reconstruction with two dimensional MR Imaging and arthroscopy. Amer. J. Roentgenol. 160 (1993) 343–345

31 Eckstein, F., H. Sittek, S. Milz, R. Putz, M. Reiser: The morphology of articular cartilage assessed by Magnetic Resonance Imaging (MRI) – reproducibility and anatomical correlation. Surg. radiol. Anat. 16 (1994) 429–438

32 Eckstein, F., H. Sittek, A. Gavazzeni, S. Milz, B. Kiefer, R. Putz, M. Reiser: Der Kniegelenksknorpel in der Magnetresonanztomographie. MR-Chondrovolumetrie (MR-CVM) mittels fettunterdrückter FLASH-3 D-Sequenz. Radiologe 35 (1995) 87–93

33 Eckstein, F., H. Sittek, S. Milz, E. Schulte, B. Kiefer, M. Reiser, R. Putz: The potential of Magnetic Resonance Imaging (MRI) for quantifying articular cartilage thickness – a methodological study. Clin. Biomech. 10 (1995) 434–440

34 Eckstein, F., H. Sittek, A. Gavazzeni, E. Schulte, S. Milz, B. Kiefer, M. Reiser, R. Putz: Magnetic Resonance Chondro-Crassometry (MR CCM): a method for accurate determination of articular cartilage thickness? Magn. Reson. Med. 35 (1996) 89–96

35 El-Koury, G. Y., R. L. Wira, R. S. Berbaum, T. L. Tope, T. U. V. Monu: MR Imaging of patellar tendinitis. Radiology 184 (1992) 849–855

36 Engel, A., P. C. Hajek, J. Kramer et al.: Magnetic Resonance knee arthrography. Enhanced contrast by gadolinium complex in the rabbit and in humans. Acta orthop. scand. 61, Suppl. 240 (1990) 1–57

37 Erickson, S. J., I. H. Cox, G. F. Correra, J. A. Strandt, L. D. Estokowski: Effect of tendon orientation on MR Imaging signal intensity: a manifestation of the „magic angle" phenomenon. Radiology 181 (1991) 389–392

38 Feller, J. F., M. Rishi, E. C. Hughes: Lipoma arborescens of the knee. MR demonstration. Amer. J. Roentgenol. 163 (1994) 162–164

39 Fisher, S. P., J. M. Fox, W. Del Pizzo, M. J. Friedman, S. J. Snyder, R. D. Ferkel: Accuracy of diagnoses from Magnetic Resonance Imaging of the knee: a multicenter analysis of one thousand and fourteen patients. J. Bone Jt Surg. 73-A (1991) 2–10

40 Fullerton, G. D., I. L. Cameron, V. A. Ord: Orientation of tendons in the magnetic field and its effect on T2 relaxation times. Radiology 155 (1985) 433–435

41 Gavazzeni, A., F. Eckstein, H. Sittek, S. Milz, E. Schulte, B. Kiefer, R. Putz, M. Reiser: Die Bestimmung der quantitativen Verteilung des hyalinen Knorpelgewebes mittels Magnetresonanztomographie. Sportorthop. Sporttraumatol. 11 (1995) 176–182

42 Gentili, A., L. L. Seeger, L. Yao, H. M. Do: Anterior Cruciate ligament tear: indirect signs at MR Imaging. Radiology 193 (1994) 835–840

43 Grover, J. S., L. W. Bassett, M. L. Gross, L. L. Seeger, G. A. M. Finerman: Posterior cruciate ligament: MR Imaging. Radiology 174 (1990) 527–530

44 Gylys-Morin, V. M., P. C. Hajek, D. J. Sartoris, D. Resnick: Articular cartilage defects: detectability in cadaver knees with MR. Amer. J. Roentgenol. 148 (1987) 1153–1157

45 Hajek, P. C., D. J. Sartoris, D. H. Neumann, D. Resnick: Potential contrast agents for MR arthrography: in vitro evaluation and practical observations. Amer. J. Roentgenol. 149 (1987 a) 97–104

46 Hajek, P. C., L. L. Baker, D. J. Sartoris, C. Neumann, D. Resnick: MR arthrography: anatomic pathologic investigation. Radiology 163 (1987 b) 141–147

47 Hayes, C. W., R. W. Swyer, W. F. Conway: Patellar cartilage lesions: in vitro detection and staging with MR Imaging and pathological correlation. Radiology 176 (1990) 479–483

48 Herman, L. J., J. Beltran: Pitfalls in MR Imaging of the knee. Radiology 167 (1988) 775–781

49 Heuck, A., B. Allgayer, H. Sittek, J. Scheidler: Oblique coronal sequences increase the accuracy of MR Imaging of the anterior cruciate ligament. Radiology 193 (1994) 290

50 Howe, J., R. J. Johnson: Knee injuries in skiing. Orthop. Clin. N. Amer. 16 (1995) 303–313

51 Iversen, B. F., J. Stürup, K. Jacobsen, K. Andersen, J. Andersen: Implications of muscular defense in testing for the anterior drawer sign in the knee. Amer. J. Sports Med. 5 (1989) 409–413

51 a Jackson, D. W., L. D. Jennings, R. M. Maywood, P. E. Berger: Magnetic Resonance Imaging of the knee. Amer. J. Sports Med. 16 (1988) 29–38

52 Janzen, D. L., C. G. Peterfy, J. R. Forbes, P. F. Tirman, H. K. Genant: Cystic lesions around the knee joint: MR Imaging findings. Amer.J. Roentgenol. 163 (1994) 155–161

53 Jelinek, J. S., M. J. Kransdorf, J. A. Utz, B. H. Berrey, J. D. Thomson: Imaging of pigmented villonodular synovitis with emphasis on MR Imaging. Amer. J. Roentgenol. 152 (1989) 337–342

54 Just, M., M. Runkel, J. Ahlers, P. Grebe, K.-F. Kreitner, M. Thelen: MR-Tomographie bei Innenbandverletzungen des Kniegelenkes. Fortschr. Röntgenstr. 156 (1992) 555–558

55 Justice, W. W., S. F. Quinn: Error patterns in the MR Imaging evaluation of menisci of the knee. Radiology 196 (1995) 617–621

56 Kapelow, S. R., L. M. Teresi, W. G. Bradley, N. R. Bucciarelli, D. M. Murakami, W. J. Mulin, J. E. Jordan: Bone contusions of the knee: Increased lesion detection with fast spin-echo MR Imaging with spectroscopic fat saturation. Radiology 189 (1993) 901–904

56 a Kaplan, P. A., R. H. Gehl, R. G. Dussault et al.: Bone Contusions of the Posterior Lip of the medial plateau (Contrecoup Injury) and associated Internal Derangements of the Knee at MRI. Radiology 211 (1999) 747–754

57 Kennedy, J. C., H. W. Weinberg, A. S. Wilson: The anatomy and function of the anterior cruciate ligament. J. Bone Jt Surg. 56-A (1974) 223–235

58 Kirsch, M. D., S. W. Fitzgerald, H. Friedman, L. F. Rogers: Transient lateral patellar dislocation: diagnosis with MR-Imaging. Amer. J. Roentgenol. 161 (1993) 109–113

59 König, H., J. Sieper, K.-J. Wolf: Rheumatoid Arthritis: Evaluation of hypervascular and fibrous pannus with dynamic MR Imaging enhanced with Gd-DTPA. Radiology 176 (1990) 473–477

60 Kornick, J., E. Trefelner, S. McCarthy, R. Lange, K. Lynch, P. Joki: Meniscal abnormalities in the asymptomatic population at MR Imaging. Radiology 177 (1990) 463–465

61 Kottal, R. A., J. B. Volger, A. Matamoros et al.: Pigmented villonodular synovitis: a report of MR Imaging in two cases. Radiology 163 (1987) 551

62 Kramer, J., R. Stiglbauer, A. Engel, L. Prayer, H. Imhof: MR Contrast Arthrography (MRA) in osteochondrosis dissecans. J. Comput. assist. Tomogr. 16 (1992) 254–260

63 Kramer, J., M. P. Recht, H. Imhof, R. Stiglbauer, A. Engel: Postcontrast MR arthrography in assessment of cartilage lesions. J. Comput. Assist. Tomogr. 18 (1994) 218–224

64 Kramer, J., A. Scheurecker, E. Mohr: Osteochondrale Läsionen. Radiologe 35 (1995) 109–116

65 Kursunoglu-Brehme, S., B. Schwaighofer, L. Gundry, C. Ho, D. Resnick: Jogging causes acute changes in the knee joint: a restudy in normal volunteers. Amer. J. Roentgenol. 154 (1990) 1233–1235

66 Lang, P., S. Grampp, M. Vahlensieck, M. Mauz, E. Steiner, H. Schwickert, A. Gindele, R. Felix, H. K. Genant: Spontane Osteonekrose des Kniegelenkes: MRT im Vergleich zur CT, Szintigraphie und Histologie. Fortschr. Röntgenstr. 162 (1995) 469–477

67 Lee, J. K., L. Yao: Tibial collateral ligament bursa: MR Imaging. Radiology 178 (1991) 855–857

68 Lee, J. K., L. Yao, C. T. Phelps, C. R. Wirth, J. Czajka, J. Lozmann: Anterior cruciate ligament tears: MR Imaging compared with arthroscopy and clinical tests. Radiology 166 (1988) 861–864

69 Lehner, K. B., H. P. Rechl, J. K. Gmeinwieser, A. F. Heuck, H. P. Lukas, H. P. Kohl: Structure, function, and degeneration of bovine hyaline cartilage: assessment with MR Imaging in vitro. Radiology 170 (1989) 495–499

70 Leutner, C., M. Vahlensieck, U. Wagner, F. Dombrowski, M. Reiser: Hochauflösende axiale Kernspintomographie arthrotomisch gesetzter Meniskusläsionen am Kniegelenk. Osteologie 2 (1993) 27

71 Lotke, P. A., M. L. Ecker: Osteonecrosis of the knee. J. Bone Jt Surg. 70-A (1988) 470–473

72 Lotysch, M., J. Minck, C. V. Crues, S. A. Schwartz: Magnetic Resonance Imaging in the detection of meniscal injuries. Magn. Reson. Imag. 4 (1986) 185

73 Lynch, T. C., J. Crues III, F. W. Morgan, W. E. Sheehan, L. P. Harter, R. Ryu: Bone abnormalities of the knee: prevalence and significance at MR Imaging. Radiology 171 (1989) 761–766

74 Lysholm, J., J. Gillquist: Arthroscopic examination of the posterior cruciate ligament. J. Bone Jt Surg. 63-A (1981) 363–366

75 McCauley, T. R., R. Kier, K. J. Lynch, P. Jokl: Chondromalacia patellae. Diagnosis with MR Imaging. Amer. J. Roentgenol. 158 (1992) 101–105

76 McLaughlin, R. F., E. L. Raber, A. D. Vallet, J. P. Wiley, R. C. Bray: Patellar tendinitis: MR Imaging features, with suggested pathogenesis and proposed classification. Radiology 197 (1995) 843–848

77 Mesgarzadeh, M., A. A. Sapega, A. Bonakdarpour, G. Revesz, R. A. Moyer, H. A. Maurer, P. D. Alburger: Osteochondritis dissecans. Analysis of mechanical stability with radiography, scintigraphy and MR Imaging. Radiology 165 (1987) 775–780

78 Mink, J. H., T. Levy, J. V. Crues III: Tears of the anterior cruciate ligament and menisci of the knee: MR Imaging evaluation. Radiology 167 (1988) 769–774

79 Mink, J. H., Al. Deutch: Occult cartilage and bone injuries of the knee: detection, classification, and assessment with MR Imaging. Radiology 170 (1989) 823–829

80 Modl, J. M., L. A. Sether, V. M. Haughton, J. B. Kneeland: Articular cartilage: correlation of histologic zones with signal intensity at MR Imaging. Radiology 181 (1991) 853–855

81 Muhle, C., J. Brossmann, M. Heller: Funktionelle MRT des Femoropatellargelenkes. Radiologe 35 (1995) 117–124

82 Munk, P. L., C. A. Helms, H. K. Genant, R. G. Holt: Magnetic resonance Imaging of the knee: current status, new directions. Skelet. Radiol. 18 (1989) 569–577

83 Nägele, M., M. F. Reiser, A. I. Vellet, P. L. Munk: Synovial structure of the knee and arthritis. In Munk, P., C. A. Helms: MRI of the Knee. Aspen, Gaithersburg 1992

84 Patten, R. M.: MRI of the postoperative knee: meniscal appearances. MRI Decisions 10 (1993) 17–25

85 Powers, T. A., T. J. Limbbird: MRI of the knee in sarcoidosis: synovial and marrow involvement. J. Comput. assist. Tomogr. 18 (1994) 313–314

86 Quinn, S. F., T. F. Brown: Meniscal tears diagnosed with MR Imaging versus arthroscopy: how reliable a standard is arthroscopy? Radiology 181 (1991) 843–847

87 Quinn, S. F., T. R. Brown, J. Szumowski: Menisci of the knee: radial MR Imaging correlated with arthroscopy in 259 patients. Radiology 185 (1992) 577–580

88 Recht, M. P., J. Kramer, S. Marcelis, M. N. Pathria, D. Trudell, P. Haghighi, D. J. Sartoris, D. Resnick: Abnormalities of articular cartilage in the knee: analysis of available MR techniques. Radiology 187 (1993) 473–478

89 Reicher, M. A., S. Hartzman, G. R. Duckwiler, L. W. Basset, L. J. Anderson, R. H. Gold: Meniscal injuries: detection with MR Imaging. Radiology 59 (1986) 753–757

90 Reiser, M., N. Rupp, B. Heimhuber, W. Haller, O. Paar, A. Breit: Bildgebende Verfahren in der Kniegelenksdiagnostik. Prakt. Sport-Traumatol. Sportmed. 4 (1985) 14–18

91 Reiser, M., N. Rupp, K. Pfändner, S. Schepp, P. Lukas: Die Darstellung von Kreuzbandläsionen durch die MR-Tomographie. Fortschr. Röntgenstr. 145 (1986) 193–198

92 Reiser, M., G. Bongartz, R. Erlemann, M. Strobel, T. Pauly, K. Gaebert, U. Stoeber, P. E. Peters: Magnetic resonance in cartilaginous lesions of the knee joint with three-dimensional gradient-echo imaging. Skelet. Radiol. 17 (1988) 465–471

93 Reiser, M. F., G. P. Bongartz, R. Erlemann, M. Schneider, Th. Pauly, H. Sittek, P. E. Peters: Gadolinium DTPA in rheumatoid arthritis and related diseases: first results with dynamic Magnetic Resonance Imaging. Skelet. Radiol. 18 (1989) 591–597

94 Reiser, M., M. Vahlensieck, H. Schüller: Imaging of the knee joint with emphasis on Magnetic Resonance Imaging. Europ. Radiol. 2 (1992) 87–94

95 Reiser, M., H.-J. Refior, A. Stäbler, A. Heuck: MRT in der Orthopädie: Gelenkdiagnostik. Orthopäde 23 (1994) 342–348

96 Reiser, M., A. Heuck, A. Stäbler: Überlegungen zur Kosten-Nutzen-Relation in der Skelettradiologie. In Buck: Radiologie – Träger des Fortschritts. Springer, Berlin 1995

97 Remig, J. W., E. R. McDevitt, P. N. Ove: Progression of meniscal degenerative changes in college football players: evaluation with MR Imaging. Radiology 181 (1991) 255–257

98 Robertson, P. L., M. E. Schweitzer, A. R. Bartolozzi, A. Ugoni: Anterior cruciate ligament tears: evaluation of multiple signs with MR Imaging. Radiology 193 (1994) 829–834

99 Ruwe, P. A., J. Wright, R. L. Randall, K. J. Lynch, P. Jokl, S. McCarthy: Can MR Imaging effectively replace diagnostic arthroscopy? Radiology 183 (1992) 335–339

100 Sanchis-Alfonso, V., V. Martinez-Sanjuan, E. Gastaldi-Orquin: The value of MRI in the evaluation of the ACL deficient knee and in the postoperative evaluation after ACL reconstruction. Europ. J. Radiol. 16 (1993) 126–130

101 Sandberg, R., B. Balkfors: Partial rupture of the anterior cruciate ligament. Clin. Orthop. 220 (1987) 176–178

102 Schweitzer, M. E., D. G. Mitchell, S. M. Ehrlich: The patellar tendon: thickening, internal signal buckling, and other MR variants. Skelet. Radiol. 22 (1993) 411–416

103 Schweitzer, M. E., D. Tran, D. M. Deely, E. L. Hume: Medial collateral ligament injuries: evaluation of multiple signs, prevalence and location of associated bone bruises, and assessment with MR Imaging. Radiology 194 (1995) 825–829

104 Shahriaree, H.: Chondromalacia. Contemp. Orthop. 11 (1985) 27–39

105 Shellock, F. G., J. H. Mink, A. L. Deutsch, J. M. Fox: Patellar tracking abnormalities: clinical experience with kinematic MR Imaging in 130 patients. Radiology 172 (1989) 799–804

106 Silverman, J. M., J. H. Mink, A. L. Deutsch: Discoid menisci of the knee: MR Imaging appearance. Radiology 173 (1989) 351–354

107 Sittek, H., A. Heuck, F. Eckstein, M. Reiser: Magnetresonanztomographie bei Traumen des Kniegelenkes. Radiologe 35 (1995) 101 – 108

108 Sittek, H., F. Eckstein, A. Gavazzeni, S. Milz, B. Kiefer, E. Schulte, M. Reiser: Assessment of normal patellar cartilage volume and thickness using MRI: an analysis of currently available pulse sequences. Skelet. Radiol. 25 (1996) 55 – 62

109 Smith, D., W. G. Totty: The knee after partial meniscectomy: MR Imaging features. Radiology 176 (1990) 141 – 144

110 Sonin, A. H., S. W. Fitzgerald, H. Friedman, F. L. Hoff, R. W. Hendrix, L. F. Rogers: Posterior cruciate ligament injury: MR Imaging diagnosis and patterns of injury. Radiology 190 (1994) 455 – 458

111 Steinbach, L. S., C. H. Neumann, D. W. Stoller, et al.: MRI of the knee in diffuse pigmented villonodular synovitis. Clin. Imag. 13 (1989) 305 – 316

112 Stoller, D. W., C. Martin, J. V. Crues, L. Kaplan, J. Mink: MR Imaging – pathologic correlations of meniscal tears. Radiology 163 (1987) 731 – 735

113 Tolin, B., A. Sapega: Arthroscopic visual field mapping at the medial meniscus: a comparison of different portal approaches. Arthroscopy 9 (1993) 265 – 271

114 Tung, G. A., L. M. Davis, M. E. Wiggins, P. D. Fadale: Tears of the anterior cruciate ligament: primary and seccondary signs at MR Imaging. Radiology 188 (1993) 661 – 667

115 Turner, D. A., M. I. Rapaport, W. D. Erwin, M. McGould, R. I. Silvers: Truncation artifact: a potential pitfall in MR Imaging of the Menisci of the knee. Radiology 179 (1991) 629 – 633

116 Tyrell, R. L., K. Gluckert, M. Pathria, M. T. Modic: Fast three-dimensional imaging of the knee: comparison with arthroscopy. Radiology 166 (1988) 865 – 872

117 Umans, H., O. Wimpfheimer, N. Haramati, Y. H. Applbaum, M. Adler, J. Bosco: Diagnosis of partial tears of the anterior cruciate ligament of the knee: value of MR Imaging. Amer. J. Roentgenol. 165 (1995) 893 – 897

118 Vahey, T. N., H. T. Bennet, L. E. Arrington, K. D. Shelbourne, J. Ng: MR Imaging of the knee: pseudotear of the lateral meniscus caused by the meniscofemoral ligament. Amer. J. Roentgenol. 154 (1990) 1237 – 1239

119 Vahey, T. N., D. R. Broome, K. J. Kayes, K. D. Shelbourne: Acute and chronic tears of the anterior cruciate ligament. Differential features at MR Imaging. Radiology 181 (1991) 251 – 253

120 Vahlensieck, M.: Schnelle und ultraschnelle Bildgebung des muskuloskelettalen Systems. Radiologe 35 (1995) 973 – 980

121 Vahlensieck, M., M. Reiser: Knochenmarködem in der MRT. Radiologe 32 (1992) 509 – 515

122 Vahlensieck, M., K. Seelos, F. Träber, J. Gieseke, M. Reiser: Magnetresonanztomographie mit schneller STIR-Technik: Optimierung und Vergleich mit anderen Sequenzen an einem 0,5-Tesla-System. Fortschr. Röntgenstr. 159 (1993) 288 – 294

123 Vahlensieck, M., F. Dombrowski, C. Leutner, U. Wagner, M. Reiser: Magnetization Transfer Contrast (MTC) and MTC-subtraction: enhancement of cartilage lesions and intracartilaginous degeneration in vitro. Skelet. Radiol. 23 (1994) 535 – 539

124 Vahlensieck, M., T. Wischer, A. Schmidt, K. Steuer, T. Sommer, E. Keller, J. Gieseke, M. Hansis, H. Schild: Indirekte MR-Arthrographie: Optimierung der Methode und erste klinische Erfahrung bei frühen degenerativen Gelenkschäden am oberen Sprunggelenk. Fortsch. Röntgenstr. 162 (1995) 338 – 341

125 Vellet, A. D., P. Marks, P. Fowler, P. H. Munro: Occult posttraumatic osteochondral lesions of the knee: prevalence, classification, and shortterm sequelae evaluated with MR Imaging. Radiology 178 (1991) 271 – 276

126 Vellet, A. D., D. H. Lee, P. L. Munk, L. Hewett, M. Eliasziw, S. Dunlavy, L. Vidito, P. J. Fowler, A. Miniasci, A. Amendola: Anterior cruciate ligament tear: prospective evaluation of diagnostic accuracy of middle- and highfield strength MR Imaging at 1.5 and 0.5 T. Radiology 197 (1995) 826 – 830

127 Virolainen, H., T. Visur, T. Kuusela: Acute dislocation of the patella: MR findings. Radiology 89 (1993) 243 – 246

128 Wacker, F., X. Bolze, H. Mellerowicz, K. J. Wolf: Diagnostik von Veränderungen des Kniegelenkes bei Leistungssportlern. Radiologe 35 (1995) 94 – 100

129 Watanabe, A. T., B. C. Carter, G. P. Teitelbaum, W. G. Bradley: Common pitfalls in Magnetic Resonance Imaging of the knee. J. Bone Jt Surg. 71-A (1989) 857 – 862

130 Weiss, K. L., H. T. Morehouse, I. M. Levy: Sagittal MR images of the knee: a low signal band parallel to the posterior cruciate ligament caused by a displaced bucket-handle tear. Amer. J. Roentgenol. 156 (1991) 117 – 119

131 Winalski, C. S., P. Aliabadi, R. J. Wright, S. Shortkroff, C. B. Sledge, B. N. Weissman: Enhancement of joint fluid with intravenously administered gadopentetate dimeglumine: technique, radionale and implications. Radiology 187 (1993) 179 – 185

132 Wright, D. H., A. A. De Smet, M. Norris: Bucket-Handle Tears of the medial and lateral menisci of the knee: value of MR Imaging in detecting displaced fragments. Amer. J. Roentgenol. 165 (1995) 621 – 625

133 Yao, L., J. K. Lee: Occult intraosseous fracture: detection with MR Imaging. Radiology 167 (1988) 749 – 751

134 Yao, L., D. Dungan, L. L. Seeger: MR Imaging of tibial collateral ligament injury: comparison with clinical examination. Skelet. Radiol. 23 (1994) 521 – 524

135 Yulish, B. S., J. Montanez, D. B. Goodfellow, P. J. Bryan, G. P. Mulopulos, M. T. Modic: Chondromalacia patellae: assessment with MR Imaging. Radiology 167 (1987) 763 – 766

Ankle and Foot

M. Steinhorn and M. Vahlensieck

8

Introduction

With many osseous elements and a complex arrangement of active and passive stabilizers, ankle and foot constitute an anatomically complex unit, accommodating the various movements of standing, walking, and running.

Apart from the knee, the ankle is the joint most frequently subjected to trauma. Often, however, the ankle becomes symptomatic without the patient recalling any trauma. Both chronic and acute complaints are often only inadequately localized and diagnosed clinically.

Since MRI achieves an exquisite visualization of both osseous and cartilaginous structures, it has become an indispensable diagnostic method.

Examination Technique

■ Patient Positioning

The patient is examined *supine* in the foot first position. The foot should be placed in a *neutral position* or in *slight plantar flexion*, with the feet held in this position by sandbags and straps. For visualization of the ligaments of the ankle, positioning in extreme dorsal or lateral position can be advantageous.

■ Coil Selection

To achieve an adequate signal for the required resolution, the examination should be conducted with an *extremity coil (knee coil)*. If a comparison of both sides is required, the two ankles can be examined together with a *head coil*. To visualize the toes, a flexible surface coil can be used.

■ Sequences and Parameters

The examination of the ankle should begin with an axial T_2-weighted SE sequence by virtue of its high anatomic resolution, followed by axial, sagittal and coronal SE, TSE and GRE sequences. It is helpful to obtain images in at least one plane using a STIR technique. Such a protocol will detect most pathologic changes. Sometimes, the protocol must be modified to accommodate specific questions and diagnostic presumptions. Specific angulations are employed to visualize ligamentous structures. The field of view (FOV) is characteristically between *120 and 160 mm^2* with a *section thickness of 3–4 mm*. Recommendations for the remaining technical parameters are found in the table in the Appendix.

The forefoot and toes are generally examined in the *axial* and *sagittal* planes. In contrast to the examination of the ankle, a *thinner section thickness of 3 mm* and a *smaller field of view of 80–100 mm* should be used.

■ Special Examination Technique

For unclear bone and soft tissue processes and for the delineation of inflammatory changes, the use of IV Gd-based contrast medium might be necessary. After administration of contrast medium, fat saturated T_1-weighted images can be obtained in addition to T_1-weighted SE sequences.

For the examination of the ligamentous structures, sequences with acquisition of a three-dimensional data set can be used to reconstruct images in any plane. Because of the lower resolution and the inferior image contrast of these reconstructed images, additional SE sequences cannot be abandoned where a definitive assessment of the ligaments is needed. The reconstructed images benefit the evaluation of the ligamentous connections and the exact geometric planning of the SE sequences.

Anatomy

■ General Anatomy

Fibula, tibia, and talus constitute the *ankle or talocrural joint*. The fibula and tibia form the ankle mortise, which is stabilized by the taut anterior and posterior tibiofibular ligaments, also referred to as the tibiofibular syndesmosis. The *joint capsule* inserts into the anterior tibia about 10 mm proximal to the joint space and at the mid portion of the talar neck. Elsewhere, it inserts near the bone–cartilage junction. Along its medial plantar surface, the talus has a deep sulcus, the sulcus tali, which forms the roof of a fat-containing space, the *sinus tarsi*. Laterally, the sinus tarsi is bordered by the inferior extensor retinaculum (Figs. 8.**1** and 8.**25**).

The *medial collateral ligament* (also known as the deltoid ligament) is divided into four fibrous cords that

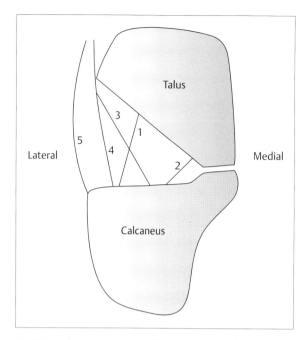

Fig. 8.**1**   Schematic drawing of the ligaments in the sinus tarsi. Coronal section (after Klein and Spreitzer).
1 = cervical ligaments
2 = interosseous talocalcaneal ligaments
3 = medial fascicle of the inferior extensor retinaculum
4 = intermediate fascicle of the inferior extensor retinaculum
5 = lateral fascicle of the inferior extensor retinaculum

arise at the tip of the medial malleolus and extend to the navicular tuberosity and by way of the talar neck and sustentaculum tali to the posterior talar process.

The *lateral collateral ligament complex* consists of three ligaments: the anterior fibulotalar ligament, the posterior fibulotalar ligament, and the fibulocalcaneal ligament. The anterior fibulotalar ligament arises at the anterior circumference of the tip of the fibular malleolus and inserts into the lateroanterior aspect of the talar neck. In dorsiflexion, it assumes an almost transverse course. This ligament is frequently divided, resists the anterior translation of the talus and, especially in plantar flexion, any varus deviation. The posterior fibulotalar ligament originates at the posterior inner margin of the fibula and extends horizontally to the posterior talar process where it inserts at the lateral tubercle. The fibulocalcaneal ligament arises near the tip of the lateral malleolus medially and runs obliquely to the lateral surface of the calcaneus. It is extra-articular and separated from the joint capsule by a fatty layer. Its primary function is to resist supination.

The *anterior extensor group* of the lower leg constitutes, in mediolateral direction, tibialis anterior, extensor hallucis longus, and extensor digitorum longus. The tendon of the tibialis anterior inserts into the plantar surface of the first metatarsal base and medial cuneiform. The tendon of the extensor hallucis longus inserts into the proximal and distal phalangeal bases of

the first toe, while the extensor digitorum longus inserts by means of four digital expansion into the middle and distal phalanges of the second to fifth toes. The *lateral extensor group* consists of the peroneus longus and brevis. The tendons of both muscles pass behind the lateral malleolus in a common synovial sheath and are held in place by the superior perioneal retinaculum. The peroneus longus forms a sling under the foot inserting into the tuberosity of the first metatarsal base and the intermediate cuneiform. The peroneus brevis inserts at the tuberosity of the fifth metatarsal base. The *superficial flexor group* constitutes the triceps, comprised of three muscles, the gastrocnemius, soleus, and the variably developed plantaris. Gastrocnemius and soleus have a common tendon, the Achilles tendon, which inserts at the posterior calcaneal tuberosity.

The *deep flexor group* includes, medial to lateral, the flexor digitorum longus, tibialis posterior, and flexor hallucis longus. In the distal third of the lower leg, the flexor digitorum longus crosses the tibialis posterior tendon, placing the latter in the most anteromedial position. Between the medial malleolus and the calcaneus, obliquely oriented fibers in the crural fascia cover and restrain the tendons (flexor retinaculum). The tarsal tunnel is bordered by the tip of the medial malleolus, the medial surface of the talus and calcaneus, and the flexor retinaculum. In the anteroposterior direction, the posterior tibialis tendon, flexor digitorum longus tendon, posterior tibial vessels, and, most posterior, the flexor hallucis longus tendon pass through the tarsal tunnel (Fig. 8.**33**).

The extensor digitorum brevis and extensor hallucis brevis arise on the *dorsum of the foot*. In the interosseous spaces between the metatarsals, the dorsal interossei are found dorsally and the plantar interossei inferiorly. The plantar muscles form three lengthwise groups, which are incompletely separated by connective tissue septa. The medial group comprises the abductor hallucis, adductor hallucis, and flexor hallucis longus, the intermediate group the flexor digitorum longus, flexor hallucis longus, flexor digitorum brevis, quadratus plantae and lumbricals, and the lateral group the abductor digiti minimi, flexor digiti minimi brevis, and opponens digiti minimi.

The *subtalar joint* is formed by the talus, calcaneus, and navicular. Anatomically, it consists of two completely distinct joint cavities separated by a joint capsule and the interosseous talocalcaneal ligament.

In the posterior joint cavity, the posterior calcaneal articular surface of the talus articulates with the posterior talar articular surface of the calcaneus, forming the talocalcaneal articulation. In the anterior joint cavity, the spherical articulating surface of the talar head and neck articulates with the articulating surface of the calcaneus and navicular, forming the talocalcaneonavicular articulation.

The long plantar ligament runs in the superficial *plantar layers*. It arises from the plantar surface of the calcaneus and extends to the second to fourth metatarsal bases across the insertion of the tendon of the peroneus longus.

■ Specific MR Anatomy

Transverse Plane (Figs. 8.**2**– 8.**4**)

Talocrural and subtalar articulations: Proximal to the talocrural joint, the transverse sections show, medial to lateral, the tendons of the tibialis anterior, extensor hallucis longus, extensor digitorum longus, and peroneus tertius.

The tendons of the tibialis posterior, flexor digitorum longus, and flexor hallucis longus are seen in the posterior compartment, from medial to lateral. The order of the tendons can be easily recalled easily, using the mnemonic Tom, Dick, and Harry (tibialis posterior, flexor digitorum longus, and flexor hallucis longus). The strongest of all tendons, the transverse ovoid Achilles tendon, is most posterior. Its posterior border is characteristically convex and its anterior border flattened.

The muscle and tendon of the peroneus brevis and, posterolateral to it, the tendon of the peroneus longus pass as the lateral muscle group behind the lateral malleolus. The anterior neurovascular bundle (anterior tibial artery and vein, deep peroneal nerve) descends posteriorly to the extensor tendons, while the posterior neurovascular bundle (posterior tibial artery and vein, tibial nerve) is seen as low signal intensity structures anteromedially to the flexor hallucis longus on the T_2-weighted image. The sural nerve is demarcated as a low signal intensity structure within the high signal fatty tissue posterior to the peroneal tendons.

Aside from the forementioned muscles, tendons, vessels, and nerves, the transverse sections at the level of the inferior tip of the lateral malleolus show segments of the deltoid ligament (the medial ligament comprising tibionavicular, anterior tibiotalar, and tibiocalcaneal ligaments). The posterior fibulotalar ligament can be delineated along its entire course as a low-signal structure, while the anterior fibulotalar and fibulocalcaneal ligaments are only visualized in segments. Visualizing their entire course requires the foot to be repositioned or different section planes.

Foot

Transverse sections through the foot at the level of the metatarsals delineate the extensor tendons as low-signal structures within the high-signal fatty tissue posterior to the bones. The interossei can be seen between the metatarsals, while the muscle bellies and the ten-

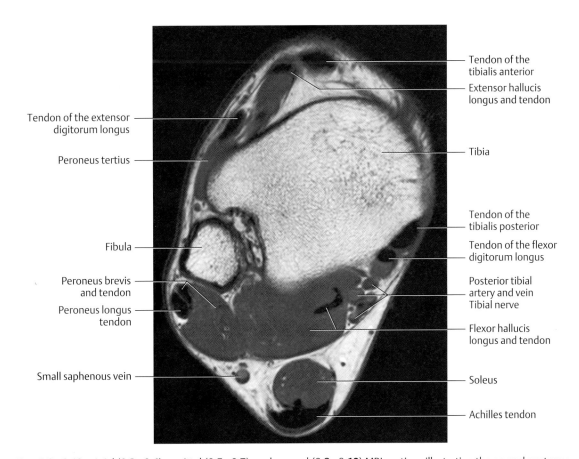

Tendon of the extensor digitorum longus

Peroneus tertius

Fibula

Peroneus brevis and tendon

Peroneus longus tendon

Small saphenous vein

Tendon of the tibialis anterior

Extensor hallucis longus and tendon

Tibia

Tendon of the tibialis posterior

Tendon of the flexor digitorum longus

Posterior tibial artery and vein
Tibial nerve

Flexor hallucis longus and tendon

Soleus

Achilles tendon

Figs. 8.**2**– 8.**10**   Axial (8.**2**– 8.**4**), sagittal (8.**5**– 8.**7**), and coronal (8.**8**– 8.**10**) MRI sections illustrating the normal anatomy.

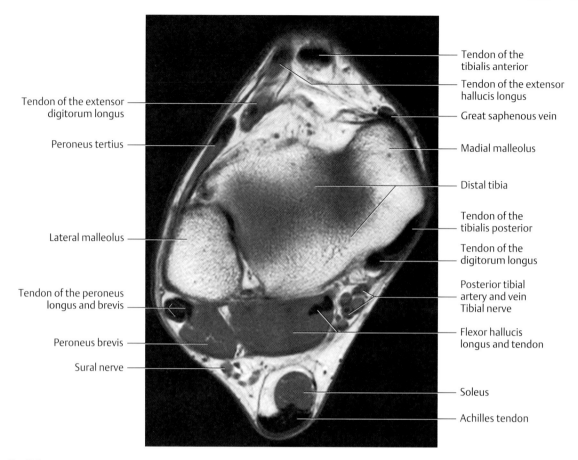

Tendon of the tibialis anterior

Tendon of the extensor hallucis longus

Great saphenous vein

Madial malleolus

Distal tibia

Tendon of the tibialis posterior

Tendon of the digitorum longus

Posterior tibial artery and vein Tibial nerve

Flexor hallucis longus and tendon

Soleus

Achilles tendon

Tendon of the extensor digitorum longus

Peroneus tertius

Lateral malleolus

Tendon of the peroneus longus and brevis

Peroneus brevis

Sural nerve

Fig. 8.**3**

dons of the abductor digiti minimi and flexor digiti minima are visualized lateral to the fifth metatarsal. Abductor hallucis, flexor hallucis brevis, tendon of the flexor hallucis longus, adductor hallucis, and tendon of the flexor digitorum longus are seen, medial to lateral, in the sole of the foot.

Sagittal Plane (Figs. 8.5– 8.7)

Talocrural and subtalar articulations: The sagittal sections delineate the longitudinal course of the long muscles of the foot. They also offer a comprehensive overview of the osseous structures that form the talocrural and subtalar articulations and are especially suitable for assessing articular surfaces including articular cartilage.

The medial sagittal sections show the tibialis posterior and flexor digitorum longus tendons, which pass behind the medial malleolus. The flexor hallucis longus runs along the posterior surface of the talus and below the sustentaculum tali of the calcaneus in the sulcus tali. On the plantar aspect, its tendon crosses under the flexor digitorum longus, sending fibrous slips to it that terminate at the distal phalanx of the second and third toes (rarely to the fourth toe).

The quadratus plantae muscle is seen on the plantar aspect of the foot arising from the plantar surface of the calcaneus and inserting along the flexor digitorum longus tendons distally.

The midsagittal sections are especially suitable for visualizing the articular surfaces of the talocrural and subtalar articulations. In both joints, the articular cartilage is delineated as a linear zone of intermediate signal intensity on the T_1-weighted image.

The subtalar articulation can be divided into an anterior and a posterior compartment, separated by the sinus tarsi. The sinus tarsi is almost completely filled by the interosseous talocalcaneal ligament, which is embedded in high-signal fatty tissue. The transected muscle and tendon of the flexor hallucis longus are seen posterior to the tibia.

The fat pad of the Achilles tendon and Achilles tendon itself are located immediately behind these structures. On the dorsum of the foot, the tibialis anterior tendon is visualized.

Sagittal sections through the distal fibula primarily visualize the longitudinal course of the peroneal tendons. The peroneus brevis tendon is located anterior to the peroneus longus tendon and continues distally to the fifth metatarsal base. The tendon of the posteriorly

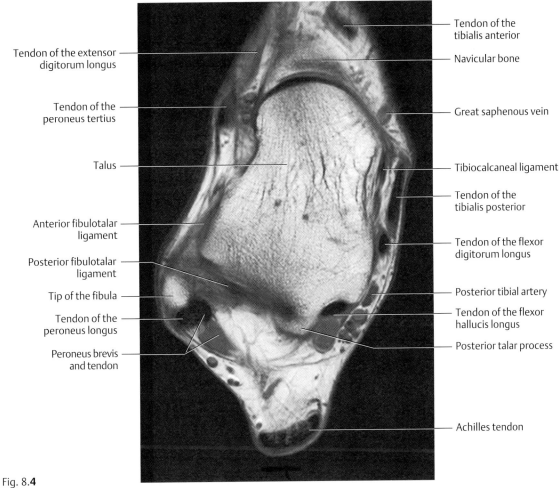

Tendon of the extensor digitorum longus

Tendon of the peroneus tertius

Talus

Anterior fibulotalar ligament

Posterior fibulotalar ligament

Tip of the fibula

Tendon of the peroneus longus

Peroneus brevis and tendon

Tendon of the tibialis anterior

Navicular bone

Great saphenous vein

Tibiocalcaneal ligament

Tendon of the tibialis posterior

Tendon of the flexor digitorum longus

Posterior tibial artery

Tendon of the flexor hallucis longus

Posterior talar process

Achilles tendon

Fig. 8.**4**

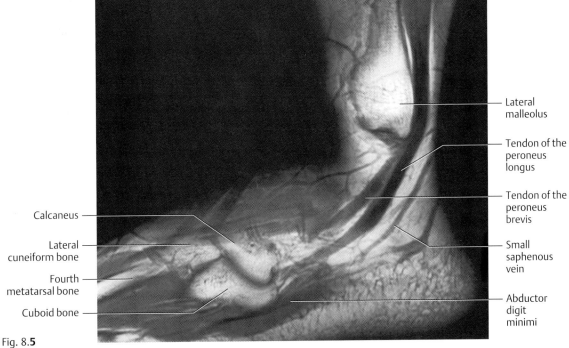

Calcaneus

Lateral cuneiform bone

Fourth metatarsal bone

Cuboid bone

Lateral malleolus

Tendon of the peroneus longus

Tendon of the peroneus brevis

Small saphenous vein

Abductor digit minimi

Fig. 8.**5**

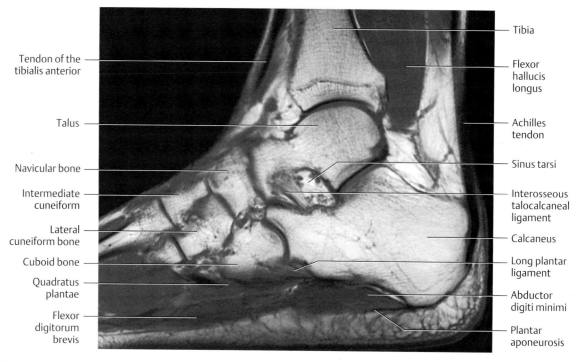

Tibia

Flexor hallucis longus

Achilles tendon

Sinus tarsi

Interosseous talocalcaneal ligament

Calcaneus

Long plantar ligament

Abductor digiti minimi

Plantar aponeurosis

Tendon of the tibialis anterior

Talus

Navicular bone

Intermediate cuneiform

Lateral cuneiform bone

Cuboid bone

Quadratus plantae

Flexor digitorum brevis

Fig. 8.**6**

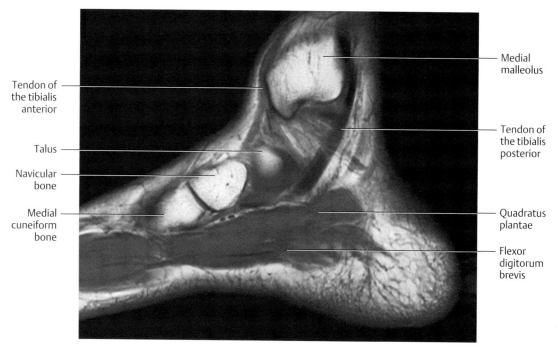

Medial malleolus

Tendon of the tibialis posterior

Quadratus plantae

Flexor digitorum brevis

Tendon of the tibialis anterior

Talus

Navicular bone

Medial cuneiform bone

Fig. 8.**7**

located peroneus longus leaves the section plane early, at the level of the lateral border of the calcaneus, and runs medially to the medial and intermediate cuneiforms.

Coronal Plane (Figs. 8.**8**– 8.**10**)

Talocrural and subtalar articulations: Coronal sections through the posterior aspect of the tibia and fibula show segments of the tibialis posterior tendon and flexor digitalis longus medial to the tibia. The flexor hallucis longus is located medial to the partially transected talus. Portions of the quadratus plantae are visualized medial to the calcaneus. The peroneal tendons are recognized as low-signal structures below the tip of the lateral malleolus.

Like the sagittal sections, the midcoronal sections allow evaluation of the talar and tibial articular surfaces and the articular cartilage. The strong posterior tibiotalar ligament is seen as low-signal structure between the medial malleolus and the medial surface of the talus. The sinus tarsi appears in the subtalar joint space,

with its high-signal fat pad and sections of the interosseous talocalcaneal ligament (Fig. 8.**30**). The cross-section of the flexor hallucis longus tendon is identified under the sustentaculum tali.

The abductor hallucis is the most medial muscle in the sole of the foot. The superficial flexor digitorum brevis and the underlying quadratus plantae are part of the intermediate muscle group.

The abductor digiti minimi is in the lateral aspect of the sole.

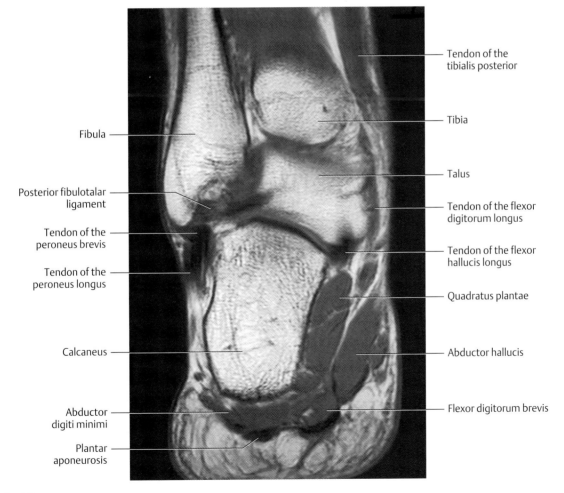

Fig. 8.**8**

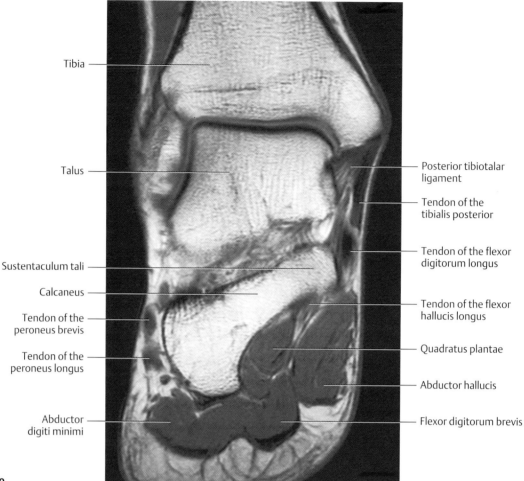

Tibia

Talus

Sustentaculum tali

Calcaneus

Tendon of the
peroneus brevis

Tendon of the
peroneus longus

Abductor
digiti minimi

Posterior tibiotalar
ligament

Tendon of the
tibialis posterior

Tendon of the flexor
digitorum longus

Tendon of the flexor
hallucis longus

Quadratus plantae

Abductor hallucis

Flexor digitorum brevis

Fig. 8.**9**

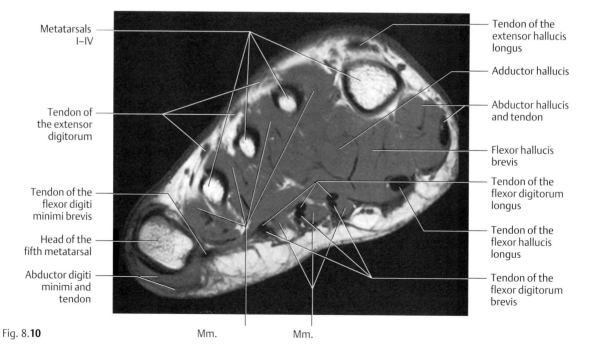

Metatarsals
I–IV

Tendon of
the extensor
digitorum

Tendon of the
flexor digiti
minimi brevis

Head of the
fifth metatarsal

Abductor digiti
minimi and
tendon

Tendon of the
extensor hallucis
longus

Adductor hallucis

Abductor hallucis
and tendon

Flexor hallucis
brevis

Tendon of the
flexor digitorum
longus

Tendon of the
flexor hallucis
longus

Tendon of the
flexor digitorum
brevis

Fig. 8.**10**   Mm.   Mm.

Disorders of the Bone

■ Osteochondral Injuries and Osteochondritis Dissecans

The talus is a common site of spontaneous or post-traumatic osteonecroses. Spontaneous osteonecrosis, osteochondritis dissecans, is usually located medially while post-traumatic osteonecrosis is frequently observed after lateral avulsion fractures. The lack of edema distinguishes an old avulsed fragment or accessory ossicle from an acute fracture or osteochondritis dissecans. Fractures and dislocations of the talus with injuries to the nutrient vessels can cause a partial or total necrosis of the talus, which shows as demineralization on conventional radiographs, following immo-

bilization, and extensive regional or total bone marrow edema on MRI (Fig. 8.**11**).

MRI is an excellent method for the early detection of osteochondral lesions of the talar articular surface. *Traumatic osteochondral injuries* are generally preceded by a severe supination injury. The lateral talar margin fractures with dorsiflexion and the medial talar margin with plantar flexion (Fig. 8.**12**).

Osteochondritis dissecans is a disease of young patients, characteristically between the ages of 20 and 40 years. This condition constitutes an avascular necrosis at the medial aspect of the talar trochlea. Its cause is not clearly known, although vascular impairment and microtrauma are frequently discussed as possible causes. The disease can be bilateral.

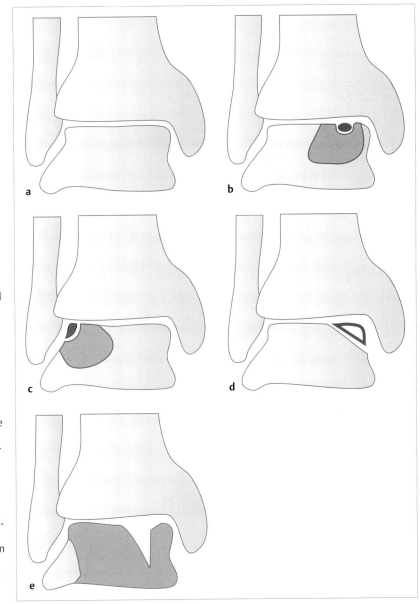

Fig. 8.**11 a–e** Avascular necrosis. Diagrammatic drawing of osteochondritis dissecans as seen in the coronal plane. **a** Normal findings. **b** Osteochondritis dissecans, characteristic location in the medial posterior third of the talar trochlea, illustrating an advanced stage. Osteochondral fragment in the crater. Surrounding perifocal edema. **c** Necrotic fragment, not dislodged, after relative recent trauma with a flake fracture typically located at the lateral talar trochlea, with localized perifocal edema. **d** Osseous fragments of the medial talar trochlea with signal intensities equal to that of bone marrow fat and without perifocal edema, representing S/P old undisplaced fracture or accessory osseous elements. **e** Extensive signal changes throughout the talus or in large areas within the talus as manifestation of total or partial talar necrosis following severed vessels in the sinus tarsi or tarsal tunnel caused by fractures or dislocations. The talar body is more frequently involved than the talar neck.

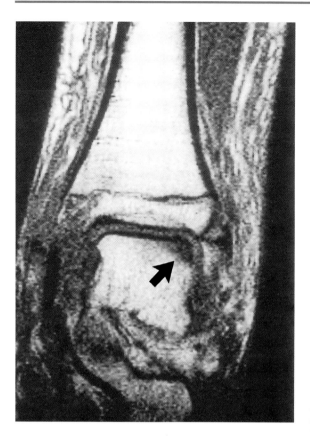

Fig. 8.**12** Osteochondral trauma of the lateral aspect of the talar trochlea, concurrent with a fracture of the medial malleolus. Subchondral decrease in signal intensity on the coronal T_1-weighted section (TR = 520 ms, TE = 20 msec) in the region of the lateral talus with intact cortex (arrow), perifocal edema with diffuse decrease in signal intensity (bone bruise). Marked decrease in signal intensity also in the region of the medial malleolus.

Sagittal and coronal sections should be selected when evaluating the talar articular surface. Osseous defects and integrity of the cartilaginous cover can be assessed on these sections. Fat suppressed imaging has been found useful for evaluating the cartilage (Fig. 8.**13**). Direct MR arthrography following intra-articular injection of contrast medium can demonstrate the extension of contrast medium from the joint space into the osseous crater. Indirect MR arthrography following intravenous injection of contrast medium and exercising of the joint also delivers contrast medium to the osseous crater. With this method, however, granulation tissue around the fragments can produce a high signal intensity and this should not be interpreted as extension of contrast medium into the cartilage defect. In our experience, the signal intensity of the enhancing granulation tissue is less than the intensity of the joint space after an adequate interval following intravenous injection (Fig. 8.**13**) (see Chapter 1).

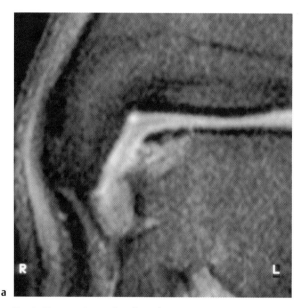

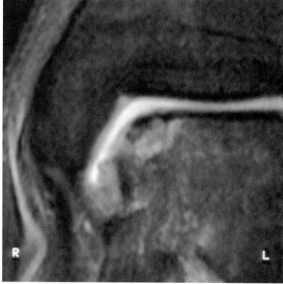

a

b

Fig. 8.**13 a–c** Osteochondritis dissecans. **a** Fat suppressed SE image (TR = 600 msec, TE = 18 msec), coronal section. Magnification. Integrity of the cartilage can be seen. **b** The indirect MRI arthrography shows no extension of contrast medium into the crater. The granulation tissue around the fragments shows faint enhancement only. **c** Indirect MR arthrography of another patient. Very high signal intensity in the osseous crater, comparable to the intra-articular signal intensity in the lateral joint space. This finding is to be interpreted as a disrupted cartilage with extension of contrast medium from the joint capsule into the osseous crater.

Fig. 8.**13 c** ▶

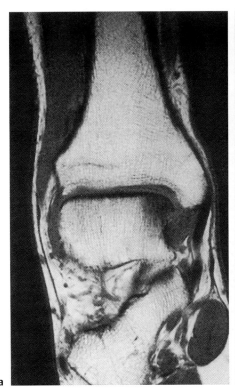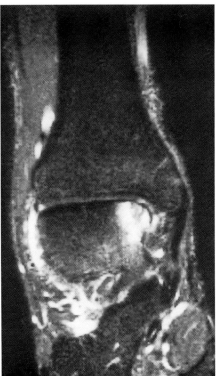

Fig. 8.**14 a, b**   Osteochondrosis dissecans, grade 1. **a** Coronal T$_1$-weighted (TR = 520 msec, TE = 20 msec) sections shows a decreased signal intensity in the subchondral bone in the region of the medial corner of the talar trochlea. **b** The STIR sequence (TR = 4800 msec, TE = 60 msec, T$_1$ = 150 msec) shows a high signal intensity of the subchondral osseous defect and reactive edema in the adjacent bone marrow. Degenerative osteoarthritis.

Nelson and co-workers (19) developed an MR classification that parallels the arthroscopic grading system and distinguishes four grades:

- Subchondral lesions of grade 1 show an intact cartilage on MRI. The osseous defect generally presents as low signal intensity on the T$_1$-weighted image. On the T$_2$-weighted image, it can have a low (sclerosis) or high (blood, joint fluid) signal intensity. A reactive bone marrow edema is frequently seen in the osseous neighborhood. It has a high signal intensity, which is best seen on STIR sequences (Fig. 8.**14**).

- The grade 2 osteochondral lesion is demarcated from the surrounding bone by a junctional zone, which can represent a reactive sclerosis or hypervascular connective tissue and consequently is of variable signal intensity. While the sclerosis is of low signal intensity on all sequences, hypervascular connective tissue shows high signal intensity on T$_2$-weighted images, which can make it difficult to distinguish it from fluid (Figs. 8.**15 a, b**). In this situation, IV contrast medium can be helpful since the hypervascular connective tissue generally shows a definite enhancement (Fig. 8.**15 c**).

- The grade 3 osteochondral lesion is surrounded by fluid that has extended from the joint space behind the lesion through fissures in the articular cartilage. Consequently, a fluid rim around an osteochondral lesion can be seen as indirect sign of a cartilaginous defect and instability (Fig. 8.**13 c**).

- The grade 4 osteochondral lesion has left the parent bone and the created defect is filled with joint fluid. The dislodged osseous fragment is characteristically seen as a loose intra-articular body, free within the joint.

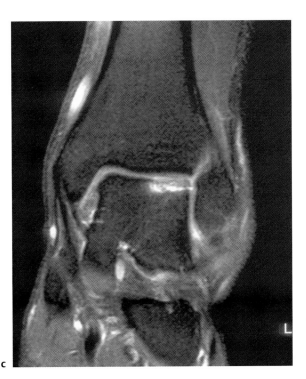

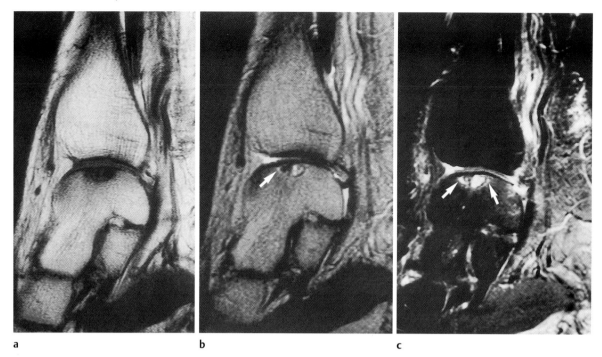

a   b   c

Fig. 8.**15a–c** Osteochondrosis dissecans, grade 2. **a** Low signal intensity in the osteochondral defect of the medial aspect of the talar trochlea on a sagittal T_1-weighted image (TR = 520 msec, TE = 20 msec). **b** The corresponding T_2-weighted section (TR = 3500 msec, TE = 80 msec) shows a definite junctional zone, exhibiting, in part, a high signal intensity (arrow). The osseous fragment also shows a high signal inten- sity posteriorly as evidence of cystic changes. **c** The contrast-enhanced fat-suppressed T_1-weighted image (TR = 150 msec, TE = 20 msec) obtained to differentiate between fluid and fibrovascular tissues shows a definite enhancement in the junctional zone (arrows) indicative of highly vascular granulation tissue.

■ Other Osteonecroses

In addition to avascular necrosis of the talar trochlea, numerous less frequent spontaneous avascular necroses of the foot skeleton are known:

- Navicular bone (Köhler I disease),
- Second metatarsal head (Köhler II disease),
- Calcaneal apophysis (Sever disease),
- Phalangeal base (Thiemann disease),
- Base of the fifth metatarsal (Iselin disease),
- Os tibiale externum (Haglund disease).

These conditions are found primarily in children and adolescents. Some types, such as the avascular necrosis of the metatarsal head, can also be observed in adults. Clinically, they may present with pain. In general, avascular necroses show an early subchondral decrease in signal intensity on the T_1-weighted image and an increase in signal intensity on the T_2-weighted image, especially on the STIR image. This can be attributed to bone marrow edema. In the course of the disease, the dominance of sclerotic changes can cause decreased signal intensity on the T_1-weighted and T_2-weighted sequences. High signal granulation tissue on T_2-weighted and T_2^*-weighted sequences indicates revascularization (29).

The junctional zone between the necrotic area and intact bone consists of two layers with an inner line of high signal intensity and an outer line of low signal intensity on T_2-weighted images, the so-called double line sign (18) (Fig. 8.16). MRI has a high sensitivity and can detect avascular necrosis before other imaging methods.

■ Stress Fractures and Occult Fractures

MRI can diagnose radiographically occult undisplaced traumatic fractures and stress fractures.

Stress fractures are fractures in healthy bone caused by repetitive microtraumas. They are characterized by an osseous break with concurrent bone repair. In the ankle and foot, they are most frequently observed in the distal tibia and fibula, calcaneus, navicular bone, and metatarsals. Characteristically, a low signal line is seen, corresponding to impacted trabecular structures and reactive bone marrow edema. It is of low signal intensity on the T_1-weighted sequences (Fig. 8.**17**). The T_2-weighted images and, particularly, STIR sequences show a high signal intensity (Fig. 8.**18**) (4). If an MRI obtained after trauma only reveals a diffuse bone marrow edema without linear decrease in signal intensity, the finding is referred to as bone bruise or trabecular microfracture (17).

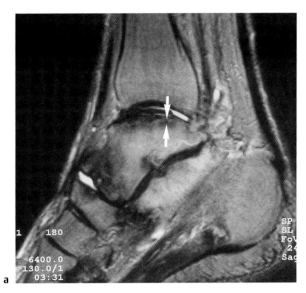

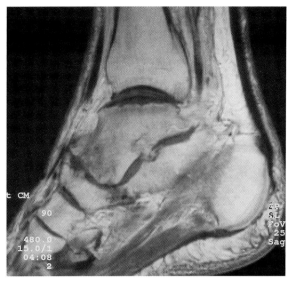

a b

Fig. 8.**16 a, b** Osteonecrosis of the talar trochlea. **a** The sagittal T$_2$-weighted sequence (TR = 6400 msec, TE = 130 msec) shows a dark bone marrow signal in the region of the talar trochlea corresponding to necrotic bone. The necrotic subchondral bone is demarcated from the remaining bone by high signal granulation tissue. The granulation tissue shows an inner line of high signal intensity and an outer line of low signal intensity (arrows), the so-called double line sign. Bone marrow edema throughout the entire talus, partially extending into the adjacent calcaneus. **b** T$_1$-weighted sequence after IV contrast medium (TR = 480 msec, TE = 15 msec) shows no enhancement of the necrotic bone and strong enhancement of the granulation tissue.

Because of the suppressed fat signal and the high signal visualization of the edema, the STIR sequence is particularly sensitive for the detection of bone bruises, occult fractures, and stress fractures.

■ Synostoses of the Tarsal Bones (Tarsal Coalitions)

Congenital synostoses (coalitions) can occur between any tarsal bones. They have an incidence of 1 – 2% and are bilateral in 50%. Different types of coalition can be observed in the same foot. They are a frequent cause of a painful flat foot in children and become symptomatic at an age when the initial cartilaginous connection (synchondrosis) between the affected bones begins to ossify. Secondary degenerative changes with increasingly painful restriction of the mobility can be prevented if the correct diagnosis is made early and the appropriate therapy, such as orthopedic support, surgical resection, or arthrodesis, is initiated.

The most frequent synostoses are between calcaneus and navicular (calcaneonavicular coalition) and between calcaneus and talus (talocalcaneal coalition). Tarsal coalitions are generally diagnosed by conventional radiography or CT. Before ossification of the synchondrosis, MRI can show a cartilaginous bridge between the affected bones. The cleft between the bones is smaller than a normal joint space and irregularly outlined. This finding is especially well seen on GRE sequences. The sections should be perpendicular to the affected joint. The ossification is completed when trabecular bone has formed and inactive fatty bone

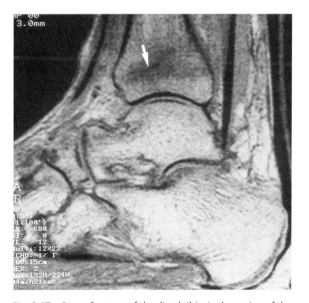

Fig. 8.**17** Stress fracture of the distal tibia. In the region of the distal tibia, the sagittal T$_1$-weighted GRE sequence (TR = 680 msec, TE = 12 msec) shows a linear, sharply outlined decrease in signal intensity corresponding to the fracture line (arrow). This is surrounded by a heterogeneous decrease in signal intensity, corresponding to reactive bone marrow edema.

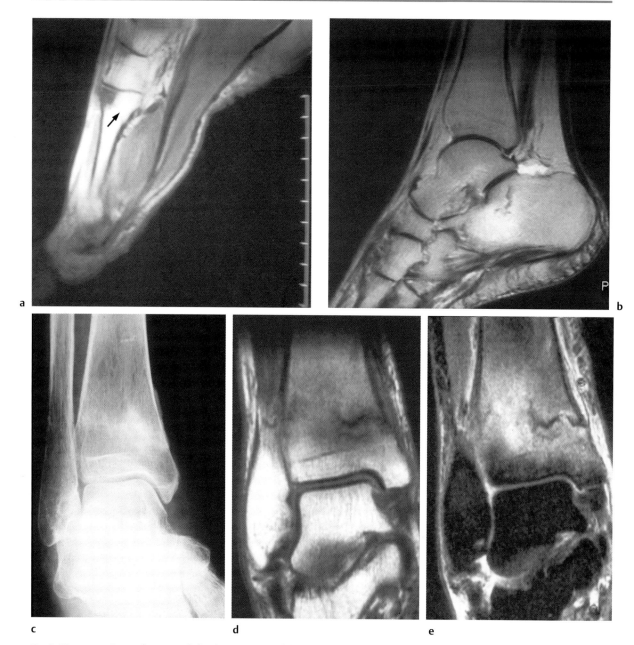

Fig. 8.**18a–e** **a** Stress fracture of the first metatarsal base with focal and linear low signal intensity edema (arrow). Sagittal T$_1$-weighted SE image. **b** Stress fracture of the calcaneus with low signal intensity fracture line and surrounding high signal intensity edema. Sagittal T$_2$-weighted TSE image. **c–e** Stress fracture of the distal tibial metaphysis. **c** Radiograph showing a band-like sclerosis and periosteal new bone formation. **d** Coronal T$_1$-weighted SE image with fracture line seen as signal void and edema as low signal intensity. **e** Coronal STIR image with signal void fracture line and high signal edema. High signal edema in the adjacent soft tissues.

marrow is seen as fat-equivalent signal intensity on MRI. A coalition that fails to ossify is referred to as a fibrous or cartilaginous coalition.

The *calcaneonavicular coalition* is a synostosis between the base of the navicular and the anterior superior calcaneus. This form of osseous bridging is best documented on oblique radiographic views. Symptoms appear between ages of 8 and 12 years. In addition to a painful flat foot, the peroneal tendons become prominent, secondary to chronic reflex-induced shortening.

The *talocalcaneal coalition* can have variable manifestations, depending on which of the three articulations (posterior, medial and anterior) between calcaneus and talus are synostosed. Synostosis of the posterior medial articulations are best evaluated on oblique axial radiographic views (ski jumper's view, Harris technique). Documenting the coalition can be difficult. The medial articulation is most frequently affected. Talocalcaneal coalition generally becomes symptomatic after the 20th year of life.

Secondary arthrodesis following infection or trauma may also show fatty bone marrow with time (Fig. 8.**19**).

Disorders of the Tendon

Tendons largely consist of dense fascicles of collagenous fibers embedded in an amorphous base substance. Because of an extremely short T_2 relaxation time, the tendons have a low signal intensity on all pulse sequences. Degenerative changes, inflammation, and partial and complete tears alter the internal structure of the tendon and render the tendon visible on MRI. The disposition of lipids secondary to degeneration and hemorrhage cause an increased intratendinous signal on the T_1-weighted image. High signal intensities on the T_2-weighted image suggest inflammatory changes or tears, depending on extent and pattern. Tendon thickening can be observed with chronic inflammatory changes, while localized thinning suggests a partial rupture.

■ Achilles Tendon

Tears of the Achilles tendon primarily occur in men between the ages of 30 and 50 years. Aside from rheumatoid arthritis and lupus erythematosus, the predisposing factors include various metabolic disorders (diabetes mellitus, gout, hyperparathyroidism, chronic renal failure), long-term corticosteroid therapy, and athletic overuse. Partial and complete ruptures occur preferentially through the zone of lowest vascularization, which is about 2–6 cm above the calcaneal insertion (25).

Most tears are readily diagnosed clinically as a palpable dehiscence of the tendon. Hemorrhage and edematous changes can be responsible for a negative palpatory finding. According to the literature the incidence of false negative clinical findings is about 25% (6, 25). For this reason the clinical examination should be supplemented by imaging, principally sonography and MRI. Sonography has the advantage of being dynamic, while MRI permits a more accurate assessment of the structural changes.

Tear

A complete tear of the Achilles tendon is characterized by a gap in the tendon, best seen in the sagittal plane. The retraction of the tendon remnants leads to a corkscrew appearance of the proximal remnant and increased buckling of the distal segment on the sagittal image (Fig. 8.**20**). Interposed fat or fluid (edema, blood) is frequently found at the site of the tear. Changes of the peritendinous tissue can be seen on axial sections.

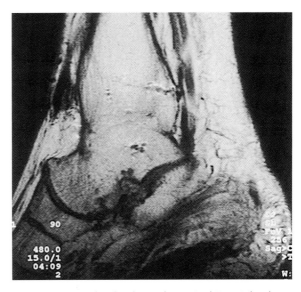

Fig. 8.**19** Surgical arthrodesis. The sagittal T_1-weighted section (TR = 480 msec, TE = 15 msec) shows a homogeneously high signal intensity in the bone marrow of the distal tibia and adjacent talus, without evidence of a residual joint space.

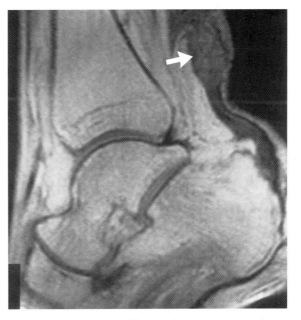

Fig. 8.**20** Complete Achilles tendon tear. Sagittal T_1-weighted sequence (TR = 600 msec, TE = 20 msec) shows thickening and buckling of the distal tendon remnant with generally increased signal intensity in the tendon (arrow).

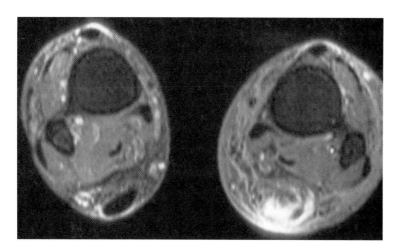

Fig. 8.**21** Complete rupture of the left Achilles tendon. Axial STIR image. The tendon is only partially discernible. Definite soft tissue swelling with accumulation of high signal intensity fluid.

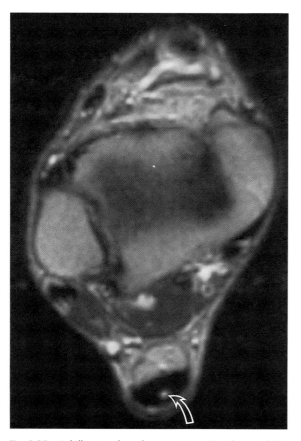

Fig. 8.**22** Achilles tendon degeneration. On the axial T_2-weighted image (TR = 3800 msec, TE = 90 msec), focally increased signal intensity within the tendon as evidence of beginning degeneration (arrow).

Blood of subacute hemorrhage shows a high signal intensity on the T_1-weighted image, while edematous and inflammatory changes exhibit a high signal intensity on the T_2-weighted image (Fig. 8.**21**).

Apart from assisting with the diagnosis, MRI provides therapeutic information since the distance between the tendon remnants determines whether conservative therapy can be expected to succeed (7). Furthermore, MRI can be used to follow those patients treated conservatively (16). Re-rupture after conservative therapy causes an intratendinous increase in signal intensity on T_1-weighted and T_2-weighted images.

Partial Tear

Partial tears are distinguished from complete tears by the detection of residual continuity on axial or sagittal sections. The tendon shows a focally increased signal intensity on the T_1-weighted image and areas of high signal intensity corresponding to blood or fluid accumulation on the T_2-weighted image. Similar findings are observed in degenerative changes or tendinitis, with neither condition reliably distinguishable from a partial tear on MRI. Partial tears often occur in the context of chronic degenerative inflammation (Fig. 8.**23**).

Tendinitis

The edematous changes occurring with tendinitis appear as focal or diffuse increases in signal intensities in the tendon on T_2 weighted, T_2^*-weighted and fat suppressed images (Fig. 8.**22**). Tendon thickening causes the anterior tendon contour to be convex on axial and sagittal images (Fig. 8.**23**). Since the Achilles tendon lacks a synovial sheath, Achilles tendinitis can be accompanied by reactive changes in the peritendinous soft tissues. IV contrast medium can improve the visualization and differentiation of inflammatory changes.

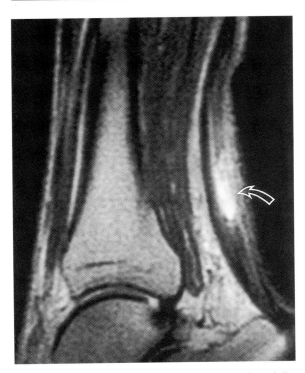

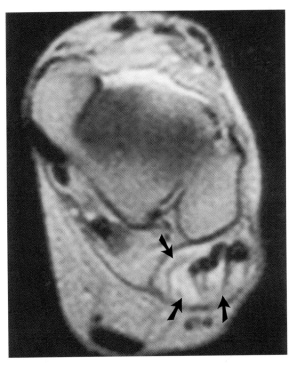

Fig. 8.**23** Tendinitis with extensive partial tear of the Achilles tendon. Diffuse increase in signal intensity within the tendon tissue on sagittal T$_2$-weighted image (TR = 3000 msec, TE = 80 msec) (arrow). Fluid-equivalent signal intensity as evidence of partial rupture. Convex anterior contour of the tendon due to edematous thickening of the tendon.

Fig. 8.**24** Chronic tenosynovitis of the peroneal tendons. The axial T$_2$-weighted section (TR = 3000 msec, TE = 80 msec) at the level of the joint space of the talocrural articulation shows fluid in the region of the cicatricially thickened tendon sheaths (arrows).

■ Peroneal Tendons

Complete or partial tears of the peroneal tendons are extremely rare. Complete tears usually affect the peroneus longus tendon at the level of the cuboid (21).

Partial tears primarily involve the peroneus brevis tendon. They are frequently associated with subluxation of the peroneal tendons and have a longitudinal morphology appearing as a longitudinal split, usually at the level of the tip of the lateral malleolus (30). On MRI, increased signal intensity is seen within the tendon giving the appearance of a longitudinal split (36).

Tendinitis generally causes diffuse thickening of the tendon, often surrounded by the fluid-filled synovial sheath and seen as increased signal intensity on the T$_2$-weighted image. This indicates an inflammatory involvement of the synovial sheath as a manifestation of tenosynovitis (Fig. 8.**24**).

Subluxation of the peroneal tendons is frequently associated with traumatic stretching or tearing of the superior peroneal retinaculum. The peroneal tendons are displaced lateroanteriorly over the tip of the lateral malleolus from their anatomic position along the posterior surface of the lateral malleolus. An absent or flat osseous groove on the outer surface of the lateral malleolus (malleolar sulcus) predisposes to such a subluxation (22).

The diagnosis can be made by MRI if the tendons are seen lateral to the lateral malleolus and not in their normal posterior location. Accompanying soft tissue edema is frequently detected. Comparison with the contralateral healthy ankle can make it easier to make the correct diagnosis (24).

■ Deep Flexor Tendons

Tibialis Posterior

The tibialis posterior tendon is an important stabilizer of the medial longitudinal arch of the foot. Tears occur primarily in women after the age of 50 years and are usually degenerative in nature. Predisposing factors are rheumatoid arthritis, long-term corticosteroid therapy and a flat foot (15).

Partial and complete tears of the tibialis posterior tendon usually occur in the region of the navicular insertion of the tendon (27). Since the diagnosis is often delayed, the site of tear is frequently suspected to be at the level of medial malleolus because of the position of the retracted tendon remnant (23). Indirect signs found with a torn posterior tibial tendon are a vertical position of the talus, an accessory navicular bone, and hypertrophy of the medial navicular tubercle (27).

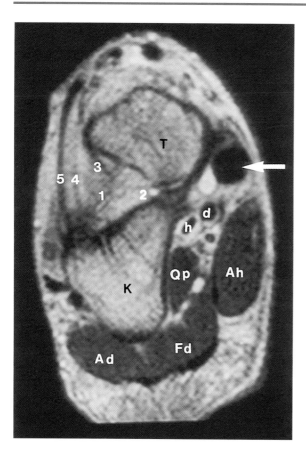

Fig. 8.**25**   Stage I tendon tear of the posterior tibialis. Definite thickening of the cross section of the tendon on the coronal T$_2$-weighted image (TR = 3000 msec, TE = 80 msec) with fluid-distended tendon sheath (arrow).
T   = Talus
C   = Calcaneus
Qp = Quadratus plantae
Ah = Abductor hallucis
Ad = Abductor digiti minimi
Fd = Flexor digitorum brevis
d   = Tendon of the flexor digitorum longus
h   = Tendon of the flexor hallucis longus
1–5 = Ligaments of the sinus tarsi:
    1 = Cervical ligament
    2 = Interossoeus talocalcaneal ligament
    3 = Medial fascicle of the medial extensor retinaculum
    4 = Intermediate fascicle of the inferior extensor
        retinaculum
    5 = Lateral fascicle of the inferior extensor retinaculum

A complete tear of the tendon produces a severe flat foot and the inability to tiptoe. Three stages of tendon tear can be distinguished on MRI:

- Stage I represents a partial tear with tendon thickening and occasional longitudinal fissures seen as lines of increased signal intensity on the T$_1$-weighted and T$_2$-weighted images. A high signal intensity fluid is generally seen in the synovial sheath on the T$_2$-weighted image (Fig. 8.**25**).
- Stage II represents a partial tear with localized narrowing of the tendon, with its cross section smaller than the cross section of the flexor digitorum longus tendon.
- Stage III refers to the complete tear with visualized tendon gap. Fluid or, if the injury is not recent, granulation tissue is found between the retracted tendon remnants (24).

An exact classification is important since the therapeutic approach will be determined by the extent and location of the injury.

Flexor Digitorum Longus

Tears of the flexor digitorum longus tendon are extremely rare and recognized by the characteristic claw-foot deformity. Tenosynovitis is more frequent and is recognized by the increased fluid content of the synovial sheaths seen on MRI.

Flexor Hallucis Longus

Partial tears, complete tears, tendinitis, and tenosynovitis of the flexor hallucis longus tendon occur primarily in ballet dancers (Fig. 8.**26**).

Since the tendon sheath frequently communicates with the joint capsule of the talocrural articulation, the fluid accumulation in the tendon sheath must be judged in relation to the size of the joint effusion.

■ Extensor Group

Tendinitis or tenosynovitis of the tibialis anterior tendon occurs predominately in chronic overuse due to running or walking downhill or in dancers. Tears, which are rare, are usually located at the level of the first tarsometatarsal articulation. Marginal osteophytes and exostoses may predispose to tendon tears as a result of friction against the tendon.

Pathologic changes of the extensor hallucis longus and extensor digitorum longus tendons are also rare. The MRI findings correspond to those of the other tendons described above.

Fig. 8.**26 a, b**   Tenosynovitis of the deep flexor tendons. **a** Before and **b** after the administration of contrast medium (axial section). Definite enhancement of the tendon sheath of the flexor hallucis longus (H), flexor digitorum longus (D), and tibialis posterior (T) (T_1-SE; TR = 450 msec, TE = 15 msec).

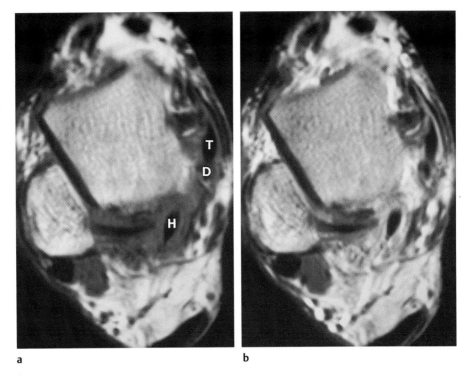

a   b

Ligamentous Injuries

■ Talocrural Articulation

In the region of the talocrural articulation, three ligament complexes are distinguished that determine stability and integrity of the joint:

- Medial collateral ligament (deltoid ligament) with four divisions (tibionavicular, tibiocalcaneal, anterior tibiotalar, and posterior tibiotalar).
- Lateral ligament, which is most frequently injured and accounts for 85% of all recurrent ligamentous tears. The underlying trauma mechanism is usually an inversion injury, which, depending on the severity, affects first the anterior tibiotalar ligament, then the fibulocalcaneal ligament and, finally, the posterior fibulotalar ligament.
- The third ligamentous complex is the tibiofibular syndesmosis, which stabilizes the ankle mortise and comprises the anterior and posterior tibiofibular ligament.

After clinical assessment, the diagnostic evaluation of an ankle sprain with possible ligamentous injury begins with radiographic views in two projections to exclude any osseous pathology. Radiographic stress views may also be obtained, but are frequently negative due to extensive post-traumatic edema and muscle spasm (31).

MRI can visualize the ligaments of the talocrural examination and determine the extent of any ligamentous injury (18, 19). Like the muscle tendons, the intact ligaments show low signal intensity on all sequences (Figs. 8.**27 a** and 8.**28 a**). Linear high signal intensity areas corresponding to intraligamentous fat deposits have been described in the tibiofibular and posterior talofibular ligaments and the deep components of the deltoid ligaments (12).

Assessment of any ligament must consider signal pattern, thickness, contour, and continuity (26), with these findings best appreciated on the T_2-weighted or $T_2{}^*$-weighted sequences. Distortions and partial tears produce an intraligamentous edema or hemorrhage and cause an increase in signal intensity on the T_2-weighted sequences. A ligamentous gap indicates a complete tear (Figs. 8.**27 b**, 8.**28 b**, and 8.**29**). Thickening or wavy contour of a ligament suggests an old trauma or a chronic injury and is frequently associated with insufficiency of the affected ligament.

For a thorough evaluation, the entire course of the ligaments should be visualized (26). By virtue of the different orientation of the individual ligaments, differently oriented sections are necessary. Because of the relatively narrow width of most ligaments, the section thickness should not exceed 3 mm.

■ Sinus Tarsi Syndrome

Together with the calcaneal sulcus, the sulcus tali forms an anatomic canal that opens laterally to form the sinus tarsi and separates the posterior subtalar joint from the talocalcaneonavicular joint. The sinus tarsi contains nerves, vessels, and ligamentous structures, embedded in fatty tissue (Figs. 8.**1**, 8.**6**, 8.**25**, and 8.**30**). The sinus tarsi is well delineated on axial and coronal sections.

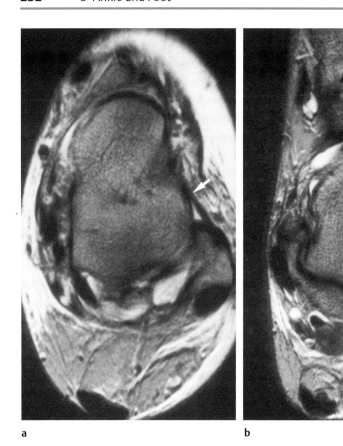

a   b

Fig. 8.**27 a, b** Visualization of the anterior
fibulotalar ligament on
axial T$_2$-weighted section
(TR = 3500 msec, TE = 110
msec). **a** The intact band
extends as a dark, low signal structure from the tip
of the fibula to the talar
neck (arrow). **b** Example of
a complete ligamentous
tear in another patient
after supination trauma,
with a high signal intensity
in the region of the original site of the ligament
and without evidence of a
continuous ligamentous
structure (T$_2$-weighted TSE
image).

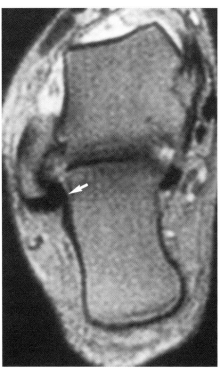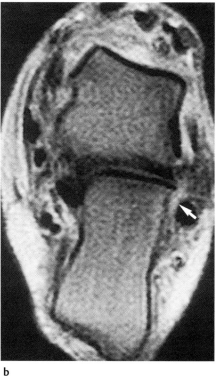

Fig. 8.**28 a, b** Visualization of the fibulocalcaneal
ligament on axial T$_2$-
weighted section (TR =
3000 msec, TE = 80 msec).
a The intact ligament extends as dark structure
medial to the peroneal
tendons (arrow).
b Complete tear of the
fibulocalcaneal ligament.
High signal intensity along
the expected course of the
tendon without evidence
of a normal ligamentous
structure (arrow).

a   b

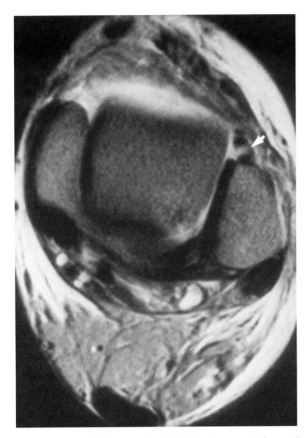

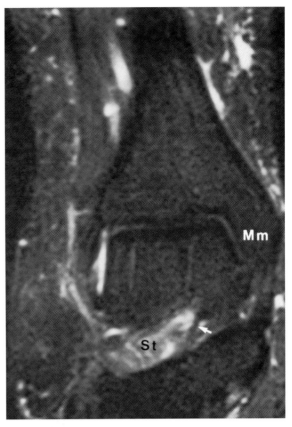

Fig. 8.**29** Tear of the anterior tibiofibular ligament. The axial T_2-weighted section (TR = 4500 msec, TE = 120 msec) shows thickening and a high signal intensity gap in the anterior tibiofibular ligament close to the fibula (arrow).

Fig. 8.**30** Sinus tarsi syndrome. This patient presented with the clinical findings of a post-traumatic sinus tarsi syndrome. The coronal STIR image (TR = 4800 msec, TE = 60 msec, TI = 50 msec) shows edematous changes in the soft tissue space of the sinus tarsi. The interosseous talocalcaneal ligament can be delineated as uninterrupted structure (arrow).
Mm = Medial malleolus
St = Sinus tarsi

The sinus tarsi syndrome occurs after supination trauma and presents as lateral foot pain, tenderness over the sinus tarsi and instability, with improvement of the complaints after local injection of an anesthetic into the region of the sinus tarsi (9). The T_1-weighted or T_2-weighted images show signal changes in the ligaments or a ligamentous gap. Moreover, non-specific inflammatory changes may be seen, with signal intensities that are low on T_1-weighted and high on T_2-weighted images (2 a). Any scar formation presents as low signal intensity on both T_1-weighted and T_2-weighted images (Fig. 8.**30**). Furthermore, synovial cysts can cause a sinus tarsi syndrome (Fig. 8.**31**). The sinus tarsi syndrome is frequently associated with a tear of the lateral collateral ligament or an injury of the tibialis posterior tendon (10, 14). If conservative therapy fails, surgical revision of the sinus tarsi may be necessary.

Diseases of the Plantar Aponeurosis

■ Plantar Fasciitis

In plantar fasciitis, chronic stress and microtrauma cause small fissures and inflammatory changes in the region of the plantar aponeurosis.

The normal plantar aponeurosis has a low signal intensity on all MRI sequences and is best seen on sagittal and coronal sections.

Berkowitz and co-workers (2) observed a significant increase in the thickness of the plantar aponeurosis in patients with plantar fasciitis in comparison with asymptomatic subjects. Areas of increased signal intensity have been occasionally observed. Edematous changes in the subcutaneous fatty tissue are less frequent. In 50% of patients, a plantar spur is encountered, which is best delineated on sagittal T_1-weighted sections (2) (Fig. 8.**32**).

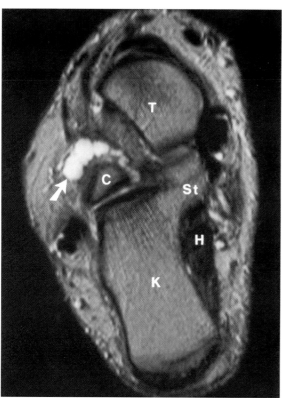

Fig. 8.**31** In this patient, the axial T₂-weighted image (TR = 3800 msec, TE = 20 msec) shows high signal cystic changes corresponding to synovial cysts (arrow) as cause of the sinus tarsi syndrome.
St = Sustentaculum tali
H = Flexor hallucis longus
Ca = Calcaneus
C = Cuboid
T = Talus

■ Plantar Fibromatosis

In plantar fibromatosis, excess fibrous connective tissue is deposited in the medial aspect of the plantar aponeurosis. In the majority of cases, a single large fibroma (approximately 20–30 mm) is found. Only 10% of cases show multiple nodules (1). MRI shows a nodular structure in the subcutaneous soft tissues of the medial sole, which exhibits a low signal intensity on T₁-weighted and T₂-weighted sequences. Some cases show areas of high signal intensity in the center of the nodules on fat-suppressed T₂-weighted sequences (35).

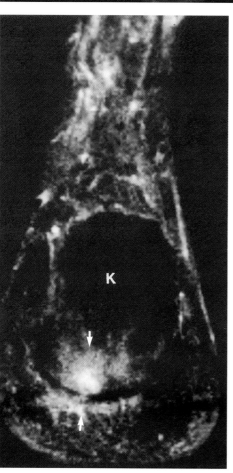

◀ Fig. 8.**32** Plantar fasciitis in the presence of a known plantar spur. The coronal STIR sequence shows a bone marrow edema of the calcaneus (upper arrow) and edematous changes above the plantar aponeurosis (lower arrow).
C = Calcaneus

Disorders of the Nerves

■ Tarsal Tunnel Syndrome

The tarsal tunnel syndrome refers to a compression neuropathy of the posterior tibial nerve or its branches in the region of the tarsal tunnel.

The roof of the tarsal tunnel is formed by the flexor retinaculum and more distally by the abductor hallucis (Fig. 8.**33**). At the level of the retinaculum, the tarsal tunnel is divided by fibrous septa into several compartments, through which muscle tendons, vessels, and nerves pass to the sole. Thus, the neural branches have little room to move if a space-occupying process develops within the tarsal tunnel.

Clinically, patients usually complain of vague, burning pain and paresthesia in the region of the sole or along the lateral foot.

Axial and coronal sections are suitable for delineating the anatomic structures of the tarsal tunnel (37). The causes of tarsal tunnel syndrome include tumor or tumor-like space-occupying lesions, ganglion cysts, varicose veins, tenosynovitis, muscle hypertrophies, accessory muscles, fibrous scars, osseous extension, or a valgus deformity of the dorsum of the foot (8).

■ Morton's Neuroma

Morton's neuroma causes a neuralgia with pain in the forefoot, characteristically between the third and fourth metatarsals, less frequently between the second and third metatarsal. Morton's neuroma is a benign pseudotumor arising from a perineural fibrosis of a plantar interdigital neural branch. The changes are best seen on axial and sagittal sections. Due to the high content of

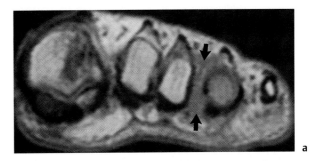

a

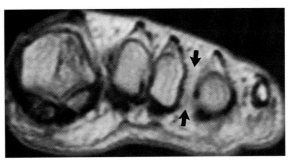

b

Fig. 8.**34 a, b** Patient with Morton's neuroma. Axial T₁-weighted images **a** before and **b** after IV contrast medium (TR = 600 msec, TE = 20 msec) show a moderately enhancing space-occupying lesion between the third and fourth metatarsals, corresponding to a perineural fibrosis of the interdigital nerve (arrows).

dense collagenous connective tissue, the tumor is isointense to hyperintense on T₁-weighted and T₂-weighted sequences. Detection and visualization of the frequently small changes can be improved by obtaining T₁-weighted fat suppressed sequences after IV contrast medium (32) (Fig. 8.**34**).

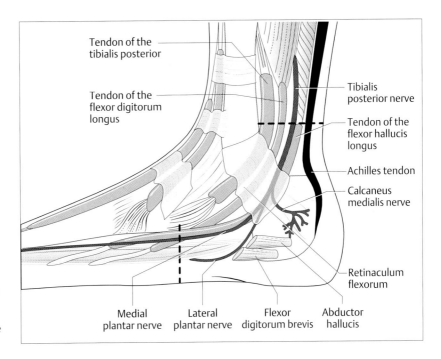

Fig. 8.**33** Drawing of the medial aspect of the foot to illustrate the anatomic situation of the tarsal tunnel (after Kerr and Frey). Dashed lines = demarcation of the tarsal tunnel.

Tendon of the tibialis posterior

Tendon of the flexor digitorum longus

Tibialis posterior nerve

Tendon of the flexor hallucis longus

Achilles tendon

Calcaneus medialis nerve

Retinaculum flexorum

Medial plantar nerve   Lateral plantar nerve   Flexor digitorum brevis   Abductor hallucis

Diabetic Foot

MRI plays a secondary role in the evaluation of osteoarthropathy of the foot caused by diabetic neuropathy. Clinical impression and conventional radiography are generally sufficient for managing the patient. For surgical planning, MRI can contribute to a more accurate determination of the extent of the osseous and soft tissue changes. Neuropathic osteoarthropathy can induce extensive signal alteration in the bone and soft tissues, usually with decreased signal intensities on T_1-weighted and T_2-weighted images. However, increased signal intensities on the T_2-weighted image may be observed. In particular, pathologic stress reactions of the bone, a frequent complication of the diabetic foot, can induce a bone marrow edema with increased signal intensity on the T_2-weighted image. Distinguishing such changes from osteomyelitis or soft tissue infection is not possible with MRI because of the similar signal pattern induced by these conditions, neither can it be achieved with other imaging methods. An indistinct outline of the area of altered signal and a perifocal fluid accumulation favors an osteomyelitis. A peripheral contrast enhancement around a liquid center suggests an abscess.

In diabetic feet, 90% of the cases of osteomyelitis arise from skin ulcerations. They are found primarily at pressure points, particularly beneath the first and fifth metatarsal heads. In comparison with other imaging methods, MRI has the highest sensitivity and specificity in diagnosing osteomyelitis in diabetic arthropathy (5, 34) (Fig. 8.**35**).

Bursitis

Acute or chronic bursitis can occur in isolation or together with inflammation of the joints or soft tissues. The diagnosis can be established clinically on the basis of tenderness and pain at the typical sites. MRI shows a fluid-filled bursa with low signal intensity on the T_1-weighted and high signal intensity on the T_2-weighted images. Hemorrhagic or proteinaceous fluid in a chronic bursitis can induce a high signal intensity on the T_1-weighted image. In chronic bursitis, the T_1-weighted image can visualize a thickened wall with increased signal intensity relative to the fluid. Bursitis as part of arthritic conditions can show small round low signal areas within the fluid-filled bursa as manifestation of synovial arthropathy with frondose growth. In the region of the talocrural articulation, the bursa anterior to the Achilles tendon at the calcaneal insertion is frequently involved (Fig. 8.**36**). This bursitis is often associated with osteophyte formation of the calcaneus (Haglund exostosis). The subcutaneous calcaneal bursa (posterior to the Achilles tendon at the level of the calcaneal insertion) and the subcutaneous bursa of the medial and lateral malleolus are less frequently involved.

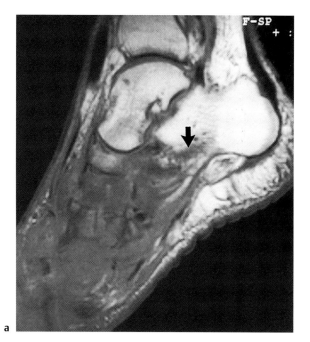

a

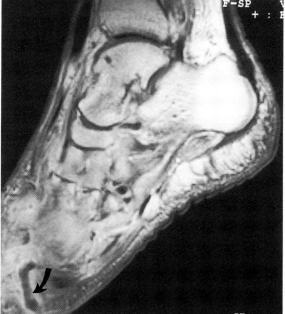

b

Fig. 8.**35 a, b**   Chronic osteomyelitis in a diabetic foot. Sagittal T_1-weighted images (TR = 500 msec, TE = 15 msec) obtained **a** before and **b** after intravenous contrast medium show a diffuse soft tissue infection and extensive osteomyelitis of the midfoot and forefoot. Early infiltration of the calcaneus (arrow). After IV contrast medium, tubular enhancement of fistulous tract in the plantar aspect of the forefoot (curved arrow).

Pitfalls in Interpreting the Images

To avoid misinterpreting MRI examinations, a few peculiarities of the signal pattern of individual anatomic structures are mentioned here.

Like the anterior cruciate ligament, the posterior tibial, fibular, and fibulotalar ligaments and the deep component of the deltoid ligament can have increased signal intensities on the T_1-weighted and T_2-weighted sequences due to fat depositions, which should not be mistaken for strains or partial tears. Similar increases in signal intensities can occur as a normal variant in the posterior tibial tendon at the insertion of the navicula (20).

Intra-articular and peritendinous fluid should not invariably be equated with pathologic changes. Specifically in the region of the posterior tendons and, in particular, around the flexor hallucis longus, large fluid accumulations can be found in asymptomatic patients. Furthermore, various compartments communicate with each other, making an exact anatomic assignment of the changes difficult (28).

On sagittal sections, the posterior tibiofibular and fibulotalar ligaments should not be mistaken for loose intra-articular bodies.

Intact tendons are normally of low signal intensities on all sequences. Depending on the orientation of the stationary magnetic field altered signal intensities can be observed, mimicking tears or inflammations. This magic angle phenomenon appears on SE and GRE sequences with short TE times if the tendon forms an angle of about 55 degrees relative to the static magnetic field. Since the altered signals disappear with longer TE times (> than 60 msec), their differentiation from pathologic changes is usually possible with the help of T_2-weighted images. Differentiation can also be assisted by repeating the examination after repositioning the patient.

The accessory ossicles and sesamoids at various sites of the foot should not be mistaken for free intra-articular bodies or avulsions. The MRI findings should always be interpreted in conjunction with conventional radiographs (12).

■ Accessory Muscles (Fig. 8.**37**)

Congenital variants of muscles are known in most regions of the body. The variations observed relate to muscle bellies and tendons, cleft formation, variants of origin and insertion as well as absence (minus variants) or supernumerary or duplicated muscle bellies (plus variants). Knowledge of these common variations is not only important to surgeons. For the diagnostic radiologist, it is particularly important to recognize accessory muscles since supernumerary muscle bellies are easily misinterpreted as space-occupying lesions. On MRI, supernumerary muscles can be recognized by the muscle-isointense signal pattern, the characteristic pennate

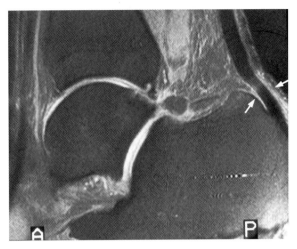

Fig. 8.**36** Bursitis involving the bursa of the calcaneal tendon and subcutaneous calcaneal bursa. Sagittal fat-suppressed SE image. A subtle high signal fluid accumulation anterior and posterior to the Achilles tendon delineates both bursae (arrows).

pattern and the fatty tissue interposed in the intramuscular fibrous tissues, as well as by the transition of the muscle into a low signal tendon. The more frequent variants are also identified by their typical location.

Accessory muscles are characteristically unilateral. The incidence of accessory muscles is not known, but appears to be low. For the lower leg and ankle region, the following three plus variants are relevant:

- Accessory soleus,
- Accessory flexor digitorum longus,
- Peroneus quartus (Fig. 8.**37**).

The *accessory soleus* refers to a third head of the normally bicapitate soleus muscle. It is anteromedial or anterotibial to the myotendinous transition of the soleus muscle, arises from the transverse fascia or posterior border of the tibia, and inserts anteromedially to the Achilles tendon at the superior surface of the calcaneus (4, 13).

MRI can demonstrate musculature in the otherwise fat-containing space anteromedial to the Achilles tendon. Clinically, this can correspond to a swelling above the heel and exercise-induced pain (33). Furthermore, a variant of a third soleal head is known, with insertion at or blending with the Achilles tendon.

The *peroneus quartus* refers to an accessory muscle in the region of the distal peroneus compartment (3). This variant of the peroneus musculature is thought to occur in 15% of the population.

The *accessory flexor digitorum longus* arises with its long head at the transverse fascia and its short head at the medial and plantar surface of the calcaneus and, after passing through the medial flexor compartment, inserts at the plantar side of the tendon of the flexor digitorum longus. The muscle bellies are small. On MRI,

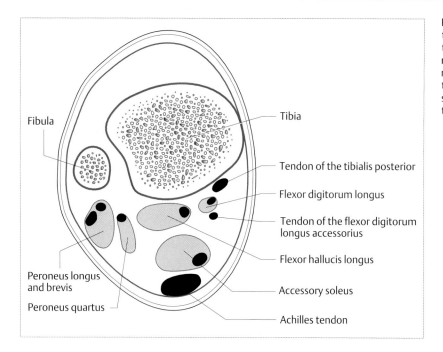

Fig. 8.**37** Schematic drawing of the axial section to illustrate the topography of the accessory muscles and their tendons in the region of the talocrural articulation (peroneus quartus, accessory soleus, and accessory flexor digitorum longus).

an otherwise unobserved tendon can be found medial to the flexor hallucis longus tendon within the medial flexor compartment.

References

1 Allen, R. A., L. B. Woolner, R. K. Ghormely: Soft tissue tumors of the sole. With special reference to plantar fibromatosis. J. Bone Jt Surg. 37-A (1955) 14–26

2 Berkowitz, J. F., R. Kier, S. Rudicel: Plantar fasciitis: MR Imaging. Radiology 179 (1991) 665–667

2a Breitenseher, M. J., J. Haller, K. C., C. Gabler, A. Kaider, D. Fleischmann, T. Helbich, S. Trattning: MRI of the sinus tarsi in acute ankle sprain injuries. J. Comput. Assist. Tomogr. 21 (1997) 274–279

3 Buschmann, W. R., Y. Cheung, M. H. Jahss: MRI of anomalous leg muscles: accessory soleus, peroneus quartus and the flexor digitorum longus accessorius. Foot and Ankle 12 (1991) 109–113

4 Faller, A.: Zur Deutung der akzessorischen Köpfe des Schollenmuskels. Anat. Anz. 93 (1942) 161–179

5 Gold, R. H., D. J. F. Tong, J. R. Crim, L. L. Seeger: Imaging of the diabetic foot. Skelet. Radiol. 24 (1995) 563–571

6 Inglis, A. E., W. N. Scott, T. P. Sculco et al.: Ruptures of the tendo achilles. J. Bone Jt Surg. 58-A (1976) 990–993

7 Keene, J. S., E. G. Lash, D. R. Fisher et al.: Magnetic Resonance Imaging of achilles tendon ruptures. Amer. J. Sports Med. 17 (1989) 333–337

8 Kerr, R., C. Frey: MR Imaging in tarsal tunnel syndrome. J. Comput. assist. Tomogr. 15 (1991) 280–286

9 Kjaersgaard-Anderson, P., K. Anderson, K. Soballe, S. Pilgaard: Sinus tarsi syndrome: presentation of seven cases and review of the literature. J. Foot Surg. 28 (1989) 3–6

10 Klein, M. A., A. M. Spreitzer: MR Imaging of the tarsal sinus and canal: normal anatomy, pathologic findings, and features of the sinus tarsi syndrome. Radiology 186 (1993) 233–240

11 Lee, J. K., L. Yao: Stress fractures: MR Imaging. Radiology 169 (1988) 217–220

12 Link, S. C., S. J. Erickson, M. E. Timins: MR Imaging of the ankle and foot: normal structures and anatomic variants that may simulate disease. Amer. J. Roentgenol. 161 (1993) 607–612

13 Loetzke, H. H., K. Trzenschik: Beitrag zur Frage der Varianten des M. soleus beim Menschen. Anat. Anz. 124 (1969) 28–36

14 Lowe, A., J. Schilero, I. O. Kanat: Sinus tarsi syndrome: a postoperative analysis. J. Foot Surg. 24 (1985) 108–112

15 Mann, R. A., F. M. Thompson: Rupture of the posterior tibial tendon causing flat foot. J. Bone Jt Surg. 67-A (1985) 556–561

16 Marcus, D. S., M. A. Reicher, L. E. Kellerhouse: Achilles tendon injuries: the role of MR Imaging. J. Comput. assist. Tomogr. 13 (1989) 480–486

17 Mink, J. H., A. L. Deutsch: Occult cartilage and bone injuries of the knee: detection, classification and assessment with MR Imaging. Radiology 170 (1989) 823–829

18 Mitchell, D. G., V. M. Rao, M. K. Dalinka et al.: Femoral head avascular necrosis: correlation of MR Imaging, radiographic staging, radionuclide imaging and clinical findings. Radiology 162 (1987) 709–715

19 Nelson, D. W., J. Di Paola, M. Colville: Osteochondritis dissecans of the talus and knee: prospective comparison of MR and arthroscopic classifications. J. Comput. assist. Tomogr. 14 (1990) 804–808

20 Noto, A. M., Y. Cheung, Z. S. Rosenberg, A. Norman, N. E. Leeds: MR Imaging of the ankle: normal variants. Radiology 170 (1989) 121–124

21 Peacock, K. C., E. J. Resnick, J. J. Thoder: Fracture of the Os peronaeum with rupture of the peroneus longus tendon: a case report and review of the literature. Clin. Orthop. 202 (1986) 223–226

22 Rosenberg, Z. S., F. Feldman, R. D. Singson: Peroneal tendon injuries: CT analysis. Radiology 161 (1986) 743–748

23 Rosenberg, Z. S., M. H. Jahss, A. M. Noto et al.: Rupture of the posterior tibial tendon: CT and surgical findings. Radiology 167 (1988) 489–493

24 Rosenberg, Z. S., Y. Cheung, M. H. Jahss: Computd tomography scan and Magnetic Resonance Imaging of ankle tendons: an overview. Foot and Ankle 8 (1988) 297–307

25 Scheller, A. D., J. R. Kasser, T. B. Quigley: Tendon injuries about the ankle. Orthop. Clin. N. Amer. 11 (1980) 801–811

26 Schneck, C. D., M. Mesgarzadeh, A. Bonakdarpour, G. J. Ross: MR Imaging of the most commonly injured ankle ligaments. Radiology 184 (1992) 499 – 512

27 Schweitzer, M. E., R. Caccese, D. Karasick, K. L. Wapner, D. G. Mitchell: Posterior tibial tendon tears: utility of secondary signs for MR Imaging diagnosis. Radiology 188 (1993) 655 – 659

28 Schweitzer, M. E., M. v. Leersum, S. S. Ehrlich, K. Wapner: Fluid in normal and abnormal ankle joints: amount and distribution as seen on MR images. Amer. J. Roentgenol. 162 (1994) 111 – 114

29 Sierra, A., E. J. Potchen, J. Moore et al.: High field Magnetic Resonance Imaging of aseptic necrosis of the talus. J. Bone Jt Surg. 68 (1986) 927 – 928

30 Sobel, M., E. F. Di Carlo, W. H. O. Bohne, L. Collins: Longitudinal splitting of the peroneus brevis tendon: an anatomic and histologic study of cadaveric material. Foot and Ankle 12 (1991) 165 – 170

31 Strong, W. B., C. L. Stanitski, R. E. Smith, J. H. Wilmore: Diagnosis and treatment of ankle sprains. Sports Med. 144 (1990) 809 – 814

32 Terk, M. R., P. K. Kwong, M. Suthar, B. C. Horvath, P. M. Colletti: Morton neuroma: evaluation with MR Imaging performed with contrat enhancement and fat suppression. Radiology 189 (1993) 239 – 241

33 Urhahn, R., K. C. Klose: Schmerzhafte präachilläre Raumforderung – MR-Diagnose. Radiologe 32 (1992) 91 – 93

34 Weinstein, D., A. Wang, R. Chambers, C. A. Stewart, H. A. Motz: Evaluation of Magnetic Resonance Imaging in the diagnosis of osteomyelitis in diabetic foot infections. Foot and Ankle 14 (1993) 18 – 22

35 Wetzel, L. H., E. Levine: Soft-tissue tumors of the foot: value of MR Imaging for specific diagnosis. Amer. J. Roentgenol. 155 (1990) 1025 – 1030

36 Yao, L., D. J. F. Tong, A. Cracchiolo, L. L. Seeger: MR findings in peroneal tendonopathy. J. Comput. assist. Tomogr. 19 (1995) 460 – 464

37 Zeiss, J., P. Fenton, N. Ebraheim, R. J. Coombs: Normal Magnetic Resonance anatomy of the tarsal tunnel. Foot and Ankle 10 (1990) 214 – 218

9 *Temporomandibular Joint*

R. Fischbach

Introduction

The temporomandibular joint (TMJ) is imaged to detect clinically suspected anomalies and dysfunctions. The role of conventional radiology is limited since only osseous changes are identified with any degree of confidence. Such changes, however, appear only late in diseases affecting this region. In the 1970s and 1980s, arthrotomography was used to diagnose diskoligamentous disorders (13, 25). CT achieves an excellent visualization of osseous changes but its sensitivity for diagnosing disorders of the disk is inadequate (11).

With the introduction of MRI, the soft tissue structures of the joint, especially the articular disc, could be imaged noninvasively. MRI has completely replaced invasive and painful arthrography and has become the modality of choice for diagnosing pathologic changes of the TMJ.

Examination Technique

■ Patient Positioning

The examination is performed with the patient supine. The patient is first examined with the mouth closed. The examination continues with the mouth open about 30 mm to achieve an adequate movement of the disk and the mandibular condyle. To keep the mouth open, adjustable jaw openers (2) can be used, or alternatively, simple dental wedges made of plastic or wood. For dynamic studies, in particular, incremental jaw openers are necessary (32).

■ Coil Selection

For the examination of the TMJ, it is essential to use a surface coil with a small diameter (5–12 cm) to achieve an adequate spatial resolution with a good signal-to-noise ratio (SNR). The coil is positioned with its center 1–2 cm anterior to the external auditory canal. Since both joints, constituting one functional unit of mastication, show an abnormality in up to 80% of TMJ disorders, the imaging should be bilateral. The simultaneous assessment of both joints can be achieved with special dual coils that are available for most units.

■ Sequences and Parameters

The examination begins with a fast T_1-weighted sequence, obtained as a localizer in the transverse plane with a body coil and a large field of view (FOV). This allows the position of the joints and the transverse axes of the condyles to be determined. On the basis of this transcondylar image, additional high-resolution sequences are planned for imaging with the mouth open and closed (Fig. 9.**1**).

The surface coils should cover a field of view of 8–12 cm. Continuous sections of 3 mm width and SE images with four signal averages are necessary for adequate detail. Decreasing the section thickness from 3 to 1.5 mm improves the delineation of the articular structures in the coronal plane (37). Thin sections are needed for visualizing complex deformities and can be obtained with 3-D-GRE techniques. With a section thickness of 3 mm, seven to nine sections are generally sufficient to encompass the entire joint.

Next, a parasagittal section is selected, with its angulation perpendicular to the long axis of the condular head, as determined from the survey image (Fig. 9.**1**). The section includes the external auditory canal, floor of the temporal fossa and the ascending mandibular ramus. The articular disk and other articular structures are best seen on the parasagittal plane. The T_1-weighted SE sequences (TR = 600 msec, TE 15–30 msec) provide a good anatomic resolution of the structure of the disk, together with good differentiation of muscle, ligaments, and bones.

Maintaining the closed mouth position is crucial for evaluating the disk position since even partial opening of the mouth can reduce a displaced disk (5, 21). As the low-signal disk is directly between the low-signal cortex of the condyle and mandibular fossa when the mouth is closed, defining configuration and signal intensity of the disk can be difficult. In these cases, delineating the disk can be improved by partially opening the mouth (5). Furthermore, an anterior displacement of the disk becomes more conspicuous with increasing translation (21). Thereafter, images are obtained with the mouth open, preferably with T_1-weighted SE sequences. Since imaging with the mouth open is primarily performed to assess the position and mobility of the disk, the number of signal averages can be lowered to shorten the acquisition time without appreciable loss of image quality. Moreover, keeping the open-mouth position for some time is uncomfortable for the patient

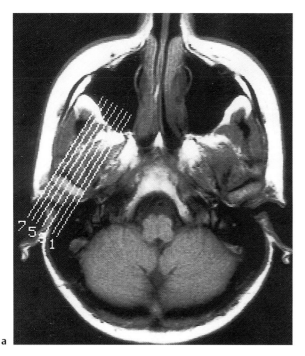
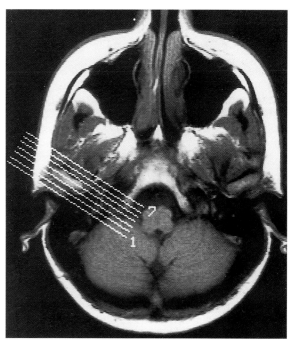

a   b

Fig. 9.**1 a, b**   Axial sections through the level of the mandibular condyles with lines indicating the **a** oblique sagittal and **b** oblique coronal sections.

and induces involuntary swallowing due pharyngeal pooling of saliva. Avoiding such introduced motion artifacts is another reason to keep the acquisition time short.

If the patient has a repositioning appliance (protrusive splint), the examination should be supplemented by a sagittal image with the repositioning appliance in place to document the reduction or adopted position of the disk.

Paracoronal sections parallel to the long axis of the condyle should be added for both joints (Fig. 9.**1**). These sections are best for assessing the degree of sideways disk displacement (14). In particular, for a disk that is not well identified on the sagittal sections, coronal sections are mandatory.

T_2-weighted SE images have inferior topographic resolution compared with T_1-weighted sequences. Because of their high tissue differentiation, T_2-weighted SE sequences (TR = 1800 – 2000 msec, TE 80 – 120 msec) are suited for detecting a joint effusion in rheumatoid or septic arthritis and after trauma (27). Furthermore, T_2-weighted images can assess the degree of disk hydration, though its clinical relevance is still undetermined (8).

If a space-occupying process is the reason for the examination, the entire region of the TMJ should be included on transverse T_2-weighted images (TR = 2000, TE 25 msec, 90 msec), supplemented by transverse and coronal T_1-weighted SE images after IV administration of Gd-DTPA at 0.1 mmol/kg body weight. Contrast-enhanced images have also been found advantageous in

diagnosing any involvement of the TMJ in rheumatoid conditions.

Special Examination Techniques

Using fast GRE sequences can clearly reduce acquisition times. Though the disk is usually well delineated on GRE images, the anatomic resolution of the surrounding structures and the disk itself is markedly inferior to SE images. Consequently, GRE images are less suitable for evaluating degenerative changes of the disk. A further disadvantage of these sequences is their sensitivity to pulsation and motion artifacts as well as to susceptibility artifacts (dental fillings).

■ **Dynamic Studies**

The fast sequences (FISP– 2 D, FFE, etc.) are suitable for obtaining dynamic motion studies with stepwise acquisition at various mandibular positions within a reasonable time frame (CINE technique) (2, 33). A disadvantage of static MR images restricted to two mandibular positions is their inability to follow the repositioning of the disk when opening the mouth, especially in cases with marked disk displacement. The dynamics and time of disk repositioning can be clinically relevant.

The use of a sequential acquisition of several mandibular positions, controlled by a mechanical mouth-opening device, can yield a pseudodynamic visualization of the movements during mouth opening by playing the individual images in a CINE loop. With examination times of less than one minute – depending on the equipment used – even the endpoints of mandibular positions can be documented. Translation, rotation, and sequence of disk reposition as well as condylar hypermobility can be assessed, particularly articular hypermobility with condylar subluxations in front of the vertex of the articular tubercle, which cannot be assessed with static MRI employing conventional SE techniques (18).

While a CINE loop displaying the motions of the TMJ is impressive, its therapeutic ramifications cannot yet be conclusively determined (1). A disadvantage of this method is the passive mouth opening, which distorts the intrinsic function. Finally, the quality of the individual images is still rather poor.

Anatomy

■ General Anatomy

The TMJ is a diarthroidal joint and constitutes the articular junction between the mandible and the temporal bone. The lentiform to ellipsoid condylar head arises from the condylar process of the mandibular ramus. Its transverse diameter exceeds its sagittal diameter. The long axis of the condyle is perpendicular to the condylar process, resulting in an anterolateral to posteromedial tilt of the axis and the articular fossa of 15 – 25 degrees relative to the frontal plane. The concave articular fossa is limited anteriorly by the articular tubercle and posteriorly by the osseous wall of the external auditory canal (Fig. 9.**2 a**). The depth of the articular fossa as well as the degree of angulation of the dorsal slope of the articular tubercle is variable.

The osseous articulating surface of the articular fossa, the articular tubercle and the mandibular condyle are covered by thin fibrocartilage. A fibrocollagenous, movable meniscus, the articular disk, divides the joint into two completely separate compartments. The upper or meniscotemporal joint cavity is larger than the lower or meniscocondylar cavity. An anterior and posterior thickening of the disk, also referred to as the anterior and posterior band, are connected by a narrow intermediate zone, giving the disk a biconcave configuration. Anteriorly, the disk is attached to the joint capsule and the superior head of the lateral pterygoid. The bilaminar region is the posterior continuation of the posterior band of the disk. It consists of two fibrous leaflets, with the superior leaflet extending into the posterior aspect of the articular fossa to insert at the Glaser fissure in front of the external acoustic canal and the lower leaflet attached at the posterior aspect of the mandibular neck together with the joint capsule.

The joint capsule is a thin, loose structure. Its attachment at the margin of the mandibular fossa of the temporal bone extends to the anterior slope of the articular tubercle. The capsule encompasses the condyle and

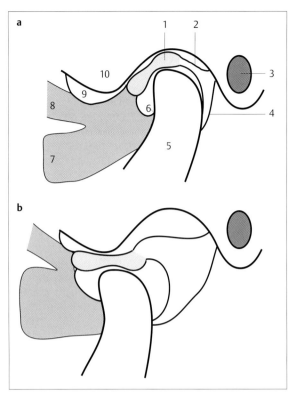

Fig. 9.**2 a, b** Diagrammatic drawing of the oblique sagittal plane with **a** closed and **b** open mouth and physiologic position of the disk. With the mouth open, the condyle reaches the apex of the articular tubercle.
1 = Disk
2 = Bilaminar region
3 = External auditory canal
4 = Joint capsule
5 = Condyles
6 = Lower synovial cavity
7 = Inferior head of the lateral pterygoid
8 = Superior head of the lateral pterygoid
9 = Upper synovial cavity
10 = Articular tubercle

attaches at the condylar neck. It is laterally and medially strengthened by fibers of connective tissue, while it is rather flaccid anteriorly and posteriorly. The sphenomandibular ligament, which is attached to the sphenoid spine of the temporal bone superiorly and to the mandibular foramen inferiorly, is medial and separate from the capsule. The stylomandibular ligament acts as a further stabilizing structure. Mandibular movements are controlled by the four masticatory muscles. The temporalis arises like a fan from the temporal fossa and inserts at the coronoid process. It is the strongest elevator of the mandible. The masseter arises from the zygomatic arch and inserts at the mandibular angle. The medial pterygoid, which extends from the pterygoid fossa to the mandibular angle, acts as the medial pendant to the masseter. These three muscles essentially function to close the mouth.

The digastric lateral pterygoid assists in all joint movements and directs the complex movements of the TMJ. Its superior head has an important role in opening the mouth. It arises medially from the greater wing of the sphenoid and extends posterolaterally to the mandibular neck, with some fibers reaching the articular disk. By virtue of the anteromedial pull of this muscle, the disk has a tendency for anteromedial displacement in the case of an anterior disk subluxation. The lower head of this lateral pterygoid arises from the lateral surface of the pterygoid plate and inserts at the mandibular condyle.

■ Specific MR Anatomy and Variants

Oblique Sagittal Plane. This plane is parallel to the ascending mandibular ramus and usually displays the condyle as a hook-shaped structure. On the T_1-weighted SE image, the low-signal cortex and the equally low-signal fibrocartilage cover of the condyle and mandibular fossa are easily distinguished from the fat-containing trabecular bone. Condyle and mandibular fossa are smoothly outlined and rounded. With the mouth closed, the condyle is centered in the mandibular fossa (Fig. 9.**2**). Owing to its composition of densely packed, intertwined fibrocartilage fibers with occasional embedded chondrocytes, the biconcave, elongated disk is delineated as a low-signal, homogeneous structure on T_1-weighted SE sequences. A slight increase in signal intensity in the posterior band is seen in more than 50% of normal disks (8) and should not be considered pathologic without concurrent changes of form or location.

With the mouth closed, the disk is located between the mandibular condyle and mandibular fossa of the temporal bone. The smaller anterior band is adjacent to the posterior slope of the articular tubercle. The thin intermediate zone is located between the anterior circumference of the condyle and the temporal articular surface (Fig. 9.**4**). The transition between the posterior band, posterior ligament, and the high-signal bilaminar zone does not deviate more than 10 degrees from a position vertically above the upper condylar pole (Fig. 9.**3**), the so-called 12 o'clock position, in 95% of asymptomatic joints (5). A position slightly more anterior is observed more frequently than a posterior one.

The bilaminar region, which consists of fibrovascular connective tissue, is attached to the posterior band and connects the disk with the posterior joint capsule. The transition between the low-signal disk and the high-signal bilaminar region is well delineated on the T_1-weighted SE image, making it easy to identify the disk. If the localization of the disk is uncertain on the SE image, the delineation of the posterior band can be improved following enhancement of the retroarticular venous plexus after administration of Gd-DTPA (28). In our experience, it is rarely necessary to administer contrast medium to determine whether the disk is displaced.

The upper layer of the bilaminar zone consists of fibroelastic tissue and is attached to temporal bone. The low signal structures occasionally seen in the bilaminar elastic fibers are attributed to the elastic fibers (12).

Function of the Temporomandibular Joint. With its two compartments, the TMJ functions as a combination of two joints. When the mouth opens, the mandibular condyle rotates in the lower joint and the disk moves forward, representing a sliding surface for the mandibular condyle. After the apex of the condyle has reached the intermediate zone of the disc, the mouth opens further by anterior translation of the upper joint, primarily promoted by the lateral pterygoid. When the mouth is fully open, the condyle has reached the apex of the articular tubercle. The disk covers the condyle in this position and its intermediate zone is placed between articular tubercle and condyle. The posterior band is now in the 2–3 o'clock position (Fig. 9.**2b**).

Oblique Coronal Plane. This plane reveals any sideways disk displacement, medially or laterally. The disk sits as low-signal structure like a cap on top of the condyles on the coronal image (Fig. 9.**4c**). Its lateral condylar attachment is normally not well delineated. The coronal image is able to document the position of the condyle and can detect abrasive denudations or marginal osteophytes of the condylar head.

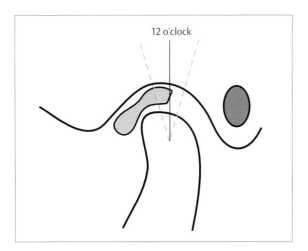

Fig. 9.**3** Schematic drawing illustrating the physiologic position of the disk. The disk is within ±10 degrees of the 12 o'clock position in 95% of normal cases.

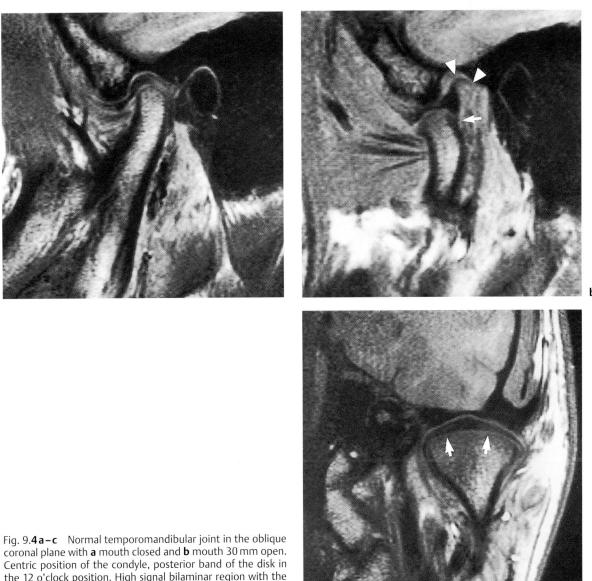

Fig. 9.**4a–c** Normal temporomandibular joint in the oblique coronal plane with **a** mouth closed and **b** mouth 30 mm open. Centric position of the condyle, posterior band of the disk in the 12 o'clock position. High signal bilaminar region with the upper (arrowheads) and lower (arrow) lamina. **c** In the oblique coronal plane, the disk sits like a cap on top of the condyle (arrows).

Disorders of the Articular Disk

Degenerative changes and internal derangement are the most frequent causes of clinical complaints of the TMJ. Internal derangement characteristically refers to anterior disk displacement. Dysfunction of the TMJ presents with clicking sounds, pain, and impaired mouth opening. It has been estimated that up to 28% of all adults have a displaced disk (30), though clinical complaints with therapeutic or diagnostic consequences are only encountered in a small proportion. In symptomatic patients, the proportion of disk displacement has been estimated to be between 66 and 80% (22, 23). Stress and mental exhaustion have been mentioned as predisposing factors for disk displacement, aside from trauma, iatrogenic hyperextension of the joints during dental or orosurgical intervention, and muscular incoordination (5, 22). Dysfunction can be caused by altered morphology and position of the articular disk due to mechanical interference with the harmonic opening and closing movements of the mandible. The internal derangement is a dynamic progressive process, the severity of which has to be judged. The most commonly applied clinical and radiologic staging has been proposed by Wilkes (38) and is summarized in Table 9.**1**.

■ Abnormal Structure and Form of the Disk

Pathologic changes of the disk are seen on MRI as abnormal morphology and signal pattern. The degenerative process begins in the posterior band at the transition to the bilaminar zone since this region takes most of the mechanical stress. Furthermore, most perforations or disk avulsions are found here (20). The normally homogeneous low signal disk can exhibit areas of increased signal intensity due to mucoid degeneration (Fig. 9.**5**) (26). Areas of decreased signal intensities are interpreted as microcalcifications (12). Frequently, signal changes are associated with loss of the normal biconcave disk configuration. Early morphologic changes present as thickening of the posterior band. The process advances with further loss of the normal disk configuration, rendering intermediate zone and disk bands indistinguishable. Clinically, these morphologic changes correlate with decreased functional elasticity (35). Severe biconcave or concentric deformities concur with chronic, irreducible disk displacement. The extent of the deformity is related to the chronicity of the disorder and can have relevant therapeutic ramifications.

Table 9.**1**   Staging criteria for internal derangements of the temporomandibular joint (after Wilkes)

	Stage I (Early stage)	Stage II (Early/intermediate stage)	Stage III (Intermediate stage)	Stage IV (Intermediate/late stage)	Stage V (Late stage)
Clinical findings	Aside from reciprocal clicking, no relevant mechanical symptoms	1–2 episodes of pain; loud clicking sounds, mechanical problems with mouth opening begin	Multiple episodes of pain, restriction of motion with sustained locking	Increase in symptoms over stage III	Grinding symptoms, episodic pain, restriction of motion with chronically impaired function
Radiologic findings	Slight forward displacement, maintained contour of the disk	Slight forward displacement, start of anatomic deformity of the disk with thickening of the posterior band	Anterior displacement with relevant deformity of the disk	Increase in disk deformity, early degenerative remodeling of the condyle and articular fossa	Gross anatomical deformity of the disk, perforation of the disk or disk attachment; gross degenerative osseous deformity with flattening of the condyle and articular tubercle, subcortical cysts
Anatomic findings	Corresponding to radiologic findings	Anterior displacement and slight deformity of the disk	Corresponding to radiologic findings	Increase in severity, osseous remodeling with osteophyte formation; multiple adhesions of the anterior and posterior recesses of the joint cavity	Corresponding to radiologic findings

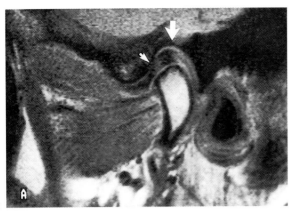

a

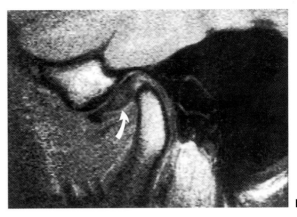

b

Fig. 9.**5 a, b**   Subtle increase in signal intensity and slight swelling of the intermediate zone (small arrow) with unremarkable disk position (large arrow). Good delineation of the bicapi-tate lateral pterygoid. **b** Partial anterior displacement of the disk with swelling and increased signal intensity of the posterior band (curved arrow).

■ Disk Displacement

Anterior Disk Displacement

Anterior disk displacements are most frequent. If the posterior disk band is anterior to the 11 o'clock position but has maintained its contact with the condyle, it is called a partial disk displacement (Fig. 9.**6**). If the disk has lost its contact with the anterior condylar pole, a complete disk displacement is present (Fig. 9.**7**). A subclassification of the partial disk displacement in to grade I and grade II has been proposed by determining the extent of the partial displacement (31) or the presence of deformities and signal alterations (8) but has no therapeutic consequence.

The distinction between a partial and complete disk displacement can be made in the mouth-closed position.

It is of great clinical relevance to document the reduction of the displaced disk into the anatomically correct position between condyle and articular tubercle during mouth opening. In partial disk displacement, generally the disk can be reduced, while this is rarely observed with complete disk displacement. Reducing the disk over the condyle with anterior mandibular translation or mouth opening is usually accompanied by an audible click. A reciprocal click may be heard or felt during mouth closure as the disk displacement recurs.

To detect the disk position on MRI, the mouth should be opened as much as possible. Because of muscle spasm or pain, very few patients can maintain maximal mouth opening long enough for an adequate MRI examination. In almost one-third of symptomatic patients with an MRI diagnosis of disk displacement without reduction, functional arthrography can document that the disk reduces when mouth opening reaches its limiting range (7).

In anterior disk displacement without reduction, the disk remains anterior to the condyle during mouth

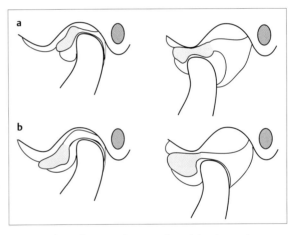

a

b

Fig. 9.**6 a, b**   Schematic drawing of partial and complete anterior disk displacements. **a** The deformed disk is anteriorly displaced, but remains in contact with the condyle. Reduction with the mouth open. **b** Complete disk displacement with failure of reduction with the mouth open. Restricted translation of the condyle.

opening where it undergoes increasing deformity. Clicks are rarely audible in these patients. The failure of reduction can be caused by the lack of restoring forces due to flaccidity of the ligamentous structures or mechanical impairment. A torn disk is rarely present. Since the anteriorly displaced disk interferes with mouth opening, the extent of the condylar translation should be further assessed. In long-standing disk displacement without reduction, the restricted mouth opening improves with time due to increasing stretching of the posterior disk attachment.

Sideways Disk Displacements

In addition to visualizing strictly anterior disk displacements, MRI can document anterolateral and anterome-

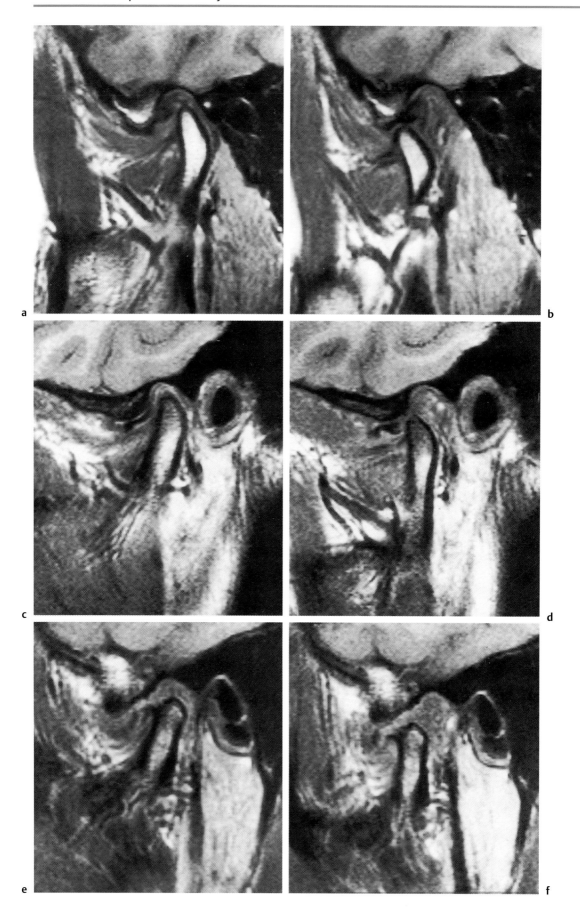

dial disk displacements as well as pure sideways disk displacements or rotations (Figs. 9.**8** and 9.**9**). The incidence of mediolateral displacements has been stated to be 26–68% (4, 6). In up to 11% of cases, a strict mediolateral displacement without concurrent anterior displacement could be observed (6). If differing disk segments are seen on the parallel sections of the parasagittal plane, a component of transverse displacement can already be diagnosed in the sagittal plane (Fig. 9.**9**). The exact assignment is easier with paracoronal sections, which display the disk in relation to the temporal articular surface and the condyle.

Posterior Disk Displacements

Displacements of the articular disk behind the 1 o'clock position are rare. Slight displacements are usually asymptomatic, while marked displacements are associated with jaw locking and pain. Eccentric posterior disk displacements occur more frequently than was thought in the past and are adequately diagnosed on cine MRI or functional arthrography (7).

Nomenclature of Disk Displacements

Aside from differentiating the disk displacement functionally by determining whether the disk reduces or not, the articular situation can be assessed by determining the direction of the disk displacement relative to the mandibular condyle (anterior, posterior, medial, lateral) and the position of the mandibular condyle (centric, eccentric) (Tab. 9.**2**). With the mouth closed, i.e., centric position of the condyle in the articular fossa and anterior displacement of the disc, it is a centric–anterior disk displacement. If the disk dislocates during mouth opening behind the condyle, it is an eccentric–posterior disk displacement. Combinations of centric and eccentric displacements are possible.

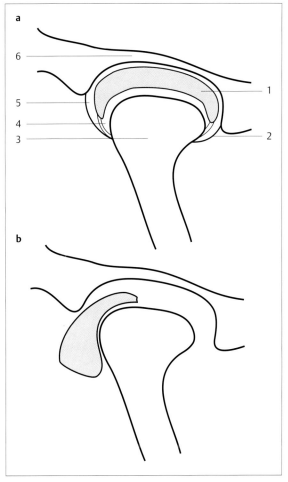

Fig. 9.**8 a, b** Schematic drawing of the oblique coronal plane with the mouth closed. **a** Normal disk position. **b** Lateral disk displacement.
1 = Disk
2 = Joint capsule
3 = Condyle
4 = Lower joint compartment
5 = Upper joint compartment
6 = Articular fossa

Table 9.**2** Discription of disk displacement

Condyle position	Extent of displacement	Direction of displacement	Reposition after mouth opening
central eccentric	partial complete	anterior anterolateral anterolateral medial lateral posterior	with reposition without reposition

◄ Fig. 9.**7 a–f** **a** Partial anterior disk displacement with retroposition of the condyle. The biconcave disk configuration is maintained and the posterior disk band swollen. **b** Reduction with the mouth open. **c** Complete anterior disk displacement. The disk is definitively anterior to the condyle. **d** With the mouth open, the deformed disk does not reduce and remains anterior to the condyle; restricted range of translation. **e** Gross deformity of the disk, degenerative flattening and anterior osteophyte of the condyle, flattened articular tubercle. **f** With the mouth open, no reduction. No recognizable continuity between disk structures and posterior disk attachment. Arthrographic confirmation of the suspected perforation.

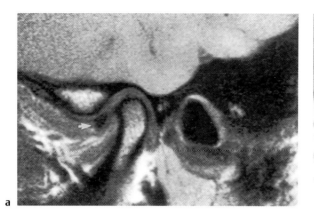

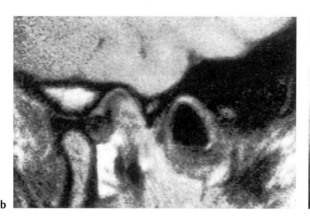

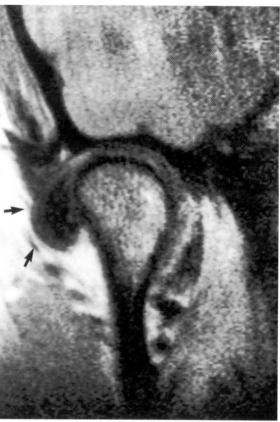

Fig. 9.**9a–c** Lateral disk displacement with reduction with the mouth open. **a** With the mouth closed, joint space narrowing with no disk seen over the condylar convexity. Low signal disk segment anterior to the condyle (arrow). **b** With the mouth open, disk in normal location and displaying an unremarkable configuration. **c** Oblique coronal plane with clearly recognizable centric late al disk displacement (arrows).

Disk Adhesions

Delicate fibrous adhesions escape detection by MRI and are only identified on double contrast arthrography and by arthroscopy (24). Extensive broad adhesions usually attach the disk to the superior joint compartment. In this situation, the superior synovial cavity is filled with a high signal tissue and the disk fails to move relative to the condyle and temporal fossa during mouth opening (Fig. 9.**10**).

Disk Perforation

MRI can detect a perforation only if the discontinuity is broad and seen on several scans (9). Perforation and friction sounds indicate advanced osteoarthritic changes, which are often combined with a disk perforation. A disk perforation should be suspected with the constellation of marked anterior disk displacement, extensive signal heterogeneities of the disk, and degenerative osseous changes of the condyle. The definitive diagnosis of a disk perforation can only be made by arthrography or arthroscopy (24, 34).

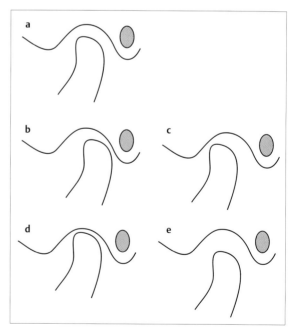

Fig. 9.**11a–e** Schematic drawing to illustrate the various malpositions of the condyle. **a** Normal position. **b** Reposition. **c** Anterior malposition. **d** Compression. **e** Distraction.

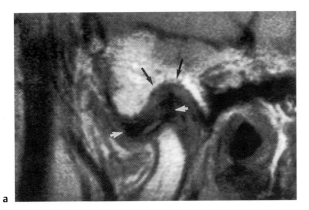

a

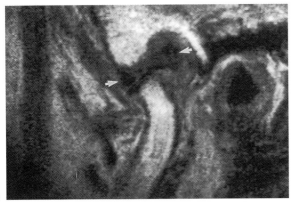

b

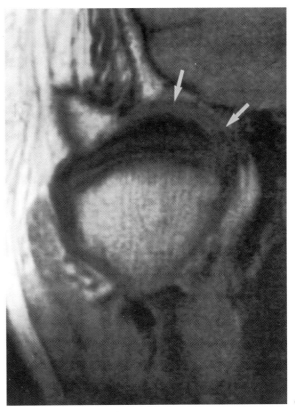

c

Fig. 9.**10a–c** Disk adhesion. **a** Heterogenously low-signal disk with swelling of the intermediate region and the posterior band (white arrows). Enlargement of the superior joint compartment (black arrows). Flattened condyle in inferoanterior malposition. **b** Mouth open without recognizable changed position of the disk (arrows) in the presence of moderate condylar translation. **c** Oblique coronal plane with visualization of the swollen disk and tissue of intermediate signal intensity detected in the upper joint compartment (arrows).

Malpositions of the Condyle

With the mouth closed the condyle is centered in the articular fossa. Deviations from this normal position are possible and easily recognized on MRI. A summary of the most frequent malpositions are shown in Fig. 9.**11**.

Arthritis and Other Synovial Disorders

■ Arthritis

An acute pyogenic infection of the TMJ can be hematogenous, secondary to local trauma or caused by spreading from adjacent structures. In addition to typical clinical inflammatory signs, a locked jaw or a pain-avoiding position of the jaw with the mouth slightly opened can be encountered. Characteristically, the T_2-weighted image detects an effusion, which can involve both or one of the joint compartments (Fig. 9.**12**). Long-standing or localized advanced processes produce extensive destruction of the osseous and diskoligamentous structures. Aside from septic arthritis, the TMJ can be affected by rheumatoid arthritis. Characteristically, rheumatoid disease involves multiple joints, with concomi-

tant changes observed in the TMJ in up to 50% of patients with rheumatoid disease. The number of symptomatic cases is clearly lower (15). MRI reveals a small effusion, which is best detected in the anterior recess, as well as deformities of the disks (flattening, fragmentation, heterogeneous signal pattern, indistinct outline), and erosions or deformities of the condyles (15). In arthritic joints, the prevalence of anterior disk displacement is increased relative to the normal population. In the past, the early changes of synovial proliferations were only detectable by arthrography and arthroscopy, but they are now easily documented on T_1-weighted SE sequences after administration of Gd-based contrast medium (29). If TMJ abnormalities associated with rheumatic diseases are suspected, closed-mouth T_1-weighted and T_2-weighted images should be supplemented by T_1-weighted images after administration of Gd-based contrast medium.

■ Synovial Chondromatosis

This rare disease affects patients after the fourth decade and is usually monoarticular. It is a benign proliferation of the synovial membrane with multiple loose or fixed cartilaginous, partially calcified nodules, obliterating

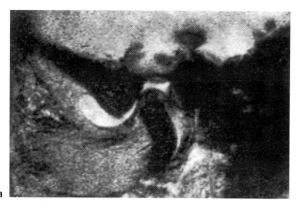
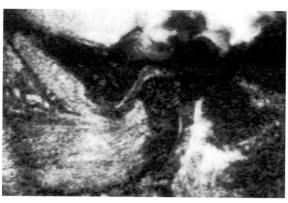

a   b

Fig. 9.**12 a, b**   **a** T$_2$-weighted GRE image (FFE) with detection of a high signal fluid accumulation in the upper joint compartment. Disk in normal position. **b** After aspiration of the pyo-   genic effusion and antibiotic therapy, only minimal residual effusion on the follow-up examination.

one or both synovial joint capsules and leading to articular dysfunction. The cortical erosions and intra-articular calcifications are best identified on CT. MRI shows an expanded joint capsule, with intra-articular low-signal nodules seen within a high-signal effusion on the T$_2$-weighted image.

Disorders of the Bone

■ Osteoarthritis

Internal derangement is considered an important predisposition to the development of degenerative changes of the TMJ. Follow-up examinations performed on diseased TMJs with disk displacement has revealed a steady progression of diskoligamentous changes and of later appearing osseous changes (38). In a study by Rao and co-workers, only half of all patients with disk displacement documented by MRI had an unremarkable configuration of the condyles (23). In this investigation, the proportion of degeneratively altered mandibular condyles was larger with irreducible disk displacements than with reducible disk displacement. Only 4% of patients with detectable osseous changes of the condyles had a normal disk position. The morphologic changes can be classified as:

- Proliferative degenerative transformation with flattening marginal osteophytes, sclerosis and subchondral cysts;
- Regressive remodeling with resultant hypoplastic condyle or small pointed articular head without relevant osteophyte formation.

Regressive remodeling is more frequently observed. Early MRI signs of condylar remodeling are decreased signal intensity on the T$_1$-weighted image and increased signal intensity on the T$_2$-weighted image due to fluid accumulation in the bone marrow as a manifestation of increased osseous activity (9). The extent of

osseous changes can have important therapeutic ramifications since the success of surgical intervention in the diskoligamentous system correlates negatively with the degree of degenerative changes of the condyles, in particular, the extent of osteophytic deformity (8).

Other, less frequent disorders of the TMJs, such as osteochondritis dissecans, avascular necrosis or hyperuricemic arthropathy, have been described (16, 26). The MRI findings are analogous to those encountered in the large joints.

Tumors

Tumors of the TMJs are only briefly mentioned here. Specific aspects of the diagnosis of tumors are dealt with in Chapter 13.

■ Benign Tumors

If cysts are present, odontogenic cysts, which arise from the dental lamina, have to be distinguished from non-odontogenic cysts. Odontogenic cysts occur in the maxilla and mandible and can reach a considerable size. T$_2$-weighted images are especially suitable for displaying the high signal content of the cyst.

A unique tumor of this region is the ameloblastoma, an epithelial odontogenic tumor arising from the ameloblast. It is an expansile tumor of high signal intensity on T$_2$-weighted images and affects the mandibular body and ramus. Another rare but mandibula-specific tumor is the calcifying epithelial odontogenic tumor (also known as Pindborg tumor). As its name suggests this lesion contains both epithelial and odontogenic components, and characteristically has intrinsic calcifications seen as signal voids on MRI.

Other benign tumors are exostoses, osteomas and lesions arising from the soft tissues of the joint, such as the synovial membrane, disk, and capsule.

In fibrous dysplasia involving the temporomandibular region, the sclerotic areas exhibit a heterogeneously low signal intensity on T_1-weighted and T_2-weighted images. The vascular fibrous areas appear less dark and enhance after administration of Gd-based contrast medium.

Neurinomas, neurofibromas and traumatic neuromas are space-occupying lesions with a low signal intensity on the T_2-weighted image and a characteristically strong enhancement after administration of Gd-based contrast medium.

■ Malignant Tumors

Malignant tumors include primary tumors of the mandible or maxilla, locally infiltrating tumors of the surrounding soft tissues arising from the oro- and nasopharynx, and metastases.

MRI should be considered as a supplemental examination after CT if better soft tissue delineation or more accurate assessment of the local extent of the lesion is indicated.

Of the sarcomas, the osteosarcoma is the most frequent tumor. Fibrosarcomas and Ewing sarcomas are considerably less frequent. Squamous cell carcinomas arising from the oro- and nasopharynx spread directly to the TMJ, infiltrating and eroding the bone. The tumor is easily identified by long T_1 and T_2 relaxation times as well as by enhancement on the T_1-weighted image following administration of Gd-based contrast medium. Infiltrations into the trabecular space present as areas of decreased signal intensity. Malignant lymphomas and other hematogenous systemic diseases can involve the TMJ.

Post-therapeutic Findings

An internal derangement is typically treated conservatively with repositioning appliances. Because of its non-invasive nature and the absence of radiation, MRI is well suited for serial examinations to follow the disk position in patients undergoing repositioning therapy (19).

The surgical therapy of internal derangement consists of arthroscopic or open disk reduction, meniscoplasty, diskectomy, and diskectomy with implantation of synthetic or autologous tissue (3, 17, 36). The results of the investigations reported so far do not show a conclusive correlation between disk position and clinical success following intervention (17, 36). In postsurgical examinations, therefore, the MRI findings should be interpreted only with knowledge of the surgery performed and the intraoperative findings and in the context of the clinical signs.

Residual or recurrent disk displacements are reliably detected on MRI. Even with clinical evidence of surgical success, disk adhesions can be expected frequently and the examination should be performed in at least two different mandibular positions.

After surgical interventions, fibrous tissue is frequently found in the joint capsule and joint space, with the fibrotic changes usually confined to the lateral joint capsule in asymptomatic joints. Postsurgical persistence of articular symptoms was found in 60% of cases with extensive fibrosis that involves the joint space and medial capsule (36). In these cases, MRI must document the extent of the lesion if additional surgery is contemplated. In 21 examined joints with autologous dermal grafts, MRI could not delineate a single graft (17). In contrast, silicone implants are recognized as smoothly outlined low-signal intensity structures.

Clinical Relevance of MRI and Comparison with Other Imaging Methods

Clinical examination is the first and most important part in the evaluation of patients with disorders of the TMJs. The imaging methods are selected on the basis of the clinical result and the clinical necessity of further evaluation. It must be the goal to document the specific morphologic changes that cause the patient's symptoms.

Conventional radiographs, including panorama views, have a low sensitivity for both osseous and soft tissue disorders.

Conventional tomography of the TMJs permits relatively accurate assessment of the osseous changes, but these findings generally represent the end stage of longstanding processes in the articular soft tissues. A negative tomographic finding does not exclude a pathologic process in the soft tissues. A high resolution CT is comparable to conventional tomography.

Arthrography of the TMJ has achieved a major role in the evaluation of internal derangements. It was introduced in the 1940 s, but achieved general acceptance in the 1980 s. Arthrography allows a good delineation of the articular disks and, moreover, can evaluate the functional changes related to disk displacement. Arthrography is also the method of choice for establishing the definitive diagnosis of a disk perforation. The only relevant alternative to arthrography is MRI.

CT is definitely inferior to MRI in the detection of soft tissue pathology. MRI is non-invasive and is less technically demanding for the examiner than arthrography. The visualization of the joint in several planes is advantageous, in particular, if medial and lateral disk displacements are considered. In patients with a previous surgical disk reduction or discectomy, MRI is superior to all other radiologic methods owing to its exquisite soft tissue visualization. Arthrography as the only other method for visualizing the articular disk can be difficult in postsurgical patients (36).

In most clinical situations, MRI is the imaging method of first choice in evaluating disorders of the temporomandibular joints (Tab. 9.**3**).

Table 9.**3**   Diagnostic steps in the evaluation of the temporomandibular joint

	Conventional radiology	Arthrotomography	CT	MRI
Disk displacement	4	2	3	1
Disk perforation		1		2
Adhesions		1		2
Arthrosis	1		2	
Arthritis	3	2	2	1
Tumors	3		1	2
Synovial chondromatosis		3	1	2
Fracture	1		2	

1   = imaging methods of highest priority
2 – 4 = imaging methods of successively lower priorities

References

1 Bell, K. A., K. D. Miller, J. P. Jones: Cine magnetic resonance imaging of the temporomandibular joint. J. craniomandib. Pract. 10 (1992) 313 – 317
2 Burnett, K. R., C. L. Davis, J. Read: Dynamic display of the temporomandibular joint meniscus by using „fast-scan" MR Imaging. Amer. J. Roentgenol. 149 (1987) 959 – 962
3 Conway, W. F., C. W. Hayes, R. L. Campbell, D. M. Laskin, K. S. Swanson: Temporomandibular joint after meniscoplasty: appearance at MR Imaging. Radiology 180 (1991) 749 – 753
4 Dolan, E. A., J. B. Vogler, J. C. Angelillo: Synovial chondromatosis of the temporomandibular joint diagnosed by Magnetic Resonance Imaging: report of a case. J. oral. max.-fac. Surg. 47 (1989) 411 – 413
5 Drace, J. E., D. R. Enzmann: Defining the normal temporomandibular joint: closed-, partially open-, and open-mouth MR Imaging of asymptomatic subjects. Radiology 177 (1990) 67 – 71
6 Duvoisin, B., E. Klaus, P. Schnyder: Coronal radiographs and videoflouroscopy improve the diagnostic quality of temporomandibular joint arthrography. Amer. J. Roentgenol. 155 (1990) 105 – 107
7 Fischbach, R., W. Heindel, Y. Lin, R. Friedrich, H. G. Brochhagen: Vergleich von Kernspintomographie und Arthrographie bei Funktionsstörungen des Kiefergelenkes. Fortschr. Röntgenstr. 162 (1995) 216 – 223
8 Helms, C. A., L. B. Kaban, C. McNeill, T. Dodson: Temporomandibular joint: morphology and signal intensity characteristics of the disk at MR Imaging. Radiology 172 (1989) 817 – 820
9 Hermans, R., J. L. Termote, G. Marchal, A. L. Baert: Temporomandibular joint imaging. Curr. Opin. Radiol. 4 (1992) 141 – 147
10 Herzog, S., M. Maffee: Synovial chondromatosis of the TMJ: MR and CT findings. Amer. J. Neuroradiol. 11 (1990) 742 – 745
11 Jend, H. H., I. Jend-Rossmann, H. J. Triebel: Computertomographie der anterioren Diskusdislokation des Kiefergelenkes. Fortschr. Röntgenstr. 146 (1987) 386 – 390
12 Katzberg, R. W., F. A. Burgener: Arthrotomographie des pathologischen Kiefergelenkes. Zweiter Teil. Fortschr. Röntgenstr. 140 (1984) 317 – 321
13 Katzberg, R. W., R. W. Bessette, R. H. Tallents, D. B. Plewes, J. V. Manzione, J. F. Schenck, T. H. Foster, H. R. Hart: Normal and abnormal temporomandibular joint: MR Imaging with surface coil. Radiology 158 (1986) 183 – 189
14 Katzberg, R. W., P. L. Westesson, R. H. Tallents, R. Anderson, K. Kurita, J. J. Manzione, S. Totterman: Temporomandibular joint: MR assessment of rotational and sideways disk displacements. Radiology 169 (1988) 741 – 748
15 Larheim, T. A., H. J. Smith, F. Aspestrand: Temporomandibular joint abnormalities associated with rheumatic disease: comparison between MR imaging and arthrotomography. Radiology 183 (1992) 221 – 226
16 Laskin, D. M.: Diagnosis of pathology of the temporomandibular joint. Radiol. Clin. N. Amer. 31 (1993) 135 – 147
17 Lieberman, J. M., J. P. Bradrick, A. T. Indresano, A. S. Smith, E. M. Bellon: Dermal grafts of the temporomandibular joint: postoperative appearance on MR images. Radiology 176 (1990) 199 – 203
18 Lin, Y., R. Friedrich, R. Fischbach: Vergleichende Untersuchung von MRT und Kontrastmittelarthrographie bei Patienten mit Kiefergelenkgeräuschen. Dtsch. zahnärztl. Z. 48 (1993) 339 – 342
19 Maeda, M., S. Itou, Y. Ishii, Y. Yamamoto, T. Matsuda, N. Hayashi, Y. Ishii: Temporomandibular joint movement. Evaluation of protrusive splint therapy with GRASS MR Imaging. Acta radiol. 33 (1992) 410 – 413
20 Norer, B., A. Pomaroli, O. Dietze: Zu den Degenerationsvorgängen am Diskus artikularis des Kiefergelenkes. Dtsch. Z. Mund-, Kiefer- u. Gesichtschir. 13 (1989) 278 – 286
21 Orwig, D. S., C. A. Helms, G. W. Doyle: Optimal mouth position for magnetic resonance imaging of the temporomandibular joint disk. J. craniomandib. Disord. 3 (1989) 138 – 142
22 Paesani, D., P. L. Westesson, M. Hatala, R. H. Tallents, K. Kurita: Prevalence of temporomandibular joint internal derangement in patients with craniomandibular disorders. Amer. J. Orthodont. 101 (1992) 41 – 47
23 Rao, V. M., A. Babaria, A. Manoharan, S. Mandel, N. Gottehrer, H. Wank, S. Grosse: Altered condylar morphology associated with disc displacement in TMJ dysfunction: observations by MRI. Magn. Reson. Imag. 8 (1990 a) 231 – 235
24 Rao, V. M., A. Farole, D. Karasick: Temporomandibular joint dysfunction: correlation of MR imaging, arthrography, and arthroscopy. Radiology 174 (1990 b) 663 – 667
25 Reich, R. H.: Zur Indikation der Arthrographie des Kiefergelenkes. Dtsch. zahnärztl. Z. 41 (1986) 36 – 42
26 Schellhas, K. P.: Internal derangement of the temporomandibular joint: radiologic staging with clinical, surgical, and pathologic correlation. Magn. Reson. Imag. 7 (1989) 495 – 515
27 Schellhas, K. P., C. H. Wilkes: Temporomandibular joint inflammation: comparison of MRT fast scanning with T1 and T2 weighted imaging techniques. Amer. J. Roentgenol. 153 (1989) 93 – 98
28 Schimmerl, S., J. Kramer, R. Stiglbauer, E. Piehslinger, R. Slavicek, H. Imhof: MRT des Kiefergelenks. Darstellbarkeit des retroartikulären vaskulären Plexus. Fortschr. Röntgenstr. 158 (1993) 192 – 196
29 Smith, H. J., T. A. Larheim, F. Aspestrand: Rheumatic and nonrheumatic disease in the temporomandibular joint: gadolinium-enhanced MR imaging. Radiology 185 (1992) 229 – 234

30 Solberg, W. K., M. W. Woo, J. B. Housten: Prevalence of mandibular dysfunction in young adults. J. Amer. dent. Ass. 98 (1979) 25 – 34

31 Vogl, T. J., D. Eberhard: MR-Tomographie Temporomandibulargelenk. Thieme, Stuttgart 1993

32 Vogl, T. J., D. Eberhard, C. Bergman, J. Lissner: Incremental hydraulic jaw opener for MR imaging of the temporomandibular joint. J. Magn. Reson. Imag. 2 (1992 a) 479 – 482

33 Vogl. T. J., D. Eberhard, P. Weigl, J. Assal, J. Randzio: Die Anwendung der „Cine-Technik" in der MRT-Diagnostik des Kiefergelenkes. Fortschr. Röntgenstr. 156 (1992 b) 232 – 237

34 Watt-Smith, S., A. Sadler, H. Baddeley, P. Renton: Comparison of arthrotomographic and magnetic resonance images od 50 temporomandibular joints with operative findings. Brit. J. oral. max.-fac. Surg. 31 (1993) 139 – 143

35 Westesson, P. L., S. L. Bronstein, J. L. Liedberg: Internal derangement of the temporomandibular joint: morphologic description with correlation to function. Oral Surg. 59 (1985) 323 – 331

36 Westesson, P. L., J. M. Cohen, R. H. Tallents: Magnetic resonance imaging of temporomandibular joint after surgical treatment of internal derangement. Oral Surg. 71 (1991) 407 – 411

37 Westesson, P. L., E. Kwok, J. B. Barsotti, M. Hatala, D. Paesani: Temporomandibular joint: improved MR image quality with decreased section thickness. Radiology 182 (1992) 280 – 282

38 Wilkes, C. H.: Internal derangement of the temporomandibular joint. Arch. Otolaryngol. 115 (1989) 469 – 477

Musculature

M. Vahlensieck and G. Layer

10

Introduction

MRI has been intensively applied to the field of myopathies and muscle physiology in recent years. Owing to its noninvasiveness, MRI can visualize new aspects of muscle physiology and anatomy. This chapter will address the specific anatomy and physiology relevant to MRI.

Examination Technique

The axial plane has been found useful for examining the musculature of the extremities. The selected field of view should encompass both legs since any asymmetry detected by comparing both sides can reveal important diagnostic information. For localized findings confined to one leg, surface coils, such as flexible rectangular coils, knee coils, and ring coils, should be used to achieve a higher resolution. T_1-weighted sequences are obtained to assess the distribution of fat and to identify fatty atrophy in chronic muscular dystrophies. A T_2-weighted sequence should be acquired to show any muscle edema either in myositis or following exercise and to discover focal areas of increased signal intensity due to tumorous or liquefying processes. Fat-suppressed STIR sequences are particularly useful for detecting edematous muscular changes. As described in Chapter 1, STIR sequences are characterized by the additive T_1/T_2-image contrast and are superior to all other sequences for the detection of edematous changes. Fat suppression can distinguish fat from blood. A distinction might be impossible otherwise since fat and blood may have high signal intensities on T_1-weighted or T_2-weighted images or both. Thus, STIR sequences as well as T_1-weighted sequences should be part of any examination of the musculature. Coronal and sagittal sections can be added to the diagnostic evaluation of the musculature whenever it is necessary to delineate the full extent of the disease process.

Specific MR Spectroscopy of the Muscles

MR spectroscopy is the only noninvasive method that can directly visualize *in vivo* concentrations of the compounds involved in energy metabolism in muscles at the cellular level. Exercise MR spectroscopy can also measure the metabolic changes during muscular exercise. However this has not yet become established in clinical practice, in part because of the complexity of the examination technique and in part because of the wide range of physiologic muscular reactions related to the different myosin filaments and various pathways of energy metabolism. Moreover, the interpretation of the measured data is still problematic. Though many investigations have proven the sensitivity of the method, a reliable assignment of the data to a particular metabolic abnormality is still lacking.

■ Basics of Energy Metabolism of the Muscles

The relevant observable metabolites in the phosphorus spectrum are phosphocreatine, inorganic phosphate, γ-, α-, β-phosphate of the nucleotide triphosphates, phosphodiester (glycerol phosphocholine and phosphoethanolamine) and phosphomonoester of phospholipid metabolism. Phosphocreatine serves as a reference substance for the changes in chemical shift of the remaining phosphorus metabolites. The changes in chemical shift of inorganic phosphates relative to phosphocreatine can be used to calculate the intracellular pH noninvasively.

The muscle cell uses ATP as the sole source of energy for its contractile force. Various pathways, which can be aerobic or anaerobic, provide the ATP for the myosin filaments. An additional reservoir of high-potential phosphoryl groups exists in the form of phosphocreatine, which is the source of energy for bursts of increased energy demands or until glycolysis takes over. The high phosphoryl transfer potential of phosphocreatine cannot be used directly to supply the energy for cellular reactions. Creatine kinase must be used to catalyze the transfer of the phosphoryl group to ADP to form ATP. The formation of ATP from phosphocreatine and the release of energy from ATP can be summarized in the following formula:

■ phosphocreatine$^2 \rightarrow$ creatine + P$_i^2$ +energy

To maintain the ATP concentration, active muscle fibers induce the hydrolysis of phosphocreatine with a decrease in the phosphocreatine level and a proportionate increase in the inorganic phosphate concentration.

Glycolysis. Glycolysis refers to the oxidation of glucose to pyruvate. For each mole of glucose, two moles of

NADH and four moles of ATP are formed. Since the phosphorylation of glucose or glucose 1-phosphate requires two moles of ATP, the conversion of glucose to pyruvate only generates a net gain of two moles of ATP. Using glycogen stored in the muscle increases the gain by 50%, with the formation of a total of three moles of ATP for each mole of glucose since the released glucose residue is already phosphorylated. The subsequent conversion of pyruvate is variable and depends on the availability of oxygen in the muscle cell. Under anaerobic conditions, so-called anaerobic glycolysis, pyruvate is catalyzed by lactate hydrogenase to form lactate. The purpose of the anaerobic conversion of pyruvate into lactate is the regeneration of the hydrogen acceptor NAD+, which is essential for maintaining glycolysis. Under aerobic conditions, so-called aerobic glycolysis, pyruvate undergoes oxidative decarboxylation and enters the citric acid cycle to form CO_2 and H_2O and to yield a total of 36 moles of ATP.

Fatty acid metabolism. After hydrolysis of triacylglycerol in the plasma, the free fatty acids are degraded into acetyl CoA in mitochondria by oxidation at the β-carbon, followed by aerobic degradation in the citric acid cycle and electron transport chain. The citric acid cycle and electron transport chain constitute the common final pathway for the metabolic intermediates of aerobic glycolysis, beta oxidation and glucogenic amino acid degradation. The oxidation of fatty acids is the most economic release of energy. The flow of electrons through the electron transport chain is coupled to the level of ATP in the inner mitochondrial membrane. This coupling assures that the oxidative phosphorylation responds to the actual energy need of the cell and represents a respiratory control since the availability of oxygen is the limiting factor. The substance preferentially metabolized by the muscle depends on both the level of activity and the type of muscle fibers. At rest, most of the energy needed is derived from the aerobic metabolic pathways. Because of the relatively low demand for ATP, even low perfusion provides an adequate supply of oxygen and fuel, and the oxidative degrada-

tion of blood glucose and fatty acids predominates. Muscular activity changes the conditions. In the early phase of active contraction, the demand for ATP increases by a many hundredfold factor compared to that at rest. However, the adaptation processes, such as vasodilation, increased cardiac output, and faster respiration, take several minutes until they improve the oxygen supply.

In the initial phase of active contraction, the muscle must cover the increased energy demand with such endogenous metabolites as phosphocreatine and glycogen that can be degraded without oxygen under anaerobic conditions. Fig. 10.1 illustrates the temporal sequence of the energy supply in muscles during exertion. Within the first few seconds, the necessary energy is delivered by the breakdown of creatine phosphate. The oxidative energy supply begins slowly and glycolysis surpasses the creatine phosphate conversion after about $1/2$ minute. After prolonged muscle exertion, the oxidative metabolic processes assume an increasingly more important role. After about 100 seconds, the proportion of anaerobic and oxidative metabolic processes is about 50% each.

Dividing the muscle fibers into type I, slow twitch muscle fibers, and type II, fast twitch muscle fibers, also correlates with the preferred metabolic pathway. While type I fibers predominantly use the aerobic metabolism and are less subject to fatigue, type II fibers primarily depend on anaerobic glycolysis and have a high contractile velocity but suffer from relatively rapid fatigue. Whether the distribution of the different muscular fiber types is genetically determined or represents adaptive processes cannot be answered definitively at present.

Exercise MR spectroscopy of phosphate metabolism is the ideal technique to study muscle physiology at rest and during exercise that occurs during athletic activities. Although biopsy is the gold standard, MRI has the advantage of being noninvasive and can be repeated as often as necessary. Numerous investigations have addressed the question whether the different types of muscle fibers are genetically determined or adaptively acquired. The discussion continues, with good arguments for each assumption. One of our own studies has shown how the use of different metabolic pathways correlates with the different fiber types constituting the muscle (5). A definite decrease in the pH value corresponded to a higher proportion of type IIb fibers and an unchanged pH value to a dominance of type I fibers. It seems that genetic factors primarily are responsible for the pattern of chemical reactions but that training can cause redistribution, even though its role might be secondary.

■ **MR Spectroscopy of Muscular Energy Metabolism**

Various disturbances of the muscular metabolism have been investigated. In particular, exercise MR spectroscopy has produced interesting and clinically relevant results.

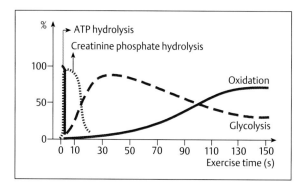

Fig. 10.**1** Time course of the energy supply in the muscle during stress.

McArdle Syndrome

This is a glycogenosis (glycogen storage disease) caused by a muscle phosphorylase deficiency. The muscle glycogen cannot be converted to glucose 1-phosphate. Exercise ^{31}P MRI spectroscopy has confirmed the theoretically expected manifestation, indicating a massive breakdown of phosphocreatine and failure of normal acidification. Infusion of glucose corrects these observed findings, with a return of the exercise-induced pH drop and considerable improvement of the muscle energy metabolism (3, 26, 33).

Phosphofructokinase Deficiency

This is involved with the conversion of fructose 1-phosphate into fructose 1,6-biphosphate. The enzyme catalyzes a step of the glycolysis. MRI spectroscopy can detect an increased PME peak, corresponding to the accumulation of fructose 1-phosphate produced as part of glycolysis. This is associated with an inadequate intracellular acidosis, attributed to impaired glycolysis with reduced production of lactic acid. Similar findings are found in patients with phosphoglyceromutase deficiency. Phosphoglyceromutase is an enzyme of glycolysis that catalyzes the shift of the phosphoryl group in the conversion of 3-phosphoglycerate into 2-phosphoglycerate (7, 32).

Respiratory Chain Defects

Considerable experience has been accumulated with spectroscopic examinations in patients with respiratory chain defects. This includes the NADH-Q reductase deficiency, repeatedly attributed to a slow recovery of phosphocreatine after exercise. A deficiency of the respiratory chain complex III (= NADH-Q reductase complex) reduces the amount of phosphocreatine and inorganic phosphorus and slows the recovery of these metabolites after exercise. Improvement of the symptoms after administration of vitamin K_3 and vitamin C, which replace the lacking reductase complex, can be documented spectroscopically (2).

Mitochondrial Myopathies

Other types of mitochondrial myopathies show abnormalities that include a decreased ratio of phosphocreatine phosphorus to inorganic phosphorus, or increased inorganic phosphorus, or both, observed in the spectrum at rest and after prolonged exercise-induced acidosis. Our extensive investigations with mitochondrial encephalomyopathies have produced variable results with MR spectroscopy. Exercise spectroscopy was found to be far superior to rest spectroscopy, which only showed a slightly lower phosphocreatine peak. Exercise spectroscopy could demonstrate myopathic changes with extraordinary sensitivity. The main findings in these patients are a delayed and incomplete decline of phosphocreatine during exercise and a slow recovery rate as well as the failure of a pH drop and the tendency to develop an alkalosis. The spectroscopic findings correlated with the severity of the disease and were as sensitive as clinical tests (22).

Muscular Dystrophies

The muscular dystrophies of Duchenne, Werdnig-Hoffmann and Kugelberg-Welander have been investigated by MR spectroscopy. An analysis of the metabolites measured spectroscopically reveals low PCr/NTP and PCr/P$_i$ ratios, an abnormally high pH and a pathologically increased phosphodiester (PDE) peak. This PDE peak increased further during muscle exercise.

Myositis

Various forms of myositis have been investigated by H–1 and P–32 spectroscopy (37).

H–1 spectroscopy provides information about the relative distribution of fat and water. Normal leg muscle contains 5–7% fat and the peaks of the fatty acids are difficult to identify on H–1 spectroscopy performed without water suppression.

Consequently, no marked changes in the fat and water peaks are seen in acute myositis. However, the T_1 relaxation times, which correspond to inflammatory and edematous tissue changes, are moderately prolonged. Chronic myositis contains areas of fatty muscular degeneration, in addition to a H–1 MR spectrum with mono- and polyunsaturated fatty acids at 5.4 ppm, with carbonyl groups at 2.3 ppm and terminal methyl groups at 1.1 ppm.

In patients with acute myositis, the P–31 spectrum shows a definite decrease in phosphocreatine relative to NTP, a normal range of the inorganic phosphate and added peaks of phosphomonoester and phosphodiester. These lines may represent phosphorylated sugars, which are metabolized in the anaerobic pathway of the glycolysis. The decrease in phosphocreatine indicates its increased hydrolysis during the synthesis of ATP. In chronic myositis, all phosphorylated metabolites are markedly decreased and the spectrum appears normal on first sight, but inorganic phosphate has essentially maintained its normal peak and, taking this into consideration, the ratio of inorganic phosphate to constant ß-NTP has increased. The decreased signal of the phosphorylated compounds is proportional to the extent of the muscular degeneration, but independent of the underlying aberration.

Anatomy

■ General Anatomy

Fig. 10.**2a–l** provides a schematic illustration of the cross-sectional anatomy of the extremities. The fasciae are outlined for easy identification of the muscle compartments, which represent the spaces along which inflammatory and necrotic muscle diseases spread. The upper arm has two compartments, the flexor and extensor compartments, which are separated by the brachial intermuscular septum. The forearm has four major compartments, the posterior and anterior extensor compartment and the deep and superficial flexor compartment, created by the antebrachial fascia and the interosseous membrane, as well as compartments for the flexor carpi ulnaris and for the flexor carpi radialis. The thigh has three major compartments, the flexor, extensor, and adductor compartment, divided by the intermuscular septa of the fascia lata. The sartorius muscle compartment is demarcated by the vastoadductorial membrane. The lower leg has four compartments: the deep and superficial flexor compartments, the anterior extensor compartment, and the peroneus compartment. These are formed by the crural fascia and its transverse intermuscular septum, anterior and posterior intermuscular septum, and the interosseous membrane.

The coloring of the muscles in Figs. 10.**2a–l** indicates the innervation and is explained below each cross-sectional diagram. In this way, the nerve supplying each muscle can easily be determined. This facilitates the distinction between neuropathy on the one hand and inflammatory myopathy on the other hand by assigning the signal changes either to a muscle compartment (the spread of inflammations and necrosis) or to the innervation territory of a particular nerve.

■ Specific MRI and Functional Anatomy

In the striated skeletal musculature, *two different types of fibers* can be distinguished:

- Type I fibers, rich in mitochondria
- Type II fibers, low in mitochondria

Type I Fibers. These are designed for slow contractions over an extended period of time. They obtain their energy through oxidation and are macroscopically red because of a high concentration of mitochondria

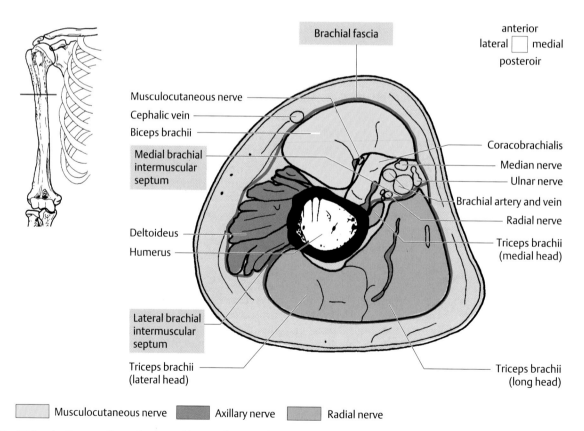

a   ☐ Musculocutaneous nerve   ■ Axillary nerve   ☐ Radial nerve

Fig. 10.**2a–l**   Cross sections of arms and legs to illustrate the muscle anatomy as seen on MRI. The muscle fasciae, which present potential spaces for the spreading of inflammatory changes, are outlined. Color coding of muscles with the same innervation to facilitate recognizing signal alterations secondary to impaired innervation (modified after Möller, T.B., E. Reif, *MR Atlas of the musculoskeletal system*. Blackwell, Wissenschaft, Berlin 1993).

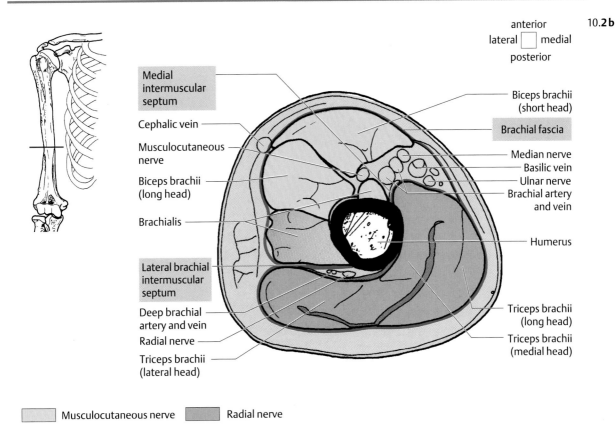

10.**2 b**

anterior
lateral ☐ medial
posterior

Medial intermuscular septum

Cephalic vein

Musculocutaneous nerve

Biceps brachii (long head)

Brachialis

Lateral brachial intermuscular septum

Deep brachial artery and vein

Radial nerve

Triceps brachii (lateral head)

Biceps brachii (short head)

Brachial fascia

Median nerve

Basilic vein

Ulnar nerve

Brachial artery and vein

Humerus

Triceps brachii (long head)

Triceps brachii (medial head)

☐ Musculocutaneous nerve   ☐ Radial nerve

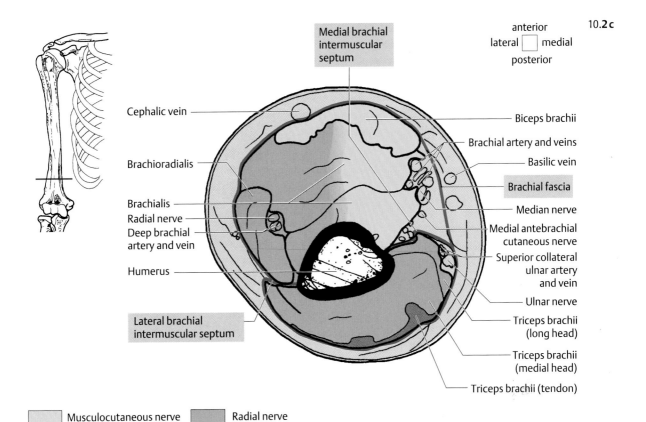

10.**2 c**

anterior
lateral ☐ medial
posterior

Medial brachial intermuscular septum

Cephalic vein

Brachioradialis

Brachialis

Radial nerve

Deep brachial artery and vein

Humerus

Lateral brachial intermuscular septum

Biceps brachii

Brachial artery and veins

Basilic vein

Brachial fascia

Median nerve

Medial antebrachial cutaneous nerve

Superior collateral ulnar artery and vein

Ulnar nerve

Triceps brachii (long head)

Triceps brachii (medial head)

Triceps brachii (tendon)

☐ Musculocutaneous nerve   ☐ Radial nerve

10.2 **d**

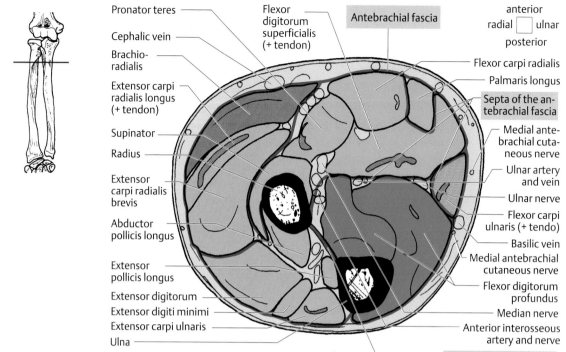

Pronator teres

Cephalic vein

Brachio-radialis

Extensor carpi radialis longus (+ tendon)

Supinator

Radius

Extensor carpi radialis brevis

Abductor pollicis longus

Extensor pollicis longus

Extensor digitorum

Extensor digiti minimi

Extensor carpi ulnaris

Ulna

Flexor digitorum superficialis (+ tendon)

Antebrachial fascia

anterior
radial ☐ ulnar
posterior

Flexor carpi radialis

Palmaris longus

Septa of the antebrachial fascia

Medial antebrachial cutaneous nerve

Ulnar artery and vein

Ulnar nerve

Flexor carpi ulnaris (+ tendo)

Basilic vein

Medial antebrachial cutaneous nerve

Flexor digitorum profundus

Median nerve

Anterior interosseous artery and nerve

Interosseous membrane

| | Radial nerve | | Radial nerve, deep branch | | Median nerve |
| | Ulnar nerve | | Interosseous palmar nerve (of the median and ulnar nerves) | | |

10.2 **e**

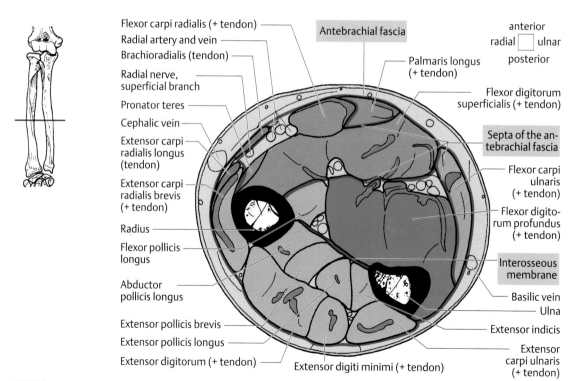

Flexor carpi radialis (+ tendon)

Radial artery and vein

Brachioradialis (tendon)

Radial nerve, superficial branch

Pronator teres

Cephalic vein

Extensor carpi radialis longus (tendon)

Extensor carpi radialis brevis (+ tendon)

Radius

Flexor pollicis longus

Abductor pollicis longus

Extensor pollicis brevis

Extensor pollicis longus

Extensor digitorum (+ tendon)

Extensor digiti minimi (+ tendon)

Antebrachial fascia

anterior
radial ☐ ulnar
posterior

Palmaris longus (+ tendon)

Flexor digitorum superficialis (+ tendon)

Septa of the antebrachial fascia

Flexor carpi ulnaris (+ tendon)

Flexor digitorum profundus (+ tendon)

Interosseous membrane

Basilic vein

Ulna

Extensor indicis

Extensor carpi ulnaris (+ tendon)

| | Radial nerve, deep branch | | Median nerve | | Interosseous palmar nerve (of the median and ulnar nerves) |
| | Median nerve, palmar interosseous branch | | Ulnar nerve | | |

10.**2f**

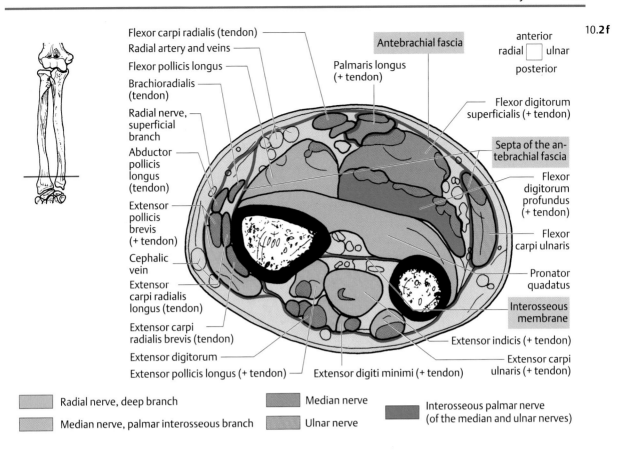

Flexor carpi radialis (tendon)
Radial artery and veins
Flexor pollicis longus
Brachioradialis (tendon)
Radial nerve, superficial branch
Abductor pollicis longus (tendon)
Extensor pollicis brevis (+ tendon)
Cephalic vein
Extensor carpi radialis longus (tendon)
Extensor carpi radialis brevis (tendon)
Extensor digitorum
Extensor pollicis longus (+ tendon)

Palmaris longus (+ tendon)
Antebrachial fascia

anterior
radial [ ] ulnar
posterior

Flexor digitorum superficialis (+ tendon)
Septa of the antebrachial fascia
Flexor digitorum profundus (+ tendon)
Flexor carpi ulnaris
Pronator quadratus
Interosseous membrane
Extensor indicis (+ tendon)
Extensor carpi ulnaris (+ tendon)
Extensor digiti minimi (+ tendon)

Radial nerve, deep branch
Median nerve, palmar interosseous branch
Median nerve
Ulnar nerve
Interosseous palmar nerve (of the median and ulnar nerves)

10.**2g**

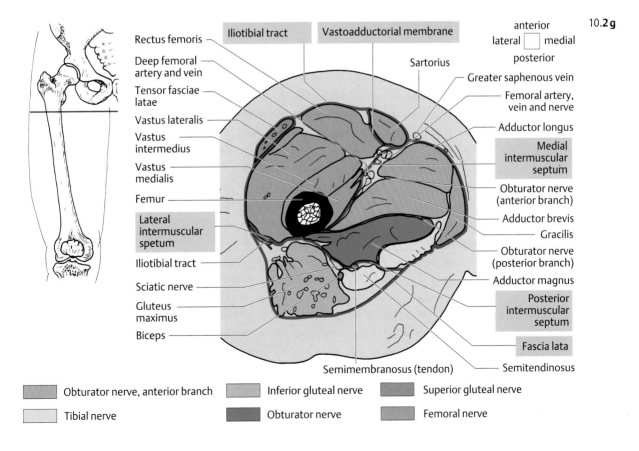

Rectus femoris
Deep femoral artery and vein
Tensor fasciae latae
Vastus lateralis
Vastus intermedius
Vastus medialis
Femur
Lateral intermuscular spetum
Iliotibial tract
Sciatic nerve
Gluteus maximus
Biceps

Iliotibial tract
Vastoadductorial membrane
Sartorius

anterior
lateral [ ] medial
posterior

Greater saphenous vein
Femoral artery, vein and nerve
Adductor longus
Medial intermuscular septum
Obturator nerve (anterior branch)
Adductor brevis
Gracilis
Obturator nerve (posterior branch)
Adductor magnus
Posterior intermuscular septum
Fascia lata
Semitendinosus
Semimembranosus (tendon)

Obturator nerve, anterior branch
Tibial nerve
Inferior gluteal nerve
Obturator nerve
Superior gluteal nerve
Femoral nerve

10.**2h**

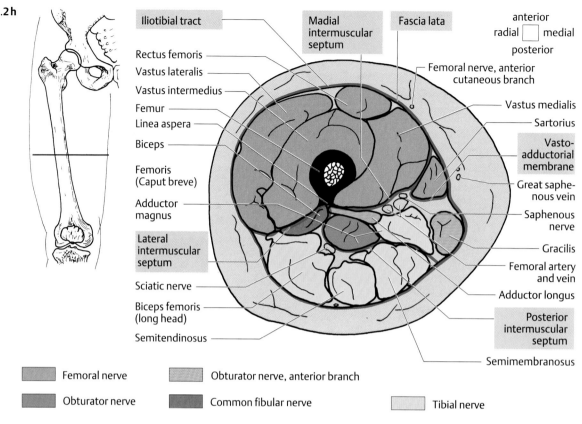

Iliotibial tract

Madial intermuscular septum

Fascia lata

anterior
radial ☐ medial
posterior

Rectus femoris

Vastus lateralis

Vastus intermedius

Femur

Linea aspera

Biceps

Femoris (Caput breve)

Adductor magnus

Lateral intermuscular septum

Sciatic nerve

Biceps femoris (long head)

Semitendinosus

Femoral nerve, anterior cutaneous branch

Vastus medialis

Sartorius

Vasto-adductorial membrane

Great saphe-nous vein

Saphenous nerve

Gracilis

Femoral artery and vein

Adductor longus

Posterior intermuscular septum

Semimembranosus

| | Femoral nerve | | Obturator nerve, anterior branch | | Tibial nerve |
| | Obturator nerve | | Common fibular nerve | | |

10.**2i**

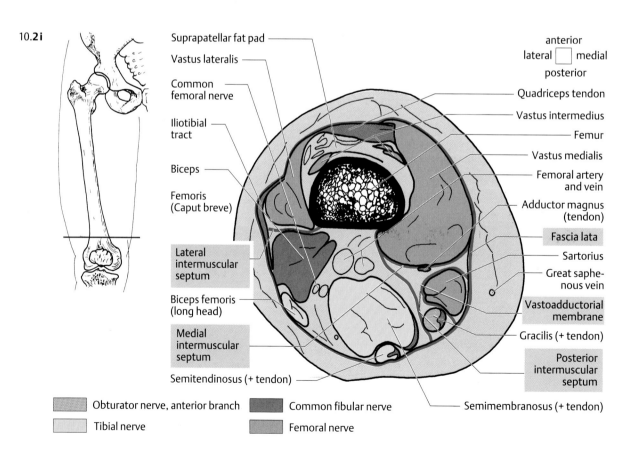

Suprapatellar fat pad

Vastus lateralis

Common femoral nerve

Iliotibial tract

Biceps

Femoris (Caput breve)

Lateral intermuscular septum

Biceps femoris (long head)

Medial intermuscular septum

Semitendinosus (+ tendon)

anterior
lateral ☐ medial
posterior

Quadriceps tendon

Vastus intermedius

Femur

Vastus medialis

Femoral artery and vein

Adductor magnus (tendon)

Fascia lata

Sartorius

Great saphe-nous vein

Vastoadductorial membrane

Gracilis (+ tendon)

Posterior intermuscular septum

Semimembranosus (+ tendon)

| | Obturator nerve, anterior branch | | Common fibular nerve |
| | Tibial nerve | | Femoral nerve |

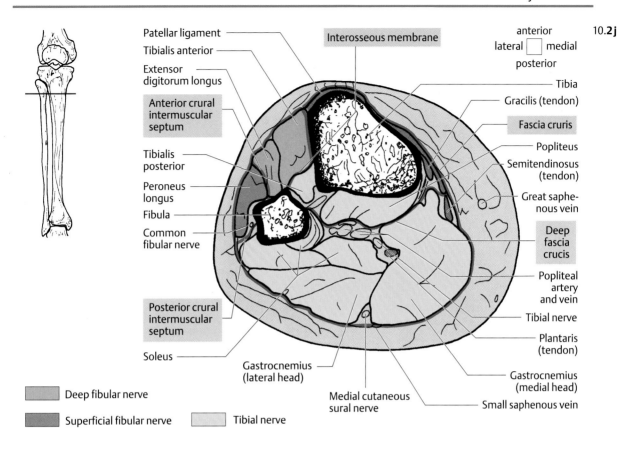

10.**2j**

anterior
lateral ☐ medial
posterior

Patellar ligament
Tibialis anterior
Extensor digitorum longus
Anterior crural intermuscular septum
Tibialis posterior
Peroneus longus
Fibula
Common fibular nerve
Posterior crural intermuscular septum
Soleus
Gastrocnemius (lateral head)
Medial cutaneous sural nerve

Interosseous membrane
Tibia
Gracilis (tendon)
Fascia cruris
Popliteus
Semitendinosus (tendon)
Great saphenous vein
Deep fascia crucis
Popliteal artery and vein
Tibial nerve
Plantaris (tendon)
Gastrocnemius (medial head)
Small saphenous vein

☐ Deep fibular nerve
☐ Superficial fibular nerve
☐ Tibial nerve

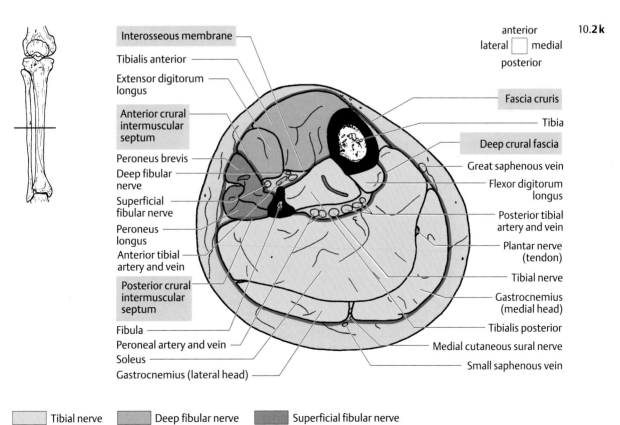

10.**2k**

anterior
lateral ☐ medial
posterior

Interosseous membrane
Tibialis anterior
Extensor digitorum longus
Anterior crural intermuscular septum
Peroneus brevis
Deep fibular nerve
Superficial fibular nerve
Peroneus longus
Anterior tibial artery and vein
Posterior crural intermuscular septum
Fibula
Peroneal artery and vein
Soleus
Gastrocnemius (lateral head)

Fascia cruris
Tibia
Deep crural fascia
Great saphenous vein
Flexor digitorum longus
Posterior tibial artery and vein
Plantar nerve (tendon)
Tibial nerve
Gastrocnemius (medial head)
Tibialis posterior
Medial cutaneous sural nerve
Small saphenous vein

☐ Tibial nerve   ☐ Deep fibular nerve   ☐ Superficial fibular nerve

10.21

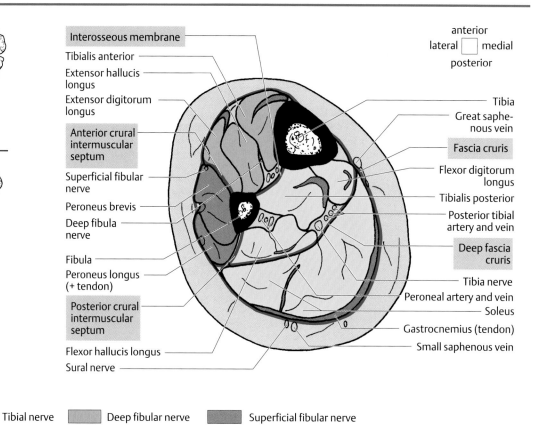

Interosseous membrane
Tibialis anterior
Extensor hallucis longus
Extensor digitorum longus
Anterior crural intermuscular septum
Superficial fibular nerve
Peroneus brevis
Deep fibula nerve
Fibula
Peroneus longus (+ tendon)
Posterior crural intermuscular septum
Flexor hallucis longus
Sural nerve

anterior
lateral ☐ medial
posterior

Tibia
Great saphenous vein
Fascia cruris
Flexor digitorum longus
Tibialis posterior
Posterior tibial artery and vein
Deep fascia cruris
Tibia nerve
Peroneal artery and vein
Soleus
Gastrocnemius (tendon)
Small saphenous vein

☐ Tibial nerve   ☐ Deep fibular nerve   ☐ Superficial fibular nerve

(Fig. 10.**3a**). Because of a dense internal structure, they are believed to have a relatively high water content. MRI shows muscles dominated by type I fibers with a relatively high signal intensity on T_2-weighted images (11).

Type II Fibers. These are designed for rapid, short, and strong contractions. They obtain their energy primarily from anaerobic glycolysis and appear macroscopically white because of a sparse internal structure (Fig. 10.**3b**). On T_2-weighted images, type II fibers have a lower signal intensity than the type I fibers.

In other animals, MRI reveals distinct differences between the fiber types. In humans, the signal differences between specific muscles of different fiber composition within the same individual are less pronounced since the different fiber types are intermingled. Distinct differences, however, are encountered between individuals. Certain muscles of high endurance athletes, such as marathon runners, have a high proportion of type 1 fibers, while peak performance athletes, such as 100 meter sprinters, have predominantly type II fibers. A significant correlation has been found between MR relaxation time and muscle fiber composition (23).

Normal muscle has a low signal intensity on T_1-weighted images, with a similarly low signal intensity on the T_2-weighted images, irrespective of the dominating fiber type of the muscle. Fibrous septations are displayed as signal voids. On fat-suppressed images, the normal musculature shows a higher signal intensity.

In healthy subjects, physiologic muscle activity induces increased perfusion of the musculature and a rise in the extracellular free water, increasing the signal intensity on the T_2-weighted images. The intensity of the signal increase depends on the type and duration of the exercise and ranges between 20 and 40% of the baseline value. Within 45–50 minutes after the end of exercise, the signal intensity normalizes with a short recovery period, probably representing the rapid normalization of vascular flow, and a slower second component related to the disappearance of extracellular water (21) (Fig. 10.**4**). When evaluating increases in signal intensity induced by physiologic exercise allowance must be made for variations in the functional anatomy of the muscle groups in question. For instance, it has been shown that 25% of subjects investigated do not use the flexor digitorum superficialis for digital flexion, but they do use it for carpal flexion. Following hand grip exercises, all the subjects investigated had increased signal intensity in flexors digitorum superficialis and profundus along with the flexor carpi ulnaris, but only 50% of them had increased signal intensity in extensor carpi ulnaris and supinator (8), indicating that exercise-induced increases in signal intensity can display a variable signal pattern.

In view of the physiologic phenomena described, MRI performed for the detection or characterization of

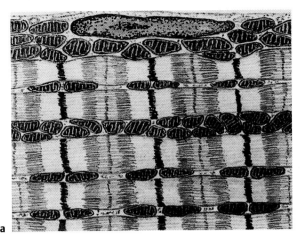

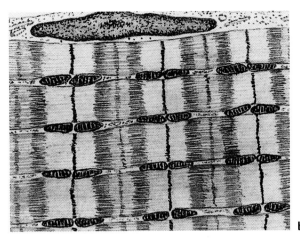

a   b

Fig. 10.**3 a, b** Types of muscle fibers, electron microscopy (from 28). **a** Type I, so-called red or dark muscle fiber, rich in large mitochondria. **b** Type II, light or white, mitochondria-deficient muscle fiber.

myopathies should not be preceded by athletic activities. Otherwise, physiologic increases in signal intensity might be mistaken for a pathologic muscle edema.

MRI Pattern of Muscular Lesions

The muscle disorders and diseases can produce certain basic patterns on MRI (Fig. 10.**5**):

- normal,
- hypertrophy,
- hypotrophy,
- atrophy,
- pseudohypertrophy,
- edema,
- necrosis,
- fibrosis.

Recognizing such muscle changes can be relevant for planning a biopsy and for monitoring the course of therapy. However, a specific diagnosis is often unattainable on MRI findings alone. Aside from recognizing the basic MRI pattern, it is necessary to determine whether the process is:

- focal, multifocal or diffuse,
- proximal, distal or bilateral,
- symmetric or asymmetric, or
- follows a centrifugal or centripetal progression.

■ Hypertrophy

Enlargement of the muscle cell, for instance through increased exercise, leads to hypertrophy. The diameter of the muscle increases without a corresponding visible alteration of the signal intensity on MRI. The intermuscular connective tissue layers are decreased in thickness, causing the intramuscular fat lines to be barely discernible. Endocrine ophthalmopathy pro-

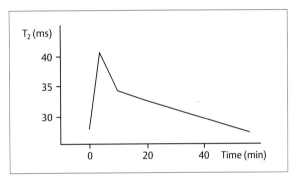

Fig. 10.**4** T_2 relaxation times of the deep and superficial flexors digitorum after hand grip exercises for 5 minutes. Rapid increase of the T_2 time within the first minute after termination of the exercise (exceeding 40%). Two phase decline in the recovery phase: rapid initial normalization (improvement of hyperemia) and slow normalization in the late phase (resorption of extracellular water) until 50 minutes after termination of the exercise (after 21).

duces the finding of extraocular muscular hypertrophy on MRI. Other examples are hypertrophy of the muscles of mastication due to teeth grinding (34) and alterations of the muscle due to hypothyroidism (11).

■ Hypotrophy

Diminution of the muscle cell secondary to decreased activity leads to hypotrophy. The diameter of the muscle is decreased but the musculature exhibits a normal signal intensity. Intermuscular connective tissue spaces are increased and filled with fat. MRI, especially the T_1-weighted image, shows an increase in high signal stripes within the muscle.

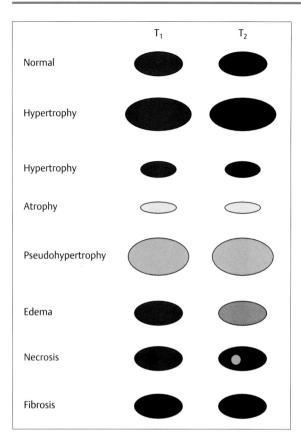

Fig. 10.**5**   MRI visualization of patterns of healthy and pathologic musculature on T_1-weighted and T_2-weighted images.

■ Atrophy

Numerous diseases and inactivity lead to the image of atrophy, with a markedly decreased cross section of the muscle. The inter- and intramuscular deposition of fat is increased, producing a diffuse to multifocal patchy increase in signal intensity on the T_1-weighted and T_2-weighted images. Since the muscle reacts in the same way to different harmful substances, numerous diseases can create the image of an atrophy:

- Late stage of denervation,
- Inflammation,
- Dystrophies,
- Necroses,
- Trauma.

Depending on the duration and intensity of the damage, the loss of muscle substance may become permanent.

■ Pseudohypertrophy

The picture of a pseudohypertrophy can be encountered in muscular dystrophies. Here, the compensatory inter- and intramuscular disposition of fat after the demise of the muscle cells can be excessive and the cross-section of the muscle increases despite a loss in lean muscle

mass. MRI shows an expanded diameter as well as a homogeneous to multifocal patchy increase in signal intensity due to intramuscular fat deposits.

■ Edema

Numerous diseases induce edema of the muscle with increased fluid accumulation in the extracellular space:

- Trauma,
- Necrosis,
- Intramuscular hemorrhage,
- Tumor,
- Polymyositis,
- Early stage of denervation,
- Other types of myositis,
- Radiation,
- Overuse.

The result is an increased signal intensity on the T_2-weighted images, especially after fat suppression. The T_1-weighted images frequently show no visible signal alteration or a subtle decrease in signal intensity. The muscle lumen is normal or can be slightly increased.

■ Necrosis

If infection, trauma or compression with ischemia has damaged the muscle severely, the resultant rhabdomyolysis can progress to necrosis. Necrosis of the muscle generally induces a focal decrease in signal intensity or no signal change on the T_1-weighted images and, on the T_2-weighted images, an increase in signal intensity. Whether the necrosis is infected (abscess), cannot be determined by the signal pattern or morphology. In this situation, the IV administration of gadolinium is helpful. A strong peripheral contrast-enhancement favors an abscess. Around the necrotic center, a broad edematous zone with corresponding signal pattern (see above) is usually seen in the adjacent soft tissues. MRI does not always achieve an exact demarcation.

■ Fibrosis

Aside from atrophy and necrosis, a chronic or very severe muscular lesion can lead to a third reaction, comprising a decrease in muscle mass and an increase in fibrous connective tissue. This relatively rare form of muscle fibrosis is found in congenital torticollis. The muscle has a reduced cross section and a decreased signal intensity on T_1-weighted and T_2-weighted images.

Neuropathy

Damage to the *peripheral nerve* from trauma, chronic or acute compression, etc. is classified by Seddon into three grades:

- Neurapraxia (grade I): Minor, regenerative damage of the nerve without electromyogram (EMG) changes of denervation potentials in the affected muscle.
- Axonotmesis (grade II): Regenerative injury of the axon and its sheath with EMG-detectable denervation potentials in the affected muscle, one to two weeks after the insult.
- Neurotmesis (grade III): Nonregenerative, total or subtotal severance of the neural fibers and their covering structures with EMG-detectable denervation potentials of the affected muscle. Neural lesions of grade II and III induce changes in the affected musculature that can be detected by MRI.

Denervation probably leads to relative shrinkage of the fibers in the affected muscle with compensatory hypertrophy of the extracellular space and subsequent prolongation of the T_1 and T_2 relaxation times (30). An irreversible denervation eventually advances to compensatory deposition of fat, which in turn reverses the prolongation of the T_1 relaxation time. These altered relaxation times add up to the following changes of the signal pattern:

Acute to Subacute Denervation. This presents as homogenous increase in signal intensities on the T_2-weighted images without additional signal changes on the T_1-weighted images. The STIR sequence is most suitable for these changes and shows a strong increase in signal intensity. The affected muscles exhibit a pattern that corresponds to the distribution of the neural branches. Thus interpreting the image rests on a thorough knowledge of the innervation pattern. Lesions affecting root, plexus, and peripheral nerve can be distinguished from the distribution pattern.

Chronic Denervation. This results in atrophy of the muscle with compensatory increase in fatty tissue. These changes lead to an increased signal intensity, which is most conspicuous on the T_1-weighted images. A moderate increase in signal intensity is seen on the T_2-weighted images, while the fat appears as areas of low signal intensity on the STIR images. Tumor compression

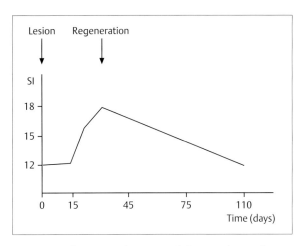

Fig. 10.**6** Relative signal intensity of the vasculature after reversible denervation (T_2-weighted MR sequences). Definite signal increase 15 days after the denervation. After regeneration over a period of more than 100 days post denervation, slow signal normalization.
SI = Signal intensity

can be one cause of a chronic progressive neural lesion. Thus, in muscle atrophies displaying a denervation pattern, the supplying nerve should be inspected along its course for any tumors (34).

Other diseases that can produce the MRI pattern of denervation include poliomyelitis (Fig. 10.**7**), diseases of the *neuromuscular junctions*, such as Eaton-Lambert syndrome, botulism, myasthenia gravis, as well as complex neurologic disorders that affect the *upper and lower neurons*, such as amyotrophic lateral sclerosis or spinal atrophy. Disorders of the upper and lower neurons generally produce symmetric signal changes.

Damage to the neurons of the anterior gray column, as found in poliomyelitis, frequently leads to unilateral paresis with corresponding MRI changes.

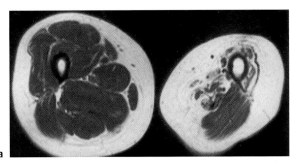
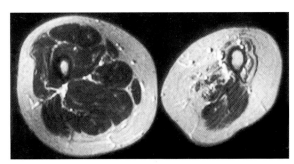

a   b

Fig. 10.**7 a, b** Status post poliomyelitis. **a** T_1-weighted SE sequence. Increased signal intensity and atrophy of muscles of the left upper thigh. The right upper thigh muscle are normal. **b** T_2-weighted SE sequence. Likewise, subtle increase in signal intensity of the residual musculature in the presence of fatty atrophy. Still discrete remnants of normal musculature in the region of the knee flexors.

Table 10.**1**   A comparison of some hereditary muscular conditions

Type	Heredity	Incidence	Age of Manifestation	Distribution Type
Duchenne	Recessive, X-chromosomal	1 : 3000	10 – 30 years	Malignant pelvic type, death before the age of 20 years
Becker	Recessive, X-chromosomal	1 : 20000	12 – 25 years	Benign pelvic type
Leyden	Recessive, autosomal	1 : 20000	5 – 15 years 30 – 40 years	Limb-girdle type with ascending or descending spread
Erb	Dominant, autosomal	1 : 200000	7 – 25 years	Facioscapulohumeral form
Welander	Dominant, autosomal	rare	40 – 60 years	Distal extremities

Myotonic Disorders

These are diseases where there is delayed muscle relaxation after contraction. They are thought to result from disturbances in the membrane of the muscle fibers or in the muscular component of the neuromuscular junction, e.g., congenital myotonia (Thomson) and dystrophia myotonica (Curshmann-Steinert). MRI shows a mixture of hypertrophy and atrophy, similar to the findings encountered with dystrophy. There are no specific changes. Unlike dystrophies, the process advances from distal to proximal. The end stage presents as atrophy with increased fat disposition (11).

Myopathies

■ Dystrophic Myopathies

The progressive dystrophic myopathies include a group of hereditary muscle diseases, which are characterized by progressive degeneration of muscle fibers and compensatory deposition of fat and fibrous tissue. Various types have been described and the most frequent are listed in Tab. 10.**1**. Etiologically, these conditions are probably a manifestation of genetically determined structural and metabolic abnormalities of the muscle cell.

The dystrophic muscular changes have MRI changes that are best seen on T_1-weighted sequences. The affected muscles show multifocal or geographic areas of increased signal intensity due to the deposited fat. Initially, the muscle volume is increased and the muscles show the picture of pseudohypertrophy. With progression of the disease, the muscle volume decreases and the muscles appear atrophic. The fat deposition in the muscle and initially also the muscle edema cause an increased signal intensity on the T_2-weighted images. The extent of intramuscular fat deposition and the degree of signal increase on MRI correlate well with the clinical stage of the disease (35).

The various, usually symmetric distribution patterns found in the affected muscles depend on the type of dystrophy and on the duration of the disease. *Duchenne muscular dystrophy* shows symmetric signal changes in the upper and lower leg, with the posterior compartments of the lower leg showing more extensive fatty infiltration than the anterior compartment. The upper leg displays only minimal changes in the gracilis, sartorius, rectus femoris, and semitendinosus (24, 35) (Fig. 10.**8**). Early in the disease, the muscles can show compensatory hypertrophy with volume increase and normal signal intensity (Fig. 10.**9**). The remaining thigh

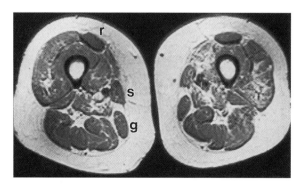
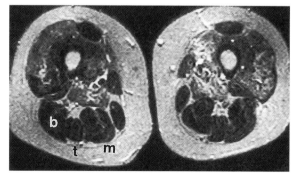

Fig. 10.**8 a, b**   Duchenne muscular dystrophy. Cross section of the thigh. **a** Proton density-weighted SE sequence. Symmetric increase in signal intensity and decrease in volume of the thigh musculature due to fat deposits and atrophy. **b** T_2-weighted SE sequence. Increased signal intensity of the thigh musculature due to fat and partial muscle edema.

b = Biceps femoris
g = Relative sparing of the gracilis, as well as knee flexors
m = Semimembranosus
r = Relative sparing of the rectus femoris
s = Relative sparing of the sartorius
t = Semitendinosus

muscles show a variable increase in signal intensity. The findings progress from proximal to distal. In the lower leg, the signal alterations occur late and tibialis anterior and posterior as well as the peronei are largely spared. Of the trunk musculature, the psoas is often normal, while longissimus and iliocostalis muscles show alterations early on (15). The extent of muscular fat deposition correlates poorly with the duration of the disease, but well with the clinically assessed severity of the muscle weakness (27).

■ Inflammatory Myopathies

Numerous conditions can underlie inflammatory myopathies (Tab. 10.2). The inflammatory changes in the muscle induce an accumulation of extracellular water. The resulting muscle edema can lead to nonspecific signal changes:

- no change or slightly reduced signal intensity on T_1-weighted images,
- increased signal intensity on T_2-weighted images, especially after fat suppression (16).

In long-standing myositis, the chronic damage of the muscle leads to atrophy of the affected muscle with compensatory increase of fatty tissue. These lipomatous transformations are only detectable after at least one year at the earliest (4). The T_1-weighted and T_2-weighted images show a multifocal, linear, or geographic increase in signal intensity. The pattern of the muscular signal alterations generally does not permit a specific diagnosis. MRI, however, can be helpful for planning a biopsy since the visualized pattern of involvement can easily distinguish an active inflammatory process from a fatty atrophy. So far, typical MRI findings have been described in idiopathic and infectious myositis and are presented here:

Polymyositis or Dermatomyositis. Published studies of patients with these types of myositis have shown that the affected muscles have diffuse signal changes, most frequently observed in the thigh muscles. The signal in-

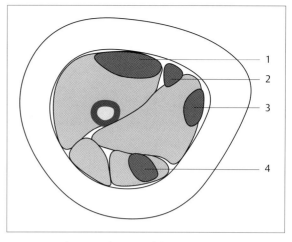

Fig. 10.**9** Schematic drawing of the cross section of the thigh (more cranial than on Fig. 10.**8**). Duchenne muscular dystrophy. Increased volume and signal intensity of the musculature (T_1-weighted and T_2-weighted contrast) due to fatty infiltration (pseudohypertrophy) (after 35).
1 = Sparing of the rectus femoris
2 = Sparing of the sartorius
3 = Sparing of the gracilis
4 = Sparing of the semitendinosus

tensity on T_2-weighted images is increased in all muscles and detected bilaterally. The increased signal intensity is different for each muscle group, with the anterior muscles, especially quadriceps and the adductor groups, most severely affected (Fig. 10.**10**) (4, 18). The signal intensity of the T_1-weighted images generally is not altered (16).

In severe cases of dermatomyositis, a T_2 signal increase can be seen in a perimuscular ('halo sign') or linear subcutaneous distribution. This is presumably the result of accompanying subcutaneous and perimuscular edema.

The signal alterations of MRI correlate with the clinical and laboratory parameters of disease activity, such as muscle weakness and elevated enzymes. Occasionally, the musculoskeletal MRI findings can persist long after normalization of the enzymes (18).

Viral Myositis. The affected muscles show a diffuse increase in signal intensity on the T_2-weighted images (17), frequently confined to one muscle group (Fig. 10.**10**). A viral myositis can be the manifestation of a systemic viral infection (e.g., influenza).

Pyomyositis. The infectious bacterial myositis results in single or multiple confluent intramuscular abscesses (Fig. 10.**11**) and predominantly involves immunosuppressed patients. Muscle enzymes can remain normal. The T_1-weighted images depict multiple, often confluent lobulated areas of decreased signal intensity (1). In rare cases, they are bordered by a high-signal rim or displayed as areas of slightly higher signal than nor-

Table 10.**2** Survey of inflammatory myopathies

Idiopathic:
- Dermatomyositis
- Polymyositis
Inclusion body myositis
Autoimmune myositis

Infectious myositis:
- Bacterial
- Viral
- Parasitic
- Mycotic
Granulomatous myositis
Paraneoplastic
Focal myositis
Myositis with vasculitis

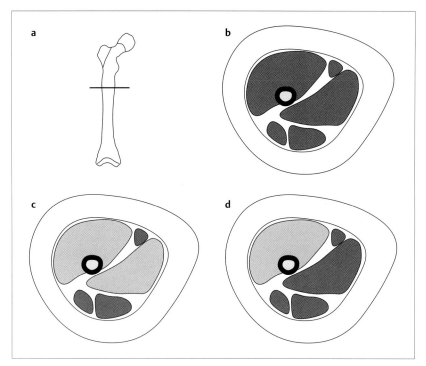

Fig. 10.**10 a–d**   Schematic drawing of the cross section of the thigh. T$_2$-weighted sequences.
a Level of the cross section. **b** Normal findings. **c** Polymyositis with increased signal intensity of quadriceps femoris, adductors, knee flexors and gluteal musculature. The increased signal intensities are homogeneous and unequally severe in the different groups.
d Viral myositis. Homogeneous increase in signal intensity confined to the quadriceps femoris.

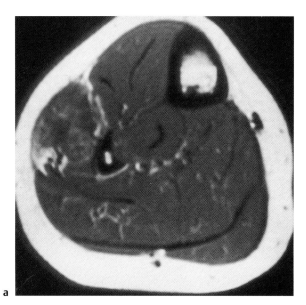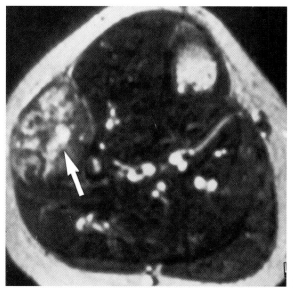

Fig. 10.**11 a, b**   Pyogenic myositis of the peroneal muscles. **a** T$_1$-weighted SE sequence. Heterogeneous signal intensity of the affected musculature with areas of decreased and increased signal intensity. **b** T$_2$-weighted SE sequence. Increased signal intensity of the affected musculature. Highly signal intense foci compatible with abscesses (arrow).

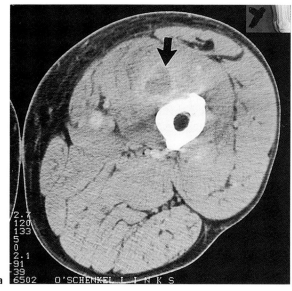

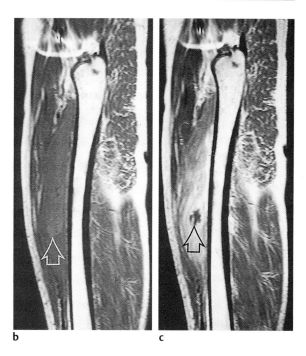

b   c

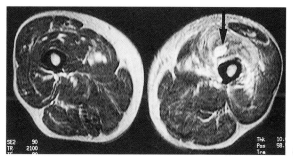

Fig. 10.**12 a–d** Pyogenic myositis of the thigh (confirmed by aspiration) four weeks after surgical stripping of the greater saphenous vein. **a** CT after injection of contrast medium shows a central ring-like enhancement along the course of the vastus intermedius as well as heterogeneity within the vastus intermedius and vastus medialis. The exact extent of the process cannot be determined. Linear thickening in the subcutaneous fatty tissues is compatible with edema. **b** On MRI, the central focus exhibits a high signal intensity in comparison with the surrounding musculature on the T_1-weighted image (sagittal section), as evidence of an accumulation of pus (arrow). **c** After injection of contrast medium, strong enhancement of the inflamed musculature surrounding a central area of no enhancement, compatible with an abscess (arrow). **d** The transverse T_2-weighted image shows the extent of the inflammation well. Accompanying reaction of the rectus femoris and vastus lateralis with discrete peripheral increase in signal intensity, as well as a central abscess (arrow).

mal muscle (Fig. 10.**12**). The cause of the high-signal rim is unknown. It could represent the accumulation of paramagnetic substances in the abscess rim (9). The surrounding musculature exhibits a normal signal intensity. The T_2-weighted image shows the abscess as high-signal focus within the musculature, which has a signal intensity that is normal or slightly increased homogeneously (Fig. 10.**12**). Peripheral enhancement is observed after IV administration of contrast medium.

Sarcoidosis. Muscular sarcoidosis is relatively rare and generally asymptomatic. Symptomatic manifestation can be nodular or diffuse. Sarcoid nodules have a high signal intensity on T_1-weighted and T_2-weighted images, often exhibiting a low-signal center. The diffuse type of sarcoid myositis is often only recognized by the MR findings of the resultant muscle atrophy (29).

■ **Muscle Changes after Radiotherapy or Local Chemotherapy**

Radiotherapy. The resultant muscular and cutaneous alterations can be visualized on MRI. About 6 weeks following radiotherapy of primary bone and soft tissues tumors with doses between 59 and 65 Gy, altered MR signal intensities were found in the musculature and skin (13). These changes consisted of increased signal intensity on T_2-weighted and STIR images as well as contrast enhancement. The radiation-induced signal alterations are sharply demarcated and follow the outline of the radiation fields. All patients in this study had a strong acute and subacute skin reaction. Radiation-induced changes are not to be mistaken for a neoplastic process. These MRI findings cannot be explained as inflammatory-edematous reaction or as increased accumulation of extracellular water. These changes can persist for up to one year following termination of the radiotherapy.

Local Chemotherapy. Changes similar to that seen after radiation can develop after local intra-arterial chemotherapy, as administered to patients with locally advanced breast carcinoma or recurrent rectum carcinoma. The exclusive administration of the chemotherapeutic agent to the tumor is rarely achieved and the inadvertent concomitant perfusion of adjacent muscle and skin can induce the same changes described above as post radiation changes. Differentiating these myositic changes from tumorous infiltration can be very difficult and limits the use of MRI for monitoring the therapeutic effect.

■ Traumatic Myopathies

Acute Overuse. Acute muscle injury on exertion is frequently observed in patients who are physically unconditioned. Injuries are primarily caused by athletic activities involving eccentric muscular action, i.e., overuse due to forced active lengthening. Concentric muscular action occurring with shortening of the muscle rarely causes muscle damage (36). The post-exercise injuries can be divided into injuries due to immediate damage (strain, contusion) and injuries due to delayed damage after 1–2 days (muscle soreness). Both types of injuries can be identified on MRI.

With *acute muscle strain*, the T_2-weighted images show a focal or heterogeneous increase in signal intensity, usually centrally located in the affected muscle. The signal changes resolve within 12 days, with a peripheral increase in signal intensity evolving after 2–3 days in many cases. This rim of increased signal intensity can extend into the perimuscular connective tissue (Fig. 10.**13**).

In *delayed onset muscle soreness* (DOMS), the T_2-weighted images show a homogeneous increase in signal intensity in the affected muscle, attributed to edematous changes (Fig. 10.**14**):

- diffuse, largely homogeneous increase in signal intensity after 1–3 days,
- the signal intensity continues to increase and reaches the maximum after 3–6 days,
- the signal changes resolve slowly within the next 10 weeks (36).

The increased signal intensities correlate poorly with the time course of the clinical symptoms. The peak signal intensity is reached when the pain improves. The increased signal intensities last considerably beyond the

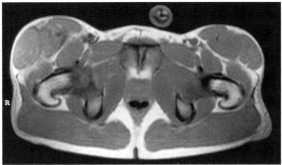

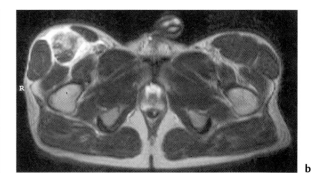

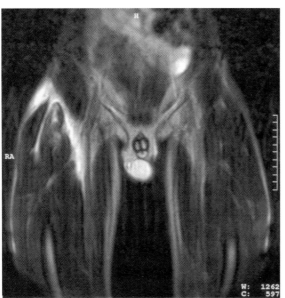

Fig. 10.**13 a–c** Partial tear and strain of the rectus femoris on the right after sports injury. **a** Axial T_1-weighted SE image. Muscle-isointense swelling with discrete central increase in signal intensity along the course of the rectus femoris as evidence of damage with hemorrhage. **b** T_2-weighted TSE image. Increased signal intensity in swollen muscle surrounded by ring-like edema as evidence of at least a severe strain. **c** Coronal T_2-weighted TSE image. Subtle wavy course and disrupted contour, suggesting a partial tear of the rectus femoris. Somewhat compromised evaluation due to motion artifact.

Fig. 10.**14a, b** Pain in the lower leg three days after intensive athletic activities. **a** Proton density-weighted SE sequence. Increased signal intensity in both heads of the gastrocnemius. **b** T₂-weighted SE sequence. Marked enhancement in both heads of the gastrocnemius. Additional perimuscular increase in signal intensity (arrows).

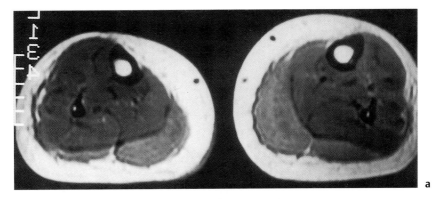

a

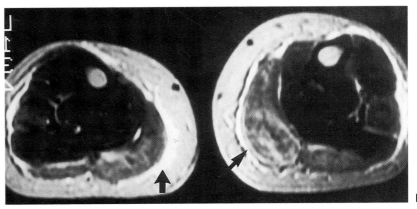

b

time of disappearance of the clinical symptoms and normalization of any possible elevated serum creatine enzyme levels.

Not all muscles in the exercised muscle group show signal alterations and only one muscle or muscle belly might be exclusively involved (9). This might be related to differential usage of the individual muscle within the overall group. Furthermore, the signal intensity is most pronounced near the insertions of the affected muscle (36). Severe cases can show extramuscular signal changes, possibly caused by microhemorrhage or extramuscular edema (Fig. 10.**14**). These extramuscular signal changes encircle the affected muscle like a ring and resemble the extramuscular changes seen with strains and ruptured fibers. Variations of functional anatomy and innervation result in a variable pattern between individuals despite comparable exercise.

Specific athletic activities predispose to injuries of certain muscles. For instance, athletes exercising their legs were found to have an involvement of the rectus femoris (so-called 'sprinter muscle') in up to 40% of all injuries (14).

The value of MRI is its contribution to the differential diagnosis of post-traumatic muscular pain. Aside from detecting exertional muscle damage, it can exclude focal hematomas or fascial herniations.

More severe injuries can cause a *partial muscle tear.* The intramuscular space created by the disrupted fibers can fill with blood or edematous fluid. This accounts for a signal pattern that might be indistinguishable from pure blood. The T₁-weighted images show a localized swelling of the muscle as well as multiple small patchy areas with slightly increased signal intensity (6). The T₂-weighted images display a localized heterogeneous area of increased signal intensity within the muscle belly (Fig. 10.**13**).

Intramuscular *hematomas* have the typical signal pattern of blood. Depending on their age, hematomas are of increased signal intensity on the T₁-weighted and T₂-weighted images, seen along the intramuscular septations and other tissue layers. Old hematomas exhibit a signal-void rim. With time, the signal intensity changes, eventually resulting in a low-signal visualization in all sequences. Aside from ferritin deposits, post-traumatic calcifications can lead to signal voids.

Complete tears can cause a large defect in the muscle, which fills with hemorrhagic fluid. The signal intensities within these defects are heterogenous and variable, primarily showing a higher signal intensity than muscles in all sequences.

Chronic Overuse. This can lead to an inflammatory reaction, usually affecting the musculotendinous transition. This 'myotendinitis' leads to a circumscribed increase in signal intensity within the affected muscle on the T₂-weighted images (Fig. 10.**15**). The typical examples are 'tennis elbow' or 'typewriter wrist.'

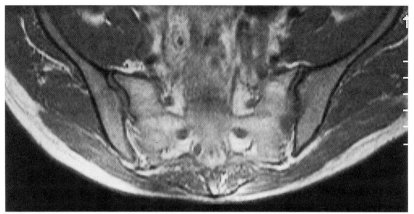

a

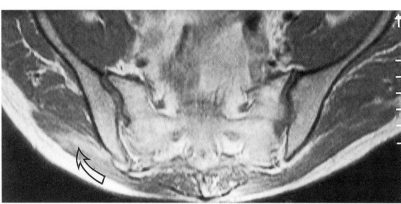

b

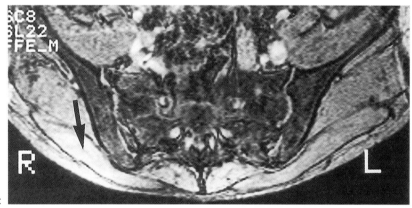

c

Fig. 10.**15 a–d** Mild tendinitis of ▶ the right gluteus maximus along its insertion at the iliac crest. This female patient complains of exercise-induced pain with relief after anti-inflammatory therapy. **a** The transverse T$_1$-weighted image shows no appreciable signal changes. **b** After injection of contrast medium, linear enhancement along the course of the gluteus maximus (arrow). **c** and **d** Transverse T$_2$-weighted (FFE) and coronal fat-saturated STIR images reveal a definite increase in signal intensity next to the attachment of the muscle (arrow).

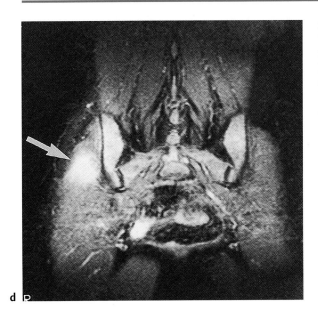

d ▷

Traumatic myositis ossificans can follow an injury of the soft tissues. Periosteal new bone formation and a soft tissue mass appear within 7–10 days after the trauma and progressively calcify within the next 2–6 weeks. Beginning at the periphery, the mass ossifies 6–8 weeks after the trauma. With maturation of this process, large areas can be transformed to fat secondary to degeneration and necrosis (31). By completion of the ossification after 5–6 months, a bizarre bone formation has developed (Fig. 10.**16**). The lesion can shrink and, though rarely, resorb. With cystic transformation of the center, an eggshell-like calcification of the soft tissues

may be observed. The signal intensity of the initial soft tissue swelling is decreased on T_1-weighted images and increased on T_2-weighted. Central calcifications cause heterogeneous areas of decreased signal intensity and ossifications appear as signal voids. Since ossification begins at the periphery, the lesions characteristically display a signal-void rim and a center with a heterogenous signal increase. Depending on the extent of fatty components, the T_1-weighted image can contain areas of increased signal intensity (Fig. 10.**17**). Fat and concentric layering are important diagnostic criteria to differentiate the lesion from para-osseous, periosteal and extra-osseous osteosarcomas, chondrosarcomas, osteomas, or chondromas.

Recently, two types of muscle injuries have repeatedly been discussed. One type is an injury of the knee flexors, including semimembranosus, semitendinosus and biceps femoris. Together with the quadratus femoris and part of the adductor magnus, these flexors are referred to as hamstring muscles and are frequently subject to sports injuries. The injury is usually proximal and encompasses the entire spectrum of possible muscle damage depending on the severity of the injury, including avulsion fractures of the ischial tuberosity or, in juveniles, apophysis. Sudden knee flexion as occurring in sprinting, basket ball playing, and weight lifting can cause such an injury (5a, 30a).

The other type is an injury involving the plantaris. This muscle is medioposterior to the medial head of the gastrocnemius and is frequently damaged by a twisting injury of the knee, as characteristically occurs in tennis (giving this injury the term 'tennis leg'), skiing and ball playing. This injury is frequently accompanied by an anterior cruciate ligament tear, bone contusion of the

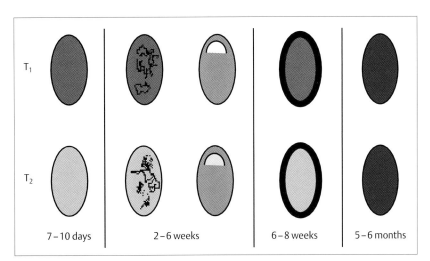

Fig. 10.**16** Traumatic myositis ossificans. Schematic drawing of the MRI findings (T_1-weighted and T_2-weighted sequences) during the 'maturation process'. Initially, 7–10 days after the trauma, the T_1-weighted image shows a dark and the T_2-weighted image a bright lesion within the paraosseous soft tissues. With time, calcifications are seen as heterogeneous signal voids and/or fat deposits as diffuse or confined areas of increased signal intensity on the T_1-weighted image and only subtle signal changes on the T_2-weighted image. After 6–8 weeks, a peripheral ossification can produce a signal-void rim. After 5–6 months, extensive ossifications are seen as signal-void areas.

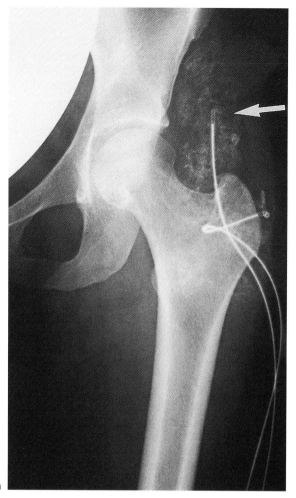

a

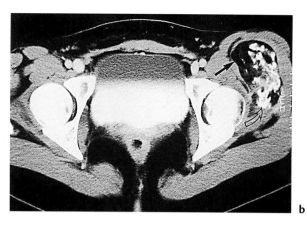

b

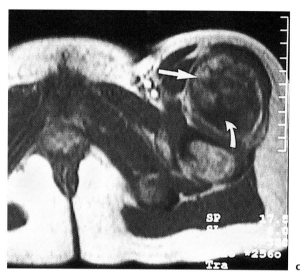

c

Fig. 10.**17 a–c**   Traumatic myositis ossificans. **a** Four weeks after the trauma, the conventional radiograph shows a swelling with extensive calcifications, as well as areas of fat density around the left hip (arrow). **b** CT shows a mass containing calcium equivalent (curved arrow) and fat equivalent (arrow) densities. **c** On MRI, the T$_1$-weighted sequence reveals a space-occupying process with very low calcium-equivalent signals (curved arrow) and high fat-equivalent signals (arrow). The fatty content indicates a mature, relatively advanced myositis ossificans.

lateral tibial plateau and an injury of the medial head of the gastrocnemius (15 a).

■ Muscle Fibrosis

Repetitive or very severe muscle trauma can lead to fibroplastic proliferation with subsequent intramuscular thickening of fibrous connective tissue. Such changes in the sternocleidomastoid fibrosis are found in congenital torticollis and are believed to be caused by mechanical factors *in utero* or obstetric complications (39). MRI shows a muscle with an altered contour and a homogeneously decreased signal intensity in all sequences.

■ Compartment Syndrome

Increased pressure within a muscle compartment, for instance after trauma or surgery, causes ischemia of the muscle. This leads to edema and, unless the edema is decompressed, to rhabdomyolysis. The T$_2$-weighted images, especially with fat suppression, show an increased signal intensity and volume of the affected compartment (e.g., tibialis anterior syndrome) (Fig. 10.**18**). The T$_1$-images may show a slightly decreased signal intensity.

■ Rhabdomyolysis

Possible causes are overuse, trauma, burns, muscle compartment syndrome, intoxication and drug overdose. Recognition of rhabdomyolysis is important due to the possible sequelae of renal failure, hyperkalemia

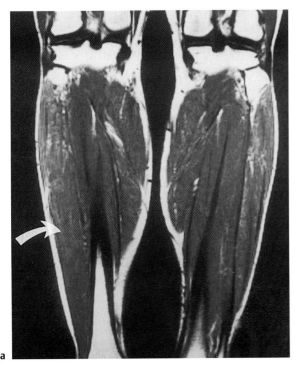

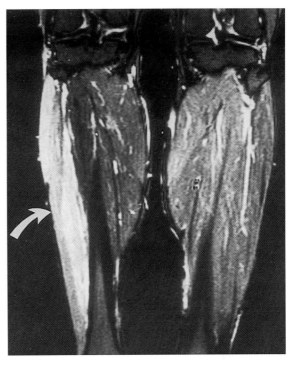

Fig. 10.**18a, b** Tibialis anterior compartment syndrome. Coronal section. a T₁-weighted SE sequence. Subtle bulging of the musculature of the right lower leg (arrow), no relevant sig-

nal changes. **b** Fat-suppressed STIR sequence. Markedly increased signal intensity in tibialis anterior, extensor hallucis longus and extensor digitorum longus (arrow).

and hypocalcemia. The affected muscles or muscle regions show a normal or homogenously decreased signal intensity on T_1-weighted images and an increased signal intensity on the T_2-weighted images (40). MRI has a very high sensitivity in detecting the muscular necrosis, approaching 100% (25). Its specificity, however, is low and other conditions with high signal intensity on T_2-weighted images must be excluded.

■ Symptomatic Myopathies

The term symptomatic myopathies includes all muscular abnormalities observed together with endocrine and metabolic diseases as well as with intoxications (Tab. 10.3). The MRI changes initially are often subtle and not yet well investigated. Persistent damage can progress to muscle atrophy.

In the myopathy of the glycogenosis type V (McArdle disease), the signal intensity is normal on the T_1-weighted images and can be slightly increased on the T_2-weighted images. The exercise-induced increase in the T_2 relaxation time, which is normally 20–40%, is markedly decreased to 0–10% (20). However, a slower increase in the signal intensity on T_2-weighted images has also been observed in some cases of mitochondrial myopathy as well as in one case of glycogenosis type VII (20).

Patients with Cushing's disease can develop an extensive symmetric muscular atrophy (11).

Table 10.**3**   Survey of symptomatic myopathies

Endocrine myopathies:
• Thyrotoxic myopathy
• Hypothyroid myopathy
• Corticosteroid-induced myopathy
Metabolic myopathies:
• Myopathy due to glycogenosis (e. g., glycogen storage disease type V: McArdle disease)
• Mitochondrial myopathy
Toxic myopathy:
• Alcoholic myopathy
• Medication-induced myopathies

Thyroid diseases can also induce muscular changes in terms of a hypertrophy, which can be observed with either hyperthyroidism (Fig. 10.**19**) or hypothyroidism. An example of an endocrine myopathy is the endocrine ophthalmopathy with muscle-isointense swelling of the extraocular muscles.

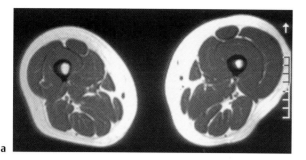

a

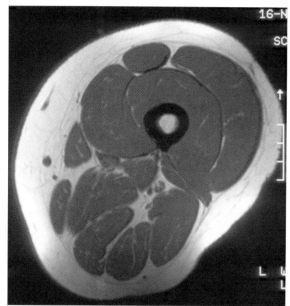

b

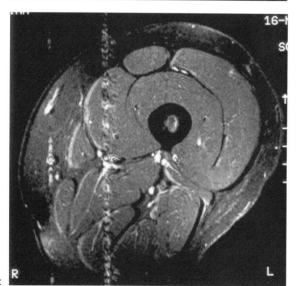

c

Fig. 10.**19 a–c**   Undetermined myopathy of a female patient with autonomous thyroid adenoma. For one year, this 40-year-old female patient had bilateral leg swelling, particularly involving the thigh and more on the left than on the right, initially progressive then alternating. A muscle biopsy performed for further evaluation did not yield a pathologic diagnosis. The muscle enzymes are within the normal range. Scintigraphic detection of an autonomous adenoma and pathologic TSH test. MRI was performed to detect or exclude edematous changes in preparation for a possible second biopsy and to check for a pseudohypertrophy with fat deposition. **a** Axial T$_2$-weighted image of both legs for comparison. Strongly developed musculature of the left thigh with the normally fat-containing septation rarefied, as seen in well-trained individuals. This female patient, however, was not engaged in athletic activities and the subcutaneous fat is disproportionally thick. **b** Axial T$_1$-weighted SE sequence. The rarefication of the intramuscular septations is clearly delineated. No fatty atrophy of the muscles. **c** Axial fast STIR sequence. No evidence of edema. Partial superimposition of pulsation artifacts. The findings are interpreted as muscle hypertrophy, predominately on the left, possibly as a manifestation of an endocrine myopathy.

Muscle Tumors

Muscle tumors are relatively rare. The rather extensive edema frequently associated with a tumor can interfere with diagnostic evaluation by MRI since the edema cannot be reliably distinguished from tumor infiltration. The tumors are discussed in Chapter 12.

Pitfalls in Interpreting the Images

Signal variations of superficial muscles. If surface coils are used, one should be aware of an artificial increase in signal intensity caused by the close vicinity of the coil. Surface coils should not have any direct skin contact. An exact position of the surface coil is especially important for spectroscopy (8).

Inversion Recovery Sequence. With inversion recovery sequences, in particular STIR sequences, the distance between the sections should be 20% of the section thickness since otherwise section-related signal variations might occur. These signal variations should not be misinterpreted as a true increase in signal intensity within the musculature. Since the STIR technique visualizes the muscles as high signal intense structures, partial volume artifacts on the coronal and sagittal sections can lead to locally increased signal intensities that should not be mistaken for pathologic changes.

Misinterpretations Due to Denervation. It should be kept in mind that increased signal intensity in the musculature seen on T_2-weighted images is a nonspecific finding encountered in a variety of conditions. Post-traumatically, muscle contusion and rhabdomyolysis must be distinguished from acute denervation. In contrast to denervation, post-traumatic changes are frequently associated with subcutaneous edema and their signal alterations fail to follow the innervation pattern of any particular nerve. Subcutaneous edema after direct trauma resolves within a few weeks, while signal alternations following denervation due to a neural lesion progress. Furthermore, interpreting an acute denervation can be difficult in the presence of anatomic variants of the innervation (19). Moreover, the neural damage follows a temporal course that does not alter the signal intensity in all muscles simultaneously. Individual muscles can be affected later. In particular, this has been observed in the ulnar territory of the musculature of the hand. An ulnar lesion first causes an increase in the signal intensity in the ulnar lumbricals and only later in the dorsal first interosseous and the adductor digiti minimi (12). This phenomenon may be caused by collateral innervation.

Clinical Relevance of MRI and Comparison with Other Imaging Methods

MRI of the musculature is characterized by a very high sensitivity. Its specificity, however, is relatively low. To obtain a definitive diagnosis, therefore, a muscle biopsy is often unavoidable. For the planning of a biopsy, the MRI images can be used to select a region that shows unequivocally pathologic signal alterations. If possible, the biopsy should be obtained from such an altered muscular region, with avoidance of necrotic or fatty areas. This approach can markedly decrease the incidence of false negative biopsies. New open MRI units and non-paramagnetic biopsy systems have simplified image-guided biopsy procedures and increased the diagnostic yield.

MRI can also be used to monitor therapies. In numerous diseases of the muscles, the signal changes correlate well with the therapeutic effects and can be even more sensitive than other examinations and laboratory tests. This can lower the number of serial EMG examinations and laboratory tests.

In comparison with competing radiologic methods, MRI has a few distinctive advantages that have made it the imaging method of choice for diagnosing muscle disorders. Owing to its high soft tissue contrast, MRI displays the muscular structures with the highest detail in comparison with other cross sectional imaging modalities. In comparison with sonography, it is more objective and less operator-dependent, making comparison of serial examinations easier. Furthermore, MRI can investigate body regions not accessible by sonography. CT has an inferior soft tissue resolution compared to MRI and is fraught with bone-induced beam hardening artifacts when applied to the diagnostic evaluation of the extremities. Furthermore, it delivers ionizing radiation. In many aspects, MRI combines the advantages of CT and sonography, without suffering from their disadvantages.

References

1 Applegate, G. R., A. J. Cohen: Pyomyositis: early detection utilizing multiple imaging modalities. Magn. Reson. Imag. 9 (1991) 187–193

2 Argov, Z., W. J. Bank, J. Maris, S. Eleff, N. G. Kennaway, R. E. Olson, B. Chance: Treatment of mitochondrial myopathy due to complex III deficiency with vitamins K3 and C: A 31 P-NMR follow-up study. Ann. Neurol. 19 (1986) 598–602

3 Argov, Z., W. J. Bank, J. Maris, B. Chance: Muscle energy metabolism in McArdle's syndrome by in vivo phosphorus Magnetic Resonance Spectroscopy. Neurology 37 (1987) 1720–1724

4 Beese, M. S., G. Winkler, V. Nicolas, R. Maas, D. Kress, K. Kunze, E. Bücheler: Diagnostik entzündlicher Muksel- und Gefäßerkrankungen in der MRT mit STIR-Sequenzen. Fortschr. Röntgenstr. 158 (1993) 542–549

5 Block, W., F. Träber, C. K. Kuhl, G. Layer, F. Zierz, H. Riuk, H. Schild: 31 PMR Spektroskopie der gesunden Wadenmuskulatur unter Belastung im Vergleich zur Biochemischen Analyse des femoralen Blutes. Fortschr. Röntgenstr. 161 (1994) 260–261

5a Brandser, E. A., G. El-Khoury, M. M. Kuthol, J. J. Callaghan, D. S. Tearse: Hamstring injuries: radiographic, conventional tomographic CT, and MR Imaging characteristics. Radiology 197 (1995) 257–262

6 Dooms, G. C., M. R. Fisher, H. Hricak, C. B. Higgins: MR Imaging of intramuscular hemorrhage. J. Comput. assist. Tomogr. 9 (1985) 908–913

7 Edwards, R. H. T., J. M. Dawson, D. R. Wilkie, D. E. Gordon, D. Shaw: Clinical use of NMR in the investigation of myopathy. Lancet I (1982) 725–732

8 Fleckenstein, J. L., L. A. Bertocci, R. L. Nunnally, R. W. Parkey, R. M. Peshock: Exercise-enhanced MR imaging of variations in forearm muscle anatomy and use: importance in MR Spectroscopy. Amer. J. Roentgenol. 153 (1989) 693–698

9 Fleckenstein, J. L., P. T. Weatherall, R. P. Parkey, J. A. Payne, R. M. Peshock: Sportsrelated muscle injuries: evaluation with MR imaging. Radiology 172 (1989) 793–798

10 Fleckenstein, J. L., D. K. Burns, F. K. Murphy, H. T. Jayson, F. J. Bonte: Differential diagnosis of bacterial myositis in AIDS: evaluation with MR Imaging. Radiology 179 (1991) 653–658

11 Fleckenstein, J. L., P. T. Weatherall, L. A. Bertocci, M. Ezaki, R. G. Haller, R. Greenlee, W. W. Bryan, R. M. Peshock: Locomotor system assessment by muscle Magnetic Resonance Imaging. Magn. Reson. Quart. 7 (1991) 79–103

12 Fleckenstein, J. L., D. Watumull, K. E. Conner, M. Ezaki, R. G. Greenlee, W. W. Bryan: Denervated human skeletal muscle: MR Imaging evaluation. Radiology 187 (1993) 213–218

13 Fletcher, B. D., S. L. Hanna, L. E. Kun: Changes in MR signal intensity and contrast enhancement of therapeutically irradiated soft tissue. Magn. Reson. Imag. 8 (1990) 771–777

14 Fornage, B. D., D. H. Touche, P. Segal, M. D. Rifkin: Ultrasonography in the evaluation of muscular trauma. J. Ultrasound Med. 2 (1993) 549–554

15 Hadar, H., N. Gadoth, M. Heifetz: Fatty replacement of lower paraspinal muscles: normal and neuromuscular disorders. Amer. J. Roentgenol. 141 (1983) 895–893

15a Helms, C. A., R. C. Fritz, G. J. Garvin: Plantaris muscle injury: evaluation with MR Imaging. Radiology 195 (1995) 201–203

16 Hernandez, R. J., D. R. Keim, D. B. Sullivan, T. L. Chenevert, W. Martel: Magnetic Resonance imaging appearance of the muscles in childhood dermatomyositis. J. Pediat. 117 (1990) 546–550

17 Hernandez, R. J., D. R. Keim, T. L. Chenevert, D. B. Sullivan, A. M. Aisen: Fat-suppressed MR Imaging of myositis. Radiology 182 (1992) 217–219

18 Hernandez, R. J., D. B. Sullivan, T. L. Chenevert, D. R. Keim: MR imaging in children with dermatomyositis: muskuloskeletal findings and correlation with clinical and labaratoy findings. Amer. J. Roentgenol. 161 (1993) 359–366

19 Jabaley, M. E., W. H. Wallace, F. R. Heckler: Internal topography of major nerves of the forearm and hand: a current view. J. Hand Surg. 5 (1980) 1–18

20 Jehenson, P., A. Leroy-Willig, E. de Kerviler, D. Duboc, A. Syrota: MR imaging as a potential diagnostic test for metabolic myopathies: importance of variations in the T2 of muscle with exercise. Amer. J. Roentgenol. 161 (1993) 347–351

21 Kerviler, E., A. Leroy-Willig, P. Jehenson, D. Duboc, B. Eymard, A. Syrota: Exercise-induced muscle modifications: study of healthy subjects and patients with metabolic myopathies with MR Imaging and P-31 spectroscopy. Radiology 181 (1991) 259–264

22 Kuhl, C. K., G. Layer, F. Träber, S. Ziers, W. Block, M. Reiser: Mitochondrial encephalomyopathy: correlation of P-31 exercise MR Spectroscopy with clinical findings. Radiology 192 (1994) 223–230

23 Kuno, S., S. Katsuta, T. Inouye, T. Anno, K. Matsumoto, M. Akisada: Relationship between MR relaxation time and muscle fiber composition. Radiology 169 (1988) 567–568

24 Lamminen, A. E.: Magnetic Resonance Imaging of primary skeletal muscle diseases: patterns of distribution and severity of involvement. Brit. J. Radiol. 63 (1990) 946–950

25 Lamminen, A. E., P. E. Hekali, E. Tiula, I. Suramo, O. A. Korhola: Acute rhabdomyolysis: evaluation with Magnetic Resonance Imaging compared with computed tomography and ultrasonography. Brit. J. Radiol. 62 (1989) 326–331

26 Lewis, S. F., R. G. Haller, J. D. Cook, R. L. Nunaly: Muscle fatigue in McArdle's disease studied by 31-P NMR: effect of glucose infusion. J. appl. Physiol. 59 (1984) 1991–1994

27 Murphy, W. A., W. G. Totty, J. E. Carroll: MRI of normal and pathologic skeletal muscle. Amer. J. Roentgenol. 146 (1986) 565–574

28 Netter, F. H.: Farbatlanten der Medizin. Band 7. Bewegungsapparat I. Thieme, Stuttgart 1992

29 Otake, S., T. Banno, S. Ohba, M. Noda, M. Yamamoto: Muscular sarcoidosis: findings at MR Imaging. Radiology 176 (1990) 145–148

30 Polak, J. F., F. A. Joresz, D. F. Adama: Magnetic Resonance Imaging of skeletal muscle: prolongation of T1 and T2 subsequent to denervation. Invest. Radiol. 23 (1988) 365–369

30a Pomeranz, S. J., R. S. Heidt: MR Imaging in the prognostication of Harmstring injury. Radiology 189 (1993) 897–900

31 Resnick, D.: Diagnosis of Bone and Joint Disorders. Saunders, Philadelphia 1995

32 Ross, B. D., G. K. Radda: Application of 31-P NMR to inborn errors of muscle metabolism. Biochem. Soc. Trans. 11 (1983) 627–630

33 Ross, B. D., G. K. Radda, D. G. Gardian: Examination of a case of suspected McArdle's syndrome by 31-P NMR. New Engl. J. Med. 304 (1981) 1338–1342

34 Schellhas, K. P.: MR Imaging of muscles of mastication. Amer. J. Radiol. 153 (1989) 847–855

35 Schreiber, A., W. L. Smith, V. Ionasescu, H. Zellweger, E. A. Franken, J. Dunn, J. Ehrhardt: Magnetic Resonance Imaging of children with Duchenne muscular dystrophy. Pediat. Radiol. 17 (1987) 495–497

36 Shellock, F. G., T. Fukunaga, J. H. Mink, V. R. Edgerton: Exertional muscle injury: evaluation of concentric versus eccentric actions with serial MR Imaging. Radiology 179 (1991) 659–664

37 Träber, F., W. A. Kaiser, G. Layer, C. Kuhl, M. Reiser: Magnetic Resonance Spectroscopy of skeletal muscle. In Baert, A. C., F. Heuck: Frontiers in European Radiology. Springer, Berlin 1993 (pp. 23–43)

38 Uetani, M., K. Hayashi, N. Matsunaga, K. Imamura, N. Ito: Denervated skeletal muscle: MR Imaging. Radiology 189 (1993) 511–515

39 Whyte, A. M., R. B. Lufkin, J. Bredenkamp, L. Hoover: Sternocleidomastoid fibrosis in congenital muscular torticollis: MR appearance. J. Comput. assist. Tomogr. 13 (1989) 163–164

40 Zagoria, R. J., N. Karstaedt, T. D. Koubek: MR Imaging of rhabdomyolysis. J. Comput. assist. Tomogr. 10 (1986) 268–270

11

Bone Marrow

M. Vahlensieck and G. Layer

Examination Technique

The imaging properties of the bone marrow in specific MRI sequences depend on the following factors:

- Distribution of red, hematopoietic active marrow and yellow marrow,
- Density of the trabecula,
- Age, gender, and anatomic region.

It is for this reason that no general examination technique can be recommended.

T_1-weighted SE Sequences. These play a fundamental role in the examination of the bone marrow. They show a high level of contrast between high-signal fatty marrow and low-signal hematopoietic marrow and pathologic lesions, with little contrast between hematopoietic marrow and pathologic lesions because of the almost equally low signal intensity.

T_2-weighted SE Sequences. In contrast to most other body regions, T_2-weighted images of the bone marrow are rarely more informative than the T_1-weighted images because of poor contrast between fatty and hematopoietic marrow. Bone containing both red and yellow marrow appears more homogenous on T_2-weighted sequences compared with T_1-weighted sequences. In addition, there is little difference in signal intensity between pathologic processes and fat containing marrow, both of which show high signal intensity on T_2-weighted images. The problem is most pronounced when TSE sequences are used since these result in higher signal intensity from fat, further reducing the contrast between pathologic lesions, with their relatively long T_2, and surrounding fatty marrow. The use of fat suppression in conjunction with T_2-weighted TSE sequences solves this problem. Bone marrow metastases may appear both hyper- and hypointense relative to surrounding healthy marrow (28).

Use of Contrast Medium. This is not necessary for the detection of pathologic bone marrow lesions in general. In individual cases, however, it can be used to further characterize a pathologic finding. Due to the increase in signal intensity in pathologic processes, the already relatively high-signal bone marrow equalizes with the enhanced, originally low-signal intensity lesion, decreasing the detection sensitivity. While marked en-

hancement suggests an acute inflammatory, post-traumatic or tumorous process, it generally cannot be used for differentiating these processes.

Opposed-Phase GRE Sequences. Opposed-phase GRE sequences are highly sensitive for the detection of red bone marrow (26). The hematopoietic bone marrow is visualized as low signal intensity or even as signal void. In part, this is due to the imaging parameters, with the phases of the fat and water protons opposed, and, in part, to susceptibility effects of iron-containing compounds in the bone marrow. A further factor must be considered when evaluating GRE images of the bone marrow. This is the appearance of susceptibility effects arising from the bony trabeculae. These cause osseous regions with a high content of trabecular bone, such as the apophyses and epiphyses, to have a lower signal intensity compared with regions of low trabecular content (52). The intensity of these effects increase with increasing echo times.

STIR Sequences. STIR images are of great value for the evaluation of pathologic lesions (19). Normal bone marrow is seen as signal void, hematopoietic bone marrow as low-signal intensity, and lesions as high-signal intensity. This technique is characterized by a high sensitivity, but a low specificity.

Chemical Shift Imaging. This method provides a quantitative basis for assessing the water and fat signal fractions within the bone marrow (49, 66). Similar to the opposed-phase GRE technique, it is based on the chemical shift between the protons of fat and water. Although this phase contrast imaging of the chemical shift cannot increase the specificity of bone marrow lesions (13), it can improve the sensitivity of MRI to bone marrow infiltrations of systemic diseases, such as found in Hodgkin disease, non-Hodgkin lymphoma or leukemia. Furthermore, by offering a quantitative assessment of the relative water fraction, it can monitor the therapy of systemic diseases, such as leukemia. Because of the additional effort of analyzing user-defined regions of interest, quantitative imaging of the chemical shift for evaluating the bone marrow has stayed in specialized referral centers.

Relaxometry. Though most pathologic lesions as well as physiologic processes of the bone marrow cause subtle alterations of the relaxation times, relaxometry has

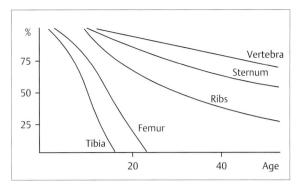

Fig. 11.**1** Age-dependent percentage of hematopoietic marrow in different bones.

not been found to be useful in evaluating the bone marrow, just as it has failed in MRI of other areas. The T_1 relaxation times can be precisely and accurately determined, for instance with spectroscopic methods using a series of inversion recovery sequences with varying inversion times (TI), but the diagnostic usefulness has not been established. Measuring T_2 relaxation times is methodically much more difficult. Because of the multifactorial nature of the T_2 relaxation times, the measurements depend on the particular method used and show considerable variation. As a result, the relaxation times between healthy bone marrow and various pathologic conditions overlap and the necessary specificity is not achieved. This is accentuated by the subtle changes related to age, gender, and location. The potential role of quantitative MRI applies to serial studies performed under identical conditions in patients undergoing myelosuppressive therapy (54).

Anatomy

■ General Anatomy

The bone marrow is the largest organ of the body. After the fourth embryonal month, the bone marrow increasingly assumes the function of *hematopoiesis* (24), and hematopoiesis occurs in all bones at birth. The need for hematopoiesis declines during childhood and more and more sections of the bone marrow become hematopoietically inactive, with fat cells replacing the hematopoietic cells. The fat cells increase in number and size. Hematopoietically active bone marrow appears red. After it has become hematopoietically inactive, it turns yellow owing to its high fat content. This conversion from hematopoietically active to hematopoietically inactive marrow begins in the distal phalanges of the hands and feet and slowly progresses centripetally (Fig. 11.**1**). Within the tubular bones, the diaphysis is converted first, followed by the distal metaphysis. The proximal metaphysis is converted last. Apophyseal and epiphyseal bone marrow contain inactive bone marrow

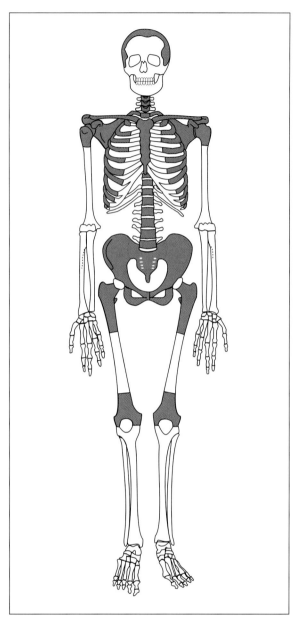

Fig. 11.**2** Hematopoietic bone marrow (black) in young adult. Fatty marrow may already predominate in the distal femoral metaphysis.

within a few months of the development of the secondary ossification centers and are hematopoietically active only for a short time (16). In the *adult* hematopoietic tissue is found in the following regions:

- proximal metaphyses of the humerus and femur,
- pelvis,
- vertebral bodies,
- sternum,
- scapula,
- calcaneus,
- calvaria (Fig. 11.**2**).

This distribution pattern is attained at about the age of 20 years, but considerable variations exist. With advancing age, the conversion of active red to inactive yellow marrow continues at a slower pace or, at least, the increase in fat in the hematopoietic marrow slows down. The percentage of fat in hematopoietically active marrow can be as high as 70% in the octogenarian (59). These changes vary and probably depend on several factors, such as disease, athletic activities, and therapies.

■ Specific MR Anatomy

The *signal intensities* in the bone marrow are determined by the proportion of its constituents, which are basically water, fat, and protein (Fig. 11.**3**). The contribution of each constituent is still not entirely understood. For instance, the relaxation of water depends on its environment and the following states with different signal characteristics can be identified:

- complex bound water,
- bound water,
- free water,
- structured water.

The state of the water in specific tissues is not exactly known.

Fat also occurs in various states with different resonance frequency, which, for instance, depends on the protons in the methyl groups and on the vicinity of double bonds in unsaturated fatty acids. Furthermore, the relaxation times of proteins are related to the state of the protein molecules in different solutions (59). It is this complexity that has so far defied any understanding of how much each individual component contributes to the signal intensity.

Hematopoietically *active (red) bone marrow* is mildly hypointense to muscle on T_1-weighted images. On T_2-weighted images, its signal intensity is slightly increased. With advancing age, the signal intensity of hematopoietic marrow shows a progressive increase on the T_1-weighted image so that it clearly exceeds that in muscle. This age-related change reflects the replacement of hematopoietic marrow by fatty marrow (see above), causing a decrease in the T_1 relaxation time and a corresponding increase in signal intensity (8).

The hematopoietically *inactive (yellow) bone marrow* has high signal intensities on T_1-weighted images, explained by its high fat content, and a slight decrease in signal intensity on T_2-weighted images. It follows the signal pattern of the subcutaneous fat. The MRI distribution of yellow marrow differs from existing macroscopic anatomical data since MRI seems to be more sensitive to the presence of microscopic fat in the marrow. Bone marrow appears as high-signal yellow marrow on MRI even if histologically it contains less than 60% fat and, in children at age 10 years, as little as 20% fat (35). Macroscopically, bone marrow becomes visibly 'yellow' only if it contains more than 80% histologic fat. These differences explain the discrepancy between the speci-

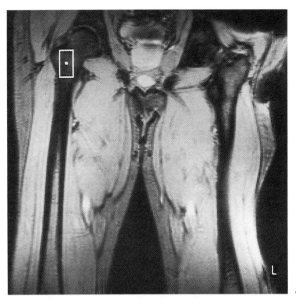

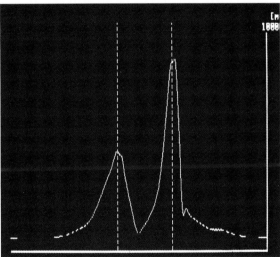

Fig. 11.**3a, b** Proton spectroscopy of hematopoietic bone marrow. **a** Volume of interest in the right femora. **b** Spectrum with high peaks of water and protein protons and a small peak of fat protons.

men-derived and MRI-derived stage of the bone marrow development.

The relative distribution of water, fat, and proteins in the bone marrow is:

- about 40% water, 40% fat, and 20% protein for hematopoietic bone marrow,
- about 15% water, 80% fat, and 5% protein for the inactive marrow.

While these numbers apply to the macroscopically distinguishable bone marrow types, the distribution is not constant, with a spectrum of values between the numbers given.

Evaluating the MRI findings requires familiarity with the various *patterns* of distribution of fatty and he-

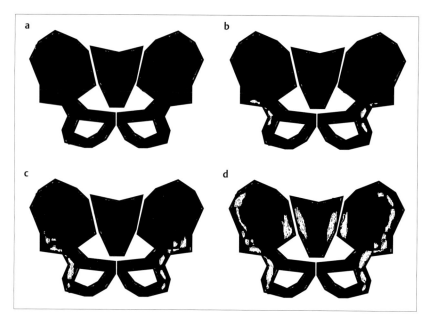

Fig. 11.**4a–d** Normal age-related distribution pattern of active and inactive bone marrow in the pelvis. **a** Hematopoietic marrow throughout the pelvis in childhood. **b** Islands of fatty marrow in the acetabular region in adolescence. **c** Islands of fatty marrow in the acetabular region and ilium in adulthood. **d** Islands of fatty marrow in the acetabulum, ilium, and along the iliosacral joints in senescence.

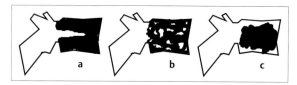

Fig. 11.**5a–c** Normal, age-related distribution pattern of active and inactive bone marrow in the vertebral bodies. **a** Predominately hematopoietic marrow with fatty marrow around the basivertebral vessels in childhood. **b** Diffusely distributed focal deposits of fatty marrow within hematopoietic marrow in adulthood. **c** Fatty marrow near the end plates in senescence.

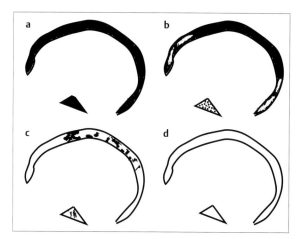

Fig. 11.**6a–d** Normal age-related distribution pattern of active and inactive bone marrow in the calvaria and clivus. **a** Exclusively hematopoietic marrow at birth. **b** Islands of fatty marrow appear in the frontal, occipital and temporal bones and in the clivus during childhood and adolescence. **c** Extensive fatty replacement with remnants of hematopoietic marrow in the parietal bone and clivus. **d** Complete fatty replacement without any hematopoietic marrow in senescence.

matopoietic bone marrow, otherwise residual hematopoietic marrow, for instance, might be mistaken for an infiltrative process. The normal age-related distribution patterns that can be recognized in important osseous regions are illustrated as schematics in Figs. 11.4– 11.10. They show no gender difference. The distribution patterns of fat and red marrow encountered can be described as follows:

- The *pelvis* can show areas of inactive marrow in the acetabulum and anterior ilium at an early age (Fig. 11.**4**) (6). With advancing age, fatty marrow appears along both sides of the sacroiliac joints.
- The *vertebral bodies* show band-like and triangular accumulations of fatty marrow near the end plates, especially in the lower lumbar spine. These findings increase with age (Fig. 11.**5**) (15). These changes might be related to the mechanical load acting on the lumbar spine. Another pattern consists of multiple small areas of fatty marrow (48). With increasing age, the signal intensity in the vertebral bodies continually increases due to diffuse deposition of fat and can exceed the intensity of the musculature. As a result, the intervertebral disks appear dark in comparison with the vertebral bodies on T_1-weighted images.
- The *calvaria* also shows a typical pattern of fat and red marrow, with fat marrow found in the occipital, temporal and frontal bones at an early age (Fig. 11.**6**). Hematopoietic marrow can persist in the parietal bone in the older patient (48). The clivus contains hematopoietic marrow at birth, with conversion to fat marrow in adulthood (41).
- The hematopoietic marrow in the *sternum and clavicle* is largely uniformly distributed (32, 69). Fat deposition is usually absent.
- The proximal *humeral metaphysis* has a predominantly homogeneous hematopoietic marrow in

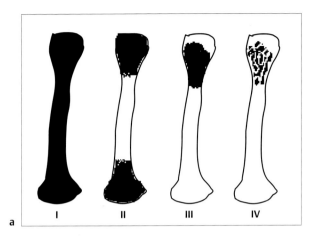

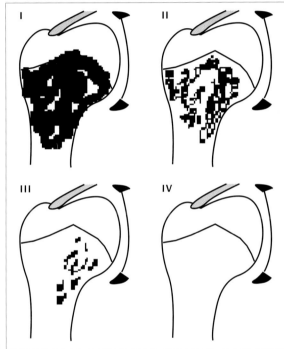

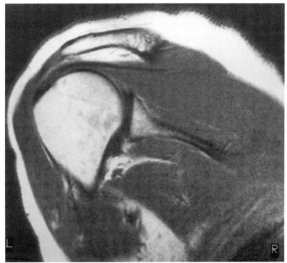

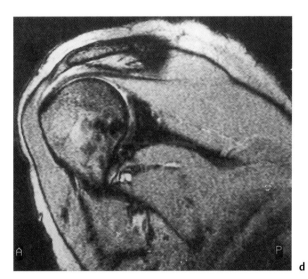

Fig. 11.**7 a–d** **a** Normal, age-related distribution pattern of active and inactive bone marrow in the humerus. **I** Hematopoietic marrow throughout the humerus. **II** Hematopoietic marrow in the proximal and distal humeral metaphyses including adjacent diaphyses in childhood. **III** Hematopoietic marrow in the proximal humeral metaphysis in adulthood. **IV** Remnants of hematopoietic marrow in the proximal humeral metaphysis in senescence. **b** Normal, age-related distribution pattern of active and inactive bone marrow in the proximal humeral metaphysis. **I** Predominately hematopoietic marrow in adolescence. **II, III** Preferentially lateral regression of hematopoietic marrow in adulthood. **IV** Few if any residues of hematopoietic marrow in senescence. **c** T_1-weighted SE sequence with preferentially medially located remnants of hematopoietic marrow seen as confluent areas of low signal intensities. **d** Visualization of hematopoietic marrow as signal void with GRE technique.

young adulthood (Fig. 11.**7 a**). With advancing age, the red marrow converts, remaining visible the longest along the medial shaft (Fig. 11.**7 b–d**) (61). Women often have more red marrow in the humerus than men. This is particularly the case with heavy smokers.

- The *scapula* shows nearly exclusively red marrow. In about 95 % of cases, however, yellow marrow confined to upper aspect of the glenoid fossa can be encountered, independent of age or gender. This may be re-

lated to mechanical factors caused by the insertion of the long biceps tendon (61) (Fig. 11.**8**). With advancing age, fatty marrow appears in the juxta-articular middle and lower glenoid areas.

- The distal *femoral metaphysis* occasionally shows a pattern of alternating linear distribution of both marrow types (Fig. 11.**9**). With advancing age, the hematopoietic marrow regresses. In the proximal femoral metaphysis, a homogeneous pattern of hemato-

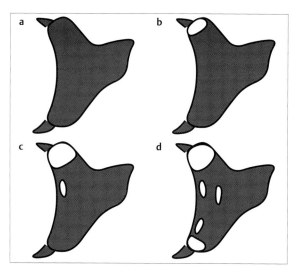

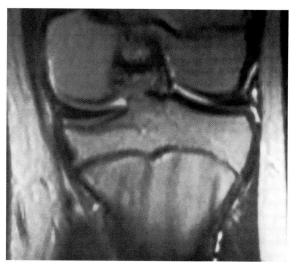

Fig. 11.**8a–d**   Bone marrow distribution pattern in the scapula. **a** Exclusive hematopoietic marrow in infancy. **b** and **c** Fatty marrow deposition in the upper aspect of the glenoid process observed in about 90% of all cases independent of age. **d** Additional areas of fatty marrow in the inferior aspect of the glenoid fossa in senescence.

Fig. 11.**9**   GRE sequence of the knee of a healthy 12-year-old boy. Linearly oriented remnants of hematopoietic marrow in the proximal tibial metaphysis.

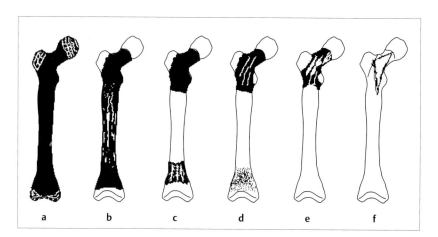

Fig. 11.**10a–f**   Normal, age-related distribution pattern of active and inactive bone marrow in the femora. **a** Hematopoietic marrow throughout the femora in childhood. The epiphyses are not yet ossified. **b** Early fatty replacement of the hematopoietic marrow in the femoral metaphysis in a child under the age of 10 years. **c** Remnants of hematopoietic marrow in the proximal and distal femoral metaphyses in adolescence until the age of 20 years. The distal metaphysis shows a striped pattern. **d** and **e** Further regression of the hematopoietic marrow with increasing age in adulthood. **f** Complete regression of the hematopoietic marrow surrounding low signal trabeculae of the proximal metaphysis in senescence.

poietic marrow is seen, which decreases in size with advancing age (34, 48). The fatty marrow progresses from the apophyses of the greater and lesser trochanter (Fig. 11.**10**).

Generalized Disorders

The disease processes that induce diffuse or multifocal changes of the bone marrow can be categorized according to the MRI pattern of the bone marrow (63). The categories include:

- conversion of fatty marrow to hematopoietic marrow with hyperplasia of the residual fraction of hematopoietic marrow (reconversion),
- marrow infiltration with regular or malignant cells,
- depletion of the hematopoietic marrow with subsequent fatty replacement,
- depletion of myeloid elements and subsequent fibrosis,
- deposition of metabolic products,
- sequelae of bone marrow transplant.

■ Reconversion, Hyperplasia

If the demand of certain diseases exceeds the capacity of the hematopoietic bone marrow, areas of inactive bone marrow are reconverted from fatty to hematopoietic marrow. This is called reconversion since it reverses the normal conversion from hematopoietic to fatty marrow during childhood. In severe or rapidly progressing conditions, hematopoietic marrow also appears in the epiphyses and apophyses. The remaining hematopoietic marrow also increases its activity and becomes hyperplastic. Marrow hyperplasia has the signal intensity of neonatal marrow and is equal to or lower than that of normal musculature. In the spine, the disk can have the same or a lower signal intensity relative to the vertebral bodies on T_1-weighted images.

The causes of reconversion and hyperplasia include conditions that

- exceed the hematopoietic ability of the normally present red marrow:
  - chronic anemia,
  - chronic infection,
  - chronic cardiac decompensation,
  - hyperparathyroidism,
  - endurance athletes (53),
  - heavy smokers (43).
- have large areas of cellular infiltration in the red marrow:
  - vertebral infiltration caused by lymphoma, plasmocytoma,
  - diffuse vertebral metastases,
  - leukemia.
- have large areas of red marrow replaced by fat:
  - chemotherapy,
  - large field radiotherapy.
- have large areas of red marrow replaced by fibrosis:
  - myelofibrosis.

Furthermore, treatment with hematopoietic growth factors can induce reconversion of initially yellow marrow to hematopoietic marrow (10), producing changes in the marrow that may simulate bone marrow involvement by tumors.

Hematopoietic hyperplasia can be an incidental finding in patients undergoing MRI for another reason and having no evidence of an underlying cause. The hyperplasia may represent hematopoietic marrow that has been reconverted by a remote and no longer identifiable process (7, 26).

To quantify the *extent* of reconversion, grading of the hematopoietic marrow in the distal femoral metaphysis has been proposed on a scale of four levels (Fig. 11.**11**) (26):

- Grade I and II indicate a low level of hematopoietic marrow. This is often encountered without apparent cause. In one study, it was a frequent finding in young obese women.
- Grade III and IV generally can be attributed to an underlying cause.

It can be difficult to differentiate foci of reconverted bone marrow in an atypical location, such as in the diaphysis of a long tubular bone, from a malignant disease process (12). Moreover, metastases within reconverted bone marrow can cause differential diagnostic problems (Fig. 11.**12**).

MRI has confirmed the marked expansion of hematopoietic bone marrow in *sickle cell disease*, with the hematopoietic hyperplasia seen as decreased signal intensity on the T_1-weighted images throughout the femur and focally in the axial skeleton (45). In sickle cell crisis with painful joints, juxta-articular foci of decreased signal intensity on the T_1-weighted image with increased signal intensity on the T_2-weighted image are consistent with acute diametaphyseal bone infarcts. Focally decreased signal intensity on T_1-weighted and T_2-weighted images indicates absence of edema and is consistent with old infarction or fibrosis.

■ Cellular Infiltration, Displacement

Increased cellularity generally causes the signal intensity to decrease on T_1-weighted images and to be the same or to increase on T_2-weighted images. GRE and

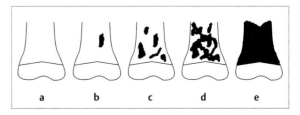

Fig. 11.**11 a–e** Schematic drawing of the various manifestations of reconverted bone marrow in the distal femora (after 26). **a** No hematopoietic marrow. **b** Focal. **c** Multifocal. **d** Confluent. **e** Complete reconversion of the marrow in distal femoral metaphysis.

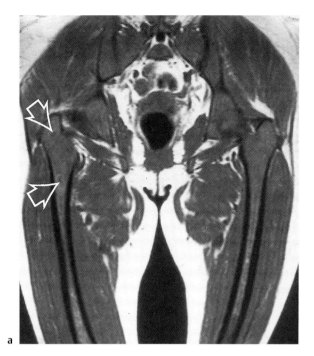

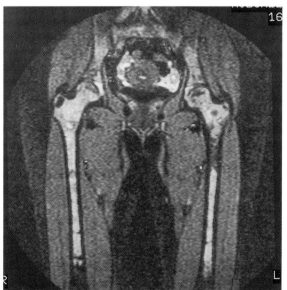

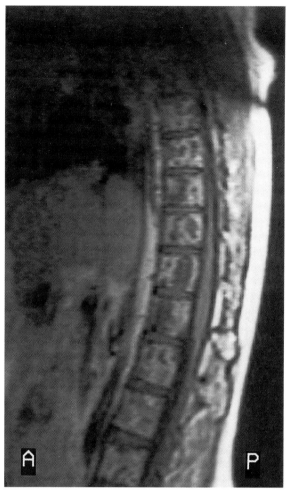

Fig. 11.**12 a–c** Extensive reconversion of the bone marrow in diffuse metastases of a medulloblastoma. **a** T_1-weighted SE sequence, coronal section through the pelvis and femora. Diffuse decrease in signal intensity in the femora and pelvis due to reconverted hematopoietic bone marrow. Occasional heterogeneity of the signal, compatible with metastases (arrows). **b** Fat-suppressed STIR sequence of the same region. High-signal visualization of the bone marrow with occasional heterogeneity of the signal. **c** Sagittal T_1-weighted SE sequence of the spine after administration of contrast medium. Diffuse metastases throughout the entire axial skeleton.

STIR sequences have a higher sensitivity in detecting these changes, which frequently increase the T_2 relaxation time.

Polycythemia

Polycythemia vera represents a clonal neoplastic proliferation of the pluripotent hematopoietic stem cells and is characterized by an increase in red cell mass and a high cell turnover.

MRI shows the increased marrow cellularity as homogeneous decrease in signal intensity on the T_1-weighted images and no change or only a slight increase in signal intensity on T_2-weighted images (17). The high cell turnover induces a reconversion of fatty to cellular marrow in the peripheral skeleton. MRI of the pelvis is especially suited for evaluating the marrow compartment and should include the spine, representative of the axial skeletal marrow, and the femora, representative of the appendicular skeletal marrow.

The MRI findings improve during treatment with phlebotomies and chemotherapy. The marrow pattern in the proximal femoral metaphysis seems to correlate well with the clinical severity as determined by established laboratory parameters (21) (Fig. 11.**13**).

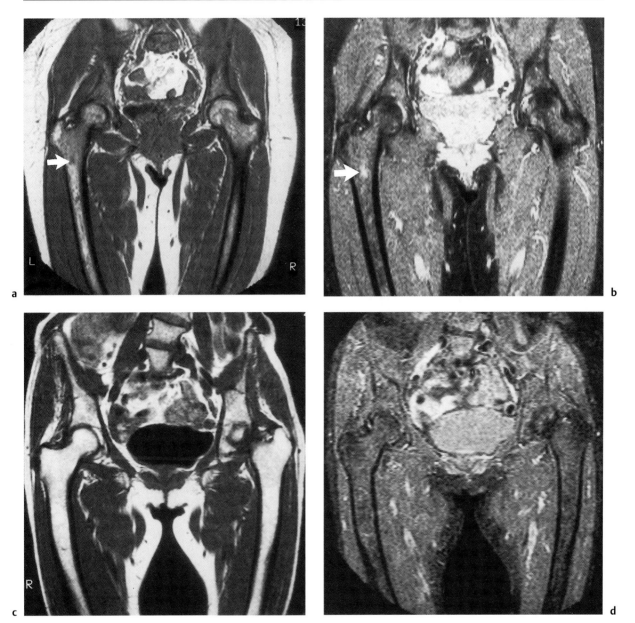

Fig. 11.**13 a–d** Two patients with polycythemia vera. **a, b** Female patient with untreated polycythemia vera and extensive polyglobulinemia. **a** T$_1$-weighted SE sequence, coronal plane. Decreased signal intensity in the femora compatible with bone marrow reconversion. Relatively low signal intensity also in the epiphysis. Remnants of normal fatty marrow in the greater trochanter and, partially, in the diaphysis. Focal decrease in signal intensity in the metadiaphyseal region compatible with a bone infarct (arrow). **b** Fat suppressed STIR sequence. In comparison with the subcutaneous fat, the femoral marrow has a relatively high signal. Focally increased signal intensity (arrow) compatible with a bone infarct. **c, d**

Female patient with polycythemia vera. Following cytostatic therapy with hydroxycarbamide, normal differential blood count. **c** T$_1$-weighted SE sequence, coronal plane. Fat-equivalent signal intensity in the entire femoral bone marrow. No physiologic remnants of hematopoietic marrow are detectable in the femoral metaphysis. In comparison to the subcutaneous fat, relatively high signal intensity of the vertebral body, compatible with low cellularity and early discrete fat replacement. **d** Fat-suppressed STIR sequence. Low signal intensity in the femora and somewhat higher signal intensity in the vertebral bodies, as evidence of remnants of hematopoietic marrow.

Malignant Diffuse Infiltrates

Leukemia. The marrow, preferentially the red marrow, is infiltrated by leukemic cells, and the increase in cellularity and proportionate decrease in fat cause a prolongation of the T_1 relaxation time with a corresponding decrease in signal intensity on the T_1-weighted images.

Leukemic infiltrates in hematopoietic bone marrow may be undetectable, unless they are surrounded by fatty bone marrow (2). In *acute lymphatic leukemia,* the mass of the lymphoblasts correlates with the T_1 relaxation time (18). Depending on the cellular composition, the T_2 relaxation time remains unchanged or increases slightly with a corresponding slight increase in signal intensity on T_2-weighted images. These MRI changes are most profound in *chronic myeloid leukemia* and *acute lymphocytic leukemia* (63). The general pattern of involvement is diffuse but can be multifocal. If malignant replacement of the hematopoietic marrow leads to hematopoietic insufficiency, hematopoietic reconversion can be observed in the yellow marrow. A differentiation between reconverted and leukemic marrow may be impossible.

Several authors have proposed using the differences between the T_1 relaxation times to stage the bone marrow involvement and to evaluate the efficacy of treatment (18, 34). Calculating the different relaxation times of leukemic and normal cells is fraught with inherent methodic difficulties.

Lymphoma. In contrast to the various leukemias, which are neoplasms of the hematopoietic stem cells and are characterized by diffuse replacement of the bone marrow by neoplastic cells, lymphomas are neoplasms of the lymphoid tissue and can arise anywhere in the body. Involvement of the bone marrow, either as primary lymphomatous disease or secondary to blood-borne dissemination, defines the prognosis and determines the best therapeutic approach. Clinical staging includes a bone marrow biopsy, which is invasive and may be falsely negative if taken from uninvolved bone. The overall incidence of bone involvement in Hodgkin disease is a matter of controversy and stated values range from 2–34%. MRI is very sensitive and demonstrates focal areas with a signal intensity that is decreased on T_1-weighted and increased on GRE and STIR images. It is not very specific and is marred by a high false positive rate, primarily caused by inflammatory infiltrates and disturbed erythropoiesis. Both conditions are associated with increased cellularity. These MRI results can be improved by considering solely focal areas as a sign of involvement and discarding large and diffuse areas as nonspecific reaction. In either case, MRI mapping of the bone marrow can be used to select the site of the biopsy.

In non-Hodgkin lymphomas, bone marrow involvement is more common and again can be focal or diffuse. The primary role of MRI in the initial diagnostic work-up consists of finding focal bone marrow changes, as described above.

Plasmocytoma. MRI can detect vertebral involvement in about 70% of all cases. In addition to a focal and multifocal pattern, a diffuse involvement can be observed in 20% of the cases. The diffuse type shows a pattern of increased cellularity with decreased signal intensity on T_1-weighted images and no or only slightly increased signal intensity on T_2-weighted images as well as increased enhancement (38) (Fig. 11.**14**). As with other bone marrow diseases with increased cellularity, the MRI findings may help confirm the response to therapy. Reinstituted fatty tissue, seen as diffuse or multifocal increase in signal intensity on the T_1-weighted images with less contrast enhancement, is regarded as evidence of successful therapy. Serial MRI might also clarify the pathogenesis of new or progressive fractures (39).

Waldenström Macroglobulinemia. This dyscrasia is marked by diffuse infiltration of the hematopoietic marrow with plasma cells and resultant increased cellularity in the presence of decreased fatty tissue. MRI shows vertebral marrow involvement in 90% of the cases with clinical evidence of a gammopathy. Depending on the cellularity, the T_1-weighted images show a decreased signal intensity, which is initially focal and becomes diffuse with progression of the disease.

The hematopoietic marrow has equal or decreased signal intensity relative to adjacent muscles, causing the intervertebral disk to appear as a structure of increased signal intensity. This change of the bone marrow is associated with increased contrast enhancement, which correlates with cellularity indices and presumably reflects the number of intramedullary abnormal plasma cells (37). These findings suggests that MRI may be valuable in staging Waldenström macroglobulinemia. The T_2-weighted images may show an increased signal intensity, but are generally normal. After successful therapy and in correlation with laboratory parameters of tumor burden, the MRI appearance of the bone marrow improves and the signal intensity of the bone marrow can return to normal, suggesting that MRI may be a noninvasive method of assessing the response to therapy (37). Focal marrow involvement is rare and believed to occur in less than 10% of the cases.

■ Hypoplasia, Fatty Replacement

Disease processes replacing hematopoietic marrow with fat must be distinguished from physiologic conversion to fatty marrow. Serial MRI examinations and awareness of physiologic processes are important to avoid misinterpretations as pathologic conditions. It is imperative to recognize the multitude of the changes in the vertebral bone marrow in conjunction with degenerative changes, such as degenerative disk dis-

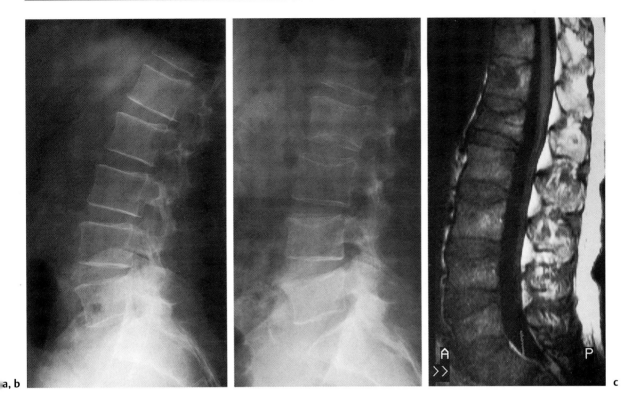

a, b

c

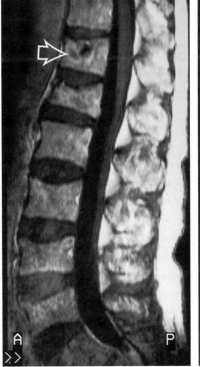

d

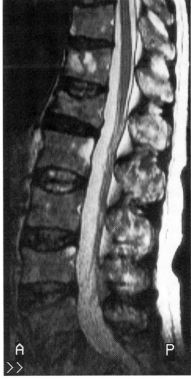

e

Fig. 11.**14 a−e**   Diffuse plasmocy-toma. **a** Lateral radiograph of the lumbar spine. Moderate mineraliza-tion. **b** Lateral radiograph of the lumbar spine, four months later. Definite progression of the demineralization and development of multiple patho-logic fractures. **c** T₁-weighted SE sequence, sagittal sections. Homo-geneous decrease in signal intensity of the vertebral bone marrow with the vertebral bodies almost equal in intensity with the intervertebral disks. Compression fractures. **d** Contrast-enhanced T₁-weighted sequence. Diffuse enhancement of the vertebral bodies. Circular en-hancement around an end plate pro-trusion (arrow) in the T12 vertebral body. **e** T₂-weighted sequence.

ease, kyphoscolioses, and osteochondrosis (14, 33). Typical vertebral changes are described in Chapter 2 on the spine.

Panmyelopathy (Aplastic Anemia)

This condition is characterized by cytopenia of the erythrocytes, leukocytes, and thrombocytes, and is thought to result from suppression of the multipotent myeloid stem cell with inadequate production or release of differentiated cell lines. The resultant decreased cellularity of the hematopoietic bone marrow is compensated for by an increase in fat. The etiology of this condition remains frequently unidentified. Drugs, viral infections, toxic substances, and hepatitis have been listed as provoking factors.

These marrow changes determine the MRI findings: homogenous increase in signal intensity in the hematopoietic marrow compartment on the T_1-weighted and T_2-weighted images, approaching the signal intensity of fat. The proximal femoral and humeral metaphyses, pelvis and lumbar spine can show a diffusely high signal intensity (20).

After successful therapy (e.g., cyclosporin A, steroids), the hematopoietically active cell nests return, largely in the marrow space of the vertebral bodies. Treated patients have multiple focal areas of low signal intensity in the spine on the T_1-weighted and T_2-weighted images (Fig. 11.**15**) (20). After complete re-covery, the MRI findings return to the normal appearance for age.

Postchemotherapy Changes

Chemotherapy causes a decrease in the number of hematopoietic cells, with compensatory increase in the fat content. MRI shows a diffuse increase in signal in all sequences. With extensive damage to the bone marrow in late stages, fibrotic changes can develop with a resultant decrease in signal intensity on all sequences.

■ Marrow Fibrosis

The marrow reacts to most toxic substances with a non-specific increase in fibrous tissue and possible calcifications. The fibrosis can be divided into:

- myeloproliferative disorders (polycythemia vera, osteomyelosclerosis, essential thrombocythemia, chronic myeloic leukemia) (Fig. 11.**16**),
- metastases,
- leukemia,
- lymphoma,
- tuberculosis,
- toxins.

In myelofibrosis, MRI shows a decreased signal intensity on all sequences (27). The signal pattern can be diffuse to patchy. The areas of the marrow uninvolved by the fibrotic changes show the imaging characteristics of their respective disease processes (see the appropriate sections).

■ Storage Diseases

Gaucher Disease

A deficiency of glucocerebrosidase, which is genetically induced, leads to the accumulation of glucocerebroside, a complex lipid, in the brain, spleen, and reticuloendothelial cells of the bone marrow, with preferential deposition in the hematopoietic compartment. Replacement of the marrow by accumulated glucocerebroside displaces functional tissue distally, giving rise to a reconversion pattern and leading to deposits in the distal marrow as well. Infiltration with Gaucher cells increases the T_1 relaxation time and shortens the T_2 relaxation time, causing low signal intensity of the affected areas on both T_1-weighted and T_2-weighted images. Depending on the distribution of the deposited glucocerebroside, the signal pattern can be heterogenous, patchy, or homogenous. Progression of the process alters the entire marrow space. Categorizing the abnormalities according to morphology and magnetic resonance properties reveals the general trend toward proximal involvement prior to distal involvement. The epiphyses are generally spared unless the marrow involvement is extensive (50).

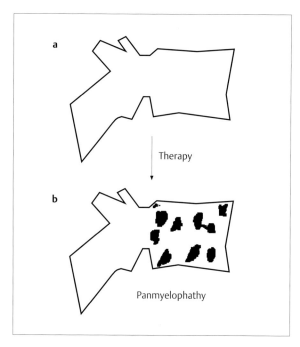

Fig. 11.**15 a, b** Distribution pattern of hematopoietic and fatty marrow in a patient with panmyelopathy (aplastic anemia). **a** Before therapy, diffusely high signal intensity due to fat. **b** After therapy, multifocal areas of decreased signal intensity due to islands of reinstituted hematopoietic tissue.

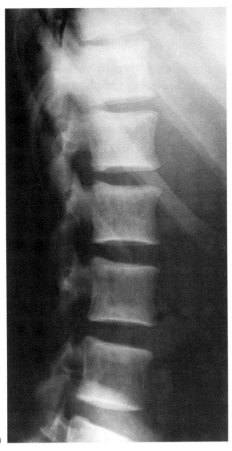

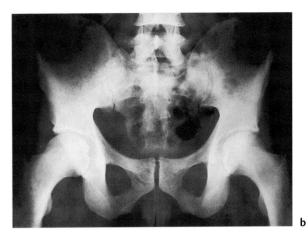

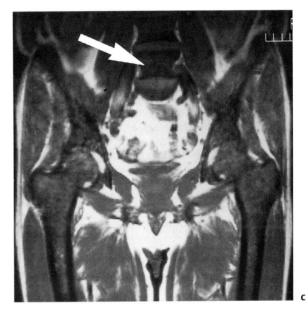

Fig. 11.**16 a – c**   Osteomyelosclerosis. **a** Lateral radiograph of the lumbar spine. Increased density of the vertebral bodies. **b** AP radiograph of the pelvis. Increased density of the visualized bones. **c** T_1-weighted SE image of the pelvis. Marked decrease in signal intensity in the vertebral body (arrow) with relatively increased signal intensity of the intervertebral disk. Decreased signal intensity in the pelvis and femora.

Bone infarcts are a frequent complication of this condition, with findings identical to those associated with infarcts in other conditions. Because of the diffuse replacement of marrow by tissue of low signal intensity, it may be difficult to detect old infarcts.

Hemosiderosis

This iron overload disorder can be primary, with the basis of excess iron accumulation obscure, or secondary, following multiple blood transfusion and hemolytic anemias (59). The iron stored in the bone marrow induces a strong decrease in signal intensity on both T_1-weighted and T_2-weighted images. The alterations are often multifocal and patchy, but can be diffuse. Excessive iron deposition can cause a nearly complete signal loss and present on MRI as 'black marrow.'

Patients with AIDS can have a diffuse to multifocally patchy decrease in signal intensity on T_1-weighted and T_2-weighted images, attributed to increased marrow accumulation of hemosiderin. These changes, which are most prevalent in the calvaria and clivus, have been identified in 50% of the patients with a fall of the CD4 count and a history of opportunistic infections or neoplasms (9).

Amyloidosis

Primary and secondary amyloidosis consists of diffuse or focal amyloid deposition in the bone marrow. MRI shows a diffuse or focal, moderate decrease in signal intensity on the T_1-weighted images, with corresponding or no signal changes on the T_2-weighted images.

■ Marrow Changes after Transplant

Bone marrow transplantation can be an option for the treatment of genetic diseases, aplastic anemia, and malignant diseases. The preparation of the patient involves high-dose chemoradiotherapy. Following this,

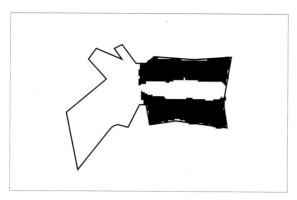

Fig. 11.**17** Band-like distribution of hematopoietic (dark) and fatty (bright) marrow in the vertebral body after bone marrow transplant.

marrow cells obtained through multiple marrow aspiration from a donor are given to the recipient by intravenous infusion. The marrow stem cells regenerate the marrow in the medullary space.

After bone marrow transplantation, the vertebral marrow exhibits characteristic changes (56). The initial changes reflect the pretransplant radiation and consist of increased signal intensity due to fat deposition. About 2 – 3 months after the transplantation, the vertebral bodies show a characteristic decrease in signal intensity along the end plates surrounding a central zone of increased signal instensity on the T_1-weighted images (Fig. 11.**17**). This *band pattern* is believed to be a reflection of the repopulation of the marrow with hematopoietic cells peripherally beneath the end plates and persistence of the fatty transformation centrally. This pattern might be determined by the vascular sinusoids, which determine the blood flow through the marrow cavity. Fat-suppressed sequences, in particular STIR images, show reciprocal changes with two peripheral zones of increased signal intensity surrounding a central zone of decreased intensity. This post-transplantation band pattern seems to persist for at least 8 – 14 months before it evolves into a homogenous pattern of normal signal intensities.

Focal Disorders

■ Edema

Bone marrow edema develops as a result of various stimuli by means of increased vascular permeability or hyperperfusion. Edema constitutes an abnormal expansion of interstitial fluid. Edema-inducing bone diseases, such as trauma, tumor, infection, and ischemia, generally cause detectable radiographic changes, such as demineralization, osseous destruction, or new bone formation. The accompanying marrow edema, which could not be imaged until the advent of MRI, can now be visualized as the only or first manifestation of an os-

seous disease process (60). MRI detects osseous pathology with a high sensitivity unsurpassed by any other imaging modalities. The interstitial fluid accumulation of the edema causes an increase in the T_1 and T_2 relaxation times. These alterations are adequately delineated on SE sequences in the majority of cases. The T_1-weighted images have an excellent negative contrast (edema dark, fat bright) and the T_2-weighted images a positive contrast (lesions bright, surrounding edema dark). The STIR images have the highest sensitivity for detecting bone marrow, with low signal intensity for normal fat tissue and high signal intensity for edema.

■ Ischemia

Whether ischemia of the bone marrow leads to a bone infarct or osteonecrosis depends on its severity, size and location. While both osseous conditions have characteristic radiographic manifestations in their late stages, they can be radiographically occult in their early stages. The accompanying edema is probably caused by reactive hyperemia. The edema has a low signal intensity on T_1-weighted images and a high signal intensity on T_2-weighted images.

Osteonecrosis

Osteonecrosis favors the subchondral region of the yellow marrow, probably related to the sparse vascularity of these regions (63). The characterizing findings and the natural course are described in other chapters on joints. Osteonecrosis of the femoral head has been most extensively investigated.

Bone Infarction

Bone infarcts favor the metadiaphyseal regions of the tubular bones, regardless of the dominating marrow type, probably related to the blood supply and vascular anatomy of the tubular bones. Predisposing conditions include hyperglobulinemia, sickle cell disease, and Gaucher disease. The infarcts can be multiple, as found, for instance, in up to 20% of cases with sickle cell disease (46).

Infarct, Early Stage. Early infarcts are seen as decreased signal intensity on T_1-weighted and increased signal intensity on T_2-weighted images, probably due to the accompanying edema (45). The signal changes are generally linear or partially geographic. They are scalloped in outline (Fig. 11.**18**). This acute stage is often painful. Acute infarcts in hyperplastic or infiltrated bone marrow may be invisible on T_1-weighted images if they are equal in signal intensity with the surrounding marrow.

Infarct, Late Stage. Old infarcts are generally calcified and the calcifications are seen as decreased signal intensity in all sequences. These low-signal areas are frequently surrounded by a signal-void rim that corre-

Fig. 11.**18 a, b** Extensive bone infarcts of the femur and tibia. **a** T$_1$-weighted SE sequence. Band-like decrease in signal intensity in the diaphysis and in the diametaphyseal transition. **b** T$_2$-weighted SE sequence showing linear and geographic areas of increased signal intensity. Small joint effusion of the knee.

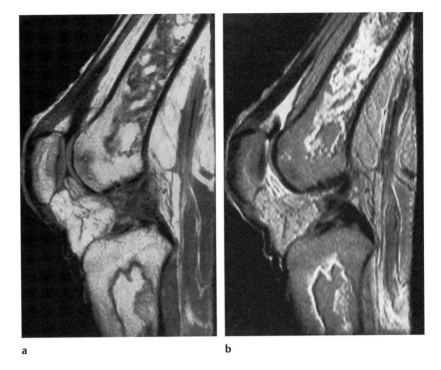

a   b

Fig. 11.**19 a, b** Transient osteoporosis of the hip. **a** T$_1$-weighted SE image. Diffuse decrease in signal intensity in the femoral metaphysis and epiphysis. The greater trochanter is spared and shows a normal fat-equivalent signal. **b** T$_2$-weighted SE sequence. Corresponding increase in signal intensity. Small joint effusion (arrow) (courtesy of Drs. P. Lang and H. K. Genant).

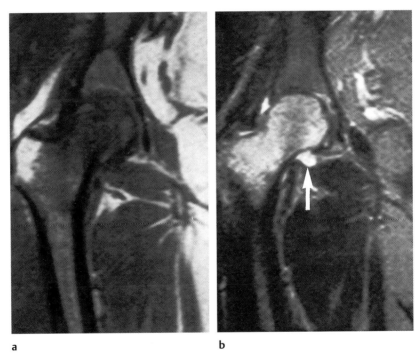

a   b

sponds to a sclerotic margin. Because of a partial blood supply to the peripheral marrow cavity, the bone infarct occasionally exhibits a peripheral line that parallels the endosteal surface of the cortex and produces a subcortical double contour, giving the appearance of 'a bone in bone.' Bone infarcts can become infected and cause osteomyelitis.

Transient Osteoporosis

Transient osteoporosis can be observed in the hip. It most likely reflects an ischemic process that induces marrow edema in the proximal femur with possible extension into the acetabulum (Fig. 11.**19**). Its etiology is not established (42). This condition, which also has been designated 'transient marrow edema syndrome,' might share a common pathophysiologic pathway with other conditions, such as reflex osteodystrophy and regional migratory osteoporosis. It has been postulated that hyperemia and increased bone metabolism might cause marrow edema and osteoporosis of the femoral epiphysis and metaphysis, occasionally extending into the acetabulum, as supported by a positive bone scan and a radiographically demonstrated moderate osteoporosis. The greater trochanter is spared. An accompanying joint effusion is common. The clinical symptoms and abnormalities on MRI regress completely within 6–12 months (1, 65). This condition is often diagnosed retrospectively by its natural course, after neoplasm and osteomyelitis have been excluded.

■ Postradiation Changes

Ionizing radiation damages the cells and supplying sinusoids and vessels. The damage is dose-related and preferentially affects the hematopoietic marrow. The initial changes are those of edema and necrosis, followed later by compensatory proliferation and hypertrophy of the fat cells. Depending on the severity of the damage to the sinusoids and connective tissue, the adipose replacement can be irreversible. The processes are quite complex, and the time sequence and severity of the changes are determined by the composition of the pre-existing bone marrow, such as the relative proportion of the differently radiosensitive mature and immature cells and the amount of adipose tissue, which is related to the patient's age, as well as by the duration, dose, and fractionation of the radiation.

Doses < 2 Gy induce no visible marrow changes on T_1-weighted images (3). Doses between 8–15 Gy produce characteristic vertebral changes on MRI (47, 57):

- During the first week of fractionated radiation, marrow edema with moderate decrease in signal intensity on T_1-weighted images, mild increase in signal intensity on T_2-weighted images and strong increase in signal intensity on STIR images.
- After the second to third week after completion of the radiation, resolution of the edema and increase in fat in the vertebral bodies, especially around the basivertebral vessels. Linear prominence of the signal from the central marrow fat or increasingly heterogeneity of the signal on the T_1-weighted images (67).
- After several weeks, extensive fatty replacement with homogeneous increase in signal intensity on the T_1-weighted image. In this late stage, possible development of a band pattern of peripheral intermediate signal intensity surrounding a persistent central increase in signal intensity (57).
- After several years, complete recovery with normal appearance of the vertebral bodies in patients treated with 30–40 Gy (3) or
- Persistent increase in signal intensity due to unchanged fat replacement of permanently ablated myeloid tissue in patients treated with 30–50 Gy (22, 23).

The visible changes are confined to areas within the radiation field (Figs. 11.**20** and 11.**21**). A distinct horizontal demarcation between normal and damaged bone marrow is often seen. Quantitative analysis, however, has been able to demonstrate a slight fat increase in areas immediately bordering the radiation field. This alteration was invisible on conventional T_1-weighted images and is attributed to scattered radiation (23). The visualization of the signal changes also depends on the magnetic field strength. On serial examinations performed following radiation therapy, images obtained with a low magnetic field detect the changes before they become visible on images obtained with a high magnetic field. For the same reason, a comparison of published findings is limited since the examinations are obtained with MRI systems operating at different magnetic field strengths. Furthermore, the studies compare groups treated with different radiation protocols. Consequently, the stated values are only to be seen as approximations.

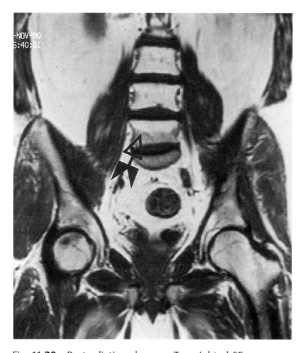

Fig. 11.**20**   Postradiation changes. T_1-weighted SE sequence, coronal section of the pelvis of a female patient, 26 months after para-aortic radiation for Hodgkin's disease. Fat-equivalent signal intensity in the superior vertebral bodies, normal signal intensity in the lower half of the L5 vertebral body, with good demarcation of the radiation field (arrow). (from Kauczor, H.U., B. Dietl: Radiologe 32 [1992] 516–522).

■ Inflammation

MRI is about as sensitive as scintigraphy in detecting osseous infections, with the sensitivities of both methods approaching 100%. Because of superior spatial resolution and high contrast visualization of the soft tissues,

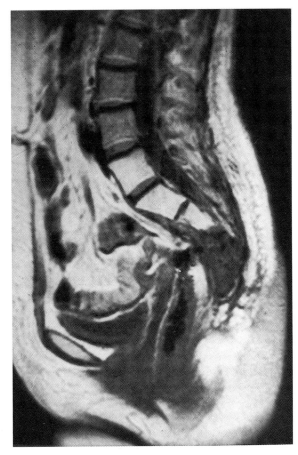

Fig. 11.**21** Postradiation changes. T_1-weighted SE sequence, sagittal section of the lumbosacral spine of a female patient, 12 months after radiation to the pelvis. Fat-equivalent signal intensity in the L5 vertebral body and sacrum. Normal signal intensities of the vertebral bodies above the radiation field.

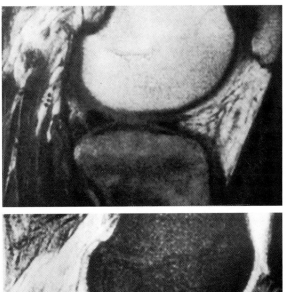

a

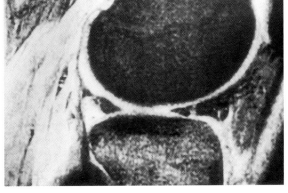

b

Fig. 11.**22 a, b** Bone marrow edema in osteomyelitis. **a** T_1-weighted SE sequence, sagittal section. Homogeneous decrease in signal intensity in the tibia. **b** T_2-weighted GRE sequence. Homogeneous increase in signal intensity in the tibia.

MRI has a greater *specificity*, which is over 90%, as opposed to the specificity of scintigraphy, which is at 65% (58, 70). Fat-suppressed imaging technique can increase the specificity as well as the conspicuity of the osseous changes further (36).

Acute Osteomyelitis

Osteomyelitic areas show decreased signal intensity on T_1-weighted and increased signal intensity on T_2-weighted images (Fig. 11.**22**), whereby the infected area may be indistinctly outlined against the surrounding bone marrow (4, 5). Intense *contrast enhancement* of the infected bone surrounded by rim enhancement characterizes the osseous findings further (36). Complications, such as soft tissue abscesses, necrotic bone, and sinus tracts, can be accurately identified by MRI (Fig. 11.**23**):

- *Sinus tracts* show a high signal intensity on T_2-weighted images, enhance and extend from the bone toward the cutaneous surface.

- *Necrotic bone* appears as homogeneous area of high signal intensity on T_2-weighted images,
- *Soft tissue extensions* demonstrate a high signal intensity in the adjacent soft tissues, most conspicuous on the T_2-weighted images.

On the basis of morphology and signal pattern alone, unenhanced MRI cannot distinguish marrow changes of acute osteomyelitis from marrow changes of osseous contusion or occult fractures. In the absence of any defining clinical findings, the *differentiation* has to rest on the natural course of the disease process. The underlying pathophysiology is probably quite similar, essentially constituting extracellular fluid accumulation due to altered vascular permeability.

Healed osteomyelitis appears as localized fat replacement within displaced hematopoietic marrow. These findings are most apparent in vertebrae.

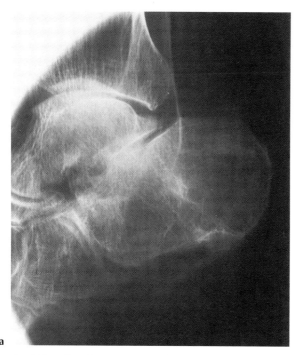

a

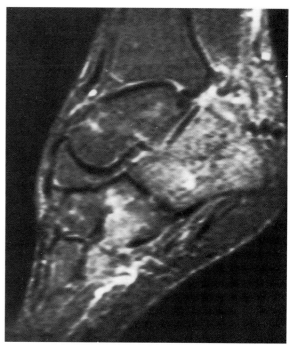

b

Fig. 11.**23 a, b**   Chronic osteomyelitis of the mid and hind foot. **a** Lateral radiograph. Diffuse osteoporosis with partially osteosclerotic and partially osteolytic areas, which are most extensive in the calcaneus. **b** Fat-suppressed STIR sequence. Increased signal intensity in the infected osseous areas. Involvement infection of the surrounding soft tissues with marked increase in signal intensity.

Chronic osteomyelitis

Active foci of chronic osteomyelitis exhibit the same signal pattern as acute osteomyelitis. The foci are generally surrounded by a sclerotic rim, which is seen as signal void that distinctly delineates the extent of the lesion. The distribution pattern of the active foci is variable and can be focal or patchy. *Sequestrated bone* appears as signal void, regardless of the selected sequence. Sinus tracts and soft tissue infections show the same signal pattern that is observed in acute osteomyelitis (30, 44). No characteristic MRI findings have yet been described for atypical manifestations of chronic osteomyelitis, such as Brodie's abscess (Fig. 11.**24**) and plasma cell osteomyelitis (Fig. 11.**25**). Chronic sclerosing osteomyelitis of Garré causes a diffuse decrease in signal intensity in all sequences.

Noninfectious Inflammations

Noninfectious inflammatory bone marrow edema can develop after arthroscopy with meniscal repair or cartilage shaving (Fig. 11.**26**). In particular, MRI can be used to diagnose and follow osteonecrosis about the knee after arthroscopic surgery (25). The signal pattern is that of marrow edema, with a signal intensity that is decreased on the T_1-weighted and increased on the T_2-weighted images.

Reflex sympathetic osteodystrophy (Sudeck disease) probably represents a dysregulation of the vasomotor sympathetic pathway with impaired vascular perfusion, frequently provoked by fractures, blunt trauma, or inflammation (51). Four stages are generally distinguished. The most important radiographic finding is a regional osteoporosis. Its appearance defines stage II and its severity increases in stages III and IV. MRI is normal in stage I and shows patchy areas of decreased signal intensity in the marrow on T_1-weighted and increased signal intensity on T_2-weighted images, corresponding to hyperemia and edema in the bone marrow (51). These changes progress in intensity and extent during stage III and rarely persist into stage IV, which is characterized by hypertrophic atrophy. Stage II and, though less pronounced, stage III show contrast enhancement in the marrow.

■ Trauma

Bone Bruises

Direct or indirect trauma to the bone can involve the bone marrow, with the severity determined by the traumatic impact. Mild marrow changes are given the generic term bone bruises and are attributed to edema, blood, and hyperemia. A precise pathogenesis still awaits histologic verification. On MRI, the bone bruises are seen as geographic (not linear) areas of decreased signal intensity on T_1-weighted and increased signal intensity on T_2-weighted images (Fig. 11.**27**). While the conventional radiograph is unremarkable, the bone scan shows increased tracer accumulation. Bone bruises resolve within 6–9 weeks, when they are no longer detectable by MRI (31).

Bone bruises are frequently observed in the juxta-articular and subchondral areas of the distal femur and proximal tibia. They often accompany ligamentous and meniscal injuries. In collateral ligament tears, a bone bruise is characteristically found in the contralateral femoral condyle, postulated to represent an impaction bone injury (31). The bone bruise can be confined to the subchondral bone. A bone bruise in the posterolateral tibial plateau or lateral femoral condyle is common in complete ACL tears following rotatory subluxation (40).

Since bone bruises heal spontaneously with rest, no further diagnostic studies or therapeutic interventions are indicated.

Fig. 11.**24 a – c** Chronic osteomyelitis with abscess formation. **a** Conventional tomography. Central radiolucency surrounded by a broad osteosclerotic rim. **b** T_1-weighted SE sequence. The central cavity is seen as low signal intensity structure (arrow), surrounded by a signal void sclerosis. **c** Fat-suppressed STIR sequence. The central cavity shows a high signal intensity (arrow).

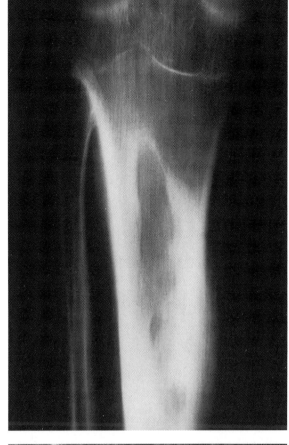

a

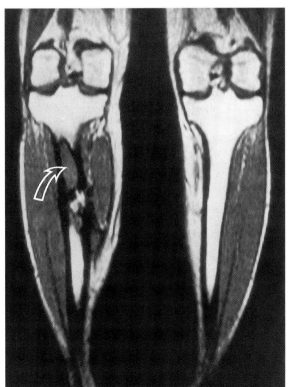

b

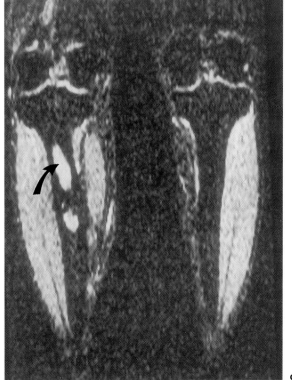

c

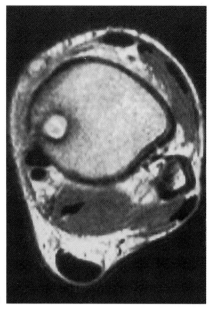
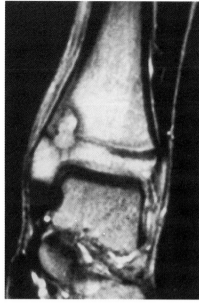

a   b

Fig. 11.**25a, b**   Plasma cell osteo-myelitis of the distal tibia. **a** Axial section. T_1-weighted SE sequence after administration of contrast medium. High-signal defect in the tibia surrounded by a signal-void rim (sclerotic border). Subtle heterogeneity of the signal in the surrounding soft tissues. **b** Coronal T_2-weighted TSE sequence. High-signal defect in the distal tibial metaphysis with extension into the epiphysis, surrounded by a thin signal-void rim.

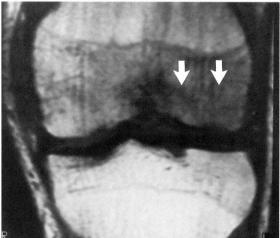

a

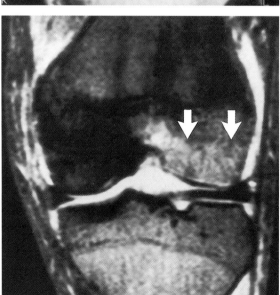

b

◀ Fig. 11.**26a, b**   Bone marrow edema of the lateral femoral condyle after arthroscopy. **a** T_1-weighted SE sequence, coronal section. Diffuse decrease in signal intensity of the femoral condyles (arrows). **b** T_2-weighted GRE sequence. Corresponding increase in signal intensity (arrows).

Occult Fractures

With increasing severity of the traumatic impact, the trabeculae can fracture or become impacted. If no radiographic changes are detected, these trabecular micro-fractures are customarily referred to as occult fractures. The bone scan is generally positive. MRI shows a linear signal void in all sequences, surrounded by an ill-defined band of decreased signal intensity on T_1-weighted and increased signal intensity on T_2-weighted images (Figs. 11.**27** and 11.**28**). Occult fractures are common around joints. They can extend to the joint space and involve the articular cartilage. These osteochondral and occult subchondral fractures can be well depicted by MRI.

Fig. 11.**28a–c**   Fracture of the femur. **a** The AP radiograph ▶ shows a break in the contour of the greater trochanter (arrow) and a short radiolucent line. Conventional tomography did not add any useful additional information. **b** T_1-weighted SE sequence. Decreased signal intensity in the right greater trochanter and lines of decreased signal intensity that extend into the metadiaphyseal region of the proximal femur (arrow). Normal curvilinear decrease in signal intensity in the left femur due to compression and tensile trabeculae, as well as remnants of hematopoietic bone marrow (open arrow). **c** T_2-weighted GRE sequence. Break in the contour of the greater trochanter (curved arrow) and linear increase in signal intensity in the metaphysis of the right femora (arrow). MRI shows the extent of the fracture better than radiography.

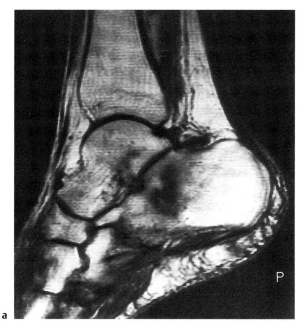
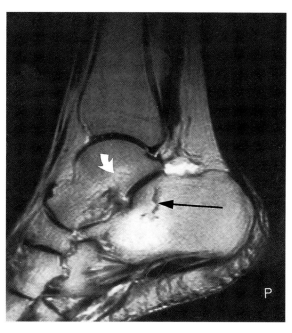

Fig. 11.**27 a, b**   S/P ankle trauma. Unremarkable radiographic examination. **a** T₁-weighted SE sequence. Focal decrease in signal intensity in the talus. Linear decrease in signal intensity in the calcaneus. **b** T₂-weighted TSE sequence. Focal increase in signal intensity in the talus, compatible with bone contusion (curved arrow). Increased signal intensity around a linear signal void, compatible with an occult fracture (arrow).

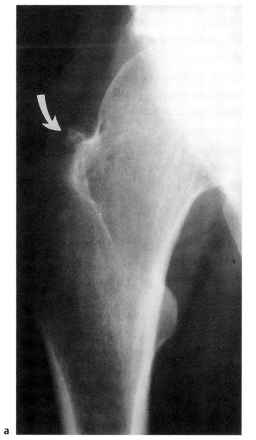
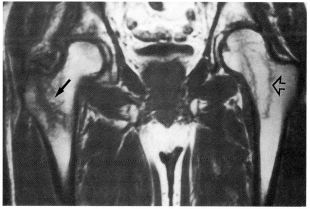
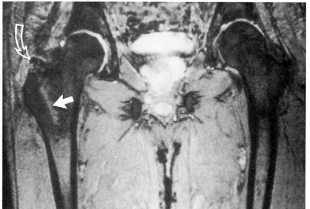

The linear signal void can be explained as dephasing artifacts along the irregular, newly created interface between trabeculae and marrow due to different susceptibility. It has also been speculated that this finding represents trabecular compression (68). The intraosseous signal of low intensity on the T_1-weighted images and high intensity on T_2-weighted images are attributed to marrow edema or hemorrhage around the trabecular fractures.

These occult fractures have a favorable prognosis, though progressive cartilage damage can occur in cases with chondral involvement. A surgical intervention is not recommended and no biopsy material is available for correlating the MRI findings with the osseous alterations. The diagnosis has to be supported by the presenting clinical findings and the spontaneous resolution.

Avulsion Fractures. A special type of occult fracture is the juxta-articular avulsion fracture. If the avulsed fragment is not, or is only minimally, dislocated, it might escape detection by conventional radiography. MRI shows a subcortical edema with low signal intensity on T_1-weighted and high signal intensity on T_2-weighted images. The fracture line or the avulsed cortical fragment has no signal and is often only indirectly visualized. A typical example of this type of injury is the avulsion fracture involving the lateral rim of the tibial plateau ('Segond fracture'), usually the result of internal rotation and varus stress injury (64).

Complete Fractures

Fractures with cortical breaks are diagnosed by the accompanying soft tissue swelling (the fracture hematoma) and marrow changes exhibiting the typical bone bruise pattern (Fig. 11.**29**), even if MRI cannot demon-

strate the cortical abnormality. Fractures that are radiographically equivocal or occult, as is frequently the case with impacted fractures of the femoral neck, can be definitively diagnosed with MRI.

Stress Fracture

Stress fractures are caused by an imbalance between the strength of the bone and the stress applied to the bone. Weakened bone (osteomalacia, osteoporosis, Paget disease) can fracture as a result of normal activity and normal bone in response to repetitive or increased load (marching, jogging, chronic cough). The characteristic radiographic changes consist of a juxtacortical transverse or oblique sclerotic band. A thin radiolucent line might be visible within this band. MRI has been found to be more sensitive in detecting stress fractures than conventional radiology and tomography. This applies especially to early stress fractures, as evidenced by positive radiographs in only 28% of scintigraphically positive and presumed early stress fractures (11). MRI can visualize the pathophysiologic changes accompanying a stress fracture, consisting of band-like signal void, generally surrounded by marrow reaction in the form of marrow edema (29, 55) (Fig. 11.**30**). The signal-void band represents trabecular microfractures and intertrabecular callus formation. Stress fractures can be associated with a subperiosteal hematoma or edema that should not be misinterpreted as bone tumor with soft tissue extension. A soft tissue edema can be present as well. The concurring signal void is the discriminating factor. The differentiation of stress fractures from occult intraosseous fractures can be difficult. Stress fractures are almost always metaphyseal or diaphyseal and occult fractures typically subchondral or epiphyseal and have a history of a single precipitating injury.

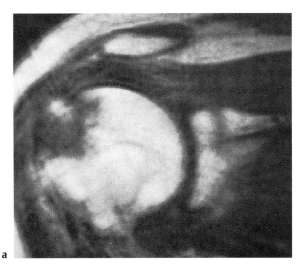

a

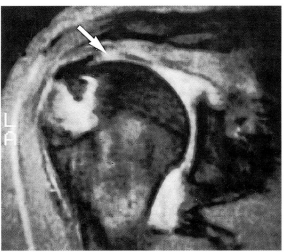

b

Fig. 11.**29a, b**   Fracture of the humeral head. **a** T_1-weighted SE sequence. Low signal defects in the humeral head and displaced fragments. **b** T_2-weighted GRE sequence. Correspond-ing high signal defect in the humeral head. Accompanying joint effusion and tear of the rotator cuff (arrow).

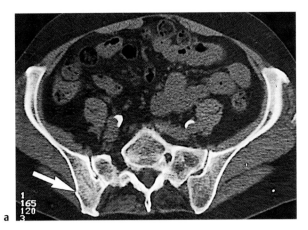
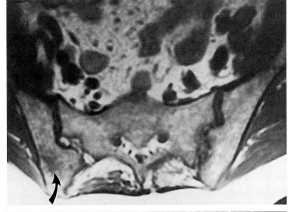
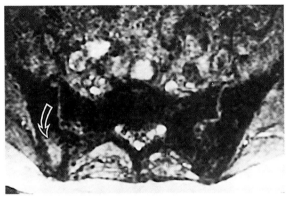

Fig. 11.**30a–c** Stress fracture of the ilium. **a** CT. Subtle break in the cortex (arrow). **b** T₁-weighted SE sequence. Partially linear decrease in signal intensity (arrow). **c** T₂-weighted GRE sequence. Corresponding increase in signal intensity (arrow).

Clinical Role of MRI and Comparison with Other Imaging Modalities

MRI displays changes at the cellular level and is well suited for imaging the bone marrow. In contrast to conventional radiology, it is not restricted to an altered osseous matrix, and in comparison with scintigraphy, it can detect many disorders with greater sensitivity. Though an abnormality seen on MRI reflects an abnormality at the cellular level, the specificity of MRI findings is often unsatisfactory, even when contrast enhancement and quantitative analysis are added. In these situations, MRI serves as screening method and the diagnosis has to be established in context with the clinical findings or by biopsy.

The most common *indications* of MRI for diagnostic evaluation of the bone marrow are:

- differential diagnosis between osteoporosis and diffuse plasmocytoma,
- staging of lymphoma,
- search and confirmation of osseous metastases,
- avascular necrosis,
- osteomyelitis,
- radiographically 'occult' fractures,
- stress adaptation.

References

1 Bloem, J. L.: Transient osteoporosis of the hip: MR imaging. Radiology 167 (1988) 753–755
2 Bohndorf, K., G. Benz-Bohm, W. Gross-Fengels, F. Berthold: MRI of the knee region in leukemic children. Part I. Initial pattern in patients with untreated disease. Pediat. Radiol. 20 (1990) 179–183
3 Casamassina, F., C. Ruggiero, D. Caramella, E. Tinacci, N. Villari, M. Ruggiero: Hematopoetic bone marrow recovery after radiation therapy: MRI evaluation. Blood 73 (1989) 1677–1681
4 Chandnani, V. P., J. Beltran, C. S. Morris, S. N. Khalil, C. F. Mueller, J. M. Burk, W. F. Bennett, P. B. Shaffer, M. S. Vasila, J. Reese, J. A. Ridgeway: Acute experimental osteomyelitis and abscesses: detection with MR imaging versus CT. Radiology 174 (1990) 233–236
5 Cohen, M. D., D. A. Cory, M. Kleiman, J. A. Smith, N. J. Broderick: Magnetic resonance differentiation of acute and chronic osteomyelitis in children. Clin. Radiol. 41 (1990) 53–56
6 Dawson, K. L., S. G. Moore, J. M. Rowland: Age-related marrow changes in the pelvis: MR and anatomic findings. Radiology 183 (1992) 47–51
7 Deutsch, A. L., J. H. Mink, F. P. Rosenfelt, A. D. Waxman: Incidental detection of hematopoietic hyperplasia on routine knee MR imaging. Amer. J. Roentgenol. 152 (1989) 333–336
8 Dooms, G. C., M. R. Fisher, H. Hricak, M. Richardson, L. E. Crooks, H. K. Genant: Bone marrow imaging: magnetic resonance studies related to age and sex. Radiology 155 (1985) 429–432
9 Eustace, S., D. McGrath, M. Albrecht, F. Fogt, B. Buff, H. E. Longmaid: Clival marrow changes in AIDS: findings at MR imaging. Radiology 193 (1994) 623–627

10 Fletscher, B. D., J. E. Wall, S. L. Hanna: Effect of hematopoetic groth factors on MR images of bone marrow in children undergoing chemotherapy. Radiology 189 (1993) 745–751

11 Greaney, R. B., F. H. Gerber, R. L. e. a. Laughlin: Distribution and natural history of stress fractures in U. S. Marine recruits. Radiology 146 (1983) 339–346

12 Gückel, F., W. Semmler, G. Brix, P. Bachert-Baumann, M. Körbling, H. Bihl, G. van Kaick: Knochenmarkveränderungen bei Morbus Hodgkin: MR-Tomographie und Chemical Shift Imaging. Fortschr. Röntgenstr. 150 (1989) 670–673

13 Gückel, F., G. Brix, W. Semmler, I. Zuna, W. Knauf, A. D. Ho, G. v. Kaick: Systemic bone marrow disorders: characterization with proton chemical shift imaging. J. Comput. assist. Tomogr. 14 (1990) 633–642

14 Hajek, P. C., L. L. Baker, J. E. Goobar: Focal fat deposition in axial bone marrow: MR characteristics. Radiology 162 (1987) 245–250

15 Hashimoto, M.: Pathology of bone marrow. Acta haematol. 27 (1962) 193–216

16 Jaramillo, D., T. Laor, F. A. Hoffer, D. J. Zaleske, R. H. Cleveland, B. R. Buchbinder, T. K. Egglin: Epiphyseal marrow in infancy: MR imaging. Radiology 180 (1991) 809–812

17 Jensen, K. E., T. Grube, C. Thomsen, P. G. Sorensen, P. Christoffersen, H. Karle, O. Henriksen: Prolonged bone marrow T1-relaxation in patients with polycythemia vera. Magn. Reson. Imag. 6 (1988) 291–292

18 Jensen, K. E., C. Thomsen, O. Henriksen, H. Hertz, H. K. Johansen, M. Yssing: Changes in T1 relaxation processes in the bone marrow following treatment in children with acute lymphoblastic leukemia. Pediat. Radiol. 20 (1990) 464–468

19 Jones, K. M., E. C. Unger, P. Granstrom, J. F. Seeger, R. F. Carmody, M. Yoshino: Bone marrow imaging using STIR at 0.5 and 1.5 T Magn. Reson. Imag. 10 (1992) 169–176

20 Kaplan, P., R. J. Asleson, L. W. Klassen, M. J. Duggan: Bone marrow patterns in aplastic anemia: observations with 1.5-T MR imaging. Radiology 164 (1987) 441–444

21 Kaplan, K. R., D. G. Mitchell, R. M. Steiner: Polycythemia vera and myelofibrosis: Correlation of MR-imaging clinical and labaratory findings. Radiology 183 (1992) 329–334

22 Kauczor, H. U., B. Dietl, K. F. Kreitner, G. Brix: Knochenmarkveränderungen nach Strahlentherapie: Ergebnisse der MR-Tomographie. Radiology 32 (1992) 516–522

23 Kauczor, H. U., B. Dietl, G. Brix, K. Jarosch, M. V. Knopp, G. van Kaick: Fatty replacement of bone marrow after radiation therapy for Hodgkin disease: quantification with chemical shift imaging. JMRI 3 (1993) 575–580

24 Kricun, M. E.: Red-yellow marrow conversion: its effect on the location of some solitary bone lesions. Skelet. Radiol. 14 (1985) 10–19

25 Kursunoglu Brahme, S., J. M. Fox, R. D. Ferkel, M. J. Friedman, B. D. Flannigan, D. L. Resnick: Osteonecrosis of the knee after arthroscopy surgery: diagnosis with MR imaging. Radiology 178 (1991) 851–853

26 Lang, P., F. Russel, M. Vahlensieck, S. Majumdar, Y. Berthezene, S. Grampp, H. K. Genant: Residuales und rekonvertiertes hämatopoetisches Knochenmark im distalen Femur. Spin-Echo und gegenphasierte Gradienten-Echo MRT. Fortschr. Röntgenstr. 156 (1992) 89–95

27 Lanir, A., L. E. Aghai, J. S. Simon, G. L. Lee, M. E. Clouse: MR imaging in myelofibrosis. J. Comput. assist. Tomogr. 10 (1986) 634–636

28 Layer, G., I. Boldt, W. Block, J. Gieseke, J. Görich, A. Steudel: T2-gewichtete Turbo-Spin-Echo-Sequenzen: sinnvolle Sequenz-Alternative in der Diagnostik von Skelettmetastasen. Zbl. Radiol. 150 (994) 138

29 Lee, J. K., L. Yao: Stress fractures: MR imaging. Radiology 169 (1988) 217–220

30 Mason, M. D., M. B. Zlatkin, J. L. Esterhai, M. K. Dalinka, M. G. Velchik, H. Y. Kressel: Chronic complicated osteomyelitis of the lower extremity: evaluation with MR imaging. Radiology 173 (1989) 355–359

31 Mink, J. H., A. L. Deutsch: Occult cartilage and bone injuries of the knee: detection, classification, and assessment with MR imaging. Radiology 170 (1989) 823–829

32 Mirowitz, S. A.: Hematopoietic bone marrow within the proximal humeral epiphysis in normal adults: investigation with MR Imaging. Radiology 188 (1993) 689–693

33 Modic, M. T., P. M. Steinberg, J. S. Ross: Degenerative disk disease: assessment of changes in vertebral body marrow with MR imaging. Radiology 166 (1988) 193–199

34 Moore, S. G., C. A. Gooding, R. C. Brasch, R. L. Ehman, H. G. Ringertz, A. R. Ablin, K. K. Matthay, S. Zoger: Bone marrow in children with acute lymphocytic leukemia: MR relaxation times. Radiology 160 (1986) 237–240

35 Moore, S. G., K. L. Dawson: Red an yellow marrow in the femur: age-related changes in appearance at MR imaging. Radiology 175 (1990) 219–223

36 Morrison, W. B., M. E. Schweitzer, G. W. Bock, D. G. Mitchell, E. L. Hume, M. N. Pathria, D. Resnick: Diagnosis of Osteomyelitis: utility of fat-suppressed contrast-enhanced MR imaging. Radiology 189 (1993) 251–257

37 Moulopoulos, L. A.: Waldenström macroglobulinemia: MR imaging of the spine and CT of the abdomen and pelvis. Radiology 188 (1993) 669–673

38 Moulopoulos, L. A., D. G. K. Varma, M. A. Dimopoulos, N. E. Leeds, E. E. Kim, D. A. Johnston, R. Alexian, H. I. Libshitz: Multiple myeloma: spinal MR imaging in patients with untreated newly diagnosed disease. Radiology 185 (1992) 833–840

39 Moulopoulos, L. A., M. A. Dimopoulos, R. Alexanian, N. E. Leeds, H. I. Libshitz: Multiple myeloma: MR patterns of response to treatment. Radiology 193 (1994) 441–446

40 Murphy, B. J., R. L. Smith, J. W. Uribe, C. J. Janecki, K. S. Hechtman, R. A. Mangasarian: Bone signal abnormalities in the posterolateral tibia and lateral femoral condyle in conplete tears of the anterior cruciate ligament: a specific sign? Radiology 182 (1992) 221–224

41 Okada, Y., S. Aoki, A. J. Barkovich, K. Nishimura, D. Norman, B. O. Kjos, R. C. Brasch: Cranial bone marrow in children: assessment of normal development with MR imaging. Radiology 171 (1989) 161–164

42 Pay, N. T., W. S. Singer, E. Bartel: Hip pain in three children accompanied by transient abnormal findings on MR images. Radiology 171 (1989) 147–149

43 Poulton, T. B., W. D. Murphy, J. L. Duerk, C. C. Chapek, D. H. Feiglin: Bone marrow reconversion in adults who are smokers. MR imaging findings. Amer. J. Roentgenol. 161 (1993) 1217–1221

44 Quinn, S. F., W. Murray, R. A. Clark, C. Cochran: MR imaging of chronic osteomyelitis. J. Comput. assist. Tomogr. 12 (1988) 113–117

45 Rao, V. M., M. Fishman, D. G. Mitchell, R. M. Steiner, S. K. Ballas, L. Axel, M. K. Dalinka, W. Gefter, H. Y. Kressel: Painfull sickle cell crisis: bone marrow patterns observed with MR imaging. Radiology 161 (1986) 211–215

46 Rao, V. M., D. G. Mitchell, M. D. Rifkin, R. M. Steiner, D. L. Burk, D. Levy, S. K. Ballas: Marrow infarction in sickle cell anemia: correlation with marrow type and distribution by MRI. Magn. Reson. Imag. 7 (1989) 39–44

47 Remedios, P. A., P. M. Colletti, J. K. Raval, R. C. Benson, L. Y. Chak, W. D. Boswell, J. M. Halls: Magnetic resonance imaging of bone after radiation. Magn. Reson. Imag. 6 (1988) 301–304

48 Ricci, C., M. Cova, Y. S. Kang, A. Yang, A. Rahmouni, W. W. Scott, E. A. Zerhouni: Normal age-related patterns of cellular and fatty bone marrow distribution in the axial skeleton: MR imaging study. Radiology 177 (1990) 83–88

49 Rosen, B. R., D. M. Fleming, D. C. Kushner, K. S. Zaner, R. B. Buxton, W. P. Bennet, G. L. Wismer, T. J. Brady: Hematologic bone marrow disorders: quantitative chemical shift MR imaging. Radiology 169 (1988) 799–804

50 Rosenthal, D. I., J. A. Scott, J. Barranger: Evaluation of Gaucher disease using magnetic resonance imaging. J. Bone Surg. 68-A (1986) 802–808

51 Schimmerl, S., H. Schurawitzki, H. Imhof, G. Canigiani, J. Kramer, V. Fialka: Morbus Sudeck-MRT als neues diagnostisches Verfahren. Fortschr. Röntgenstr. 154 (1991) 601 – 604

52 Sebag, G. H., S. G. Moore: Effect of trabecular bone on the appearance of marrow in Gradient-Echo imaging of the appendicular skeleton. Radiology 174 (1990) 855 – 859

53 Shellock, F. G., E. Morris, A. L. Deutsch, J. H. Mink, R. Kerr, S. D. Boden: Hematopoietic bone marrow hyperplasia: high prevalence on MR images of the knee in asymptomatic marathon runners. Amer. J. Roentgenol. 158 (1992) 335 – 338

54 Smith, S. R., C. E. Williams, J. M. Davies, R. H. T. Edwards: Bone marrow disorders: characterization with quantitative MR imaging. Radiology 172 (1989) 805 – 810

55 Stafford, S. A., D. I. Rosenthal, M. C. Gebhardt, T. J. Brady, J. A. Scott: MRI in stress fracture. Amer. J. Roentgenol. 147 (1986) 553 – 556

56 Stevens, S. K., S. G. Moore, M. D. Amylon: Repopulation of marrow after transplantation: MR imaging with pathologic correlation. Radiology 175 (1990 a) 213 – 218

57 Stevens, S. K., S. G. Moore, I. D. Kaplan: Early and late bone marrow changes after irradiation: MR evaluation. Amer. J. Roentgenol. 154 (1990 b) 745 – 750

58 Unger, E., P. Moldofsky, R. Gatenby, W. Hartz, G. Broder: Diagnosis of osteomyelitis by MR imaging. Amer. J. Roentgenol. 150 (1988) 605 – 610

59 Unger, E. C., T. B. Summers: Bone marrow. Top. Magn. Reson. Imag. 1 (1989) 31 – 52

60 Vahlensieck, M., M. Reiser: Knochenmarködem in der MRT. Radiology 10 (1992) 509 – 515

61 Vahlensieck, M., B. Lattka, H. M. Schmidt, H. Schild: Bone marrow distribution in the shoulder girdle: age correlated pattern analysis using MRI and cadaver dissections. SMR 13 (1994)

62 Vellet, A. D., P. H. Marks, P. J. Fowler, T. G. Munro: Occult posttraumatic osteochondral lesions of the knee: prevalence, classification, and short-term sequelae evaluated with MR imaging. Radiology 178 (1991) 271 – 276

63 Vogler, J. B., W. A. Murphy: Bone marrow imaging. Radiology 168 (1988) 679 – 693

64 Weber, W. N., C. H. Neumann, J. A. Barakos, S. A. Petersen, L. S. Steinbach, H. K. Genant: Lateral tibial rim (segond) fractures: MR imaging characteristics. Radiology 180 (1991) 731 – 734

65 Wilson, A. J., W. A. Murphy, D. C. Hardy, W. G. Totty: Transient osteoporosis: transient bone marrow edema? Radiology 167 (1988) 757 – 760

66 Wismer, G. L., B. R. Rosen, R. Buxton, D. D. Stark, T. J. Brady: Chemical shift imaging of bone marrow: preliminary experience. Amer. J. Roentgenol. 145 (1985) 1031 – 1037

67 Yankelevitz, D. F., C. I. Henschke, P. H. Knapp, L. Nisce, Y. Yi, P. Cahill: Effect of radiation therapy on thoracic and lumbar bone marrow: evaluation with MR imaging. Amer. J. Roentgenol. 157 (1991) 87 – 92

68 Yao, L., J. K. Lee: Occult intraosseous fracture: detection with MR imaging. Radiology 167 (1988) 749 – 751

69 Zawin, J. K., D. Jaramillo: Conversion of bone marrow in the humerus, sternum, and clavicle: changes with age on MR images. Radiology 188 (1993) 159 – 164

70 Zynamon, A., T. Jung, J. Hodler, T. Bischof, G. K. Schulthess: Das Magnetresonanzverfahren in der Diagnostik der Osteomyelitis. Fortschr. Röntgenstr. 155 (1991) 513 – 518

12 Bone and Soft-Tissue Tumors

P. Lang, M. Vahlensieck, J. O. Johnston and H. K. Genant

General Section

Before the introduction of cross-sectional imaging, primary bone tumors were diagnosed and categorized by conventional radiography and tomography. Even today, after CT and MRI have become part of the standard armamentarium in the clinical work-up, conventional radiography remains the method of choice for the initial diagnostic evaluation of bone tumors. In many cases, the radiographic findings allow a histopathologic diagnosis. It is often difficult to visualize tumors of the scapula, ribs, vertebra and pelvis by conventional radiography (91).

Today, MRI has become one of the diagnostic foundations in the diagnosis of malignant tumors of the skeleton. MRI is superior to CT because:

- MRI has a superior soft tissue contrast,
- MRI allows direct multiplanar imaging,
- MRI allows a better characterization of tissue owing to the different signal pattern of different tissues for individual sequences.

MRI is more accurate than other imaging methods for staging bone and especially soft-tissue tumors (11, 34, 108). Furthermore, MRI can reveal tumor infiltration of the neurovascular bundle better than CT (11, 108).

This chapter will present the current MRI methods available for delineating bone and soft-tissue tumors. Staging, tissue-specific imaging findings, changes secondary to chemotherapy and radiotherapy, and detection of tumor recurrences as well as characteristic findings of specific tumors will be discussed.

■ Coils, Sequence Protocols

The first sequence should be acquired with a body coil to allow adequate assessment of the proximal and distal extent of the lesion and to assure visualization of the tumor in its entirety. The examination with the body coil will also include any possible proximal or distal skip lesions (Fig. 12.**1** and Tab. 12.**1**).

Depending on the size of the lesion, the examination is continued with a surface coil, a torso phased-array coil, or circumferential coil. To achieve a high spatial resolution, the field of view should be small, though large enough to encompass the entire tumor including any tumorous infiltration of the vessels, nerves, and muscles.

To search for vertebral metastases, a phased-array spinal coil should be applied to examine the entire spine. A torso phased-array coil or a body coil should be selected for the metastatic evaluation of the pelvis or both upper and lower extremities.

■ Comparison between Benign and Malignant Tumors

Many of the criteria used in conventional radiology and CT for determining the malignant potential of a bone tumor are also applicable to MRI. Benign tumors generally are sharply delineated from adjacent bone marrow and surrounding soft tissues (73, 108), whereas most malignant tumors have an indistinct margin and the tendency for local infiltration (73).

A sharp, smooth, well-defined low-signal border indicates that the tumor is most likely benign (108). But

Table 12.**1**   UCSF Protocol for sequences for bone and soft tissue tumors

Sequence	Section Level	TR	TE	FOV	Section Thickness	Skip	Echo Train Length	NEX	Matrix	Options
SE	1. axial	600	min	min	5	1		2	256 × 192	NP
FSE	2. axial	3500	60	min	5	1	8	2	256 × 192	Fat sat, NP
SE	3. cor/sag	600	min	min	4	1		2	256 × 192	NP
FMPIR	4. cor/sag	3500	55	min	4	1	8	2	256 × 256	TI = 120, NP
SE – post Gd	5. axial	600		min	5	4	1	2	256 × 192	Fat sat, NP
SE – post Gd	6. cor/sag	600	min	min	4			2	256 × 192	NP

cor	Coronal	FSE	Fast or turbo spin echo	sag	Sagittal
Fat sat	Fat saturation	Gd	Gadolinium	SE	Spin echo
FMPIR	Fat multiplanar inversion recovery	NEX	Number of excitations	TI	Inversion time
FOV	Field of view	NP	No phase wrap	min	Minimal

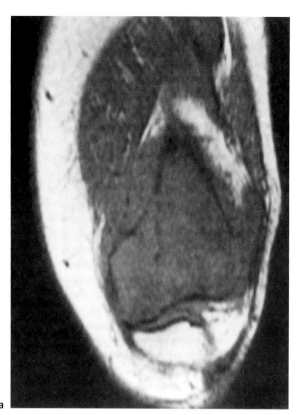

this finding is in no way specific since such a well-defined interface can also be encountered in malignant lesions (108).

Petasnik and co-workers (1886) reported that most benign tumors have a homogeneous signal intensity equal to or less than that of muscle on the T_1-weighted images and greater than that of muscle on the T_2-weighted images, with the exception of neural tumors and hemangiomas, which can appear homogeneous on the T_1-weighted images and heterogeneous on the T_2-weighted images. Most malignant tumors are homogeneous and of decreased signal intensity on the T_1-weighted images, but show a definite heterogeneity on the T_2-weighted images (73). Based on these findings, a homogeneous signal intensity on the T_2-weighted image would indicate a benign lesion. This subjective assessment of the signal pattern, however, is of limited value in distinguishing benign from malignant lesions. While it might suggest the nature of the tumor, its specificity is inadequate.

Measurement of the T_1 and T_2 relaxation times of benign and malignant lesions shows overlap and is unreliable in distinguishing between the two types of tumor (73, 108).

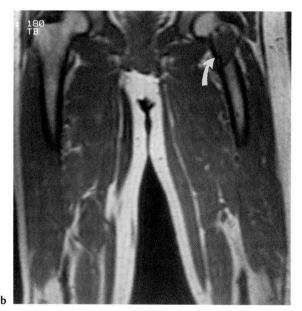

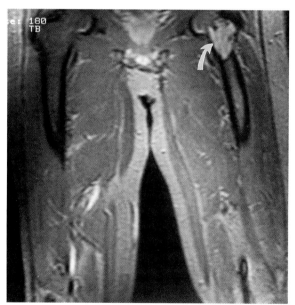

Fig. 12.**1 a–c**   Osteogenic sarcoma with osseous metastases (skip lesion). **a** T_1-weighted image. Low-signal primary lesion in the distal femur. **b** T_1-weighted image. Low-signal metastasis (arrow) in the proximal femur. **c** T_1-weighted image. High-signal metastasis (arrow) in the proximal femur.

Erlemann and co-workers (26) stated that dynamic MRI with rapid sequential image acquisition after intervenous bolus injection of Gd-DTPA might improve the distinction between benign and malignant tumors (Fig. 12.**2**). In their study of 69 patients with bone or soft-tissue tumors, the slope of the enhancement-time curve after injection of Gd-DTPA was greater than 30% in 84.1% of the malignant tumors and less than 30% in 72% of the benign tumors (26). While these results indicate that dynamic Gd-DTPA-enhanced imaging provides valuable information as to the malignant potential of a tumor, a biopsy is still needed because of the considerable overlap between the values for benign and malignant tumors (26).

Verstraete and co-workers (103) also investigated the slope of the time-intensity curve of dynamic contrast-enhanced imaging and calculated the maximal enhancement rate within the first minute after injection using a linear curve-fitting algorithm. The steepest slope of the time-enhancement curve was calculated for all pixels and displayed on a gray scale in a new computer-composed first pass image with the same matrix. The value of each pixel corresponds spatially to the first pass slope value, with high intensities indicating a steep enhancement slope and low intensities a shallow enhancement slope after injection of Gd-DTPA. This computer-composed parametric image correlated well with the tissue vascularization and perfusion, but a considerable overlap existed between values for malignant and vascular benign tumors, such as eosinophilic granuloma, giant cell tumor and osteoid osteoma. These parametric images, however, provide useful information by depicting viable tissue, which can be helpful in monitoring the tumor during chemotherapy and delineating any necrosis or surrounding inflammatory changes.

■ Characteristic Signal Intensity Pattern

Some of the tissues found histologically in tumors of the musculoskeletal tissue can be identified on the basis of their signal pattern. For instance, fat within in a tumor, as found in lipoma (Fig. 12.**3**), liposarcoma or even vertebral hemangioma, is characterized by a high signal intensity on T_1-weighted and an intermediate to high signal intensity on T_2-weighted images (Tab. 12.**2**). Chronic fibrotic scar tissue produces a low signal intensity in all sequences (Tab. 12.**2**) (75). Likewise, sclerotic bone, as found frequently in osteosarcoma, exhibits a low signal intensity in all sequences. Cystic, fluid-filled areas of the tumor generally show a low signal intensity on the T_1-weighted images and a high signal intensity on the T_2-weighted images, without any appreciable enhancement after administration of paramagnetic contrast medium (15). A cyst, however, can have a high signal intensity on T_1-weighted images if it contains proteinaceous material or methemoglobin after recent hemorrhage. Tumors characterized by a preferentially short T_1 relaxation time, i.e., high signal intensity on T_1-weighted images, are listed in Tab. 12.**3** (Figs. 12.**3** and 12.**4**). These characterizing signal findings often narrow the differential diagnosis. In addition, the presence of fluid levels can add valuable information (Tab. 12.**4**).

■ Staging

The choice between limb-saving procedure and amputation is determined by the aggressiveness and local spread of the tumor (5, 33, 71, 86). The staging system described by Enneking has proved helpful in the assessment of primary bone or soft-tissue tumors as to their prognosis, treatment, and recurrence rate (23). The staging system for tumors is based on:

- histologic grade of malignancy G (G_0 = benign, G_1 = low-grade malignant, G_2 = high-grade malignant),

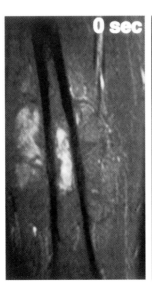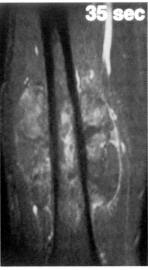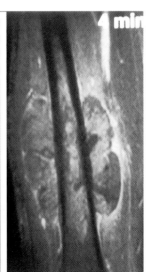

Fig. 12.**2** Osteosarcoma. Representative case of dynamic MRI with images generated at intervals of 3.5 seconds. The images obtained before (0 sec) and at 35 seconds and 4 minutes after bolus injection of contrast medium are shown. Aggressive tumor with rapid enhancement, which is characteristic of most malignant lesions.

Table 12.**2**   Signal intensities of normal and neoplastic tissue with various sequences   ▶

	SE T$_1$	SE T$_2$	FSE T$_2$	GRE „T$_1$"	GRE T$_2$*
Normal Tissue:					
• Yellow bone marrow	High	Intermediate to high	High	High	Low to intermediate [1]
• cortical bone	Low	Low	Low	Low	Low
• Muscle	Low	Intermediate to high	Intermediate to high	Low	Intemediate
• Ligaments	Low	Low	Low	Low	Low
• Tendons	Low	Low	Low	Low	Low
• Vessels	Low	Low	Low or high [2]	Low, intermediate, high [2]	Low, intermediate, high [2]
• Nerves	Low	Low to intermediate	Low to intermediate	Low	Intermediate
• Subcutaneous fat	high	Intermediate to high	Intermediate to high	High	Intermediate
Pathologic Tissue:					
• Intraosseous tumor	Low, intermediate	High, intermediate	High, intermediate	Low, intermediate	High [5]
• Extraosseous tumor	Low, intermediate	High, intermediate	High, intermediate	Low, intermediate	High [5]
• Fat containing tumor	High	Intermediate to high	Intermediate to high	High	Intermediate
• Tumor sclerosis	Low	Low	Low	Low	Low [3]
• Tumor cyst	Low	High	High	Low	High
• Hemorrhage – acute (deoxyhemoglobin)	Low	High	High	Low	High
• Hemorrhage – 4 weeks old (methemoglobin)	High	High	High	High	High
• Hemorrhage – old (hemosiderin)	Low	Low	Low	Low [3]	Low [3]
• Peritumerous edema	Low	High	High	Low	High

[1]   Caused by heterogeneous magnetic susceptibility along trabecula/marrow interface (see text)
[2]   Depends on flow direction and velocity, direction of phase encoding and distance from the entry section
[3]   In many cases with irregular, cauliflower-like appearance due to heterogeneous magnetic susceptibility with corresponding artifacts
[4]   In some cysts with peripheral enhancement corresponding to viable tumor or vessels at wall
[5]   Except for tumors that are largely fibrous or sclerotic
FSE   Fast spin echo
GRE   Gradient echo
SE   Spin echo
STIR   Short-tau-inversion-recovery

Table 12.**3**   Tumors with short T$_1$ relaxation times

Fat-containing tumors
• Lipoma
• Liposarcoma
• Hemangioma

Tumors with methemoglobin
• Telangiectatic osteosarcoma
• Hemorrhagic metastases
• Malignant tumors after chemotherapy or radiotherapy
• Pseudotumor in Hemophilia
• Lymphangioma
• Arteriovenous malformation
• Melanotic metastases of malignant melanoma

Table 12.**2**   (Continued)

STIR	SE „T_1" Post-contrast	GRE „T_1" Post-contrast
Low	High	High
Low	Low	Low
Low to medium	Low to medium	Low to medium
Low	Low	Low
Low	Low	Low
Low or high	Low	Low
Low	Low	Low
Low	High	High
High[5]	High	High
High[5]	High	High
Low	High	High
Low	Low	Low
High	Low[4]	Low[4]
High	Low	Low
High	High	High
Low	Low	Low[3]
High	High	High

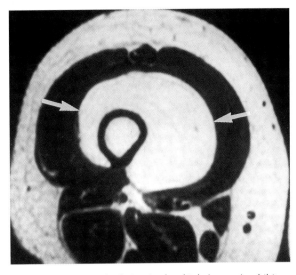

Fig. 12.**3**   Lipoma. The lesion in the thigh (arrows) exhibits a signal of high, fat-equivalent intensity on the T_1-weighted image.

Table 12.**4**   Tumors with fluid levels

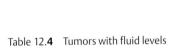

- Aneurysmatic bone cyst
- Chondroblastoma
- Osteoblastoma
- Giant cell tumor
- Osteogenic sarcoma
- Metastases
- Malignant tumors after chemotherapy or radiotherapy
- Abscess

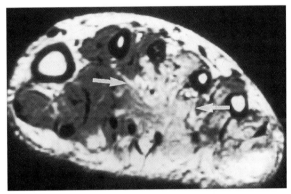

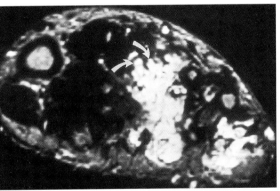

Fig. 12.**4a, b**   Hematoma. **a** T_1-weighted image. High-signal lesion in the forefoot (arrows), probably reflecting blood products and fat. **b** T_2-weighted image. The high signal intensity of the lesion persists. Dilated vascular structures are visible (curved arrows).

Table 12.**5**   Surgical approach to musculoskeletal neoplasms related to stage

Stage according to Enneking	Resection	Amputation
Benign		
• 1 (inactive)	Intracapsular	Subtotal
• 2 (active)	Extracapsular (en-bloc resection inside the reactive zone)	Marginal
• 3 (aggressive)	Wide (including safety margin through normal tissue outside the reactive zone)	Wide
Malignant		
• I (low-grade malignant)	Wide	Wide
• II (high-grade malignant)	Radical (complete removal of the involved compartments, thus often including the joint)	Radical

Table 12.**6**   Recurrence rates in % of musculoskeletal neoplasms: surgical margin versus Enneking stages (not further categorized) (from Netter, F.H.: The CIBA Collection of Medical Illustrations. Volume 8 : Musculoskeletal System, Part II. CIBA-GEIGY Corporation, West Caldwell, NJ 07006)

Surgical Margin	Stage						
	Benign			**Malignant**			
	1	2	3	IA	IB	IIA	IIB
Intracapsular margin (dissection through the reactive zone and tumor capsule)	0	30	70	90	90	100	100
Marginal margin (dissection through the reactive zone outside the capsule)	0	0	50	70	70	90	90
Wide margin (dissection through healthy tissue outside the reactive zone)	0	0	10	10	30	30	50
Radical margin (removal of tumor and its entire natural compartment)	0	0	0	0	0	10	20

- local extent T (T_0 = intracapsular, T_1 = extracapsular but still within the compartment, T_2 = extracapsular with compartmental escape),
- presence of metastases M (M_0 = no metastases, M_1 = detectable metastases).

The G, T, and M score is then used to determine the stage (Fig. 12.**5**).

Enneking's staging system does not apply to the staging of leukemias, myelomas, Ewing sarcoma or metastases. This method of staging bone and soft-tissue neoplasms has to be separated from the assessment of growth rate of bone tumors on the basis of the radiographic destruction pattern as proposed by Lodwick. MRI contributes to the accuracy of the staging through its ability to delineate the tumor in relationship to compartmental borders and neurovascular bundles.

Initial surgical procedures include limb-saving resection and amputations with four basic surgical margins (Tab. 12.**5**). The surgical planning takes into account the tumor stage and the recurrence rate of the tumor in relation to the surgical margin (Tab. 12.**6**).

Intramedullary Involvement

MRI is clearly superior to CT in determining the intramedullary extent of the tumor (1, 11, 12, 13, 34, 41, 57, 58, 70, 73, 91–95, 108). Gillespy and co-workers (34) compared the ability of CT and MRI to assess the intramedullary extension of bone tumors and correlated the sectional images with macroslides of the surgical specimens. The average difference between CT and macroslides was 16.5 mm ± 10.7 mm, and the average difference between MRI and macroslides 4.9 mm ± 4.3 mm. Much of the difference between MRI and macroslides was attributed to comparing MRI planes with different macroslides. When identical planes of section were compared in a subgroup of five patients, the average difference was 1.8 mm ± 1.6 mm (34).

Bloem and co-workers (11) prospectively evaluated the relative value of CT, MRI and bone scintigraphy in

Fig. 12.**5**   Staging of the musculoskeletal neoplasms after Enneking (after Netter). **Stages 1 – 3:** Histologically benign (G_0) with variable clinical and biologic behavior

Benign

Stage 1: Remains stationary or heals spontaneously with indolent clinical course. Well encapsulated (T_0).

Bone tumor

Soft-tissue tumor

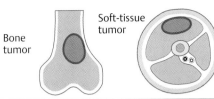

Stage 2: Active disease. Progressive symptomatic tumor growth. Remains intracapsular. Limited by natural boundaries, which are frequently deformed (T_0).

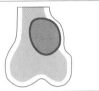

Stage 3: Agressive disease. Agressive growth not limited by capsule or natural boundaries. May penetrate cortex or compartment boundary. Higher recurrence rate (T_1–T_2).

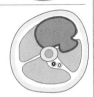

Malignant

Stage I: Histologically low grade (G_1). Well differentiated, few mitoses, moderate nuclear atypia. Tends to recur locally. Moderate radioisotope uptake.

IA — Intraosseous or intracompartmental (T_1)

IB — Extraosseous or extracompartmental; penetrates cortex or compartment boundaries (T_2)

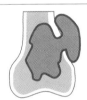
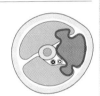

Stage II: Histologically high grade (G_2). Poorly differentiated, high cell-to-matrix ratio, many mitoses, severe nuclear atypia, necroses, neovascularity. Permeative osteolytic destruction. Intense radioisotope uptake. Higher incidence of metastases.

IIA — Intraosseous or intracompartmental (T_1)

IIB — Extraosseous or extracompartmental; penetrates cortex or compartment boundaries (T_2)

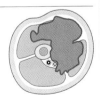

Stage III: Metastatic stage. Regional or remote metastases (viscera, lymph nodes, bones).

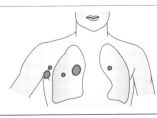
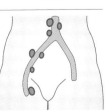

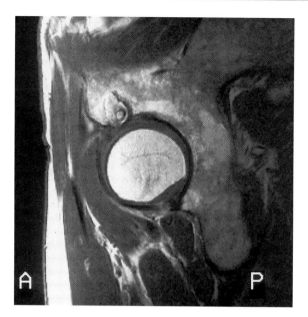

Fig. 12.**6** Oblique sagittal contrast-enhanced SE image of a tumor in the acetabulum with intra-articular extension. The cartilage of the acetabular roof is infiltrated, but the joint space and the cartilage covering the femoral head are still spared. This high resolution image could prove the intra-articular extension. The tumor shows heterogeneous enhancement. Reconverted bone marrow throughout the acetabulum is a normal finding in a 65-year-old patient. (See Chapter 11.)

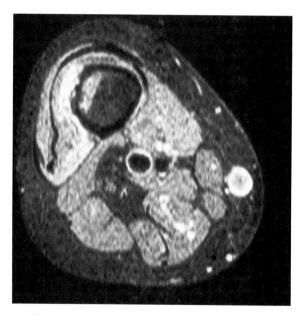

Fig. 12.**7** Metastasis in the femoral shaft. Axial fat-suppressed STIR image. Low-signal residual bone marrow, high-signal intraosseous tumor component, destroyed cortex, high-signal extraosseous tumor component. Despite relatively low spatial resolution, good delineation of the cortical destruction.

local tumor staging in comparison to the findings at dissection of the resected specimen. MRI had a nearly perfect correlation with the histopathologic specimen (r = 0.99), while CT had a lower correlation (r = 0.86). The prediction of intraosseous tumor length with bone scintigraphy was poor (r = 0.56). MRI seems to be clearly superior to CT. Since most surgeons resect the tumor with a wide margin of 5 – 6 cm, both MRI and CT may be adequate for surgical planning (75, 81).

Epiphyseal Involvement

Epiphyseal involvement is better predicted with MRI than with conventional radiography (69). Norton and co-workers observed epiphyseal extension on the pathologic specimen in 12 of 15 consecutive patients with long bone osteosarcoma and nonfused epiphyses. Plain radiography detected the epiphyseal involvement in only nine cases while MRI was accurate in identifying epiphyseal involvement in all 12 patients.

Intra-articular Involvement

It is not certain whether MRI is superior to CT in detecting joint involvement. Bloem and co-workers (11) showed that CT and MRI are equally accurate and specific, with a specificity above 90%. Aisen and co-workers (1) and Zimmer and co-workers (108) found MRI to be occasionally more accurate but comparable in the majority of cases (Fig. 12.**6**).

Unfortunately the presence of a joint effusion in the joint adjacent to the tumor is not a reliable sign of joint involvement. However, the absence of the joint effusion is a good indicator of no intra-articular invasion of the tumor.

Cortical Destruction, Periosteal Reaction

Several studies have reported the superiority of conventional radiography and CT over MRI for the evaluation of cortical destruction, tumor calcifications and ossifications and for the detection of periosteal or endosteal reaction (7, 75, 89, 90, 91, 108). The high radiodensity of the periosteal osseous reaction and osteoblastic areas is associated with a low concentration of resonating protons and resultant low signal intensity on MRI, accounting for the difficulty in visualizing these changes on MRI. However, the majority of studies reporting this aspect are several years old and were performed with low field strengths and obsolete coil technology.

Zimmer and co-workers (108) demonstrated that cortical destruction as well as periosteal and endosteal new bone formation can be identified by MRI (Fig. 12.**7**). GRE sequences can increase the sensitivity of MRI for the detection of subtle sclerotic changes (Fig. 12.**8**) since, in contrast to the SE image formation, the image is acquired without a rephasing pulse. Consequently, the heterogeneous magnetic susceptibility of focal sclerotic areas produces a signal loss. This signal loss can be used

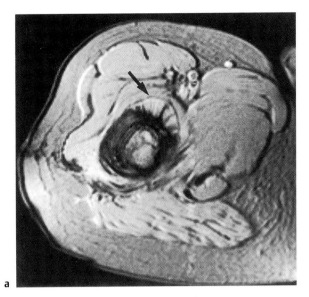
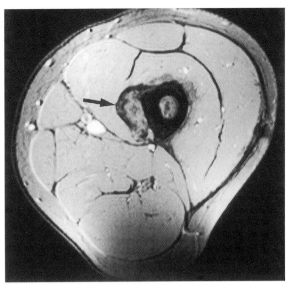

a   b

Fig. 12.**8 a, b**   Periosteal reaction of malignant bone tumor on
GRE image. Axial section. **a** Osteosarcoma of the femur with
spiculated bone formation producing a sunburst appearance
(arrow). **b** Ewing sarcoma of the femur. Laminated periosteal

reaction overlying the extraosseous tumor component
(arrow). A short echo time (TE = 9 msec) can sharply delineate
the calcium-containing periosteal reaction, despite the increased susceptibility of the measuring sequence.

to improve the delineation of focal sclerosis or periosteal reaction.

Soft-tissue Extension

Both CT and MRI can delineate the soft tissue mass of a
primary soft tissue or bone tumor. Since normal soft tissues and the soft tissue components of either tumor
often have the same radiodensity, CT largely has to rely
on indirect signs to determine soft extension, such as
obliterated intermuscular fatty septa and displaced
neighboring structures. The limited separation of intrinsically different soft tissue structures can be improved by adding intravenous injection of contrast medium to the CT examination (59, 82, 96), exploiting the
differences in tissue enhancement. Even with contrast
enhancement, however, CT does not achieve the discriminating tissue contrast of MRI and remains inferior
to MRI in delineating the extent of soft tissue lesions
(73).

   In summary, MRI is clearly superior to unenhanced
and enhanced CT for the determination of the soft-
tissue extent of primary tumors of the bone and soft tissues. The major reason is the greater contrast between
normal and abnormal tissue offered by MRI (1, 108).

Involvement of Neurovascular Bundles

MRI is also superior to CT in exhibiting the relationship
between tumor and neurovascular bundle and in demonstrating any neurovascular involvement (Fig. 12.**9**) (1,
11, 73, 75, 108). Bloem and co-workers (11) reported a
sensitivity, specificity, and accuracy of 33%, 93%, and

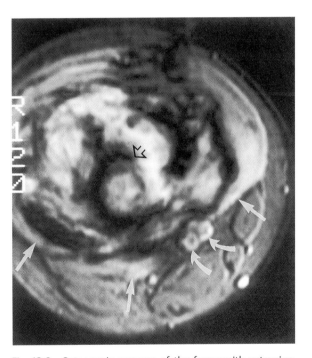

Fig. 12.**9**   Osteogenic sarcoma of the femur with extension
toward vascular structures. $T_2{}^*$-weighted GRE image shows
tumor compression (straight arrows) on the popliteal artery
and vein (curved arrow), but no encasement. The tumor has
caused extensive cortical destruction (open arrow).

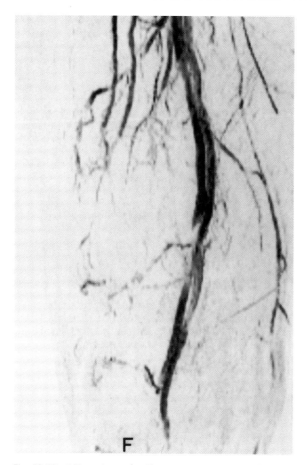

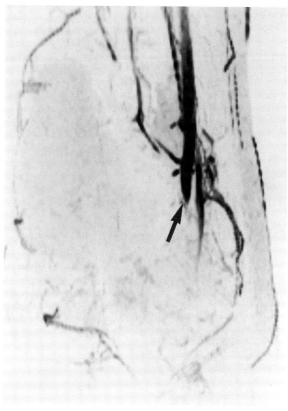

Fig. 12.**10**   MR angiography. The osteogenic sarcoma (not visible in this display) has displaced the popliteal artery and vein medially. The vessels are still patent and not encased by the tumor.

Fig. 12.**11**   MR angiography. A patient with an osteogenic sarcoma that has encased and compressed adjacent vessels, leading to lack of visualization of the vessels distal to the tumor (arrow).

82% for CT and 100%, 98%, and 98%, respectively, for MRI.

In some instances, the use of intravenous Gd-DTPA obscures the differentiation of tumor from adjacent fat (82). On unenhanced T_1-weighted images, the tumor is characteristically of low signal intensity and clearly separated from the surrounding high signal fat. After enhancement, the tumor increases in signal intensity and may be less well differentiated from fatty tissue (26, 82).

MR angiography is especially well suited to delineate tumor displacement (Fig. 12.**10**) or encroachment and encasement (Fig. 12.**11**) of the vessels (52).

Differentiation between Peritumoral Edema and Extraosseous Tumor

Both viable tumor and peritumoral edema exhibit a high signal intensity on post-contrast T_1-weighted images. Pettersson and co-workers (76) obtained conventional T_1-weighted images after administration of Gd-DTPA on five patients with soft-tissue tumors and found

strong enhancement in the tumor and in the peritumoral edema. Using a similar technique, Hanna and co-workers (38) observed a strong enhancement in viable tumor, granulation tissue and peritumoral edema.

Dynamic post-contrast MRI following intravenous bolus injection has emerged as a promising method for the differentiation of extraosseous tumor from perineoplastic edema. Lang and co-workers (53) obtained sequential images with an acquisition time of 3.5 seconds per image after bolus administration of contrast medium (Fig. 12.**12**). Using an exponential-fitting algorithm, the slope values of the contrast enhancement-time curves were calculated pixel-by-pixel and displayed as gray values in a computer-generated slope image (Fig. 12.**13**). The high temporal resolution and exponential fitting for calculating the initial slopes provided good differentiation between viable tumor and extraosseous edema. The initial slope values of viable extraosseous tumor and muscle infiltrated by tumor were 20% and more than those for perineoplastic edema (53). Since the computer-generated slope images define the margins of the lesion accurately, they

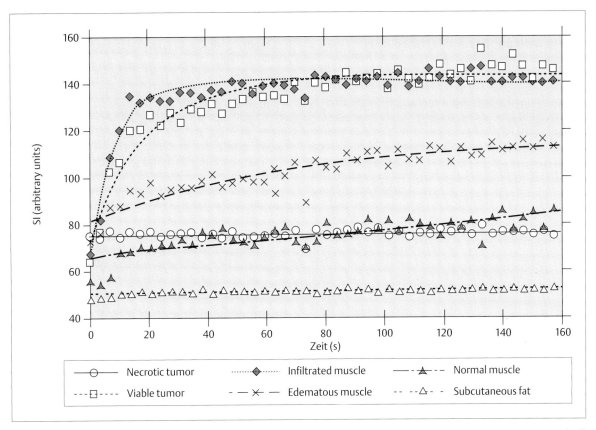

Fig. 12.**12** Contrast enhancement-time curve. Dynamic MRI can differentiate viable tumor and muscle infiltrated by tumor from edematous muscles and peritumoral edema. The slope value of the contrast enhancement-time curve is markedly greater for neoplastic tissue than for normal tissue (after 53).

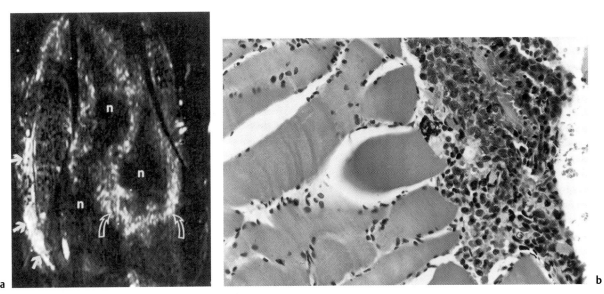

Fig. 12.**13 a, b** Computer-generated spatial mapping of the enhancement rate. **a** The gray scale is used to express the slope value of the enhancement rate, with bright areas indicating high initial slope values as found in aggressive tumor (curved arrows) or infiltrated muscles. Gray areas indicate a low initial slope value as found in perineoplastic edema (Fig. 12.**12**). The medial muscles show a bright area suspicious for tumor infiltration (arrows). **b** The photomicrograph confirms infiltrating tumor cells between the muscle fibers (after 53).
n necrosis

appear especially useful for preoperative planning of limb-sparing surgery. This technique might also play a role in monitoring the effect of chemotherapy.

Differentiation between Viable and Necrotic Tumor

MRI performed after intravenous administration of contrast medium can differentiate viable from necrotic tumor. Except for hypovascular tumors, viable tumors have a strong contrast enhancement. Necrotic areas within a tumor generally have no contrast enhancement and remain of low to intermediate signal intensity after administration of contrast medium (26, 51) (Fig. 12.**14**). It should be kept in mind, however, that the clinically available Gd-based complexes are low-molecular and, due to their small size, might diffuse into the areas of tumor necrosis by way of the extracellular space.

Traditionally, the clinical findings, such as a local soft-tissue swelling, determined the biopsy sites, with the inherent risk of obtaining a tissue sample from a necrotic area. Identifying the areas of viable tumor by dynamic contrast-enhanced MRI can help select the most suitable biopsy site (26, 51).

■ Monitoring the Effect of Therapy

It is highly desirable to know the response of tumors to chemotherapy considering the high morbidity of chemotherapy and the need to abandon an ineffective therapeutic regimen in favor of alternative regimens. It is difficult to measure the therapeutic response solely by clinical means. Clinical parameters of tumor response, such as local soft tissue swelling or hyperthermia, correlate poorly with histologic responses (45, 105). Furthermore, conventional radiography, angiography, CT and scintigraphy, all of which have been used to measure the response to chemotherapy in the past, are poor predictors with a specificity of around 50% (15, 84).

MRI is more sensitive and can provide morphologic as well as quantitative information of the chemotherapy effect. The morphologic findings of a therapeutic effect are:

- Decrease in tumor volume,
- Improved delineation of the muscle and intermuscular fatty septa,
- Appearance of cystic areas in the tumor matrix (44, 71).

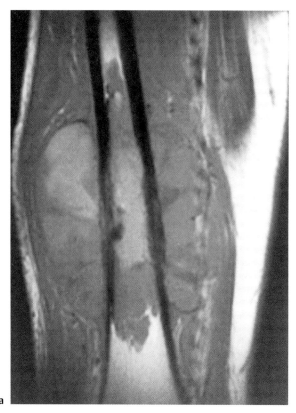
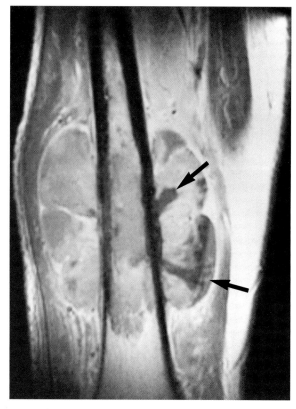

a

b

Fig. 12.**14a, b**   Osteogenic sarcoma with viable and necrotic components. **a** T₁-weighted pre-contrast MRI. The tumor in the distal femur has a predominately homogeneous low-signal intensity. **b** T₁-weighted post-contrast MRI. Large areas of the tumor show an intense enhancement corresponding to viable tissue. Necrotic areas fail to enhance and remain of low-signal intensity (arrows).

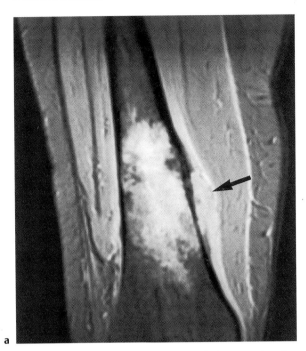
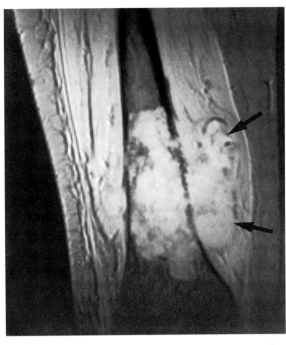

a

b

Fig. 12.**15 a, b** Osteogenic sarcoma before and after chemotherapy. **a** T_2^*-weighted GRE image. The tumor has a high signal intensity. Only a small extraosseous component is seen on this image obtained before chemotherapy (arrow).

b T_2^*-weighted GRE image. The extraosseous component has increased in size on this image obtained after chemotherapy (arrows). The intramedullary tumor has also grown. These interval changes indicate a chemotherapy failure.

An increase in tumor volume indicates an unfavorable response to chemotherapy (Fig. 12.**15**), while progressive calcifications along the periphery as well as in the central areas of an osteosarcoma are a sign of good response (17, 64). The perineoplastic edema decreases with a favorable tumor response (44, 71). Osteogenic sarcomas are frequently surrounded by a dark rim, corresponding to a layer of dense collagenous fibers that are continuous with the periosteum on the histologic examination. With a favorable tumor response, this dark rim can become thicker due to a decrease in the perineoplastic edema (71).

Pan and co-workers (71) discerned four major postchemotherapy patterns based on the MRI appearance of the tumor. A *dark pattern* was characterized by predominant areas of low and intermediate signal intensity on the T_1-weighted and T_2-weighted images. This reflected a good therapeutic response with small foci of residual tumor. A *mottled or speckled pattern* was characterized by a predominant area of intermediate intensity on the T_1-weighted image and a high intensity with interspersed areas of low-signal intensity on the T_2-weighted images. This pattern also corresponded to generally low levels of residual viable tumor. A *homogeneous pattern* was characterized by a predominant area of intermediate intensity on the T_1-weighted and high intensity on the T_2-weighted images and distinguished from the previous pattern by the absence of mottling. The homogeneous areas corresponded to macroscopic quantities of residual viable tumor. The *cystic pattern* was characterized by areas of intermediate intensity on T_1-weighted and high intensity on the T_2-weighted images, with a distinct multicystic or bubbly appearance. The finding also indicated a high proportion of residual viable tumor along the periphery of cysts (71).

Holscher and co-workers (44) demonstrated a significant correlation between poor pathologic response and increase in the high signal intensity of the extraosseous tumor component on serial T_2-weighted images (r = 0.57, p = 0.02). A chemotherapy-induced high T_2-weighted signal may also represent necrosis, cystic hemorrhagic areas or fibroblastic repair tissue (60).

A decrease in the signal intensity of the extraosseous component on T_2-weighted images correlated with a satisfactory therapy response (44). MacVicar and co-workers (60) found microscopic clusters of viable tumor in areas of both low and high signal intensity after treatment and concluded that MRI is unreliable for excluding active disease but suitable for providing qualitative evidence of chemotherapeutic effect by assessing the change in signal intensity.

Erlemann and co-workers (27) were able to demonstrate that dynamic MRI with rapid GRE sequences obtained after the bolus injection of Gd-DTPA can be used for assessing the response to preoperative chemotherapy. A drop in the slope value of the enhancement-time curve by at least 60% relative to the baseline value indicated a response to the therapy. Nonresponders generally had a drop of less than 60% (27). Similar findings have been reported by Fletcher and co-workers and by Hanna and co-workers (28, 29, 39, 40, 77).

Van der Wounde and co-workers (100) reported that remnant viable tumor was often located at the margins of the tumor or subperiosteally. The viable tumor areas showed early enhancement and rapid wash-out on dynamic MR images (100).

MR angiography might supplement the assessment of chemotherapeutic response. Decreased neovascularity is observed in patients who respond to therapy and persistent or even increased neovascularity in nonresponding patients (52, 54).

■ Recurrent Tumor and Postoperative Fibrosis or Edema

The differentiation between local recurrence and changes induced by surgery, chemotherapy, or radiotherapy can be difficult. Nodular lesions with low-signal intensity on T_1-weighted and high-signal intensity on T_2-weighted images are suspicious for recurrence (16, 35, 78, 101). Additional suspicious findings are a mass effect, infiltrative extension into the surrounding soft tissues and osseous destruction. In patients who underwent radiotherapy, lesions of high-signal intensity on the T_2-weighted image can be seen in active tumor as well as in radiation-induced inflammatory changes (101). Other causes of an increased T_2-weighted signal are listed in Tab. 12.**7**.

Areas of homogeneous, low signal intensity on T_1-weighted images that show no appreciable increase in signal intensity on the T_2-weighted images and lack any focal or nodular components generally reflect chronic sequelae following surgery, chemotherapy, or radiation therapy. Similar findings might be observed in rare cases of malignant fibrous histiocytomas with predominant fibroblastic component, precluding any reliable differentiation (78).

Reuther and colleague (78) compared CT and MRI for evidence of tumor recurrence. The sensitivity was 57.5% and the specificity 96.3% for CT, and 82.5% and 96.3%, respectively, for MRI, indicating that MRI is more sensitive for the detection of tumor recurrence (78). Postsurgical scars generally show an edema-equivalent signal up to 6 months after surgery, with a few cases ex-

hibiting edema with corresponding high signal intensity on T_2-weighted images for a much longer period after surgery. In these cases, a recurrence cannot be diagnosed unless this finding is associated with a space-occupying effect. These cases may benefit from evaluation by MTC since scar tissue, as opposed to malignant and most benign tumors (less than 25%), has a very high MTC effect (exceeding 50%) (see Chapter 1) (Fig. 12.**16**) (99).

Specific Section

Depending on the tissue of origin, numerous benign and malignant bone and soft-tissue tumors are distinguished (Tab. 12.**8**, page 324). Imaging alone rarely affords a definitive differentiation or classification. Though conventional radiography remains of great value, primarily due to its well-established criteria based on experience gathered over many years, MRI can add to the preoperative prediction of the histologic diagnosis, in addition to its contribution to tumor staging. The current state of clinical usefulness of MRI in evaluating and characterizing different tumor entities will be presented in the remaining sections of this chapter.

■ Malignant Bone Tumors

Osteosarcoma

Osteosarcomas comprise 20% of all primary malignant bone tumors, occurring most frequently between the ages of 10 to 15 years. The most common sites are the metaphyses of the long tubular bones, most frequently involving distal femur, proximal tibia, and humerus.

MRI is clinically most useful in the detection of intramedullary skip lesions, which occur in 25% of cases (Fig. 12.1), and for displaying the true extent of the bone marrow and soft tissue involvement (13, 94, 108). Dense sclerotic tumor components have a low signal intensity on T_1-weighted and T_2-weighted images. Cortical destruction and extensive perineoplastic edema are common (85) (Fig. 12.**9**).

The tumor is characteristically surrounded by a rim of low signal intensity on T_1-weighted and T_2-weighted images, corresponding to the periosteal reaction. Cystic and necrotic changes as well as fluid levels are frequently observed after chemotherapy (43).

Preoperative chemotherapy is administered to control micrometastases and to reduce the size and extent of the primary tumor as well as the peritumoral edema. Joint-saving surgery is generally attempted, but amputations are still often necessary. MRI is especially useful to follow patients undergoing chemotherapy. In case of an inadequate response, the chemotherapeutic regimen can be changed to offer the patient another chance of eliminating micrometastases and improving the prognosis. MRI is also well suited for detecting local tumor recurrence.

Table 12.**7**   Causes of high signal intensity at T_2-weighted imaging after treatment for musculoskeletal neoplasms (after 72)

- Tumor recurrence
- Residual perineoplastic edema
- Postsurgical changes: edema, hematoma, seroma, hemostatic packing material, granulation tissue (up to 6 months after surgery)
- Postradiation inflammatory changes
- Fat necrosis
- Atrophic muscle (e. g., denervation due to surgical trauma)
- Intercalary bone graft

Fig. 12.**16a–h** **a–d** Follow-up examinations after surgical removal of a malignant fibrous histiocytoma of the lower leg, axial plane. **a** GRE sequence. **b** MTC image. **c** T$_1$-weighted SE sequence. **d** Fat suppressed STIR sequence. Scar formation of the skin with marked decrease in signal intensity induced by the MTC pulse. Low signal visualization on the T$_1$-weighted image, high signal visualization on the fat-suppressed STIR image. This signal pattern of the scar on the T$_1$-weighted and fat suppressed image is also observed in tumors. The strong MT effect, however, favors a scar. **e–h** Follow-up after surgical removal of a leiomyosarcoma of the lower leg, axial plane. **e** GRE sequence. **f** MTC sequence. **g** MTC subtraction image. **h** Fat-suppressed STIR sequence. The cutaneous scar formation shows a markedly decreased signal intensity on the MTC image. The decrease in signal intensity is almost as pronounced as that found in the musculature. The MTC subtraction image accentuates this effect and displays scar and musculature as bright structure. The fat-suppressed STIR image shows a high-signal visualization of the scar. This signal pattern is uncharacteristic and can also be observed in tumor tissue.

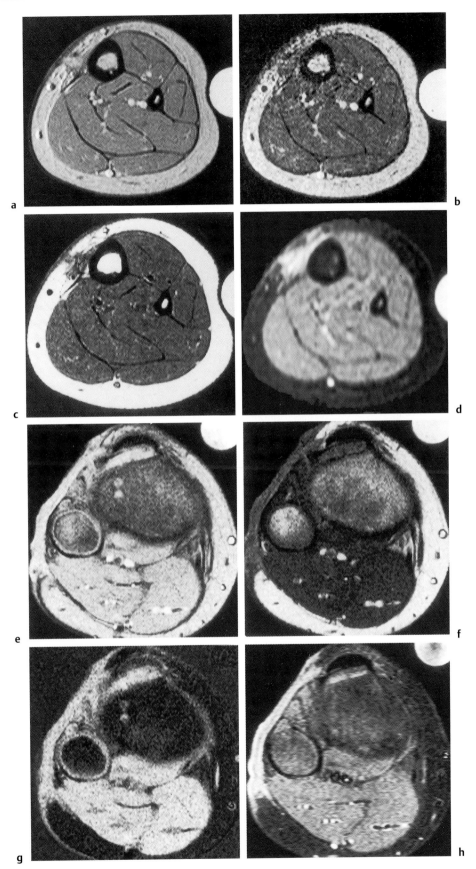

Table 12.**8** Primary musculoskeletal neoplasms (usual presenting Enneking stage in brackets) (modified from Netter, F.H.: The CIBA Collection of Medical Illustrations. Volume 8 : Musculoskeletal System, Part II. CIBA-GEIGY Corporation, West Caldwell, NJ 07006 [p. 118])

Tissue Type	Benign Tumors	Malignant Tumors
Bone tumors		
• Osseous	Osteoid Osteoma (2) Osteoblastoma (2–3) Osteoma (1)	Classic osteosarcoma (IIB) Parosteal osteosarcoma (IA) Periosteal osteosarcoma (IIA)
• Cartilaginous	Enchondroma (2) Exostosis (2) Periosteal chondroma (2) Chondroblastoma (2–3) Chondromyxoid fibroma (2–3)	Primary chondrosarcoma (IIB) Secondary chondrosarcoma (IA)
• Fibrous	Nonossifying fibroma (1–2) Desmoplastic fibroma (2–3) Fibrous dysplasia (NA) Ossifying fibroma (2–3)	Fibrosarcoma of bone (IIB) Malignant fibrous histiocytoma (IIB)
• Reticulo-endothelial	Eosinophilic granuloma (NA) Hands-Schüller-Christian disease (NA) Abt-Letterer-Siwe disease (NA)	Ewing's sarcoma (IIB) Reticulum-cell sarcoma (IIB) Myeloma (III)
• Vascular	Aneurysmal bone cyst (2) Hemangioma of the bone (2)	Angiosarcoma (IIB) – Hemangioendothelioma (IA) – Hemangiopericytoma (IA)
• Unknown	Solitary bone cyst (NA) Giant-cell tumor in bone (2–3)	Giant-cell sarcoma (IIB) Chordoma (IB) Adamantinoma (IA)
Soft-tissue tumors		
• Osseous	Myositis ossificans (NA)	Extraosseous osteosarcoma (IIB)
• Cartilaginous	Chondroma (2) Synovial chondromatosis	Extraosseous chondrosarcoma (IB)
• Fibrous	Fibroma (1–2) Fibromatosis (3)	Fibrosarcoma (I–IIB) Malignant fibrous histiocytoma (IIB)
• Synovial	Pigmented villonodular synovitis (2)	Synovial sarcoma (IIB)
• Vascular	Hemangioma (2–3)	Angiosarcoma (IIB) – Hemangioendothelioma (IB) – Hemangiopericystoma (IB)
• Fatty	Lipoma (1) Angiolipoma (3)	Liposarcoma (IA)
• Neural	Neurinoma (2) Neurofibroma (2–3)	Neurosarcoma (IIB) Neurofibrosarcoma (IIB)
• Muscular	Leiomyoma (2) Rhabdomyoma (2–3)	Leiomyosarcoma (IIB) Rhabdomyosarcoma (IIB)
• Unknown	Giant-cell tumor of the tendon sheath (2)	Epithelia sarcoma (IB) Clear cell sarcoma (IB) Mesenchymoma (IIB) Undifferentiated sarcoma (IIB)

NA = Enneking staging not applicable

Osteosarcomas characteristically arise in the intramedullary cavity. However, variants exist and from this central location the following entities can be distinguished histologically, radiographically, and prognostically:

• parosteal (juxta-articular) osteosarcoma with a lower grade of malignancy, growing primarily between cortex and musculature and only later infiltrating the intramedullary cavity,

• periosteal osteosarcoma with crater-like cortical erosion, growing along the outer surface of the cortex, macroscopically dominated by a chondroid matrix and also eliciting a periosteal reaction,

• telangiectatic osteosarcoma, appearing as predominantly osteolytic tumor with blood-filled pseudocysts and resembling an aneurysmal bone cyst.

On the basis of the dominating histologic differentiation, a distinction is made between osteoblastic (about 50% of the cases), chondroblastic (about 25%), and fibroblastic (about 25%) types. The radiographic features add a distinction between mixed, osteolytic and osteoblastic types (30). The osteosarcoma arising in pagetic bone is a separate entity.

Ewing Sarcoma

This is a highly malignant tumor, primarily occurring in children and arising in the intramedullary reticuloendothelial system. The Ewing sarcoma comprises about 10% of all primary bone tumors. In 90% of patients, it occurs between the ages of 5 and 30 years, with a peak incidence between the ages of 5 and 15 years. The Ewing sarcoma tends to originate in the lower skeleton, with two-thirds of the tumors affecting the pelvis, sacrum, femur, and tibia. The clinical manifestations can be dominated by fever and local signs of inflammation, resembling the findings of osteomyelitis.

In long bones the Ewing sarcoma most frequently occurs in metadiaphyseal or diaphyseal regions and, in contrast to a neuroblastoma, accompanied by local soft tissue swelling. Sclerotic areas can be observed in the intramedullary component but rarely in the soft tissues. The primary tumor is treated with radiation and chemotherapy, followed by resection according to some protocols. The main role of MRI is in staging and monitoring therapy. In some cases, MRI demonstrates a low signal thickening and lamination of the overlying periosteum corresponding to the radiographic onion-skin finding (Fig. 12.**17**).

Chondrosarcoma

Chondrosarcoma is the third most common primary malignant bone tumor, accounting for about 20% of these tumors. It usually occurs after the age of 45 years. Secondary osteosarcomas arise from pre-existing benign cartilaginous tumors, such as an osteochondroma or enchondroma. About 45% of the tumors are in long tubular bones although the pelvis is another common site (Fig. 12.**18**). Low signal calcifications are frequently encountered in the cartilaginous matrix (Fig. 12.**19**). The tumors frequently exhibit a scalloped contour on the T_2-weighted image, and may show a delicate ring-and-arc pattern of enhancement on the T_1-weighted image (32). The combination of these findings is highly specific for low-grade chondrosarcomas (19).

Aside from the classic, centrally or eccentrically located chondrosarcoma, the following variants are determined by cell type and location:

- undifferentiated high-grade chondrosarcoma with often barely recognizable anaplastic chondroid structure; the tumor is relatively aggressive; few calcifications;

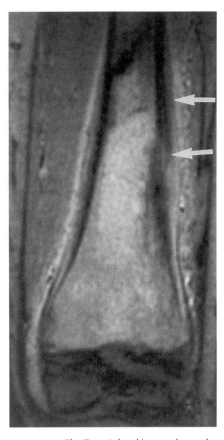

Fig. 12.**17**   Ewing sarcoma. The T_2-weighted image shows the intermedullary component of the lesion as area of moderate signal intensity. Cortex and periosteum appear thickened and partly laminated (arrows) corresponding to the onion-skin periosteal reaction seen on conventional radiographs.

- clear cell chondrosarcoma (chordochondral sarcoma) with interspersed clear cells; low-grade malignant tumor; few calcifications resembling those in chondroblastoma;
- juxta-articular low-grade chondrosarcoma, arising from the surface of the bone with well-differentiated cartilage and at times difficult to classify as malignant tumor; it has a tendency for late metastatic dissemination and contains exuberant calcifications.

Fibrosarcoma and Malignant Fibrous Histiocytoma

These malignant tumors have an even age distribution from the second to the seventh decade. The tumor usually affects the ends of the long tubular bones (Fig. 12.**20**). MRI lacks any characterizing findings, but can delineate the extent of intraosseous and extraosseous disease and may be used to monitor the response to chemotherapy (91).

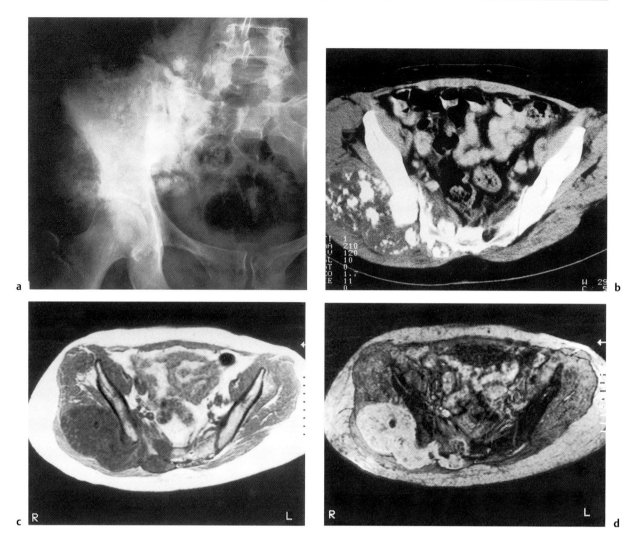

Fig. 12.**18a–d**   Chondrosarcoma of the pelvis. **a** Radiograph with ill-defined osseous destruction and soft tissue calcifications in projection of the right ilium. **b** CT. Osseous destruction and extensive calcifications in the tumor matrix of the large soft tissue component. **c** Axial T_1-weighted SE image with hy- pointense tumor containing multifocal signal voids caused by calcifications. **d** T_2^*-weighted GRE image. The tumor has a high signal intensity with multifocal signal voids. Clear demarcation of the tumor infiltration in the ilium and sacrum.

Angiosarcoma

The MRI presentation of the more aggressive vascular tumors, such as the angiosarcoma, hemangioendothelioma, and hemangiopericytoma, is similar (68), though often nonspecific. The presence of vascular structures supports the diagnosis. MRI can provide adjunct information for the diagnosis and for staging and therapeutic monitoring.

Primary Lymphoma

Primary lymphoma of bone, a rare entity, is usually located in the metaphysis and epiphysis of the long bones of the extremities. Primary osseous lymphoma characteristically has a heterogeneous signal pattern on T_2-weighted images. Areas of low signal intensity on the

T_2-weighted image may represent intratumoral fibrosis (87).

■ Benign Bone Tumors

Giant Cell Tumor

Giant cell tumors (osteoclastomas) occur in the long tubular bones, usually in the distal femur or proximal tibia, but can be found in the sacrum, and have a predilection for men between the ages of 20 and 40 years. The tumor arises in the epiphysis and can extend into the metaphysis. Owing to its distinctive radiographic features, it is generally diagnosed on conventional radiographs. MRI is performed to determine the extent of the lesion. It can be aggressive and break into the neighboring joint. In the knee, the articular involve-

Fig. 12.**19 a, b** Chondrosarcoma.
a T$_1$-weighted image demonstrates
the lesion in the distal femur. Occasional low-signal calcifications are
visible in the chondroid matrix
(arrows). **b** Macroscopic specimen
with longitudinal section through
the tumor.

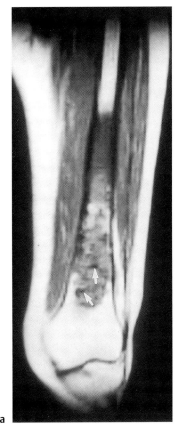

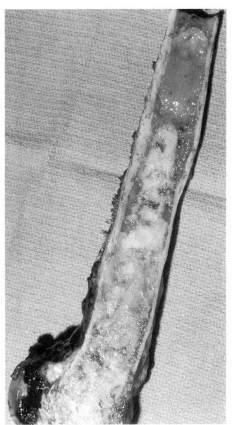

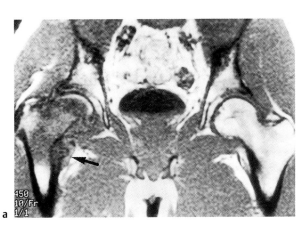

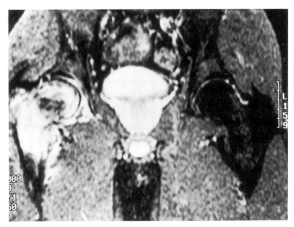

Fig. 12.**20 a, b** Malignant fibrous histiocytoma. **a** T$_1$-
weighted image. The tumor in the proximal femur has a low
signal intensity. Visualization of both intramedullary and extraosseous (arrow) component. **b** T$_2$-weighted image. The lesion has a high signal intensity. Articular extension with effusion.

ment extends from the osseous origin of the cruciate
ligaments. Clinically, the patient complains of local
pain. Joint effusion develops after erosion into the joint
space. MRI shows a sharply outlined tumor, usually displaying a low signal intensity on the T$_1$-weighted image
(Fig. 12.**21**). On the T$_2$-weighted image, the giant cell
tumor can be heterogeneous with areas of decreased

and increased signal intensity (95). Hemosiderin
deposits are common and appear as low signal intensity
on both T$_1$-weighted and T$_2$-weighted images (2). The
tumor tends to recur, and detecting recurrent tumor is
the major role of MRI. The cardinal findings of a locally
recurrent tumor are:

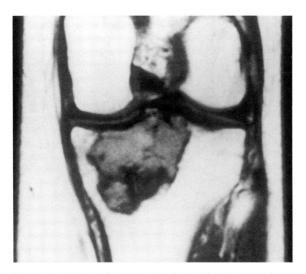

Fig. 12.**21**   Giant cell tumor. The T_1-weighted image shows the low signal lesion in the epiphysis, characteristically abutting the joint space. The tumor has also spread to the metaphysis. Signal-void tumor components representing hemosiderin deposits.

- resorption of the autogenous bone packed in the curettaged original lesion. However, this may also occur with infection,
- progressive osteolytic destruction.

■ Fibrous Bone Tumors

Fibrous Dysplasia

This condition represents a disordered maturation of bone with formation of immature fibrous tissue and is included in the tumor-like bone lesions. The process causes bone expansion and displaces normal bone. It affects adolescents and young adults, and can be monostotic or polyostotic. The polyostotic form may be part of a recognized syndrome (e.g., Albright syndrome: polyostotic fibrous dysplasia in young girls, associated with café-au-lait spots and sexual precocity). The monostotic type preferentially involves the proximal femur, proximal tibia, mandible and ribs. The lesions are largely in the metaphysis and diaphysis. The polyostotic type involves the long tubular bones and the short tubular bones of the hands and feet as well as the pelvis, and may be limited to one side of the skeleton.

The limited strength of the fibrous bone as well as pathologic fractures can produce severe deformities, especially in affected long tubular bones.

Conventional radiographs show a lesion of ground glass texture surrounded by a sclerotic rim, local deformity and coarse trabecular pattern representing remodeled trabeculae.

MRI shows a matrix of homogeneous, low signal intensity on the T_1-weighted image and, in the majority of cases, a homogeneous, high signal intensity on the T_2-weighted image (Fig. 12.**22**). In about one-third of cases, the signal intensity can be lower than or equal to muscle on the T_2-weighted images. Sclerotic rim and coarse trabeculations appear as signal-void in all sequences. Fractures and formation of secondary bone cysts lead to a more heterogeneous image pattern.

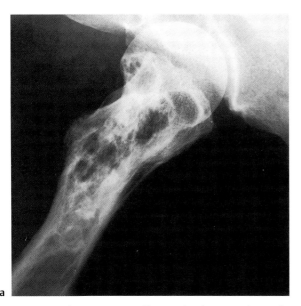

a

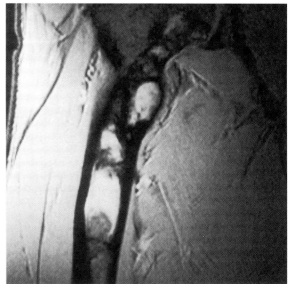

b

Fig. 12.**22 a, b**   Monostotic fibrous dysplasia involving the metadiaphyseal region of the femur. **a** Radiograph showing confluent osteolysis, sclerotic rims, and trabecular thickening.

b Coronal $T_2{}^*$-weighted GRE image. The process is dominated by homogeneous areas of high signal intensity, interrupted by signal-void sclerotic rims and thickened trabecular plates.

Nonossifying Fibroma (Benign Fibrous Cortical Defect, Fibroxanthoma)

This developmental aberration of the periosteal-formed cortex produces a fibrous lesion intermixed with fibroblasts, giant cells, and xanthomatous cells, usually in the metaphysis of the distal femur or distal tibia.

The lesion appears in childhood and adolescence and heals by ossification after completion of bone growth. On conventional radiographs, it is seen as an eccentric intracortical or extracortical lesion with trabeculations and a thin sclerotic rim. The radiographic pattern is pathognomonic. After healing, there may be residual focal sclerosis.

The MRI pattern is variable and depends on the age of the lesion. In the early stages, the defect is seen in a typical location as an area of slightly increased intensity on the T_1-weighted image (high proportion of lipid-laden xanthomatous cells) and low signal intensity on the T_2-weighted image .(hemosiderin, fibrous tissue). After healing is complete, the remaining sclerotic areas are seen as low signal intensity or signal void in all sequences. Subsequent resorption of the sclerosis equalizes the signal with the signal in the surrounding yellow bone marrow. The signal intensity pattern can be quite heterogeneous (65).

Desmoplastic Fibroma (Desmoid)

The desmoid tumor of bone predominantly involves the long tubular bones of young adults. The tumor appears aggressive (usually Enneking 3). Conventional radiographs can at times display large, sharply outlined, trabeculated osteolytic lesions, frequently with cortical erosions and soft tissue infiltrations.

MRI shows a nonspecific signal pattern, with low signal intensity on T_1-weighted and high signal intensity on T_2-weighted images (65).

Intraosseous Lipoma

These benign tumors present with MRI findings similar to those of soft tissue lipomas. The typical sites for the formation of intraosseous lipomas are the calcaneus and femoral neck. They have a high signal intensity on the T_1-weighted and intermediate to high signal intensity on T_2-weighted images. Fat necrosis with focal calcifications and variable degree of cyst formation can be observed (10, 66) (Fig. 12.**23**).

Eosinophilic Granuloma

This tumor-like lesion is characterized by a histiocytic infiltration of the bone marrow. Hand-Schüller-Christian disease and Letter-Siwe syndrome are different expressions of the same disease. Eosinophilic granuloma

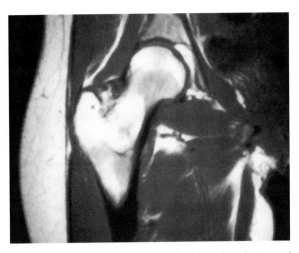

Fig. 12.**23** Intraosseous lipoma in the femoral neck. Coronal T_1-weighted SE image. High-signal space-occupying lesion with a central cystic component of low signal intensity. The tumor is surrounded by the low signal intensity of the residual hematopoietic bone marrow. Fatty marrow of equal intensity is seen in the greater trochanter, proximal femoral epiphysis, and the partially visualized diaphysis.

usually affects children, adolescents, and young adults, with a preponderance for males. It is more often unifocal than multifocal. The condition commonly affects the skull, mandible, spine, ribs, and long tubular bones, less often clavicle, pelvis, and scapula. It is almost never encountered in the bones of the hand and feet. Clinically, it presents with local pain, swelling, low-grade fever, elevated sedimentation rate, and, in its early stage, peripheral eosinophilia. Curettage is curative in the majority of cases. Eosinophilic granuloma develops through four different histopathologic stages (20) and this leads to a wide range of imaging features. The entire radiographic spectrum of bone destruction can be encountered, with correspondingly various MRI findings. Descriptively, an initial, intermediate and late phase can be distinguished (8). The initial phase is dominated by diffuse, indistinctly outlined osseous infiltration, accompanied by marrow edema, cortical destruction and periosteal reaction. This is followed by resolution of the marrow edema and a less aggressive appearing osseous process. In the late phase, the lesion is well-demarcated with no or only minimal marrow edema or soft tissue component.

The signal pattern is nonspecific, with decreased to slightly increased signal intensity on the T_1-weighted and increased to strongly increased signal intensity on the T_2-weighted images. The lesion shows strong enhancement.

Favored manifestations of the eosinophilic granuloma are the vertebra plana, beveled lesion in the skull due to a different extent of involvement of the external and internal table, central sequestra with a signal void on all sequences and soft tissue involvement, especially in the initial stages (Fig. 12.**24**).

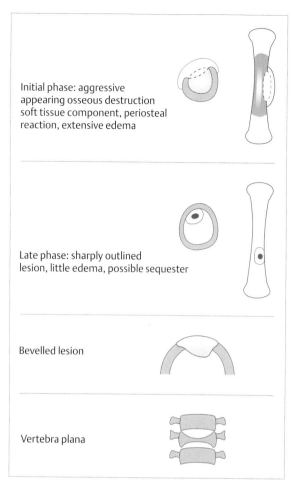

Initial phase: aggressive appearing osseous destruction soft tissue component, periosteal reaction, extensive edema

Late phase: sharply outlined lesion, little edema, possible sequester

Bevelled lesion

Vertebra plana

Fig. 12.24 A few characteristic features of the eosinophilic granuloma, depending on activity phase and location.
Initial phase: aggressive
apparent osseous destruction,
soft tissue component, periosteal reaction, extensive edema
Late phase: sharply outlined lesion,
little edema, possible sequestrum
Beveled lesion
in the calvaria
Vertebra plana

Finding a sequestrum raises a differential diagnosis of the following entities:

- osteomyelitis,
- fibrosarcoma,
- osteoid osteoma,
- intraosseous lipoma,
- eosinophilic granuloma,
- lymphoma.

If the eosinophilic granuloma is encountered in its early stage, osteomyelitis and Ewing sarcoma must be considered in the differential diagnosis.

■ Cartilaginous Bone Tumors

Chondroma (Enchondroma and Exostosis)

The enchondroma is a common benign bone tumor, observed in all age groups, and generally asymptomatic. It is usually located in the metaphysis of the long bones and is attributed to proliferated rests of epiphyseal cartilage. The tumor matrix consists of mature hyaline cartilage with characteristic lacunae, partially circular in arrangement. Their favored sites are the tubular bones, especially the short tubular bones of the hands and feet. Less common sites are the pelvis, with a purported greater rate of malignant transformation, and the scapula. The tumors are usually solitary, but can be multiple as part of hereditary syndromes (enchondromatosis, Ollier disease) with a higher risk of becoming malignant. A malignant transformation must be suspected clinically with the onset of new pain, scintigraphically with a sudden increase in the uptake of bone-specific tracer on serial bone scans, and radiographically with increasing blurring and heterogeneity of the lesion, cortical erosions, periosteal reaction, and so-called intracortical crests due to atypical ossifications.

Radiographically, the active early stage presents as well-circumscribed oval radiolucent lesion that expands and thins the cortex with scalloping of its endosteal surface. The cortical expansion can be pronounced (enchondroma protuberans). The inactive late stage is characterized by nodular or stippled calcifications of the chondroid matrix. It lacks the scalloped calcific rim that is typical of a bone infarct, its principal differential diagnostic consideration. The lesion shows increased tracer uptake on the bone scan.

On MRI, the enchondroma exhibits a characteristic finding determined by the scalloped outline of the chondroid matrix (Fig. 12.**25**):

- the T_1-weighted image demonstrates a slightly heterogeneous, predominantly low-signal lobulated lesion, with signal bands that probably represent residual fat,
- the T_2-weighted image shows a heterogeneous, predominantly high-signal lobulated lesion,
- the post-contrast image shows enhancement of scalloped margins and curvilinear septa (ring-and-arc pattern) between the non-enhancing cartilage matrix (3),
- all sequences depict punctate and circular signal voids representing calcifications of the chondroid matrix.

Another manifestation of the chondroma is the *parosteal or juxtacortical chondroma.* It arises from the periosteum of the long bones and produces a saucer-like erosion and sclerosis of the underlying outer cortex. Chondroid calcifications are rare. They may present as palpable painful swelling in adolescents and young adults. A typical location is the insertion of the deltoid muscle at the humerus (Fig. 12.**26**). MRI shows the typi-

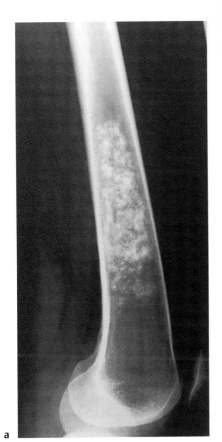

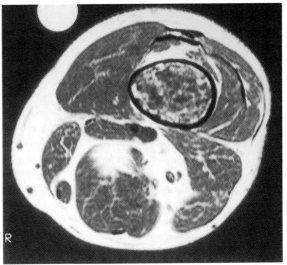

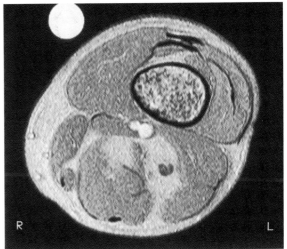

Fig. 12.**25 a–c** Enchondroma of the femur, inactive (latent phase), in an asymptomatic 50-year-old patient. **a** Radiograph with a discrete radiolucency, cortical scalloping and extensive punctate and coarse matrix calcifications. **b** T_1-weighted axial SE image. The tumor has largely a low signal intensity. It contains signal-void calcifications and high-signal residual fatty marrow, with partially circular and partially linear arrangement. Subtle cortical scalloping. **c** T_2^*-weighted GRE image. Heterogeneous tumor with high-signal matrix and punctate areas of signal-void calcifications.

cal finding of a chondroid matrix with displacement of the adjacent soft tissues.

Chondroblastoma

This relatively rare epiphyseal tumor tends to occur in the femur, humerus and tibia, although the foot, most often talus or calcaneus, accounts for 10% of the involved sites. It is usually painful. About 90% of chondroblastomas are encountered between the ages of 5 and 25 years. Chondroblastomas typically present as well-defined, round, lobulated lesions that are not larger than 5–6 cm. They can extend into the metaphyses, but involve the adjacent joint. The signal intensity is low on T_1-weighted and heterogeneous on T_2-weighted im-

ages. The heterogeneity with low-signal areas on the T_2-weighted image is attributed to a chondroid matrix with fibrous stroma and calcifications. Perineoplastic marrow edema, cortical expansion and periosteal reaction with an overlying soft edema suggest an aggressive lesion (Enneking 3) (Fig. 12.**27**).

Chondromyxoid Fibroma

This uncommon asymptomatic tumor typically occurs in adolescents and presents as an eccentric lesion in the metaphysis of long tubular bones. Its matrix is composed of varying proportions of chondroid, fibrous and myxoid tissue. Calcifications are generally absent. MRI does not display the typical findings of a chondroid

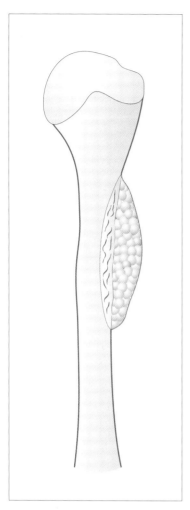

Fig. 12.**26**   Periosteal chondroma in the region of the deltoid insertion of the humerus, coronal schematic drawing. Tumor along the humeral surface with cortical impression and erosion, as well as cartilaginous matrix.

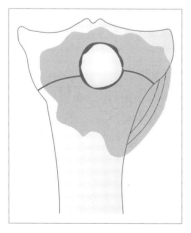

Fig. 12.**27**   Highly aggressive chondroblastoma (Enneking stage 3) in the tibial epiphysis. Coronal schematic drawing. Metaphyseal intrusion, bone marrow edema, periosteal reaction, soft tissue edema.

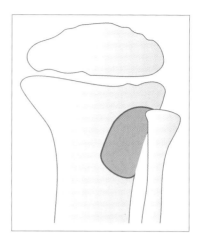

Fig. 12.**28**   Chondromyxoid fibroma in a child. Coronal schematic drawing. Smoothly delineated tumor without bone marrow or soft tissue edema in the tibial metaphysis.

matrix. The MRI features are not diagnostic with decreased signal intensity on T_1-weighted and increased signal intensity on T_2-weighted images (Fig. 12.**28**).

Osteochondroma

The osteochondroma (synonymous with ecchondroma or cartilage capped exostosis) is a common benign tumor, which is either developmental or acquired after trauma or irradiation. Osteochondromas can be solitary or multiple, and 70–80% are diagnosed before the age of 20 years. They frequently arise from the metaphyses of long tubular bones, but can affect the pelvis and scapula. By identifying the cartilage cap of the exostosis and the continuity of the exostotic cortex and medullary space with the cortex and medullary space the bone, MRI displays the characteristic morphologic features of osteochondromas (Fig. 12.**29**) (46). Typically the cartilaginous cap measures less than 1 cm in thickness. Where the cartilage cap is thicker than 2 cm consideration must be given to the possibility of malignant transformation with the development of a chondrosarcoma. It is important to consider that the cartilage cap is usually thicker in younger patients before cessation of bone growth (56). In the adult the cap may even be absent. Other signs of malignant transformation include associated bone destruction or erosion and soft tissue invasion.

Multiple osteochondromas have a higher risk of malignant transformation. Whenever an osteochondroma becomes painful or begins to enlarge, the development into a chondrosarcoma must be considered. Benign osteochondromas rarely cause local pain, unless they become large enough to press on adjacent structures, for instance, on a bursa with resultant bursitis. Most osteochondromas are palpated as a nontender bony mass adjacent to a joint. Osteochondromas grow outward pointing away from the nearest joint and can

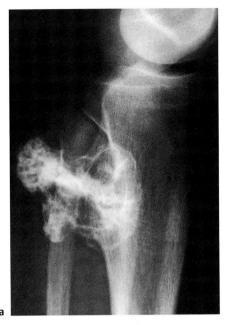

a

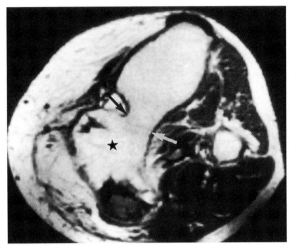

b

Fig. 12.**29 a, b** Osteochondroma (ecchondroma or exostosis). **a** The conventional radiograph shows a partially sclerotic lesion arising on a stalk from the proximal tibia. **b** T₁-weighted image. The lesion (*) is seen in the posteromedial soft tissues. An important characteristic finding is the continuation of the tibial bone marrow into the lesion (arrow).

be broad-based or pedunculated. They are readily diagnosed radiographically. The cartilage cap is effectively evaluated by MRI. Multiple exostoses are observed as a manifestation of the syndrome of hereditary cartilaginous exostoses or diaphyseal aclasia, with a predilection of the exostoses around the knee and in the pelvis. It can be associated with considerable deformities.

MRI readily shows that both the cortex and medullary cavity of the exostosis are continuous with those of the bone from which the exostosis arises. On T₁-weighted images the cap is usually of intermediate intensity, but on T₂-weighted sequences the cap is of homogeneous high intensity corresponding to hyaline cartilage elsewhere.

◼ Aneurysmal Bone Cyst

In 80% of cases, this tumor occurs in patients younger than 20 years, and typically involves the metaphyses of the long tubular bones and the posterior vertebral elements, but it can be observed in the pelvis. Histologically, the tumor consists of blood-filled spaces that are lined by granulation tissue, osteoid and multinucleated giant cells. Calcifications may be present. The tumor expands and erodes the cortex. The pathogenesis is not clear. One theory postulates vascular proliferations following hemorrhage into a primary tumor, such as giant cell tumor, chondroblastoma, nonossifying fibroma, and chondromyxoid fibroma, as well as unicameral bone cyst, fibrous dysplasia, fibrous histiocytoma, eosinophilic granuloma and malignant tumors. The underlying condition can involute completely or remain

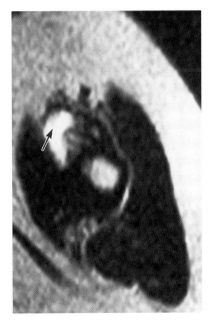

Fig. 12.**30** Exostosis of the humerus. Axial T₂-weighted TSE image. The cortical region of the stalk is transected and visualized as low-signal structure. Its central lumen (not visualized) contains fatty bone marrow. A large cartilaginous cap is visualized as high signal structure (arrow).

detectable by tissue remnants. Most patients typically complain of swelling and moderate pain. Curettage of the lesion is adequate as initial treatment. Recurrences should be aggressively treated with radical surgical ex-

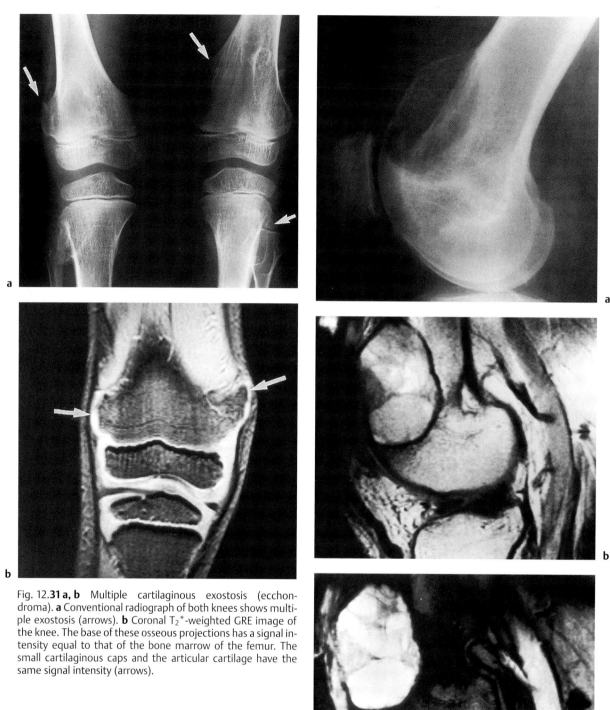

Fig. 12.**31 a, b** Multiple cartilaginous exostosis (ecchondroma). **a** Conventional radiograph of both knees shows multiple exostosis (arrows). **b** Coronal $T_2{}^*$-weighted GRE image of the knee. The base of these osseous projections has a signal intensity equal to that of the bone marrow of the femur. The small cartilaginous caps and the articular cartilage have the same signal intensity (arrows).

cision although embolization may have a role either on its own or in combination with surgery.

On MRI, the aneurysmal bone cyst typically has a rim of low signal intensity and multiple central areas with a wide range of signal intensities on T_1-weighted and T_2-weighted images, often with fluid-fluid levels in well-defined cystic cavities. The layering of different intensities probably reflects intracystic hemorrhage of different ages (6, 108) (Fig. 12.**32**). The aneurysmal bone cyst shows intense enhancement after intravenous injection of contrast medium.

Fig. 12.**32 a–c** Aneurysmal bone cyst. **a** The conventional radiograph shows a lytic lesion in the distal femur. **b** The T_1-weighted image shows the lesion to be heterogeneous with high and low signal components. **c** The T_2-weighted image shows multiple, delicate septations in the otherwise high signal lesion.

■ Unicameral Bone Cyst

The unicameral bone cyst is a cystic cavity filled with a yellow transparent fluid and lined with a membrane. It typically occurs in the long bones of children 3–14 years of age. Its pathogenesis is not known. It is most frequently recognized after fracture following a minor trauma. It originates next to the epiphysis and migrates further into the diaphyses with longitudinal bone growth. The active phase is followed by the inactive or latent phase with separation of the cyst from the cartilage. It is the inactive phase that is diagnosed as a large well-demarcated diaphyseal cyst in adolescents older than 14 years. Unicameral bone cysts may be multiple. The differential diagnosis includes fibrous dysplasia and aneurysmal bone cyst. Curettage and introduction of bone chips is generally the treatment of choice. Injection of corticosteroids has been advocated. The recurrence rate of cysts treated in the latent stage is lower than that of cysts treated in the active stage.

MRI demonstrates a cystic appearance, with a smooth low-signal or signal-void rim surrounding the fluid-filled cavity of low signal intensity on T_1-weighted and high signal intensity on T_2-weighted images. Contrast enhancement is not observed. Gas may accumulate in the cyst and is detected as an air-fluid level. Diagnostic evaluation by MRI is not necessary in the majority of unicameral bone cysts.

■ Hemangioma

The hemangioma is a benign vascular tumor, often seen as an incidental finding in middle-aged patients. It tends to occur in the vertebral bodies (see Chapter 1), skull and facial bones. The typical MRI findings consist of increased signal intensity on both T_1-weighted and T_2-weighted images. The increased signal intensity on the T_1-weighted image is attributable to the fatty component of the hemangioma, while the increased signal intensity on the T_2-weighted image is not easily characterized and remains a matter of speculation (80). Postcontrast images show enhancement.

MRI may be valuable for determining the aggressiveness of vertebral hemangiomas in patients with spinal cord and nerve root compression. It has been hypothesized that vertebral hemangiomas with a predominantly fatty stroma and a high signal intensity on the T_1-weighted image represent an inactive form and those with a predominantly soft-tissue stroma and a low signal intensity on the T_1-weighted image, an aggressive form with potential to compress the spinal cord (42, 55).

■ Osteogenic Tumors

Osteoid Osteoma

The osteoid osteoma is an osteoid-producing lesion, which is generally not larger then 1.5 cm. Because of its small size, it has also been called a confined or small osteoblastoma. It has a predilection for the long tubular bones, especially of the lower extremities. The bones of the hands and feet as well as the posterior vertebral elements are less frequently affected sites. In principle, any bone can be involved. The lesion is most frequently seen in the 10 to 35 year age group. Patients typically complain of pain that is worse at night and relieved by aspirin. The vertebral location can induce muscle spasm and secondary scoliosis.

The osteoid osteoma follows a natural evolution characterized by different degrees of activity: early phase, intermediate phase, and late phase with growth arrest and possible spontaneous regression.

The imaging findings of the osteoid osteoma are determined by its activity as well as by the specific bone it involves and the site of involvement in that bone. Four different types can be distinguished on the basis of the skeletal location:

Cortical Type. This comprises 80–90% of all osteoid osteomas and is by far the most common manifestation. The center of the tumor (nidus) is in the cortex and appears as localized radiolucency less than 1.5 cm in diameter. It can contain linear, punctate, or coarse calcifications. Radiographic identification of the nidus may require tomography. Finding the nidus is clinically relevant since the nidus must be resected in its entirety for curative treatment without risk of recurrence. Two separate nidal radiolucencies can occur, but this is rare. In the absence of calcifications, the nidus has a decreased signal intensity on T_1-weighted and an increased signal intensity on T_2-weighted images. The signal intensities around the nidus correlate with the extent of the sclerotic response in the surrounding bone. Before complete mineralization, MRI might display the reactive sclerosis at a higher signal intensity than normally mineralized trabeculae. This reactive sclerosis is the most conspicuous radiographic finding. It can involve the cortex of the long bone eccentrically or circumferentially (Fig. 12.**33a**). The completely mineralized reactive sclerosis is seen as signal void on MRI and is indistinguishable from a nidus that is calcified. MRI may show an accompanying marrow edema as well as a soft tissue edema with enhancement after injection of contrast medium (4, 36, 37, 106) (Fig. 12.**34**), indicating an active lesion.

Some debate exists as to the relative merits of CT and MRI as diagnostic tools for osteoid osteoma. While MRI readily demonstrates the accompanying marrow edema, it is less accurate in detecting the nidus and, since edema is a non-specific finding, many argue that CT is the modality of choice for imaging this lesion.

Medullary (Trabecular) Type. This type is observed less frequently. The nidus is located in medullary spongiosa (femoral neck, carpal and tarsal bones) and surrounded by a moderate, asymmetric sclerotic rim. The calcification is often most dense centrally, creating a

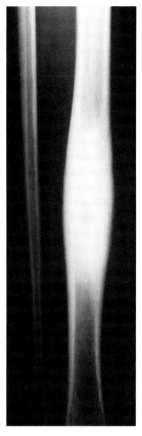

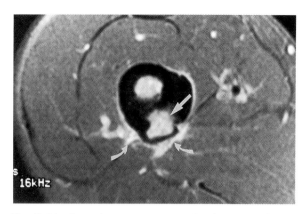

Fig. 12.**34** Osteoid osteoma. T_2-weighted image. The intracortical nidus has a high signal intensity (arrow). Discrete high-signal edema is seen in the adjacent soft tissues (curved arrows).

target configuration. Radiographs show a large round calcification up to 2 cm in diameter, surrounded by a thin radiolucent rim. MRI displays the central calcifications as signal void and its surrounding thin rim as decreased signal intensity on T_1-weighted and increased signal intensity on T_2-weighted images. Extensive edema is observed in the adjacent bone marrow. Lesions close to the articular surface induce a reactive synovitis with effusion and synovial proliferations.

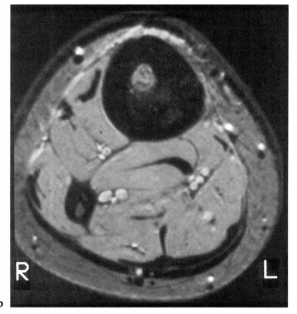

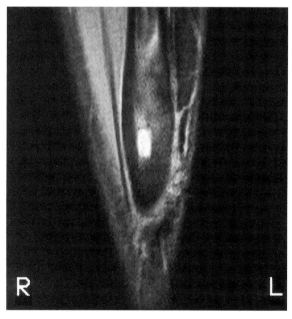

Fig. 12.**33 a–c** Cortical osteoid osteoma. S/P resection of the nidus. **a** Radiograph. Marked residual fusiform sclerosis involving the entire tibial circumference. Central surgical defect. **b** Axial T_2^*-weighted GRE image. The sclerosis appears as signal void. No soft tissue or bone marrow edema of this postsurgi-cally inactive process. **c** Coronal STIR image. The sclerotic area is seen as signal void and the smoothly delineated surgical defect as high signal area. No edematous changes. In summary, no evidence of recurrence.

Subperiosteal Type. This is an extremely rare type. The nidus is subperiosteal in location and does not induce a reactive sclerosis, but a periosteal ossification. This can be accompanied by a reactive edematous soft tissue swelling with corresponding MRI findings.

Intra-articular Type. This type is located in an intra-articular (or juxta-articular) osseous segment. Its synovial inflammatory response may lead to findings that suggest inflammatory joint disease by conventional radiography and MRI. Involvement of the epiphyseal plate can interfere with normal bone growth.

Surgical resection of the entire nidus or spontaneous regression lead to slow resolution of the reactive sclerosis. If new edematous changes are seen in the bone or soft tissues on follow-up MRI examinations, a recurrence is likely (Fig. 12.**33**).

Osteoblastoma

The osteoblastoma is an osteoid-producing tumor that is closely related to the osteoid osteoma. It is larger than 1.5 cm in diameter and has been called a giant osteoid osteoma. It has a predilection for the vertebral bodies, but can occur in the long tubular bones and, in principle, in any skeletal region. It is generally found in the 10 to 30 years age group, sharing the same age distribution as the osteoid osteoma. Moreover, osteoblastoma and osteoid osteoma share the same features on both conventional radiography and MRI, except for the somewhat more aggressive appearance of the osteoblastoma. Osteoblastoma stage 3 has been referred to as a pseudo-malignant osteoblastoma. In comparison with the osteoid osteoma, the osteoblastoma is usually accompanied by a lesser degree of reactive sclerosis. Clinically, it is generally asymptomatic, but if pain occurs, it is inadequately relieved by aspirin. Osteoblastomas may calcify entirely and can be associated extensive soft tissue and marrow edema with corresponding MRI findings.

Osteoma

This entity is formed by mature, densely sclerotic bone in the skull and facial bones (from which it protrudes into the paranasal sinuses), trabecular bone (bone island, enostosis) and juxta-articular, para-osseous region with extension into the soft tissues. It is characterized by its high radiodensity on conventional radiography and signal void on MRI.

■ Malignant Soft-Tissue Tumors

Most malignant soft-tissue tumors have indistinct margins and often infiltrate the surrounding structures (73). Most malignant lesions are heterogeneous on T_2-weighted images (73). Invasion of neighboring bone and encasement and infiltration of neurovascular bundles favor malignancy, but can be seen in benign lesions (49, 62, 63, 73). On T_1-weighted images, malignant lesions have a variable signal pattern, but the signal intensity is generally lower than fat. On T_2-weighted images, the signal intensity of most malignant lesions is increased relative to muscle (73). The malignant fibrous histiocytoma, however, can have a low signal intensity on the T_2-weighted image.

Malignant Fibrous Histiocytoma

Malignant fibrous histiocytoma can arise in soft tissues as well as in bone, and is the most common malignant soft-tissue tumor in adults. The average patient age is 50 years (20). It has a high recurrence rate (up to 45%). Multiple histologic variants are recognized. The most important variants are composed of histiocytic, fibromatous or xanthomatous cells (22). The malignant fibrous histiocytoma exhibits a low to intermediate signal intensity on T_1-weighted and a heterogeneous high signal intensity on T_2-weighted images (61, 62) (Fig. 12.**35**). The signal changes are not specific for malignant fibrous histiocytoma. If the fibromatous cells predominate, the tumor can take on a low signal intensity on the T_2-weighted image (91, 93). The tumor shows a relatively strong, heterogenous enhancement. Intratumoral necroses are common.

Liposarcoma

The liposarcoma is a frequent malignant tumor in adults, with the greatest incidence between the ages of 40 and 60 years. They tend to occur in the extremities and retroperitoneum, where they are notorious for developing into large tumors. They are divided into four variants, with the grade of malignancy inversely proportional to the amount of fat in the cytoplasmic vacuoles and proportional to the number of polymorphic cells (97):

- *well differentiated liposarcoma*, low-grade malignancy, predominantly atypical lipocytes, resembling a lipoma, traversed by fibrous septa,
- *myxoid liposarcoma* (Fig. 12.**36**), the most common subtype (40–50% of all liposarcomas), low-grade malignancy, predominantly lipoblasts of different degrees of maturity, myxoid ground substance,
- *round cell liposarcoma*, high-grade malignancy, hypercellular,
- *pleomorphic liposarcoma*, high-grade malignancy, bizarre pleomorphic cells.

Hypercellular, high-grade malignant tumors can be devoid of any normal fat cells and are indistinguishable from other soft tissue sarcomas by MRI. Well-differentiated liposarcomas show no or only little contrast enhancement. Moreover, the well-differentiated liposarcoma is well-circumscribed and can easily be mistaken for a benign lipoma (48, 50). The other variants are indistinctly outlined. The undifferentiated high-grade malignant liposarcoma shows intense contrast en-

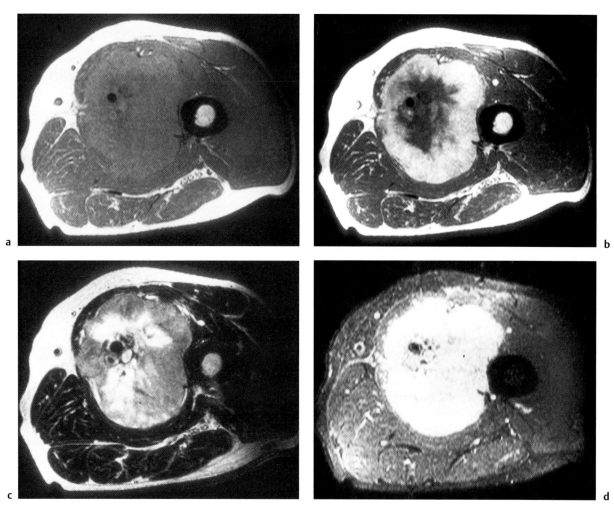

Fig. 12.**35 a–d**   Malignant fibrous histiocytoma of the thigh. Axial plane. **a** T$_1$-weighted SE image showing the tumor to be of low signal intensity, slightly more intense than the muscula-ture. **b** Heterogeneous enhancement. **c** T$_2$-weighted TSE image. Heterogeneous high-signal tumor. **d** Fat-suppressed STIR image. Tumor encasement of a central vessel.

hancement, with a heterogeneously mottled to circular pattern (97). Newly appearing necrotic areas suggest ongoing dedifferentiation of the tumor. Myxoid and necrotic areas have a high signal intensity on T$_2$-weighted images.

Liposarcomas have a high recurrence rate.

Synovial Sarcoma

This malignant tumor arises from the soft tissues and mimics the histology of synovial tissue. However, it does not arise from the synovial lining of the joint capsule and less than 10% are intra-articular. It usually occurs in young adults. It grows slowly and tends to involve the lower extremity. Metastases and local recurrence after resection are frequent. Extensive calcifications, which typically occur along the periphery, are found in one-third of patients.

The MRI signal pattern is nonspecific, with decreased signal intensity on T$_1$-weighted and increased

signal intensity on T$_2$-weighted images. Morphologically, the tumor is lobulated and smoothly outlined, has septations, and contains fluid levels due to hemorrhage.

Angiosarcoma

Angiosarcomas are rare and frequently arise on the basis of chronic lymphedema (see 'Differential diagnosis of the swollen extremity by MRI' in the Appendix, page 377) as so-called Stewart-Treves Syndrome after mastectomy. Specific MRI criteria have not been established.

■ Benign Soft-Tissue Tumors

Lipoma

Lipomas are benign soft-tissue tumors. They typically have a high signal intensity on T$_1$-weighted (Fig. 12.**37**) and an intermediate to high signal intensity on T$_2$-

weighted (Fig. 12.**3**) images, corresponding to the signal pattern of fat-containing tissue (75). The tumor is generally homogeneous in both sequences. It is encapsulated and can be septated. The possibility of a liposarcoma must be raised if the signal pattern is heterogeneous or the tumor outline indistinct.

Lipomas generally occur in the subcutaneous fat tissue (superficial lipomas), but can be found in deeper soft tissue structures (deep lipomas) (67 a), in muscles (intramuscular and intermuscular lipomas), in bone (intraosseous lipoma), and in the periosteum (periosteal or para-osseous lipoma), as well as together with fibrous (fibrolipoma) or vascular (angiolipoma) proliferations. Lipomatosis refers to a neoplastic or possibly drug-induced (corticosteroids) reactive space-occupying proliferation of adipose tissue. It can arise in several regions of the body, including mediastinum, abdomen, pelvis, or spinal canal (epidural lipomatosis) (Fig. 12.**38**) (98). Epidural lipomatosis can lead to neurologic deficits and can involve the thoracic as well as the lumbar spinal canal. In contradistinction to lipomas, lipomatosis is not encapsulated.

One further entity that is recognized is the atypical lipoma. This appears similar to (and may be impossible to differentiate radiologically from) a low grade liposarcoma. It contains a large amount of fatty tissue but will contain some areas of poorly defined non-fatty material. While these lesions behave benignly and do not metastasize, they do have a great propensity to recur after surgery. They may rarely undergo sarcomatous transformation.

Intramuscular Myxoma

The intramuscular myxoma is a benign mesenchymal lesion (24) and most commonly occurs in patients between the ages of 50 and 70 years. The pathologically altered fibroblasts produce an excess amount of mucopolysaccharides and lack the capability of producing normal collagen. Intramuscular myxomas most frequently occur in the thigh, but can be found at other sites, such as shoulder, upper arm, and buttocks (24). A notable incidence of associated fibrous dysplasia has been observed in some patients with multiple intramuscular myxomas (24). The intramuscular myxoma is sharply marginated within the muscle (47, 74, 96). Its signal intensity is lower than that in normal muscle on T_1-weighted images and strongly increased on T_2-weighted images, comparable to the signal pattern of a cyst. Unlike a cyst, however, the myxoma shows heterogeneous enhancement after intravenous injection of contrast medium (74). Myxoid tissue can also be produced by other tumors, such as myxoid liposarcoma, myxoid chondrosarcoma and myxoid malignant fibrous histiocytoma, but also by ganglion cells, and finding myxoid tissue in biopsy material is not diagnostic of an intramuscular myoma. A neurinoma is a differential diagnostic consideration of the MRI pattern. A less common variant is the juxta-articular myxoma which, apart

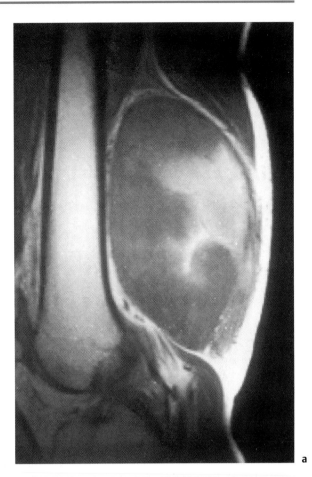

a

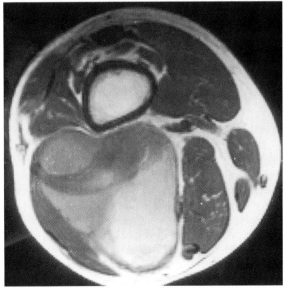

b

Fig. 12.**36 a, b** Myxoid liposarcoma. **a** Sagittal T_1-weighted image. Fat-equivalent, high-signal intensity in the posterior aspect of the tumor. The anterior aspect of the tumor shows a low-signal intensity. This marked heterogeneity suggests the diagnosis of a myxoid liposarcoma. **b** The axial T_1-weighted image confirms the fat-containing, high-signal portion and the heterogeneous low-signal areas in the tumor.

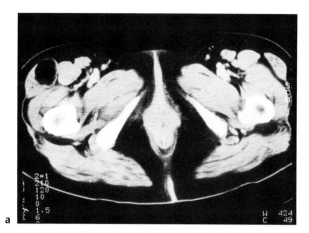

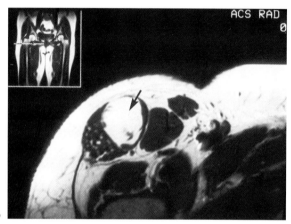

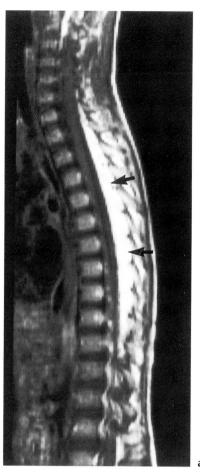

Fig. 12.**37 a, b**   Intramuscular lipoma of the tensor fascia latae. **a** CT showing a hyperdense space-occupying lesion in the enlarged muscle. **b** Axial T$_1$-weighted SE image showing a high-signal space-occupying lesion in the muscle (arrow).

from it location, appears similar to the intramuscular form.

Desmoid (Extra-abdominal Desmoid, Aggressive Fibromatosis)

Extra-abdominal desmoids arise in the fibrous tissue of muscles, fasciae and aponeurosis, and tend to occur in the thigh, upper arm, and buttock. The age of the patients is generally between 15 and 40 years (79). Desmoids are poorly demarcated and characteristically grow aggressively and infiltrate neighboring structures. They can be multicentric, but do not metastasize. The lesion often has a paucity of cells, which are interspersed in dense collagenous fibers. Recurrence after local resection is common (between 25% and 68%) (79). The major role of MRI consists of determining the extent of the desmoid and its relationship to the neurovascular bundles. MRI can also be used for the early detection of recurrent disease.

The cellular areas of the desmoid have homogeneously low signal intensity on the T$_1$-weighted

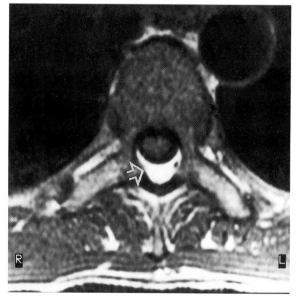

Fig. 12.**38 a, b**   Thoracic epidural lipomatosis. **a** Sagittal T$_1$-weighted SE image in an adolescent. High-signal fat accumulation with space-occupying effect in the epidural space of the thoracic spinal canal (arrows). The patient had clinical signs of cord compression. **b** Axial T$_1$-weighted SE image in an adult. Crescentic accumulation of fat (arrow) with indentation of the dural sac.

image, about equal to or lower than the signal intensity in muscle, but can have a high signal intensity in the presence of a large myxoid and adipose component. On the T_2-weighted image, the cellular areas exhibit a homogeneously high signal intensity. The fibrous fascicles of the tumor appear quite variable as linear or nodular signal void on the T_1-weighted and T_2-weighted images. The MRI findings are multifarious and not specific, but if the fibrous fascicles are prominent, the correct diagnosis can be suggested. (Fig. 12.**39**) (102).

Aside from its extra-abdominal manifestation, aggressive fibromatosis can encountered as abdominal or intra-abdominal disease. An additional small group of superficial fibromatosis includes

- palmar fibromatosis (Dupuytren contracture),
- plantar fibromatosis (Ledderhose disease),
- penile fibromatosis (plastic induration of the penis, Peyronie disease).

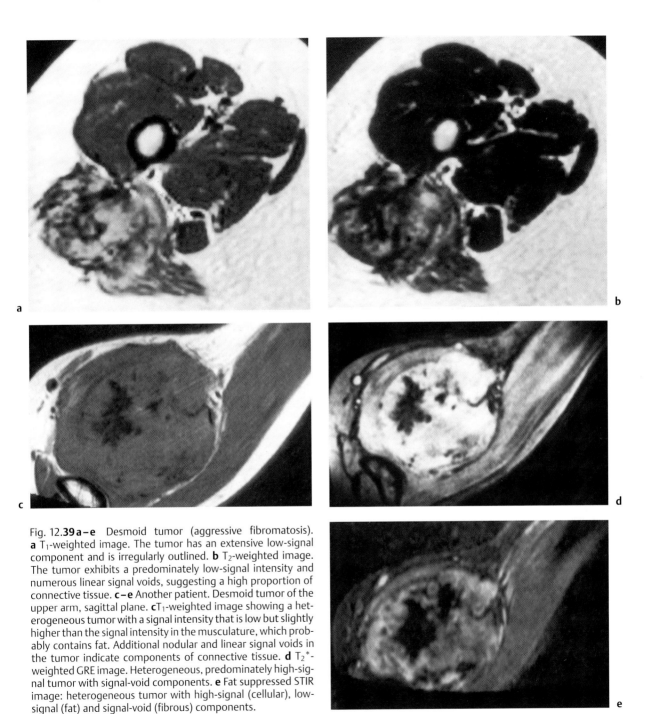

Fig. 12.**39a–e** Desmoid tumor (aggressive fibromatosis). **a** T_1-weighted image. The tumor has an extensive low-signal component and is irregularly outlined. **b** T_2-weighted image. The tumor exhibits a predominately low-signal intensity and numerous linear signal voids, suggesting a high proportion of connective tissue. **c–e** Another patient. Desmoid tumor of the upper arm, sagittal plane. **c** T_1-weighted image showing a heterogeneous tumor with a signal intensity that is low but slightly higher than the signal intensity in the musculature, which probably contains fat. Additional nodular and linear signal voids in the tumor indicate components of connective tissue. **d** T_2^*-weighted GRE image. Heterogeneous, predominately high-signal tumor with signal-void components. **e** Fat suppressed STIR image: heterogeneous tumor with high-signal (cellular), low-signal (fat) and signal-void (fibrous) components.

Vascular Tumors: Hemangioma, Angiomatosis, Hemangioendothelioma, Lymphangioma, Angiolipoma

Hemangiomas occur in the skin and subcutaneous tissues (25) as well as in deep soft tissues, and tend to be located in the extremities. Hemangiomas in children usually involve the skeletal musculature (18, 25) and can be associated with muscle atrophy (14, 107). While most hemangiomas are sharply demarcated, they can incorporate the entire extremity (angiomatosis). A clear distinction between capillary and cavernous variants is often impossible (25). The hemangiomas show a high signal intensity on both T_1-weighted and T_2-weighted images when compared with normal muscle (Figs. 12.**4a, b**) (107). Slow flow or pooling of blood, thrombosis, occluded vessels, and various amounts of fat can account for deviations from the high signal intensity in either sequence (107). Dilated vessels are characteristically seen as serpiginous high-signal structures (Fig. 12.**40**). GRE sequences may visualize flowing blood as high signal density, depending on the direction of blood flow (21). T_1-weighted and T_2-weighted images can visualize fibrotic areas as low signal intensities.

Hemangiomas characteristically contain phleboliths (Fig. 12.**41**), which appear as signal void on all sequences.

Hemangiomas show intermediate to intense enhancement.

The hemangioendothelioma (hemangiopericytoma) is a semi-malignant variant with a high incidence of malignant transformation (Fig. 12.**41**). The imaging findings for lymphangiomas are indistinguishable from those of hemangiomas.

The angiolipoma has a heterogeneous signal pattern with areas of increased signal intensity on T_1-weighted and T_2-weighted images (75) (Fig. 12.**42**). Both sequences show areas of recent hemorrhage as high signal intensity. Structures resembling vessels are commonly visualized.

Schwannoma (Neurinoma, Neurilemoma) and Neurofibroma

Schwannomas and neurofibromas occur in all age groups, but are most frequently observed at ages between 20 and 50 years (25). Schwannomas are typically solitary while neurofibromas may be solitary or multiple. The latter is the case in neurofibromatosis (Recklinghausen disease) especially in patients with Recklinghausen disease. A variant of the neurofibroma is the plexiform neurofibroma (also termed giant neurofibroma), arising from large nerve trunks in patients with peripheral neurofibromatosis and creating a large wormlike mass (elephantiasis neuromatosa). Schwannomas of the upper extremity typically involve the flexor region along the large nerves. They grow slowly and are freely movable, but not along the axis of the nerve from which they arise. Most schwannomas and neurofibromas show a slightly heterogeneous distribution of intermediate signal intensity on the T_1-weighted image and, typically, a very high signal intensity on the T_2-weighted images, occasionally quite heterogeneously distributed (88). The heterogeneity may be attributable to hypocellular and hypercellular areas as well as to necrotic and fibrotic areas. MRI often delineates a low-signal capsule. Schwannomas are typically round or ovoid in outline (Fig. 12.**43**) and tend to occur in the subcutaneous tissue with indentation of adjacent muscle or neighboring large nerves. MRI cannot reliably distinguish a malignant nerve sheath tumor from its benign counterpart (88). Tumors may be primary malignant, arising from intrinsically malignant perineural cells, or secondary malignant due to transformation of a benign neurofibroma. A sudden onset of rapid growth is suspicious for malignant transformation, although this is rare in a solitary neurofibroma.

In many cases of benign neurofibroma and schwannoma the lesion exhibits a characteristic 'target' appearance on T_2-weighted images with a high signal rim

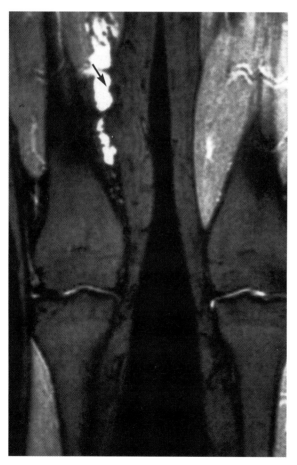

Fig. 12.**40** Hemangioma of the right thigh. Coronal fat-suppressed STIR image. The tumor is seen as high-signal serpiginous lesion between subcutis and musculature (arrow).

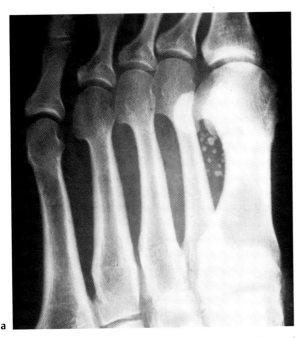

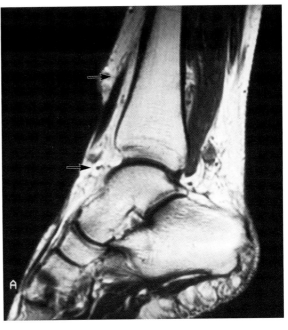

a

b

Fig. 12.**41 a, b** Hemangiopericytoma of the lower leg and foot. **a** Radiograph of the forefoot with phleboliths between the first and second toes. **b** Contrast-enhanced SE image, sagittal section. Several enhancing nodular tumors (arrows).

peripherally and a low signal center. This is thought to be due to fibrocollagenous tissue being surrounded by peripheral myxomatous tissue.

The terminology is variable and inconsistent. Different terms, such as malignant schwannoma, malignant neurilemoma and nerve sheath fibrosarcoma, have been applied to designate malignant tumors of the peripheral nerves. The imaging criteria of malignancy include large size, indistinct outline, infiltration of surrounding structures and severe heterogeneity. Clinically, the combination of peripheral denervation, muscle atrophy, and soft-tissue mass along a major nerve should raise the possibility of a nerve sheath tumor.

Pigmented Villonodular Synovitis

This condition basically represents a chronic inflammatory tumor. The knee is the most frequent site, but any joint can be involved. The patient complains of intermittent pain and swelling. Radiographs show soft-tissue tumor with possible osseous erosions. The T_1-weighted image demonstrates a tumor of heterogeneous, intermediate signal intensity or of decreased signal intensity relative to skeletal muscle. The T_2-weighted image shows a heterogeneous, low signal intensity, largely reflecting hemosiderin deposits.

Giant Cell Tumor of Tendon Sheath

Giant cell tumors of the tendon sheath are histologically identical to pigmented villonodular synovitis seen in

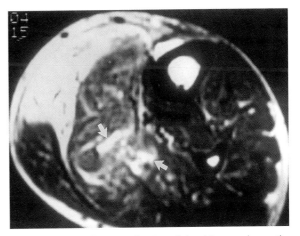

Fig. 12.**42** Angiolipoma. The T_2-weighted image shows the tumor to be of high signal intensity. In addition, vascular structures of high signal intensity are visualized (arrows).

joints, composed of fibrous tissue, hemosiderin deposits, histiocytes, macrophages and giant cells (25). They correspond to a nodular chronic inflammation of the synovial sheath and preferentially involve the flexor tendons of the fingers. The condition is not typically painful, but can be accompanied by exercise-induced pain. The recurrence rate after resection is 9–20%. Malignant transformation can occur. The lesion presents as low-signal intensity along the involved tendon sheath on the T_1-weighted image and is heterogeneous on the T_2-weighted image (83). Low-signal areas corre-

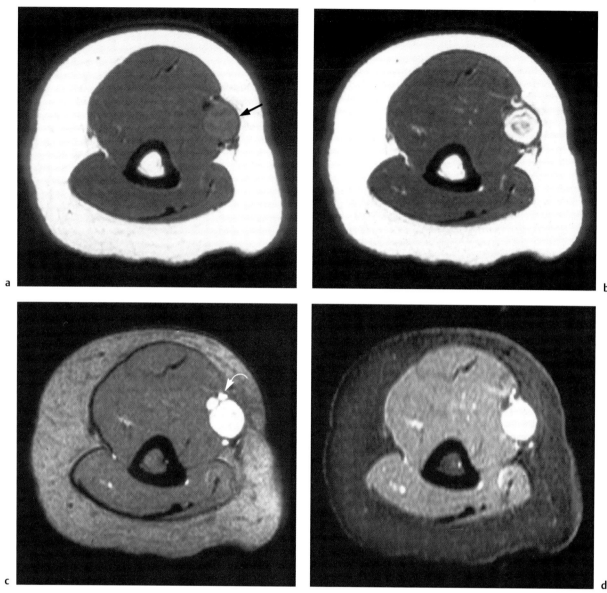

Fig. 12.**43 a – d**   Schwannoma of the upper arm. The tumor is peripherally located between subcutis and musculature next to vessels. It is round and encapsulated (arrow). Axial plane. **a** T$_1$-weighted SE image. The tumor has a low signal intensity and contains a few heterogeneous areas. **b** Contrast-enhanced image. Intense enhancement with central heterogeneity. **c** T$_2$*-weighted GRE image. **d** Fat-suppressed STIR image. High-signal visualization with minimal heterogeneities. Displaced vessels (curved arrow in **c**).

spond to fibrotic areas or hemosiderin deposits, while high-signal areas reflect inflamed synovial tissue (83).

Myogenic Tumors

Myogenic tumors can arise from striated (skeletal) or smooth musculature (Tab. 12.**9**). The signal pattern is nonspecific with decreased signal intensity on T$_1$-weighted and increased signal intensity on T$_2$-weighted images. A myogenic tumor is suspicious for malignancy if it presents as a soft-tissue lesion with the typical malignant criteria, such as indistinct outline, signal heterogeneity, and high growth rate, as well as large size.

■ Metastases

Secondary malignancies comprise the majority of malignancies encountered in the bones and soft tissues, with osseous metastases seen far more frequently than cutaneous and other soft tissue metastases. Without further addressing the epidemiology of bone and soft-

Table 12.**9** Summary of myogenic tumors

Smooth musculature

Benign:
- Leiomyoma (cutaneous and deep)
- Angiomyoma (vascular leiomyoma)
- Epithelial leiomyoma (benign leioblastoma)
- i. v. Leiomyomatosis
- Disseminated peritoneal leiomyomatosis

Malignant:
- Leiomyosarcoma
- Epithelial leiomyosarcoma (malignant leiomyosarcoma)

Striated musculature

Benign:
- Adult rhabdomyoma
- Genital rhabdomyoma
- Fetal rhabdomyoma

Malignant:
- Rhabdomyosarcoma (embryonal, alveolar, pleomorphic, mixed)
- Ectomesenchymoma

tissue metastases, the MRI findings and their differential diagnostic considerations will be reviewed here.

Osseous metastases have a low *signal intensity* on T_1-weighted and a high signal intensity on T_2-weighted images, and enhance after administration of contrast medium. The sequences sensitive for detecting metastases are the fat-suppressed STIR sequence and contrast-enhanced sequences (particularly using a subtraction technique, which depicts the enhancement as areas of increased signal intensity), as well as T_1-weighted sequences for metastases in the hematopoietic inactive yellow marrow.

In contrast, hemorrhagic metastases and melanotic metastases from a malignant melanoma can have a high signal intensity on the T_1-weighted image. The more common amelanotic metastases of the malignant melanoma have a uncharacteristic signal pattern. Predominantly osteoblastic metastases exhibit a signal of low intensity in all sequences. Necrotic areas have a fluid-equivalent signal and do not enhance.

Morphologically, metastases present as round, relatively well-circumscribed space-occupying lesions first and progress to ill-defined lesions due to increasing edema. Vertebral metastases commonly induce a pathologic signal pattern throughout the vertebral body. Pathologic fractures are generally well delineated by radiography, conventional tomography, or CT, but are also visualized as cortical deformity or break on MRI. Metastases with multifocal tiny deposits as in carcinomatosis or diffuse involvement as in plasmocytoma (see Chapter 2) produce a diffuse signal pattern of the involved region or vertebra. MRI is well suited for evaluating extraosseous extension with infiltration of the adjacent soft tissues by virtue of the superior display of soft tissue changes. For instance, MRI may find the vertebral metastases responsible for neurologic deficits by dem-

onstrating extravertebral tumor in the spinal canal or intervertebral foramina.

MRI cannot assess the static strength of metastatically altered bone. The assessment of the mineral base needed for the bone to withstand compression load and tensile strain rests on radiographic modalities, which directly visualize the calcium content of the bone. Morever, MRI is disadvantaged by the edema-induced signal changes, which cannot be distinguished from the underlying metastatic tumor and interfere with the assessment of the tumor mass. MRI may be helpful in distinguishing vertebral collapse secondary to metastatic deposits from insufficiency fractures such as seen in osteoporosis (see Chapter 13).

In *differential diagnosis,* the following factors favor metastases:

- advanced patient age,
- multiple osseous lesions,
- known malignancy,
- increase in size and number within a short interval,
- preferential location of osseous sites with hematopoietically active, red bone marrow (increased perfusion).

Schmorl's nodes of the vertebral body must be distinguished from early metastases. Schmorl's nodes are indentations of the end plates and are characterized by location, surrounding sclerosis, and absent or only faint contrast-enhancement, as well as by a stable appearance in comparison with previous and subsequent examinations (this emphasizes the importance of locating old examinations for comparison whenever possible). Hemangiomas of the vertebral bodies are identified by their fat-equivalent signal pattern on T_1-weighted and T_2-weighted images. Only occasionally can distinguishing vertebral hemangiomas from melanotic metastases of a malignant melanoma pose a differential diagnostic problem. Bone cysts are brighter than metastases on T_1-weighted images and do not enhance.

In summary: MRI is very sensitive in detecting metastases and should be employed whenever conventional radiography or bone scans are suspicious for metastases or do not adequately explain the clinical findings, such as pain or elevated alkaline phosphatase, especially in patients with a malignant tumor that has the propensity for bone metastases. Early and purely osteolytic metastatic lesions can escape radiographic as well as scintigraphic detection, and might only be detectable by MRI.

Cutaneous and other soft tissue metastases are rare. Because of its exquisite soft-tissue contrast, MRI is superior to radiography, sonography, and CT for the evaluation of soft-tissue changes. In the absence of visible or palpable findings, MRI is indicated for the search of suspected soft-tissue metastases. Visible cutaneous changes and palpable soft-tissue tumors can be assessed as to extent and infiltration. If the MRI findings are inconclusive in the clinical context of a known primary tumor, histologic confirmation of the nature of the soft-tissue changes is necessary.

References

1 Aisen, A. M., W. Martel, E. M. Braunstein, K. I. McMillin, W. A. Phillips, T. F. Kling: MRI and CT evaluation of primary bone and soft-tissue tumors. Amer. J. Roentgenol. 146 (1986) 749–756

2 Aoki, J., K. Moriya, K. Yamashita et al.: Giant cell tumors of bone containing large amounts of hemosiderin: MR-pathologic correlation. J. Comput. assist. Tomogr. 15 (1991) 1024–1027

3 Aoki, J., S. Sone, F. Fujioka, K. Terayama, K. Ishii, O. Karakida, S. Imai, F. Sakai, Y. Imai: MR of enchondroma and chondrosarcoma: rings and arcs of Gd-DTPA enhancement. J. Comput. assist. Tomogr. 15 (1991) 1011–1016

4 Assoun, J., G. Richardi, J. J. Railhac et al.: Osteoid osteoma: MR Imaging versus CT. Radiology 191 (1994) 217–223

5 Baker, H. W.: The surgical treatment of cancer. Cancer 43 (1979) 787–789

6 Beltran, J., D. C. Simon, M. Levy, L. Herman, L. Weis, C. F. Mueller: Aneurysmal bone cysts: MR Imaging at 1.5 T. Radiology 158 (1986) 689–675

7 Beltran, J., A. M. Noto, D. W. Chakeres, A. J. Christoforidis: Tumors of the osseous spine: staging with MR Imaging versus CT. Radiology 162 (1987) 565–569

8 Beltran, J., F. Aparisi, L. M. Bonmati, Z. S. Rosenberg, D. Present, G. C. Steiner: Eosinophilic granuloma: MRI manifestations. Skelet. Radiol. 22 (1993) 157–161

9 Berquist, T. H.: Magnetic Resonance Imaging of musculoskeletal neoplasms. Clin. Orthop. 244 (1989) 101–118

10 Blacksin, M. F., N. Ende, J. Benevenia: Magnetic Resonance Imaging of intraosseous lipomas: a radiologic-pathologic correlation. Skelet. Radiol. 24 (1995) 37–41

11 Bloem, J. L., A. H. Taminiau, F. Eulderink, J. Hermans, E. K. Pauwels: Radiologic staging of primary bone sarcoma: MR imaging, scintigraphy, angiography, and CT correlated with pathologic examination. Radiology 169 (1988) 805–810

12 Bohndorf, K., M. Reiser, B. Lochner, W. Féaux de Lacroix, W. Steinbrich: Magnetic Resonance Imaging of primary tumors and tumor-like lesions of bone. Skelet. Radiol. 15 (1986) 511–517

13 Boyko, O. B., D. A. Cory, M. D. Cohen, A. Provisor, D. Mirkin, G. Paul DeRosa: MR Imaging of osteogenic and Ewing's sarcoma. Amer. J. Roentgenol. 148 (1987) 317–322

14 Buetow, P. C., M. J. Kransdorf, R. P. Moser, J. S. Jelinek, B. H. Berrey: Radiologic appearance of intramuscular hemangioma with emphasis on MR Imaging. Amer. J. Roentgenol. 154 (1990) 563–567

15 Carrasco, C. H., C. Charnsangavej, K. Raymond et al.: Osteosarcoma: angiographic assessment of response to preoperative chemotherapy. Radiology 170 (1989) 839–842

16 Choi, H., D. G. K. Varma, B. D. Fornage, E. E. Kim, D. A. Johnston: Soft-tissue sarcoma: MR Imaging vs sonography for detection of local recurrence after surgery. Amer. J. Roentgenol. 157 (1991) 353–358

17 Chuang, V. P., R. Benjamin, N. Jaffe et al.: Radiographic and angiographic changes in osteosarcoma after intraarterial chemotherapy. Amer. J. Roentgenol. 139 (1982) 1065–1069

18 Cohen, E. K., H. Y. Kressel, T. Perosio et al.: MR Imaging of soft-tissue hemangiomas: correlation with pathologic findings. Amer. J. Roentgenol. 15 (1988) 1079–1081

19 De Beuckeleer, L., A. De Schepper, F. Ramon, J. Somville: Magnetic Resonance Imaging of cartilaginous tumors: a retrospective study of 79 patients. Europ. J. Radiol. 21 (1995) 34–40

20 DeSchepper, A. M. A., F. Ramon, E. VanMarck: MR Imaging of eosinophilic granuloma: report of 11 cases. Skelet. Radiol. 22 (1993) 163–166

21 Dumoulin, C. L.: Flow imaging. In Budinger, T. F., A. R. Margulis: Medical Magnetic Resonance. A Primer-1988. Society of Magnetic Resonance in Medicine, Berkeley 1988 (pp. 85–108)

22 Edeiken, J., M. Dalinka, D. Karasick: Bone tumors and tumor-like conditions. In Edeiken, J., M. Dalinka, D. Karasick: Roentgen Diagnosis of Diseases of Bone, Vol. 1. Williams & Wilkins, Baltimore 1990 (pp. 33–574)

23 Enneking, W. F.: Staging of musculoskeletal neoplasms. Skelet. Radiol. 13 (1985) 183–194

24 Enzinger, F. M.: Intramuscular myxoma: a review and follow-up study of 34 cases. Amer. J. clin. Pathol. 43 (1985) 104–110

25 Enzinger, F. M., S. W. Weiss: Soft Tissue Tumors. Mosby, St. Louis 1988 (pp. 719–728)

26 Erlemann, R., M. F. Reiser, P. E. Peters et al.: Musculoskeletal neoplasms: static and dynamic Gd-DTPA-enhanced MR Imaging. Radiology 171 (1989) 767–773

27 Erlemann, R., J. Sciuk, A. Bosse et al.: Response of osteosarcoma and Ewing sarcoma to preoperative chemotherapy: assessment with dynamic and static MR Imaging and skeletal scintigraphy. Radiology 175 (1990) 791–796

28 Fletcher, B. D.: Response of osteosarcoma and Ewing sarcoma to chemotherapy: imaging evaluation. Amer. J. Roentgenol. 157 (1991) 825–833

29 Fletcher, B. D., S. L. Hanna, D. L. Fairclough, S. A. Gronemeyer: Pediatric musculoskeletal tumors: use of dynamic, contrast-enhanced MR Imaging to monitor response to chemotherapy. Radiology 184 (1992) 243–248

30 Freyschmidt, J., H. Ostertag: Knochentumoren. Springer, Berlin 1988

31 Frouge, C., D. Vanel, C. Coffre, D. Couanet, G. Contesso, D. Sarrazin: The role of Magnetic Resonance Imaging in the evaluation of Ewing sarcoma. A report of 27 cases. Skelet. Radiol. 17 (1988) 387–392

32 Geirnaerdt, M. J., J. L. Bloem, F. Eulderink, P. C. Hogendoorn, A. H. Taminiau: Cartilaginous tumors: correlation of gadolinium-enhanced MR Imaging and histopathologic findings. Radiology 186 (1993) 813–817

33 Gilbert, H. A., A. R. Kagan, J. Winkley: Management of soft-tissue sarcoma of the extremities. Surg. Gynecol. Obstet. 139 (1974) 914–918

34 Gillespy, T. D., M. Manfrini, P. Ruggieri, S. S. Spanier, H. Pettersson, D. S. Springfield: Staging of intraosseous extent of osteosarcoma: correlation of preoperative CT and MR Imaging with pathologic macroslides. Radiology 167 (1988) 765 to 767

35 Glazer, H. S., J. K. T. Lee, R. G. Levitt et al.: Radiation fibrosis: differentiation from recurrent tumor by MR Imaging. Radiology 156 (1985) 721–727

36 Goldman, A. B., R. Schneider, H. Pavlov: Osteoid osteomas of the femoral neck: report of four cases evaluated with isotopic bone scanning, CT, and MR Imaging [see comments]. Radiology 186 (1993) 227–232

37 Greenspan, A.: Benign bone-forming lesions: osteoma, osteoid osteoma, and osteoblastoma. Clinical, imaging, pathologic, and differential considerations. Skelet. Radiol. 22 (1993) 485–500

38 Hanna, L. S., H. L. Magill, D. M. Parham, L. C. Bowman, B. D. Fletcher: Childhood chondrosarcoma: MR Imaging with Gd-DTPA. Magn. Res. Imag. 8 (1990) 669–672

39 Hanna, S. L., D. M. Parham, D. L. Fairclough, W. H. Meyer, A. H. Le, B. D. Fletcher: Assessment of osteosarcoma response to preoperative chemotherapy using dynamic FLASH gadolinium-DTPA-enhanced Magnetic Resonance mapping. Invest. Radiol. 27 (1992) 367–373

40 Hanna, S. L., W. E. Reddick, D. M. Parham, S. Gronemeyer, J. S. Taylor, B. D. Fletcher: Automated pixel-by-pixel mapping of dynamic contrast enhanced MR Images for evaluation of

osteosarcoma response to chemotherapy: preliminary results. JMRI 3 (1993) 849–853

41 Harle, A., M. Reiser, R. Erlemann, P. Wuisman: The value of Nuclear Magnetic Resonance Tomography in staging of bone and soft tissue sarcomas. Orthopäde 18 (1989) 34–40

42 Heredia, C., J. M. Mercader, F. Graus et al.: Hemangioma of the vertebrae: contribution of Magnetic Resonance to its study. Neurologia 4 (1989) 336–339

43 Holscher, H. C., J. L. Bloem, M. A. Nooy, A. H. Taminiau, F. Eulderink, J. Hermans: The value of MR Imaging in monitoring the effect of chemotherapy on bone sarcomas. Amer. J. Roentgenol. 154 (1990) 763–769

44 Holscher, H. C., J. L. Bloem, M. A. Nooy, A. H. Taminiau, F. Eulderink, J. Hermans: The value of MR Imaging in monitoring the effect of chemotherapy on bone sarcomas. Amer. J. Roentgenol. 154 (1990) 763–769

45 Jurgens, H., U. Exner, H. Gadner et al.: Multidisciplinary treatment of Ewing's sarcoma of bone. Cancer 61 (1988) 23–32

46 Keigley, B. A., A. M. Haggar, A. Gaba, B. I. Ellis, J. W. Froelich, K. K. Wu: Primary tumors of the foot: MR Imaging. Radiology 171 (1989) 755–759

47 Kilcoyne, R. F., M. L. Richardson, B. A. Porter et al.: Magnetic Resonance Imaging of soft-tissue masses. Clin. Orthop. 228 (1988) 13–22

48 Kransdorf, M. J.: Malignant soft-tissue tumors in a large referral population: distribution of diagnoses by age, sex, and location. Amer. J. Roentgenol. 164 (1995) 129–134

49 Kransdorf, M. J., J. S. Jelinek, R. J. Moser et al.: Soft-tissue masses: diagnosis using MR Imaging. Amer. J. Roentgenol. 153 (1989) 541–547

50 Kransdorf, M. J., J. M. Meis, J. S. Jelinek: Dedifferentiated liposarcoma of the extremities: imaging findings in four patients. Amer. J. Roentgenol. 161 (1993) 127–130

51 Lang, P., C. A. Gooding, J. J. Johnston, G. Honda, W. Rosenau, H. K. Genant: What is the preferable imaging sequence for bone tumors in children (YOUNG INVESTIGATOR'S AWARD, SOC. PED. RADIOL.). The Society for Pediatric Radiology, Seattle, Washington, 12. – 15. 5. 1993. SPR.

52 Lang, P., S. Grampp, M. Vahlensieck et al.: Primary bone tumors: value of MR angiography for preoperative planning and monitoring response to chemotherapy. Amer. J. Roentgenol. 165 (1995) 135–142

53 Lang, P., G. Honda, T. Roberts et al.: Musculoskeletal neoplasm: perineoplastic edema versus tumor on postcontrast MR Images with spatial mapping of instantaneous enhancement rates. Radiology 197 (1995) 831–839

54 Lang, P., M. Vahlensieck, K. Matthay et al.: Monitoring neovascularity and response to chemotherapy in osteogenic and Ewing sarcoma using magnetic resonance angiography. Med. Pediat. Oncol. 26 (1996) 329–333

55 Laredo, J. D., E. Assouline, F. Gelbert, M. Wybier, J. J. Merland, J. M. Tubiana: Vertebral hemangiomas: fat content as a sign of aggressiveness. Radiology 177 (1990) 467–472

56 Lee, J. K., L. Yao, C. R. Wirth: MR Imaging of solitary osteochondroma: report of eight cases. Amer. J. Roentgenol. 149 (1987) 557–560

57 Lee, Y. Y., T. P. Van: Craniofacial chondrosarcomas: imaging findings in 15 untreated cases. Amer. J. Neuroradiol. 10 (1989) 165–170

58 Lee, Y. Y., T. P. Van, C. Nauert, A. K. Raymond, J. Edeiken: Craniofacial osteosarcomas: plain film, CT, and MR findings in 46 cases. Amer. J. Roentgenol. 150 (1988) 1397–1402

59 Lukens, J. A., R. A. McLeod, F. H. Sim: Computed Tomographic evaluation of primary osseous malignant neoplasm. Amer. J. Roentgenol. 139 (1982) 45–48

60 MacVicar, A. D., J. F. Olliff, J. Pringle, C. R. Pinkerton, J. E. Husband: Ewing sarcoma: MR Imaging of chemotherapy-induced changes with histologic correlation. Radiology 184 (1992) 859–864

61 Mahajan, H., E. E. Kim, Y. Y. Lee, H. Goepfert: Malignant fibrous histiocytoma of the tongue demonstrated by magnetic resonance imaging. Otolaryngol. Head Neck Surg. 101 (1989) 704–706

62 Mahajan, H., E. E. Kim, S. Wallace, R. Abello, R. Benjamin, H. L. Evans: Magnetic Resonance Imaging of malignant fibrous histiocytoma. Magn. Reson. Imag. 7 (1989) 283–288.

63 Mahajan, H., J. G. Lorigan, A. Shirkhoda: Synovial sarcoma: MR Imaging. Magn. Reson. Imag. 7 (1989) 211–216

64 Mail, J. T., M. D. Cohen, L. D. Mirkin, A. J. Provisor: Response of osteosarcoma to preoperative intravenous high-dose methotrexate chemotherapy: CT evaluation. Amer. J. Roentgenol. 144 (1985) 89–93

65 Mandell, G. A., H. T. Harcke, S. K. Kumar: Fibrous lesions of the extremities. Topics Magn. Reson. Imag. 4 (1991) 45–55

66 Milgram, J. A.: Intraosseous lipomas. Clin. Orthop. 231 (1988) 277–302

67 Morton, D. L., F. R. Eilber, C. M. Townsend, T. T. Grant, J. Mirra, T. H. Weisenburger: Limbsalvage from multidisciplinary treatment approach for skeletal and soft-tissue sarcoma of the extremity. Ann. Surg. 184 (1976) 268–278

67 a Mugel, T., M. Ghossain, C. Guinet, J. Buy, D. Vadrot: MR and CT findings in a case of hibernoma of the thigh extending into the pelvis. Europ. Radiology 8 (1998) 476–478

68 Murphey, M. D., K. J. Fairbairn, L. M. Parman, K. G. Baxter, M. B. Parsa, W. S. Smith: From the archives of the AFIP. Musculoskeletal angiomatous lesions: radiologic-pathologic correlation. Radiographics 15 (1995) 893–917

69 Norton, K. I., G. Hermann, I. F. Abdelwahab, M. J. Klein, L. F. Granowetter, J. G. Rabinowitz: Epiphyseal involvement in osteosarcoma. Radiology 180 (1991) 813–816

70 O'Flanagan, S. J., J. P. Stack, H. M. McGee, P. Dervan, B. Hurson: Imaging of intramedullary tumour spread in osteosarcoma. A comparison of techniques. J. Bone Jt Surg. 73 (1991) 998–1001

71 Pan, G., A. K. Raymond, C. H. Carrasco et al.: Osteosarcoma: MR Imaging after preoperative chemotherapy. Radiology 174 (1990) 517–526

72 Panicek, D. M., L. H. Schwartz, R. T. Heelan, J. F. Caravelli: Nonneoplastic causes of high signal intensity at T2-weighted MR Imaging after treatment of musculoskeletal neoplasm. Skelet. Radiol. 24 (1995) 185–190

73 Petasnick, J. P., D. A. Turner, J. R. Charters, S. Gitelis, C. E. Zacharias: Soft-tissue masses of the locomotor system: comparison of MR Imaging with CT. Radiology 160 (1986) 125–133

74 Peterson, K. K., D. Renfrew, R. M. Feddersen, J. A. Buckwalter, G. Y. El-Khoury: Magnetic Resonance Imaging of myxoid containing tumors. Skelet. Radiol. 20 (1991) 245–250

75 Pettersson, H., T. Gillespy, D. J. Hamlin et al.: Primary musculoskeletal tumors: examination with MR Imaging compared to conventional modalities. Radiology 164 (1987) 237–241

76 Pettersson, H., J. Eliasson, N. Egund et al.: Gadolinium-DTPA enhancement of soft-tissue tumors in Magnetic Resonance Imaging – preliminary clinical experience in 5 patients. Skelet. Radiol. 17 (1988) 319–323

77 Reddick, W. E., R. Bhargava, J. S. Taylor, W. H. Meyer, B. D. Fletcher: Dynamic contrast-enhanced MR Imaging evaluation of osteosarcoma response to neoadjuvant chemotherapy. JMRI 5 (1995) 689–694

78 Reuther, G., W. Mutschler: Detection of local recurrent disease in musculoskeletal tumors: Magnetic Resonance Imaging versus Computed Tomography. Skelet. Radiol. 19 (1990) 85–90

79 Rock, M. G., D. J. Pritchard, H. M. Reiman, R. A. McLeod: Extraabdominal demoid tumor. Mayo Clin. Tumor Rounds 7 (1984) 141–147

80 Ross, J. S., T. J. Masaryk, M. T. Modic, J. R. Carter, T. Mapstone: Vertebral hemangiomas: MR Imaging. Radiology 165 (1987) 165–169

81 Seeger, L. L., J. J. Eckardt, L. W. Bassett: Cross-sectional imaging in the evaluation of osteogenic sarcoma: MRI and CT. Semin. Roentgenol. 24 (1989) 174–184

82 Seeger, L. L., B. E. Widoff, L. W. Bassett, G. Rosen, J. J. Eckardt: Preoperative evaluation of osteosarcoma: value of gadopentetate dimeglumine-enhanced MR Imaging. Amer. J. Roentgenol. 157 (1991) 347–351

83 Sherry, C. S., S. E. Harms: MR evaluation of giant cell tumors of the tendon sheath. Magn. Reson. Imag. 7 (1989) 195–201

84 Shirkoda, A., N. Jaffe, S. Wallace et al.: Computed Tomography of osteosarcoma after intraarterial chemotherapy. Amer. J. Roentgenol. 144 (1985) 95–99

85 Shuman, W. P., R. M. Patten, R. L. Baron, R. M. Liddell, E. U. Conrad, M. L. Richardson: Comparison of STIR and spin-echo MR Imaging at 1.5 T in 45 suspected extremity tumors: lesion conspicuity and extent. Radiology 179 (1991) 247–252

86 Simon, M. A., W. F. Enneking: The management of soft-tissue sarcomas of the extremities. J. Bone Jt Surg. 58 A (1976) 317–327

87 Stiglbaur, R., I. Augustin, J. Kramer, H. Schurawitzki, H. Imhof, T. Radaszkiewicz: MRI in the diagnosis of primary lymphoma of bone: correlation with histopathology. J. Comput. assist. Tomogr. 16 (1992) 248–253

88 Stull, M. A., R. P. Moser, M. J. Kransdorf, G. P. Bogumill, M. C. Nelson: Magnetic Resonance appearance of peripheral nerve sheath tumors. Skelet. Radiol. 20 (1991) 9–14

89 Sundaram, M.: Radiographic and Magnetic Resonance Imaging of bone and soft-tissue tumors and myeloproliferative disorders. Curr. Opin. Radiol. 3 (1991) 746–751

90 Sundaram, M., D. J. McDonald: The solitary tumor or tumorlike lesion of bone. Topics Magn. Reson. Imag. 1 (1989) 17–29

91 Sundaram, M., R. A. McLeod: MR Imaging of tumor and tumorlike lesions of bone and soft tissue. Amer. J. Roentgenol. 155 (1990) 817–824

92 Sundaram, M., M. H. McGuire, Z. F. Schajowic: Soft-tissue masses: histologic bases for decreased signal (short T2) on T2-weighted images. Amer. J. Roentgenol. 148 (1987) 1247–1251

93 Sundaram, M., M. H. McGuire, F. Schajowicz: Soft-tissue masses: histologic basis for decreased signal (short T2) on T2-weighted MR images. Amer. J. Roentgenol. 148 (1987) 1247–1250

94 Tehranzadeh, J., W. Mnaymneh, C. Ghavam, G. Morillo, B. J. Murphy: Comparison of CT and MR Imaging in musculoskeletal neoplasms. J. Comput. assist. Tomogr. 13 (1989) 466–472

95 Tehranzadeh, J., B. J. Murphy, W. Mnaymneh: Giant cell tumor of the proximal tibia: MR and CT appearance. J. Comput. assist. Tomogr. 13 (1989) 282–286

96 Totty, W. G., W. A. Murphy, J. K. T. Lee: Soft-tissue tumors: MR Imaging. Radiology 160 (1986) 135–141

97 Uhl, M., T. Roeren, B. Schneider, G. W. Kauffmann: MRT der Liposarkome. Fortschr. Röntgenstr. 165 (1996) 144–147

98 Vahlensieck, M., L. Solymosi, G. Reinheimer, C. Buchbender, M. Reiser: Ätiologie, Symptomatik, Diagnostik und Therapie der spinalen epiduralen Lipomatose. Akt. Neurol. 20 (1993) 1–4

99 Vahlensieck, M., F. Träber, R. deBoer, U. Schlippert, H. Schild: Magnetization-Transfer-Contrast (MTC): Vergleich maligner und benigner Erkrankungen des Stütz- und Bewegungsapparates. Radiologe 35 (1995) 100 (abstract)

100 van der Woude, H. J., J. L. Bloem, K. L. Verstraete, A. H. M. Taminiau, M. A. Nooy, P. C. W. Hogendoorn: Osteosarcoma and Ewing sarcoma after neoadjuvant chemotherapy: value of dynamic MR Imaging in detecting viable tumor before surgery. Amer. J. Roentgenol. 165 (1995) 593–598

101 Vanel, D., M. J. Lacombe, D. Couanet, C. Kalifa, M. Spielmann, J. Genin: Musculoskeletal tumors: follow-up with MR Imaging after treatment with surgery and radiation therapy. Radiology 164 (1987) 243–245

102 VanKints, M. J., T. A. Tham, D. Vroegindeweij, A. J. Erp: MRI findings in aggressive fibromatosis. Europ. J. Radiol. 16 (1993) 230–232

103 Verstraete, K. L., Y. De Deene, H. Roels, A. Dierick, D. Uyttendaele, M. Kunnen: Benign and malignant musculoskeletal lesions: dynamic contrast-enhanced MR Imaging – parametric „first-pass" images depict tissue vascularization and perfusion. Radiology 192 (1994) 835–843

104 Weatherall, P. T., G. E. Maale, D. B. Mendelsohn, C. S. Sherry, W. E. Erdman, H. R. Pascoe: Chondroblastoma: classic and confusing appearance at MR Imaging. Radiology 190 (1994) 467–474

105 Winkler, K., G. Beron, G. Delling et al.: Neoadjuvant chemotherapy of osteosarcoma: result of a randomized cooperative trial (COSS-82) with salvage chemotherapy based on histological tumor response. J. clin. Oncol. 6 (1988) 329–337

106 Woods, E. R., W. Martel, S. H. Mandell, J. P. Crabbe: Reactive soft-tissue mass associated with osteoid osteoma: correlation of MR Imaging features with pathologic findings. Radiology 186 (1993) 221–225

107 Yuh, W. T. C., M. H. Kathol, M. A. Sein, S. Ehara, L. Chiu: Hemangiomas of skeletal muscle: MR findings in five patients. Amer. J. Roentgenol. 149 (1987) 765–768

108 Zimmer, W. D., T. H. Berquist, R. A. McLeod et al.: Bone tumors: Magnetic Resonance Imaging versus Computed Tomography. Radiology 155 (1985) 709–718

13 Osteoporosis

S. Grampp, M. Vahlensieck, P. Lang, and H. K. Genant

Introduction

Numerous techniques are currently available for diagnosing osteoporosis and osteoporotic fractures and for measuring osseous density and fracture risk (19). Most methods use ionizing radiation and calculate the bone mineral density (BMD) from the measured radiation absorption. In recent years, MRI has been used for diagnosing osteoporosis, with emphasis on visualizing osteoporotic deformities and fractures. *High resolution techniques* have been used to depict the internal osseous structures in order to make statements about their abnormalities in osteoporosis. Furthermore, the relaxation times *(relaxometry)* have been quantified to diagnose osteoporosis and to monitor its course (36a, 42a, 46a, 49a). Such quantification generally measures the effective T_2 time (T_2^*), sometimes expressed as its reciprocal value ($1/T_2^*$). So far, MRI cannot deliver the required low reproducibility of less than 2% as achieved by other quantitative osteoporotic methods. This chapter presents the MRI evaluation of osteoporosis by discussing imaging and relaxometry separately.

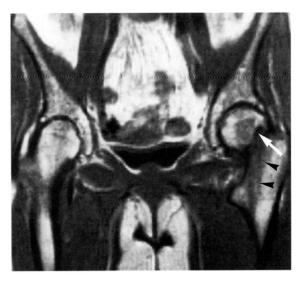

Fig. 13.**1**   MRI of the hip 8 hours after fracture of the femoral neck in a 76-year-old patient. The coronal GRE image shows a subcapital fracture line of low signal intensity (white arrow) with adjacent areas of moderate to low signal intensity (black arrowheads), corresponding to edema or hemorrhage.

MR Imaging of Osteoporosis

■ Osteoporotic Fractures

MRI can diagnose fractures that are undetectable on radiographs. Such radiologically *occult fractures* are relatively common in old osteoporotic patients. The detection of occult fractures of the proximal femur with MRI has been documented in several studies (12, 33, 38, 40, 52). MRI characteristically delineates the fracture line as markedly decreased signal intensity, surrounded by bone marrow edema. These changes are attributed to focal hyperemia and edema, impacted osseous trabeculae and reparative processes. MRI can diagnose osteoporotic insufficiency fractures of the pelvis, sacrum, hips and long tubular bones with a sensitivity that is at least comparable to and, according to some studies, even greater than scintigraphy (4, 5, 34). This is especially true during the few days following trauma (Fig. 13.1), when the findings of the bone scan often are still inconclusive.

MRI also makes a great clinical contribution by its ability to distinguish osteoporotic compression fractures of vertebral bodies from pathologic compression fracture due to underlying malignancy (1, 2, 42, 50, 53). *Pathologic tumor-related fractures* induce an abnormal signal pattern in the affected vertebral bodies (18, 35, 37), often accompanied by a convex deformity of the anterior and posterior margins of the vertebral bodies. The adjacent vertebral bodies frequently harbor metastases and show corresponding foci that have a low signal intensity on T_1-weighted and a high signal intensity on the T_2-weighted images. *Osteoporotic fractures*, in contrast, frequently show band-like signal changes, adjacent and parallel to the end plates. The nondeformed portions of the vertebral body exhibit a normal signal pattern (Fig. 13.**2**). Neighboring nonfractured vertebral bodies generally display a normal signal intensity in the bone marrow. For the differentiation between osteoporotic and pathologic vertebral compression fractures, MRI has a higher sensitivity than bone scintigraphy and a higher specificity than CT (1, 2, 50).

Some studies have suggested that a distinction between osteoporotic and malignant vertebral collapse can be achieved with intravenous administration of contrast medium (9, 22). Osteoporotic vertebral collapse shows enhancement that is linear and parallel to

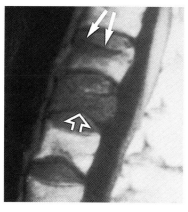 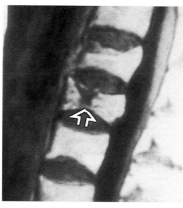

a b

Fig. 13.**2 a, b** Osteoporotic vertebral compression fractures. **a** Sagittal T_1-weighted image several days after the fracture. The L1 vertebral body shows a biconcave deformity (open arrow) and a low-signal marrow. In addition, the superior end plate of the T12 vertebral body is indented and shows a low signal intensity (arrows). **b** Sagittal T_1-weighted SE image several months after the fracture. Normalization of the signal pattern in the T12 vertebral body. The small area of decreased signal intensity in the L1 vertebral body (open arrow) corresponds to focal sclerosis.

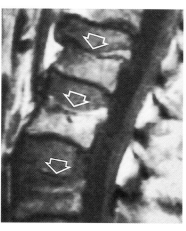 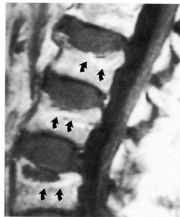

a b

Fig. 13.**3 a, b** Osteoporotic compression fracture before and after administration of contrast medium. **a** The precontrast sagittal T_1-weighted SE image shows several compression fractures (open arrows) involving the L2–L4 lumbar vertebral bodies. **b** After administration of contrast medium, there is linear enhancement (curved arrows) parallel to the fracture lines in the affected vertebral bodies. This pattern is characteristic of osteoporotic fractures.

the fracture line (Fig. 13.**3**), while malignant collapse generally shows patchy enhancement.

MRI has a limited ability to distinguish between *acute traumatic* and *osteoporotic insufficiency fractures* since either fracture produces localized signal changes caused by bleeding and reparative processes. Marked osseous deformity together with dislocated fragments is more often seen after acute trauma, while finding other collapsed vertebral bodies with a normal marrow signal pattern favors an osteoporotic origin.

The altered signal pattern of the bone marrow induced by a non-neoplastic fracture generally returns to normal within several months and only a deformed vertebral body remains.

■ High Resolution Imaging of the Trabecular Pattern

Besides measuring trabecular density and width, MRI can produce high resolution images that visualize the trabecular microstructure. After appropriate modification of the computer programs, standard MRI systems can generate images with a resolution of $78 \times 78 \times 300\,\mu m$ for the finger phalanges (24) and of

$78 \times 78 \times 700\,\mu m$ for the distal radius (Fig. 13.**4**) and calcaneus (32).

Postprocessing using CT-derived techniques of image analysis (1, 8, 13, 24, 25, 36, 51) can yield quantitative parameters, such as the proportion of bone in a two-dimensional section, the average trabecular thickness, the number of trabecular branches and their preferred spatial orientation. When interpreting these parameters, one must be aware of erroneous calculations due to misregistrations introduced by incorrect separation of bone and marrow components, relatively limited spatial resolution or partial volume effects. Aside from these methods, additional techniques for image and structure analysis are available but will not be discussed in detail since they are largely still investigational. They include morphological granulometry (6), calculation of fractal elements (32), and wavelet processing (46). It is hoped that the quantitative analysis of the osseous morphology may predict the fracture risk better than the quantitative measurement of the bone density.

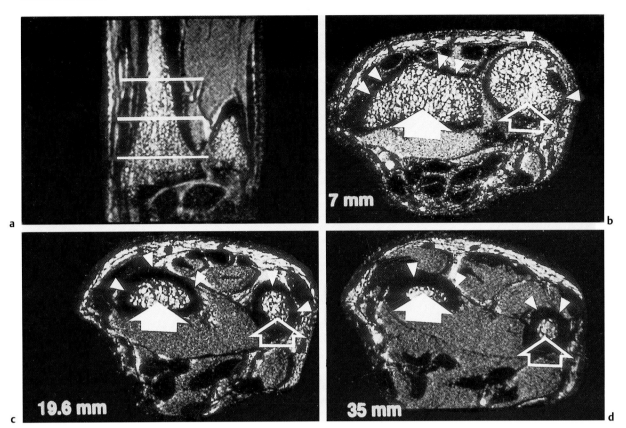

Fig. 13.**4a–d**   Visualization of the distal radius with a 1.5 T-Signa MRI system (General Electric, Milwaukee, USA). High resolution imaging with a T_2-weighted water presaturated GRASS sequence with sagittal thickness of 700 μm and a spatial resolution of 156 μm. **a** Coronal section through the distal forearm and wrist. The levels of the axial sections are marked as white lines on the coronal image. **b** Axial section about 7 mm distal to the cortical end plate of the radius (average T_2^* relaxation time in twelve healthy subjects = 18.02 msec [20]). **c** Axial section about 20 mm distal to the cortical end plate of the radius (T_2^* time = 21.20 msec). **d** Axial section about 35 mm distal to the cortical end plate of the radius (T_2^* time = 32.50 msec). Trabecular bone in the radius (closed arrow), ulna (open arrow), and cortex of both bones (arrowheads).

MR Relaxometry

Because of the low proportion of free electrons, *cortical bone* cannot emit an MR signal that can be registered. The relaxation times are not measurable or extremely short.

The *trabecular bone* is different. In addition to the lattice of osseous trabeculae, it contains numerous cells and fat as part of the bone marrow. The MR signal emitted from the bone marrow is primarily determined by its cellular and adipose components and has a high intensity due to the abundance of fat in the yellow bone marrow as opposed to the hematopoietic red bone marrow. The feasibility of MRI for the quantitative assessment of osteoporosis depends on the contribution of the number, distribution and thickness of the osseous trabeculae (the *bone density*) to the relaxation time of the bone marrow signal. Furthermore, it has to be addressed whether an altered strength or elasticity, expressed as Young's modulus of elasticity, affects the relaxation times and can be a measure of the fracture risk.

Numerous investigations have addressed these questions. Measuring the relaxation times within trabecular spaces and correlating their variations with the trabecular bone density revealed no significant variations of the T_1 and T_2 *relaxation times,* indicating no significant contribution of the bone density to the relaxation rates of bone marrow (31). The elasticity coefficient may only have a limited effect on the T_2 relaxation time (46a).

The situation is different for the effect of bone density and elasticity coefficient on the *effective T_2-(T_2^*) time,* which is markedly affected by both. The T_2^* time is sensitive to the distribution of the magnetic field, which is locally heterogeneous due to the abrupt susceptibility changes along the interfaces between trabeculae and marrow space. Since such interfaces dominate the trabecular bone, it follows that changes of the intertrabecular distance and trabecular width introduce local magnetic field heterogeneity with resultant changes of the T_2^* time (Fig. 13.**5**).

Increased trabecular density causes a faster decay with resultant shorter T_2^* times; decreased trabecular

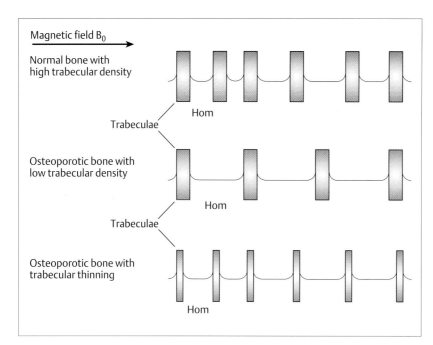

Fig. 13.**5** Increase in the homogeneous magnetic field due to low trabecular density and trabecular thinning in comparison to normal bone. This induces an increase in the T_2^* time in osteoporotic trabecular bone.

density, as found in osteoporosis or with aging, causes a slower decay with resultant longer T_2^* times. Currently, measuring the T_2^* relaxation times seems to be the most promising approach to quantitative evaluation by MRI. As expected, these parameters are age-dependent, with increasing age showing a prolongation of the T_2^* time in lumbar vertebrae at a rate of about 0.3 msec/year in premenopausal women and up to 0.9 msec/year in postmenopausal women. Moreover, a significant difference in T_2^* times was found in the lumbar spine when normal subjects (15.8 + 2.5 msec) were compared with osteoporotic patients (18.8 + 2.8 msec) (46a, 49a). This has been confirmed in other studies of the lumbar spine (healthy subjects: 13.4 + 1.9 msec, osteoporotic patients: 19.9 + 3.8 msec) (16).

The poor *reproducibility* of measuring T_2^* remains an important concern. So far, no variations of less than 7% have been achieved for either short or long times (29, 30). This can be attributed to several factors. The T_2^* time usually is measured with GRE sequences. Several measurements are made with different echo times and the T_2^* time is calculated from signal intensities, which are registered within a certain region of interest according to the following formula:

$$I(TE) = Io \times exp\,(-TE/T_2^*)$$

Since a rephasing pulse is lacking, GRE sequences are sensitive not only to changes of the T_2^* time but also to the phase effects introduced by the different bone marrow components (see Chapter 11). Echo time and field strength show a considerable influence on the phase effects (36a). Consequently, the T_2^* time is not only determined by the bone density but also by the composition of the bone marrow, which can be quite variable. Other problems are the lack of any methodical standards for selecting the regions of interest (20) and just simple MRI artifacts. Several solutions have been proposed to solve these problems and are part of current research. One approach consists of minimizing the phase effects by restricting the measurements to peripheral sites with purely adipose bone marrow, as found in the calcaneus and radius. Some studies found a significant correlation between bone density measured by peripheral quantitative CT and the T_2^* time (21). The advantages and disadvantages of measuring the bone density at peripheral sites will not be discussed further. Another proposed solution uses fat suppression or so-called water images for calculating the T_2^* time, which is promising but time-consuming. Moreover, spectroscopy can be used to determine the T_2^* time. Other methods, such as interferometry and MAGSUS (simultaneous assessment of the MAGnetic field and SUSceptibility), are mentioned here only for the sake of completeness (42a).

Current Role of Relaxometry

Conventional MRI can be quite helpful in the differential diagnosis of osteoporotic fractures and has been established for this indication. The high resolution methods for mapping the microstructure are still investigational and require further advancement before they can compete with the rapidly advancing quantitative CT. Quantifying the T_2^* time has shown promising results *in vivo* as well as *in vitro*, and the ongoing advances in computer hardware and software can be expected to improve the reproducibility of the measurements. This will promote the role of MRI in the differential diagnosis of osteoporosis by providing morphologic information (e.g., the presence of edema) together with valuable quantitative information.

References

1 Allgayer, B., E. Flierdt, A. Heuck, M. Matzner, Pl. Lukas, G. Luttke: NMR Tomography compared to skeletal scintigraphy after traumatic vertebral body fractures. Fortschr. Rontgenstr. 152 (1990) 677–681

2 Baker, L. L., S. B. Goodman, I. Perkash, B. Lane, D. R. Enzmann: Benign versus pathologic compression fractures of vertebral bodies: assessment with conventional spin-echo, chemical-shift, and STIR MR Imaging. Radiology 174 (1990) 495–502

3 Black, D., S. R. Cummings, H. K. Genant, M. C. Nevitt, L. Palermo, W. Browner: Axial and appendicular bone density predict fractures in older women. J. Bone Mineral Res. 8 (1992) 633–638

4 Blomlie, V., H. H. Lien, T. Iversen, M. Winderen, K. Tvera: Radiation-induced insufficiency fractures of the sacrum: evaluation with MR Imaging. Radiology 188 (1993) 241–244

5 Brahme, S. K., V. Cervilla, V. Vint, K. Cooper, K. Kortman, D. Resnick: Magnetic Resonance appearance of sacral insufficiency fractures. Skelet. Radiol. 19 (1990) 489–93

6 Chen, Y., E. R. Dougherty, S. M. Totterman, J. P. Hornak: Classification of trabecular structure in Magnetic Resonance Images based on morphological granulometries. Magn. Reson. Med. 29 (1993) 358–370

7 Chevalier, F., A. M. Laval-Jeantet, M. Laval-Jeantet, C. Bergot: CT image analysis of the vertebral trabecular network in vivo. Calcif. Tiss. int. 51 (1992) 8–13

8 Chung, H., F. W. Wehrli, J. L. Williams, S. D. Kugelmass: Relationship between NMR transverse relaxation, trabecular bone architecture, and strength. Proc. nat. Acad. Sci. 90 (1993) 10250–10254

9 Cuenold, C., J. Laredo, V. Chicheportiche: Vertebral collapses: distinction between porotic and malignant causes on MR Image before and after Gd-DTPA enhancement. Radiology 177 (P) (1990) 240

10 Cummings, S. R., J. L. Kelsey, M. C. Nevitt, K. J. O'Dowd: Epidemiology of osteoporosis and osteoporotic fractures. Epidemiol. Rev. 7 (1985) 178–208

11 Davis, C. A., H. K. Genant, J. S. Dunham: The effects of bone on proton NMR relaxation times of surrounding liquids. Invest. Radiol. 21 (1986) 472–477

12 Deutsch, A. L., J. H. Mink, A. D. Waxman: Occult fractures of the proximal femur: MR Imaging. Radiology 170 (1989) 113–116

13 Durand, E. P., P. Rüegsegger: Cancellous bone structure: analysis of high-resolution CT Images with the run-length method. J. Comput. assist. Tomogr. 15 (1991) 133–139

14 Ford, J. C., F. W. Wehrli: In vivo quantitative characterization of trabecular bone by NMR interferometry and localized proton spectroscopy. Magn. Reson. Med. 17 (1991) 543–551

15 Ford, J. C., F. W. Wehrli, H. Chung: Magnetic field distribution in models of trabecular bone. Magn. Reson. Med. 30 (1993) 373–379

16 Funke, M., H. Bruhn, R. Vosshenrich, O. Rudolph, E. Grabbe: Bestimmung der T_2^*-Relaxationszeit zur Charakterisierung des trabekulären Knochens. Fortschr. Röntgenstr. 161 (1994) 58–63

17 Glazel, J. A., K. H. Lee: On the interpretation of water Nuclear Magnetic Resonance relaxation times in heterogeneous systems. J. Amer. chem. Soc. 96 (1974) 970–978

18 Godersky, C., R. K. Smoker, R. Knutzon: Use of Magnetic Resonance Imaging in the evaluation of metastatic spinal disease. Neurosurgery 21 (1987) 676–680

19 Grampp, S., M. Jergas, C. C. Glüer, P. Lang, P. Brastow, H. K. Genant: Radiological diagnosis of osteoporosis: current

methods and perspectives. Radiol. Clin. N. Amer. 31 (1993 a) 1133–1145

20 Grampp, S., S. Majumdar, M. Jergas, Y. Huang, H. K. Genant: In vivo precision of bone marrow MR relaxation time. Europ. Radiol. 3 (1993) 108 (abstract)

21 Grampp, S., S. Majumdar, M. Jergas, P. Lang, H. K. Genant: In vivo estimation of bone mineral density in the radius using Magnetic Resonance and Peripheral Quantitative Computed Tomography. Radiology 189 (P) (1993 c) 283

22 Hosten, N., K. Neumann, C. Zwicker, P. Schubeus, A. Kirsch, D. Huhn, R. Felix: Diffuse Demineralisation der Lendenwirbelsäule. Fortschr. Röntgenstr. 159 (1993) 264–268

23 Ito, M., K. Hayashi, M. Uetani, Y. Kawahara, M. Ohki, M. Yamada, H. Kitamori, M. Noguchi, M. Ito: Bone mineral and other bone components in vertebrae evaluated by QCT and MRI. Skelet. Radiol. 22 (1993) 109–113

24 Jara, H., F. W. Wehrli, H. Chung, F. C. Ford: High-resolution variable flip angle 3D MR Imaging of trabecular microstructure in vivo. Magn. Reson. Med. 29 (1993) 528–539

25 Jensen, K. S., L. Mosekilde, L. Mosekilde: A model of vertebral trabecular bone architecture and its mechanical properties. Bone 11 (1990) 417–423

26 Lang, P., R. Fritz, S. Majumdar, M. Vahlensieck, C. Peterfy, H. K. Genant: Hematopoietic bone marrow in the adult knee: spin-echo and opposed-phase gradient-echo MR Imaging. Skelet. Radiol. 22 (1993) 95–103

27 Lang, P., H. K. Genant, S. Majumdar: Bone marrow disorders. In: Chan Genant, L.: MRI of the Musculoskeletal System. Saunders, Philadelphia 1994

28 Majumdar, S.: Quantitative study of the susceptibility differences between trabecular bone and bone marrow: computer simulations. Magn. Reson. Med. 22 (1991) 101–110

29 Majumdar, S., H. K. Genant: In vivo relationship between marrow T_2^* and trabecular bone density determined with a chemical shift-selective asymmetric spin-echo sequence. J. Magn. Reson. Imag. 2 (1992) 209–219

30 Majumdar, S., D. Thomasson, A. Shimakawa, H. K. Genant: Appearance of bone marrow in the presence of trabecular bone: quantitation of the susceptibility effects and correlation with bone density. Radiology 177 (P) (1990) 128–129

31 Majumdar, S., D. Thomasson, A. Shimakawa, H. K. Genant: Quantitation of the susceptibility difference between trabecular bone and bone marrow: experimental studies. Magn. Reson. Med. 22 (1991) 111–127

32 Majumdar, S., A. Gies, M. Jergas, S. Grampp, H. Genant: Quantitative measurement of trabecular bone structure using high resolution gradient echo imaging of the distal radius. Proc. Soc. Magn. Reson. Med. 12 (1993) 455

33 Matin, P.: The appearance of bone scans following fractures, including immediate and long term studies. J. nucl. Med. 20 (1979) 1227

34 Meyers, S. P., S. N. Wiener: Magnetic Resonance Imaging features of fractures using the short tau inversion recovery (STIR) sequence: correlation with radiographic findings. Skelet. Radiol. 20 (1991) 499–507

35 Modic, M. T., T. J. Masaryk, D. Paushter: Magnetic Resonance Imaging of the spine. Radiol. Clin. N. Amer. 24 (1986) 229–245

36 Mosekilde, L.: Age-related changes in vertebral trabecular bone architecture-assessed by a new method. Bone 9 (1988) 247–250

36a Parizel, P. M., B. van Riet, B. van Husselt, S. van Geothem, L. Hauwe: Influence of magnetic field strength on T_2^* decay and phase effects in gradient echo MRI of vertebral Bone marrow. JCAT 19 (1995) 465–471

37 Porter, B. A., A. F. Shields, D. O. Olson: Magnetic Resonance Imaging of bone disorders. Radiol. Clin. N. Amer. 24 (1986) 269–289

38 Quinn, S. F., J. L. McCarthy: Prospective evaluation of patients with suspected hip fracture and indeterminate radiographs: use of T_1-weighted MR Images. Radiology 187 (1993) 469–471

39 Ricci, C., M. Cova, Y. S. Kang, A. Yang: Normal age-related patterns of cellular and fatty bone marrow distribution in the axial skeleton: MR Imaging study. Radiology 177 (1990) 83

40 Rizzo, P. F., E. S. Gould, J. P. Lyden, S. E. Asnis: Diagnosis of occult fractures about the hip. Magnetic Resonance Imaging compared with bone-scanning. J. Bone Jt. Surg. 75-A (1993) 395–401

41 Rosenthal, H., K. R. Thulborn, D. I. Rosenthal, B. R. Rosen: Magnetic susceptibility effects of trabecular bone on Magnetic Resonance bone marrow imaging. Invest. Radiol. 25 (1990) 173–178

42 Sartoris, D., P. Clopton, A. Nemcek, C. Dowd, D. Resnick: Vertebral-body collapse in focal and diffuse disease: patterns of pathologic processes. Radiology 160 (1986) 479–483

42a Schick, F., D. Seitz, S. Machmann, O. Lutz, C. D. Claussen: Magnetic resonance bone densitometry: comparison of different methode based on susceptibility. Invest. Radiol. 30 (1995) 254–265

43 Sebag, G. H., S. G. Moore: Effect of trabecular bone on the appearance of marrow in gradient-echo imaging of the appendicular skeleton. Radiology 174 (1990) 855–859

44 Sugimoto, H., T. Kimura, T. Ohsawa: Susceptibility effects of bone trabeculae. Quantification in vivo using an asymmetric spin-echo technique. Invest. Radiol. 28 (1993) 208–213

45 Tanaka, Y., T. Inoue: Fatty marrow in the vertebrae. A parameter for hematopoietic activity in the aged. J. Gerontol. 31 (1976) 527–532

46 Tasciyan, T., M. Schweitzer: Bone density MR Images via wavelet processing. Proc. Soc. Magn. Reson. Med. (1993) 417

46a Wehrli, F. W.: Osteoporosis. Proc. Soc. Magn. Reson. Med. 12 (1992) 115

47 Wherli, F. J., J. C. Ford, J. G. Haddard, M. Attie, F. S. Kaplan: Can quantitative MR Imaging help diagnose osteoporosis? J. Magn. Reson. Imag. 3 (1993) 175

48 Wehrli, F. W., T. G. Perkins, A. Shimakawa: Chemical shift induced amplitude modulations in images obtained with gradient refocussing. Magn. Reson. Imag. 5 (1987) 157–158

49 Wehrli, F. W., J. C. Ford, M. Attie, H. Y. Kressel, F. S. Kaplan: Trabecular structure: preliminary application of MR interferometry. Radiology 179 (1991) 615–621

49a Wehrli, F. W., S. C. Ford, S. G. Haddad: Osteoporosis: clinical assessment with quantitative MR imaging in diagnosis. Radiology 196 (1995) 631–641

50 Wiener, S. N., D. R. Neumann, M. S. Rzeszotarski: Comparison of magnetic resonance imaging and radionuclide bone imaging of vertebral fractures. Clin. nucl. Med. 14 (1989) 666–670

51 Wu, Z., H. Chung, F. Wehrli: Sub-voxel tissue classification in NMR microscopic images of trabecular bone. Proc. Soc. Magn. Reson. Med. (1993) 451

52 Yao, L., J. K. Lee: Occult intraosseous fracture: detection with MR imaging. Radiology 167 (1988) 749–751

53 Yuh, W. T., C. K. Zachar, T. J. Barloon, Y. Sato, W. J. Sickels, D. R. Hawes: Vertebral compression fractures: distinction between benign and malignant causes with MR Imaging. Radiology 172 (1989) 215–218

14 *Sacroiliac Joints*

M. Bollow and J. Brown

Introduction

The evaluation of the sacroiliac joints begins with conventional radiography (24, 28, 40). The wide variations in interpreting radiographs of the sacroiliac spine (41, 54, 103), both in the same observer and between different observers, have made it necessary to add other imaging examinations. Depending on availability and preference, the traditional choice has been between bone scintigraphy, conventional tomography, and CT. Scintigraphy is marked by a high sensitivity (36, 77, 84), but its initially high expectation could not be fulfilled because of low specificity (26, 37, 45, 53). Conventional tomography (27, 74, 105) and CT (13, 16, 32, 38, 99, 102), in contrast, have a high sensitivity and a high specificity. Since scintigraphy, conventional tomography, and CT are associated with radiation exposure and deliver a relatively high dose to pelvic organs, especially to the female gonads, they were often used restrictively for the initial diagnostic work-up in children with sacroiliac complaints and for following young patients with known rheumatoid arthritis of the sacroiliac joints.

MRI offers imaging without ionizing radiation for diagnosing inflammatory, degenerative, septic, traumatic, and neoplastic changes of the sacroiliac joints.

Examination Technique

Using an optimal field strength of 1.5 T and a body array coil or a body coil, the patients are examined supine with the legs elevated. The initial acquisition is obtained in the sagittal plane with the following parameters: TR = 200 msec/TE = 15 msec, matrix [MA] = 128 × 128, FOV = 400 mm, number of sections [No] = 5, section thickness [SL] = 8 mm, image averaging = acquisition [Ac] = 1. This is followed by oblique axial sections that are angulated 30–40 degrees to the body axis and parallel to the long axis of the sacrum (Fig. 14.**1**). T$_1$-weighted SE sequences (TR = 500 msec/TE = 15 msec, MA = 256 × 256, FOV = 220–300 mm, No = 12, SL = 5 mm, Ac = 2, acquisition time about 4 minutes) and T$_2$-weighted (TR = 125 msec/TE = 12 msec, flip angle = 30 degrees, MA = 256 × 256, FOV = 220–300 mm, No = 12, SL = 5 mm, Ac = 4, acquisition time about 4 minutes) are used. To avoid artifacts, the signal processing uses a left-to-right phase-encoding gradient.

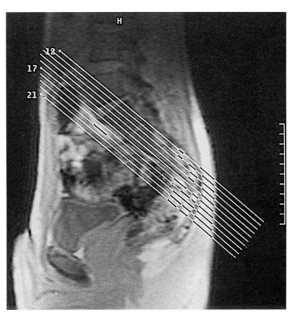

Fig. 14.**1** Sagittal scout view with markings of ten oblique axial sections parallel to the longitudinal axis of the sacrum, nearly perpendicular to the sacroiliac joint surfaces (Fig. 14.**3**).

After selection of a representative section through the center of the joint, a dynamic study can be obtained with a T$_1$-weighted opposed phase GRE sequence (TR = 50 msec/TE = 12 msec, flip angle = 70 degrees, MA = 256 × 256, FOV = 220–300 mm, No = 1, SL = 5 mm, Ac = 4). By averaging 4 acquisitions per image, it will take 50 sec to acquire this sequence (delay time 2 sec). After an interval of 52 sec (delay time 2 sec), the dynamic study is obtained with eight repetitions and a total acquisition time of 7 minutes. Between the first and second measurements, 0.1 mMol Gd-DTPA/kg body weight is injected as a bolus through an indwelling catheter and flushed with a 0.9% NaCl solution.

Quantitative Evaluation. The dynamic acquisition is quantitatively evaluated by measuring the signal intensity of circular (1–10 mm^2) or user-drawn regions of interest (ROIs) placed over the articular cartilage, joint capsule and periarticular bone marrow. The ROIs are optimally placed over the areas of maximum enhancement, which are selected by subtracting the pre-contrast image from the last post-contrast image. An enhancement-time curve is obtained for the cavity and capsule of each sacroiliac joint as well as for the respective subchondral iliac and sacral bone marrow, and is used for calculating the percentage of maximal enhancement above the pre-contrast signal intensity, the enhancement factor F_{enh}, and the rate of enhancement, the enhancement slope S_{enh}:

$$F_{enh} (\%) = (SI_{max} - SI_{pre}) \times 100/SI_{pre},$$
$$S_{enh} (\%/min) = (SI_{max} - SI_{pre}) \times 100/(SI_{pre} \times T_{max}).$$

SI_{pre} corresponds to the pre-contrast signal intensity and SI_{max} to the curve point of the peak post-contrast signal intensity before entering the plateau. T_{max} is the time interval in minutes from the injection of contrast medium to SI_{max}.

Anatomy

■ General Anatomy

The sacroiliac joints are composed of two parts, the true joint and a strong retroarticular ligamentous attachment between the two bones (Fig 14.**2**). The true joint, a synovial joint, comprises the anteroinferior half to two-thirds of the joint. The articular surfaces are covered with cartilage and separated by a joint space. The exclusively hyaline cartilage layer of the sacral surface measures about 3 mm in thickness and the mixed hyaline and fibrocartilage layer of the iliac surface only 1 mm. The relative thickness of the overlying cartilage explains why disease processes tend to involve the iliac subchondral bone first. Posterosuperiorly the retroarticular space between the ilium and sacrum contains adipose and loose connective tissue. Through this run strong interosseous ligaments joining the two bones together. There is no overlying cartilage covering the bony surfaces at this point. The joint is further strengthened anteriorly by anterior sacroiliac ligaments and posteri-

orly by the sacrospinous and sacrotuberous ligaments. The sacroiliac joint is innervated by dorsal branches of the S1 and S2 spinal nerves (28, 27). The dorsal ligaments also receive dorsal branches of the S3 and S4 spinal nerves. After leaving the dorsal sacral foramina, the dorsal branches of the S1 –S4 spinal nerves pierce the dorsal ligamentous complex, give off tiny branches to the sacral origin of the gluteus maximus and continue as medial cunial branches to the skin. The sacroiliac joints receive their vascular supply from branches of the iliolumbar artery, lateral sacral arteries, and superior and inferior gluteal arteries (28).

■ Specific MRI Anatomy

Within the posterosuperiorly located retroarticular space, MRI (1, 8, 9, 10, 42, 75) shows punctate areas of low-signal intensities amidst high-signal tissue (Fig. 14.**3**), corresponding to interosseous ligaments traversing adipose connective tissue. The synovial compartment of the sacroiliac joint, which is anterior and extends inferiorly, has a characteristic morphology on MRI: the T_1-weighted images display the ilial and sacral cartilage as a smoothly outlined, homogeneous structure of intermediate signal intensity along the signal-void subchondral cortex. Owing to its fat content, the periarticular bone marrow has an intermediate to high signal intensity (34). The articular cartilage is visualized as a relatively smoothly delineated, homogeneous structure of high signal intensity on the $T_2{}^*$-weighted GRE images and is distinguished by its high contrast relative to the subchondral and juxta-articular regions on the opposed-phase images. The joint space may be partially visualized (Fig. 14.**4**) between the 3 mm thick sacral and 1 mm thick iliac cartilage layer. Small triangular signal voids on the iliac side of the anterior joint space (Fig. 14.**4**) represent physiologic hyperostoses of the ilium, most likely as adaptation to the localized

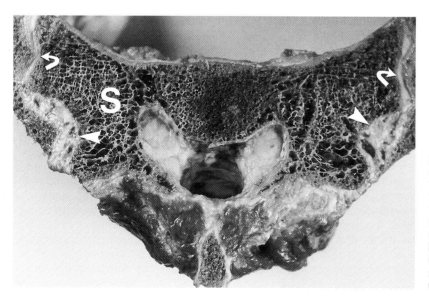

Fig. 14.**2** Transverse section of an anatomic specimen of the pelvis at the level of the first sacral element: the sacroiliac joints are formed by the lateral masses of the sacrum (S) and by the ilium. The joint is composed of the anteroinferiorly located synovial compartment (curved arrows) and the postero-superior located fibrous retroarticular space (arrowheads).

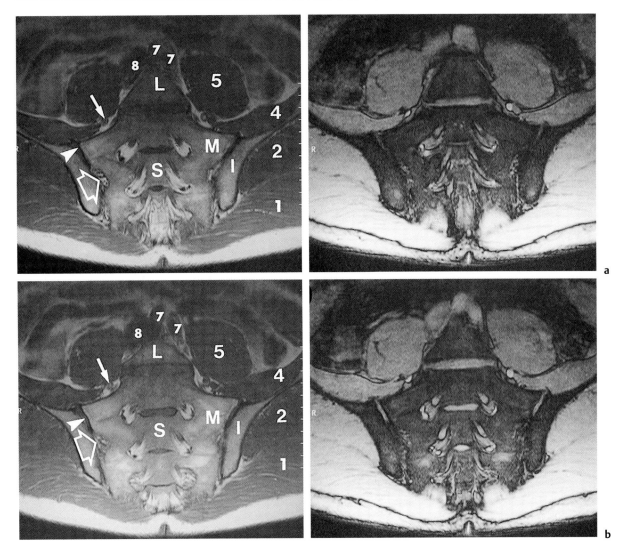

Fig. 14.**3 a–f**   The MR anatomy of a 34-year-old male subject, as seen on T_1-weighted images (left) and corresponding $T_2{}^*$-weighted images (right), cranial (section level 14 in Fig. 14.**1**) to caudal (section level 19 in Fig. 14.**1**), using contiguous 5 mm sections.

1 = Gluteus maximus
2 = Gluteus medius
3 = Gluteus minimus
4 = Iliacus
5 = Psoas
6 = Piriformis
7 = Common iliac artery
8 = Common iliac vein
9 = Inferior gluteal artery and vein
C = Coccyx
I = Ilium
L = L5 vertebral body
M = Sacral lateral mass
S = Sacrum with four sacral elements and four neural foramina with visualization of the nerve roots S1 –S4

Asterisks = Sacral plexus: the sacral branches S1 –S3 exit the sacral foramina anteriorly and, together with the lumbosacral trunk (portion of the fourth and fifth lumbar branches), form the sacral plexus, from which the sciatic nerve arises as the major nerve.
Arrows = Femoral nerve
Curved arrows = Median sacral artery
Angulated arrows = Inferior paraglenoid sulcus (synonym: juxta-articular sulcus): insertion of the fibrous anterior joint capsule at the ilium and sacrum; a superior sulcus is less frequently visualized.
Open arrows = Fibrous compartment of the sacroiliac joints: fatty retroarticular space traversed by low signal interosseous ligaments.
Arrowheads = Synovial cartilage compartment of the sacroiliac joints, seen as intermediate signal intensity on T_1-weighted images and high signal intensity on T_2-weighted images; the caudal sections show low signal defects corresponding to the joint space.

Fig. 14.**3**   (Continued) ▶

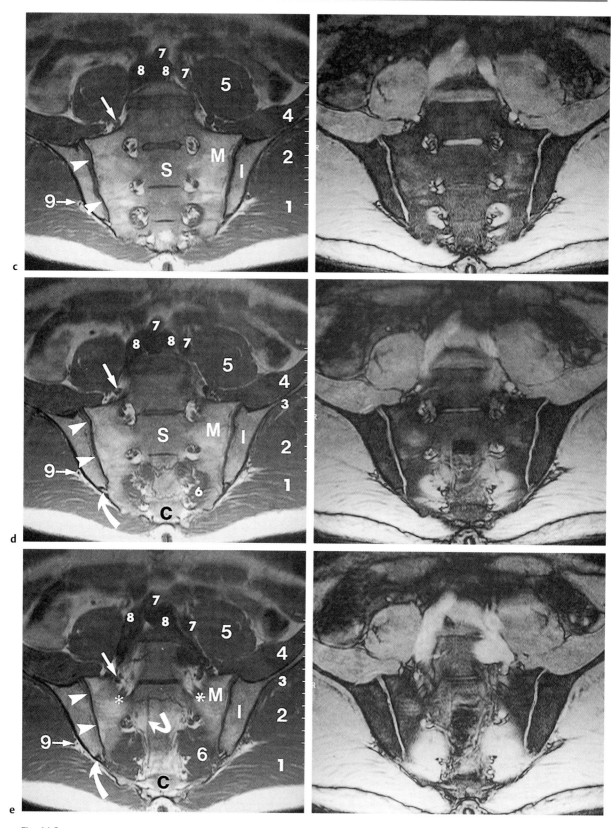

Fig. 14.**3c–e**

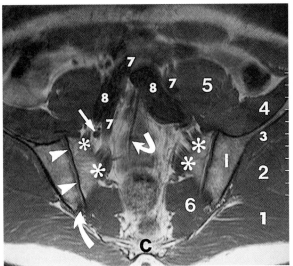
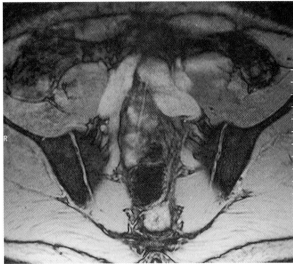

Fig. 14.**3 f**

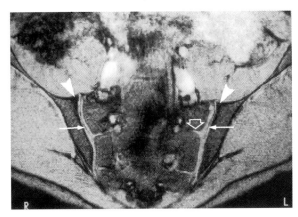

Fig. 14.**4** Normal MR anatomy of the sacroiliac joints in a 14-year-old boy (pre-contrast T_2^*-weighted GRE sequence TR = 125 msec, TE = 12 msec, flip angle = 30 degrees). The joint space is seen bilaterally as a low-signal line (arrows). Physiologic triangular hyperostotic area of the ilium bilaterally (arrowheads). The epiphyseal junctions of the sacral alae (open arrows) show partial ossification medially.

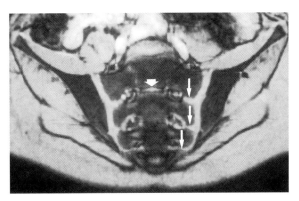

Fig. 14.**5** Normal MR anatomy of the sacroiliac joints of a 10-year-old boy (pre-contrast T_2^*-weighted GRE sequence TR = 125 msec, TE = 12 msec, flip angle = 30 degrees): Broad cartilaginous junctions (arrows) of the joints to the disk remnants of the sacrum (small thick arrow). These junctions correspond to the segmental apophyses, which arise from the costal ossification centers of the sacral segments S1 through S3 and are incorporated into the sacral ala.

weight load on the sacroiliac joints in the upright position.

Children have a different MRI morphology of the sacroiliac joints than adults. In children under the age of 16 years, a cartilaginous connection exists between the sacroiliac joints and the neural foramina of the sacral alae at the level of the sacral disk spaces (Fig. 14.**5**). These connections correspond to cartilaginous lines between the conjoined epiphyseal ossification centers of the S1 –S3 costal elements (28, 63). After fusion with the corresponding transverse processes, they form the sacral alae. The S1 and S3 costal ossification centers are incorporated in the articular surface of either sacral ala.

This ossification process of the epiphyses of the lateral sacral elements is not completed until late adolescence. The articular cartilage of normal sacroiliac joints is avascular and nourished by diffusion. It lacks any relevant contrast enhancement on dynamic Gd-enhanced studies using the opposed-phase technique (8, 9, 10). The enhancement-time curves of normal bone marrow in the adult sacrum and ilium even show a phase-related initial decrease in signal intensity of about 20% followed by a slow return to the original values (12). After administration of contrast medium, the joint capsule, which is obscured by isointense surrounding structures on the pre-contrast image, can be seen in

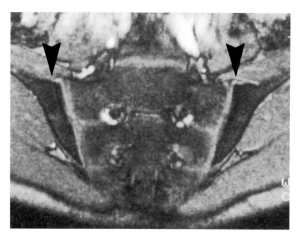

Fig. 14.**6** Normal anatomy of a 12-year-old boy (post contrast T₁-weighted GRE sequence TR = 50 m sec, TE = 12 m sec, flip angle = 70 degrees): After administration of contrast medium, the joint capsule is seen as a delicate linear enhancement (arrowhead). The anterior capsule can extend for several centimeters along the iliac periosteum.

children as delicate linear structure due to enhancement (Fig. 14.**6**). No enhancement is generally observed in adults.

Inflammatory Rheumatoid Conditions

■ Classification and Clinical Findings

Spondyloarthropathy. Patients with known or suspected seronegative spondyloarthropathy constitute the largest group, some 95%, of all patients referred for MRI evaluation of the sacroiliac joints. Seronegative and

HLA-B27-associated spondyloarthropathy (Fig. 14.**7**) is a heterogenic clinical entity of undetermined etiology (33, 64, 107). It includes well-defined subcategories, such as ankylosing spondylitis (23, 69, 70), psoriatic arthropathy (62, 101), arthropathy associated with chronic inflammatory intestinal diseases (enterocolic spondyloarthropathy) (88), reactive arthritis (e.g., Reiter syndrome) and unclassified spondyloarthropathy (33, 107). *Ankylosing spondylitis* is the most frequent and most characteristic spondyloarthropathy (23, 28, 69, 70). This chronic inflammatory systemic disease consists of an array of destructive and proliferative changes involving the axial skeleton, eventually leading to complete ankylosis. In 99% of the patients, ankylosing spondylitis begins with radiographic changes of the sacroiliac joints (28). To establish the diagnosis of ankylosing spondylitis in the presence of sacroiliitis, at least one of the three modified New York criteria must be present (69) (inflammatory spinal pain, limited motion in the lumbar spine, limited chest expansion) together with definite radiographic evidence of sacroiliitis that is higher than grade 2 and bilateral or higher than grade 3–4 and unilateral. The inflammatory sacroiliitis is consistently bilateral and symmetrical in ankylosing spondylitis and usually bilateral and asymmetric in *psoriatic arthropathy. Reactive arthritis* invariably presents with unilateral inflammatory involvement. In rare cases, radiographic changes of inflammatory sacroiliitis can be seen in rheumatoid arthritis (22, 28), Behçet disease (80), Lyme arthritis (97), and collagenous diseases (28), such as systemic lupus erythematosus, polyarteritis nodosa, polymyositis, dermatomyositis, and progressive scleroderma. Erosions, subchondral sclerosis and joint space narrowing including ankylosis of the sacroiliac joints frequently develop in so-called neurogenic paraosteoarthropathies (28) as part of hemi-, para-, and tetraplegia and rarely in metabolic diseases:

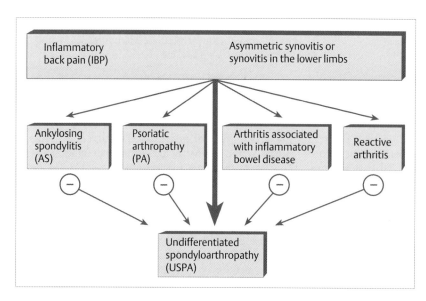

Fig. 14.**7** Diagnostic diagram of seronegative spondyloarthropathy on the basis of criteria proposed by the European Spondylarthropathy Study Group.

gout, articular chondrocalcinosis (pseudogout), polychondritis, ochronosis, Gaucher disease, multicentric reticulohistiocytosis (lipoid dermatoarthritis), primary and secondary hyperparathyroidism, and Cushing disease (28).

Juvenile-Onset Spondyloarthropathy. New data suggest that juvenile-onset spondyloarthropathy is the second most frequent chronic inflammatory joint disease in children and adolescents after juvenile rheumatoid arthritis (17, 49, 57, 59, 60, 98). It is characterized by predominantly inflammatory changes of the lumbar spine and, usually unilateral, sacroiliitis. As in its adult counterpart, this entity includes juvenile onset ankylosing spondylitis (15), reactive arthritis (58), psoriatic arthropathy (62, 101), arthritis associated with inflammatory bowel disease (71), and unclassified spondyloarthropathy (56).

Ankylosing Spondylitis (3, 29, 30). This can be seen as a special manifestation of spondyloarthropathy (Fig. 14.**8**). The reactions that induce the 'variegated picture' (28, 30) of erosions, subchondral sclerosis, and interarticular ankylosing buds fade in the second half of life. 'The ossification of the sacroiliac joint capsule and anterior sacroiliac ligaments dominates at this stage' (30).

Typical Clinical Presentation of Spondyloarthropathy. Spondyloarthropathies are characterized by synovitis, primarily involving the lower limbs, and so-called 'inflammatory back pain' (Fig. 14.**7**), which is defined as insidious onset of pain at rest and improved with exercise.

■ MRI Findings

Subchondral Sclerosis (Figs. 14.**9** and 14.**10**). This is seen as a rim of low signal intensity or signal void on all sequences and shows no contrast enhancement. During the early stages, the sclerotic changes are primarily on the iliac side and appear only later in the disease on the sacral side. With progression of the sclerosis, the joint space becomes increasingly indistinct. Further progression of the sclerosis leads to irregular joint space narrowing and eventually to ankylosis. Histopathologically, the sclerosis represents new bone formation as a reaction to persistent inflammation (14).

Juxta-articular Fat/Accumulation (Figs. 14.**9** and 14.**10**). The juxta-articular bone marrow shows a patchy to diffuse accumulation of fat replacing active hematopoietic marrow. More fat is deposited in the iliac than in the sacral juxta-articular bone marrow, generally commensurate with the degree of chronicity. The deposited fat has a high signal intensity on the T_1-weighted and an intermediate signal intensity on the T_2*-weighted images. With progressing chronicity, the fat tends to spread more diffusely and crosses the former joint space after complete ankylosis of the joint.

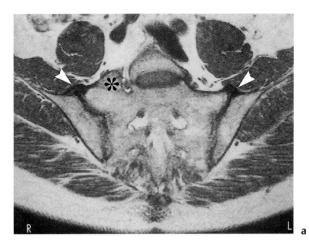

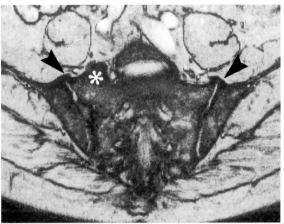

Fig. 14.**8 a, b**   **a** T_1-weighted image (TR = 500 msec, TE = 15 msec, flip angle = 90 degrees) and **b** T_2*-weighted image (TR = 125 msec, TE = 12 msec, flip angle = 30 degrees). In a 57-year-old man with a five-year history of inflammatory back pain. The images are at the level of the transition of the retroarticular space to the synovial joint compartment, which is transected anteriorly and posteriorly (see anatomy, Fig. 14.**3**). Visualized bilateral ossification of the anterior joint capsule and the anterior sacroiliac ligaments (arrowhead). No relevant enhancement of either joint or joint capsule. Incidentally noted is a hemisacralization of the L5 vertebra on the right (asterisk). In addition to senile spondyloarthropathy, hyperostotic spondylosis should be considered in the differential diagnosis.

Erosions (Figs. 14.**10**– 14.**12**). These enhance and show low signal intensity on the T_1-weighted and a high signal intensity on the T_2*weighted images before administration of contrast medium. They interrupt the subchondral cortex and represent extensions of the joint space. Large (> 2 mm) or confluent erosions appear as so-called pseudo-widening of the joint space. Immunohistologic studies have documented that destructive pannus-like infiltrates fill the erosions (14).

Juxta-articular Osteitis (Figs. 14.**10**– 14.**12**). The juxta-articular bone marrow, which has a low signal intensity on unenhanced T_1-weighted and intermediate signal

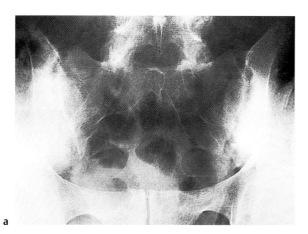

a

Fig. 14.**9 a–c**   **a** Radiograph of a 27-year-old patient with known ankylosing spondylitis for 10 years. The sacroiliac joints are bilaterally ankylosed. **b** The T_1-weighted image (TR = 500 msec, TE = 15 msec, flip angle = 90 degrees) shows a bizarre formation of decreased signal intensity along the previous joint space (arrowheads), representing sclerotic replacement of the original articular cartilage. Generalized periarticular fat accumulations (asterisks) extend over large areas into the previous joint space. **c** Pre-contrast T_2*-weighted image (TR = 125 msec, TE = 12 msec, flip angle = 30 degrees) at the same level as in **a**: Cartilage-equivalent tissue of the original joint is no longer detectable. The sclerotic substitution (arrows) appears as low-signal intensity or signal void. The generalized periarticular fat accumulation (asterisks) exhibits an intermediate signal intensity.

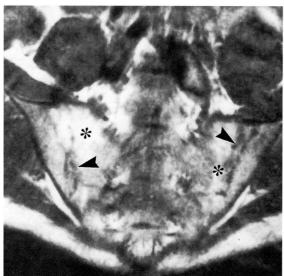

b

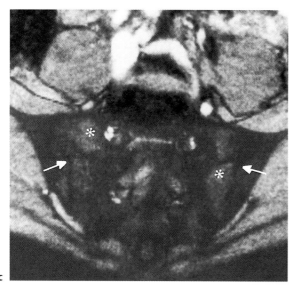

c

Fig. 14.**10 a–f**   **a** CT (5 mm section) of a 22-year-old female ▶ patient with known ankylosing spondylitis for two years and complaining of severe back pain: the sacroiliac joints show symmetric subchondral sclerosis of moderate severity (asterisks) as well as occasional erosions (arrows). **b** T_1-weighted SE sequence (TR = 500 msec, TE = 15 msec, flip angle = 90 degrees): subchondral signal void (asterisk) involving both sacroiliac joints, as well as juxta-articular decrease in signal intensity in the upper third of the left joint, obliterating the articular borders (arrowhead). In addition, areas of high signal intensity corresponding to periarticular fat accumulations (f). **c** T_1-weighted image of the dynamic GRE sequence using single section technique (TR = 50 msec, TE = 12 msec, flip angle = 70 degrees) before injection of contrast medium: the subchondral sclerosis (asterisks) is seen as signal void and the periarticular fat accumulations (f) as structures of high to intermediate signal intensity. **d** Post-contrast image of the dynamic GRE sequence (TR = 50 msec, TE = 12 msec, flip angle = 70 degrees): contrast enhancement in both joint spaces, erosions (arrows), left joint capsule (open black arrow) and juxta-articular and periarticular areas (arrowhead). By virtue of the high intensity and steep enhancement slope, these areas are to be interpreted as osteitis. **e** An enhancement factor of 158 % (129 pre-

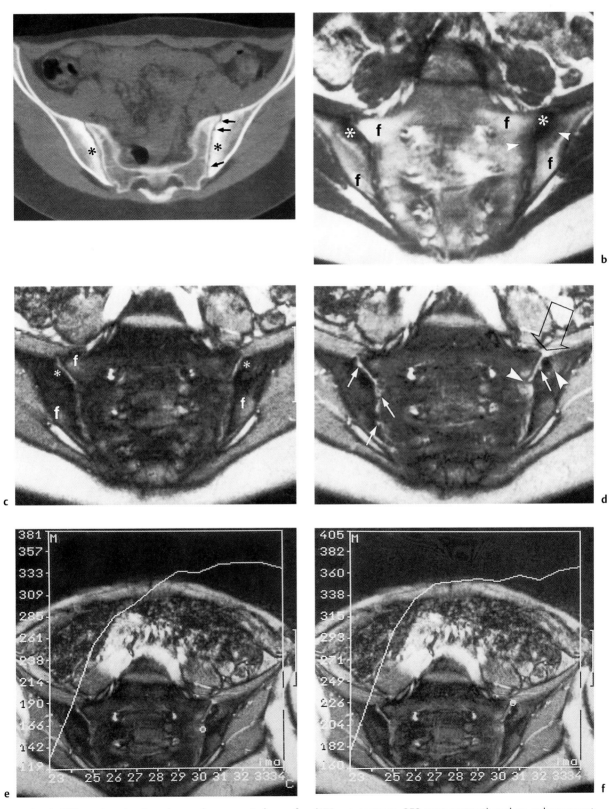

contrast, 333 post-contrast) and an enhancement slope of 38%/minute (administration of contrast medium at 24, maximum signal intensity at 29, T_{max} = 4.17 minutes) could be calculated from the time-intensity curve of an ROI placed over the middle third of the left joint. **f** An enhancement factor of 100%

(176 pre-contrast, 352 post-contrast) and an enhancement slope of 40%/minute (administration of contrast medium at 24, maximum signal intensity at 27, T_{max} = 2.5 minutes) could be calculated from a time-intensity curve of an ROI placed over the left joint capsule.

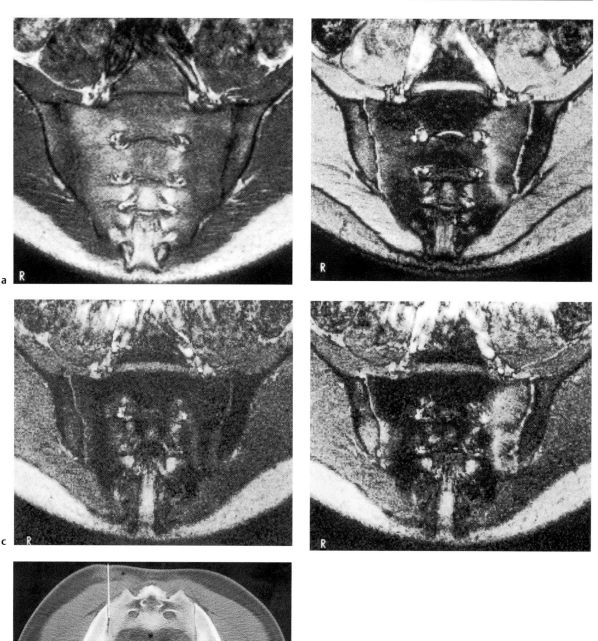

Fig. 14.**11 a–g**   A 16-year-old patient who had complained of 'hip pain' since age 14. Both hips were unremarkable on sonography and MRI. The pre-contrast T_1-weighted image (TR = 500 msec, TE = 15 msec, flip angle = 90 degrees) shows an indistinct articular outline caused by subchondral and juxta-articular decrease in signal intensity. Signal-void subchondral sclerosis or high-signal periarticular fat accumulations are absent. **b** The T_2*-weighted image (TR = 125 msec, TE = 12 msec, flip angle = 30 degrees) at the same level reveals an irregular articular con- tour, caused by multiple small erosions. The juxta-articular and periarticular bone marrow shows ill-defined areas of increased signal intensity bilaterally. **c** Pre-contrast T_1-weighted image of the dynamic GRE sequence using single section technique (TR = 50 msec, TE = 12 msec, flip angle = 70 degrees). **d** Post-con- trast dynamic GRE sequence (TR = 50 msec, TE = 12 msec, flip angle = 70 degrees): both joint spaces, including erosions, cap- sule and juxta-articular and periarticular bone marrow spaces, show a mean increase in signal intensity of 200 % after adminis- tration of contrast medium. **e**   CT- guided puncture for corti- costeroid instillation bilaterally (only shown on the left), fol- lowed by bilateral core biopsy for histologic examination.

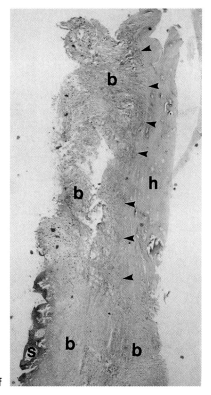

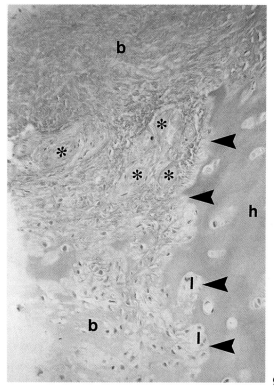

f Photomicrograph, original magnification × 40, Goldner stain and **g** Photomicrograph, original magnification × 100, Goldner stain: the tissue core represents the cartilage–bone interface of the left sacroiliac joint. A hypercellular collagenous connective tissue (b) is seen in the marrow space of the bone between the trabeculae (s) and hyaline articular cartilage (h), primarily derived from active local connective tissue cells. Numerous vessels (asterisks) are found within this collagenous con-

nective tissue. The destructive character of this pannus is apparent from the indistinct transitional zones between connective tissue and hyaline articular cartilage (arrowheads) and has caused lacunae (l) in the cartilage tissue. Activated chondrocytes with enlarged halos are seen in the hyaline cartilage. Osseous interface and columnar cartilage layer have been consumed by the subchondrally growing pannus.

intensity on T_2^*-weighted images in juxta-articular osteitis, shows a steep enhancement slope and a high enhancement factor after injection of contrast medium. Bone marrow edema, which has to be considered in the differential diagnosis, demonstrates a markedly slower rate of enhancement (shallower enhancement slope). As opposed to erosions, the areas of osteitis do not interrupt the continuity of the subcortical cortex on MRI. Ahlström and co-workers (1) have also described comparable signal changes and interpreted them as 'early inflammatory changes in sacroiliitis in the subchondral structures.' This interpretation concurs with the histopathologic correlation of our own MRI investigations performed on patients with early stages of sacroiliitis (Fig. 14.**11**). This is corroborated by histopathologic studies of a Japanese group (90), which revealed 'subchondral inflammatory granulation tissue with cartilaginous and osseous metaplasia' and by Dihlmann's (31) description of a 'subchondral chondroid aggressively proliferating metaplasia.' The strong contrast enhancement can be attributed to the neovasculature in the pannus tissue (Fig. 14.**11 f–g**).

Pathologic Capsular Enhancement (Figs. 14.**10** – 14.**12**). In contradistinction to physiologic enhancement, this is enhancement in a thickened joint capsule with a high enhancement factor and a steep enhancement slope. The pericapsular tissues are spared or, at most, show a subtle edema. The capsular enhancement continues into the joint space. This signal pattern may reflect the inflammation adjacent to the capsular insertion described by Dihlmann and co-workers (31).

■ Index of Chronicity and Activity

MRI Chronicity Index. Based on the results of a prospective study of 125 patients (10) and a prospective study of 66 patients undergoing serial MRI examinations to evaluate therapeutic efficacy (11), the MRI chronicity index of sacroiliitis was defined from unenhanced images:

- *Grade 0:* No chronic inflammatory changes (Fig. 14.**12**).
- *Grade 1:* Mild subchondral sclerosis without sclerosis-induced blurring of the joint space, with or

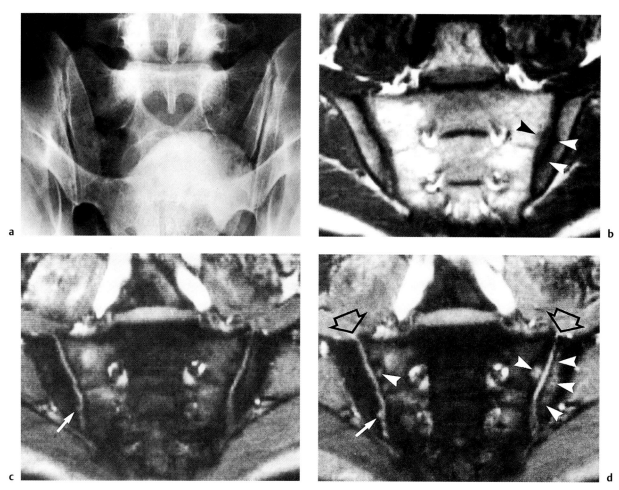

Fig. 14.**12 a–d** **a** Unremarkable radiograph of a 40-year-old patient who complained of severe back pain for half a year. **b** The T₁-weighted image (TR = 500 msec, TE = 15 msec, flip angle = 90 degrees) shows a juxta-articular decrease in signal intensity on the left (arrowheads). **c** Pre-contrast image of the dynamic GRE sequence in single section technique (TR = 50 msec, TE = 12 msec, flip angle = 70 degrees): the sacroiliac joints are smoothly outlined and normal in width. In the lower third of the right sacroiliac joint, however, an erosion is seen on the iliac side (arrow). The sacral bone marrow shows fatty con-

version commensurate with the patient's age. **d** Post-contrast image of the dynamic GRE sequence (TR = 50 msec, TE = 12 msec, flip angle = 70 degrees): increased signal intensity in the joint space bilaterally, in the erosion on the right (arrow), in the anterior joint capsule bilaterally (open arrows), and in a localized juxta-articular region on the right, as well as in the juxtaarticular and periarticular bone marrow on the left (arrowheads). In view of the measurably steep enhancement slope and strong enhancement factor, these changes of the bone marrow are to be interpreted as subchondral osteitis.

without juxta-articular fat accumulation or fewer than two erosions.
- *Grade 2:* Moderate subchondral sclerosis with sclerosis-induced blurring of less than one third of the joint space, with or without juxta-articular fat accumulation or more than two discrete erosions without confluence (Fig. 14.**11**).
- *Grade 3:* Severe subchondral sclerosis obscuring more than one third of the joint space, with or without juxta-articular fat accumulation or pseudowidening of the joint space (normal width of the joint space 4 ± 0.5 mm) due to confluent erosions or circumscribed 'ankylosing buds' of less than one-fourth of the joint space (Fig. 14.**10**).

- *Grade 4:* Definite ankylosis exceeding one-fourth of the joint space (14.**9**).

MRI activity index. Based on contrast enhancement, an MRI activity index of the sacroiliac joints has been defined (10, 11):
- *Grade X:* $F_{enh} \leq 25\%$: no inflammatory activity,
- *Grade A:* $F_{enh} > 25 \leq 0\%$: moderate inflammatory activity (latent sacroiliitis),
- *Grade B:* $F_{enh} > 70\%$: severe inflammatory activity (florid sacroiliitis).

A linear correlation has been found between a subjective back pain index and the enhancement factor. Florid stages of sacroiliitis are frequently accompanied by juxta-articular osteitis or capsulitis. These alterations can even be seen in very early stages of sacroiliitis before any changed articular contour is apparent on MRI (10, 11). In these cases, the activity of the sacroiliitis is solely determined by the enhancement factor of the juxta-articular osteitis or capsulitis. The diagnosis of an inflammatory rheumatoid sacroiliitis can be considered established when an activity index of A or B or a chronicity index of 2 was calculated. A chronicity index of 1 can be found in degenerative sacroiliitis, especially next to the anterior and posterior capsular insertions.

Degenerative Changes

In general, MRI is not indicated for evaluating degenerative sacroiliitis (28) (Fig. 14.**13**) or the hyperostotic sacroiliitis (28, 29) that is part of diffuse idiopathic skeletal hyperostosis *(DISH)*. However, MRI may be necessary to distinguish these conditions from senile spondyloarthropathy.

Osteitis Condensans Ilii

It can be difficult to differentiate the radiographic findings of unilateral or bilateral osteitis condensans ilii from inflammatory rheumatoid sacroiliitis. Osteitis condensans ilii is an entity of unknown origin, characterized by radiographically visualized ovoid to triangular sclerosis of the ilium (Fig. 14.**14**). Recently, it has been attributed to 'stress adaptation' of the ilium induced by gravitational increase in weight load due to the upright position (30). The iliac sclerosis abuts but does not alter the joint space. In contrast to the spondyloarthropathies, osteitis condensans ilii is not associated with the HLA-B27 antigen (94). CT can unequivocally differentiate between an inflammatory rheumatoid sacroiliitis and an osteitis condensans ilii (79). MRI shows the sclerotic areas as low signal structures on the T_1-weighted and T_2-weighted images next to the normally appearing sacroiliac joints. Dynamic MRI reveals increased enhancement in iliac sclerosis.

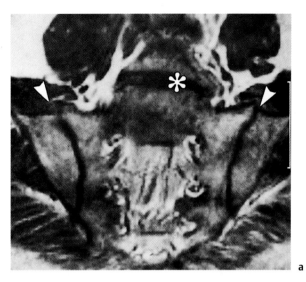

a

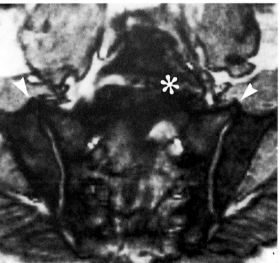

b

Fig. 14.**13 a, b**   **a** T_1-weighted image (TR = 500 msec, TE = 15 msec, flip angle = 90 degrees) and **b** T_2^*-weighted image (TR = 125 msec, TE = 12 msec, flip angle = 30 degrees): 56-year-old woman with pseudoradicular symptoms for 8 years. Besides degenerative changes in the L5/S1 disk (asterisks), both sacroiliac joints show anterior osteophytes, which contain marrow-like signals on the T_1-weighted image (arrowheads). The sacroiliac joints are normal in width and smoothly outlined. After administration of contrast medium, no enhancement in the joints or joint capsule.

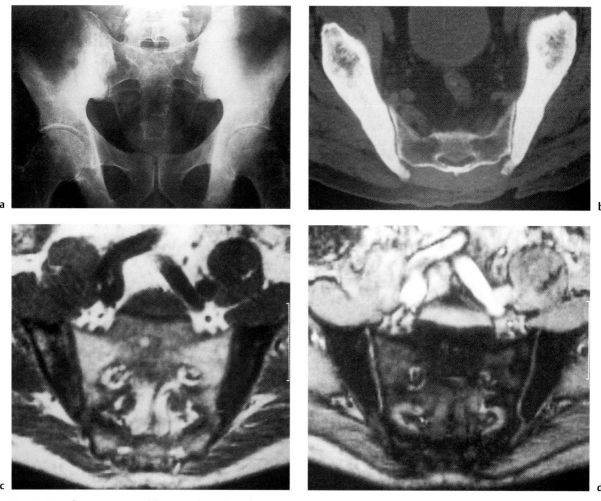

Fig. 14.**14a–d** **a** A 64-year-old man with moderately severe pseudoradicular symptoms. The radiograph shows extensive bilateral sclerosis in projection of the SI joints. **b** CT unequivocally assigns the sclerosis to the ilium bilaterally. The sacrum and sacroiliac joints are unremarkable. **c** T_1-weighted image (TR = 500 msec, TE = 15 msec, flip angle = 90 degrees) and **d** T_2*-weighted image (TR = 125 msec, TE = 12 msec, flip angle = 30 degrees): the T_1-weighted and T_2-weighted images show the iliac sclerosis as low signal intensity. The sacroiliac joints are normal in width and smooth outline, best appreciated on the T_2-weighted image.

Infectious Sacroiliitis

Septic sacroiliitis, which is generally unilateral and presents in about half of the cases in the acute stage and in about half of the cases in the subacute to chronic stage (2, 4, 19, 21, 25, 35, 39, 55, 68, 76, 89, 98), frequently leads to progressive immobilizing symptoms with referred pain in the back, pelvis, hip and even abdomen. Localizing the *clinical* findings to the sacroiliac joints can be challenging. Infectious sacroiliitis generally arises from hematogenous spread, with a skin infection often serving as the source of infection. Trauma and pregnancy are predisposing factors.

Infectious sacroiliitis was rarely described before 1970, but a steady increase in the number of cases has been reported in intravenous drug addicts since then

(43, 46, 48, 81), with *Pseudomonas aeruginosa, Staphylococcus aureus,* and streptococci the most common *etiologic agents.* The acute form of pyogenic sacroiliitis presents with high temperature is caused primarily by *Staphylococcus aureus,* streptococci, and *Enterobacter,* while the subacute and chronic form often has a paucity of symptoms and is largely due to mycobacteria and *Brucella.* The average time interval between onset of symptoms and diagnosis is from 7 days for the acute form to more than 6 weeks for the subacute form. A positive blood culture is rare. Conventional radiographs are often normal during the initial 2–4 weeks (21, 25, 35, 46, 48, 67, 72, 89). *Bone scans* have been advocated as offering the strongest diagnostic contribution, but were found to be still negative within the first week in 23% of cases with acute sacroiliitis. The *CT findings* (5, 18, 20, 73, 82, 83) of infectious sacroiliitis (Fig. 14.**15**) include

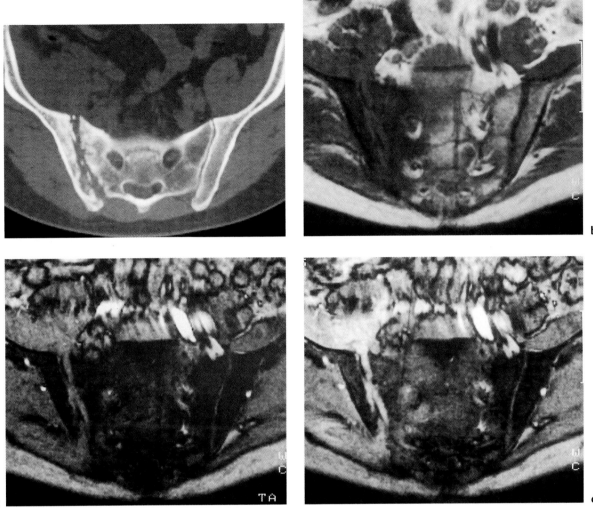

Fig. 14.**15a–d** **a** 58-year-old patient with a right staphylococcal septic sacroiliitis secondary to hematogenous spread from panaritium. The CT shows loss of the subchondral cortex and a widened joint space due to bone destruction with intra-articular sequestra, as well as anterior and posterior soft tissue thickening of the iliopsoas and gluteal musculature. The left sacroiliac joint is unremarkable. **b** T_1-weighted SE sequence (TR = 500 msec, TE = 15 msec, flip angle = 90 degrees), **c** Pre-contrast image of the dynamic T_1-weighted GRE sequence (TR = 50 msec, TE = 12 msec, flip angle = 70 degrees). **d** Post-contrast image of the dynamic T_1-weighted GRE sequence (TR = 50 msec, TE = 12 msec, flip angle = 70 degrees): the right sacroiliac joint exhibits an intermediate signal intensity on the T_1-weighted image. The periarticular decrease in signal intensity extends diffusely anteriorly to the iliopsoas musculature and posteriorly to the gluteal musculature, as well as to the sacral and iliac bone marrow. After administration of contrast medium, strong enhancement of the widened joint and the surrounding infiltrations. Intravascular sequestra are clearly delineated after administration of contrast medium.

blurring or obliteration of the subchondral interface, decreased attenuation of the subchondral bone matrix, subchondral sclerosis and erosions, widening or narrowing of the joint space, sequestrations and gas formation as well as anterior—less frequently posterior—soft tissue abscesses. Soft tissue edema and abscesses induce periosteal reaction and thickening of adjacent muscles. The morphologic CT criteria of an early sacroiliitis with a still negative bone scan has been observed as early as 36 hours after the onset of symptoms.

The *MRI findings* are as follows (18, 51, 65, 67, 85, 104) (Fig. 14.**15**): The signal intensity of the joint is low on T_1-weighted and high on T_2-weighted images. The signal changes extend diffusely into the iliopsoas muscle and into the sacral and iliac bone marrow, without a clear demarcation from surrounding structures. The sacroiliitis is accompanied by joint effusion with joint space widening and, as evidence of extra-articular extension, by osseous, periosteal, and muscular edema and abscess formation with strong contrast enhancement. Also observed are non-enhancing intra-articular fragments consistent with sequestration. Sequestra are not clearly delineated before administration of contrast medium. Inflammatory rheumatoid ar-

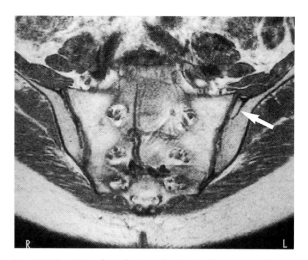

Fig. 14.**16**   Osteophyte fracture line in the ilium, extending to the sacroiliac joint (arrow). This occult undisplaced fracture was not visualized on the radiographic examination obtained two years earlier following a fall.

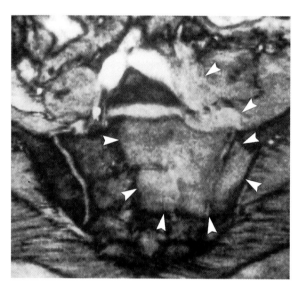

Fig. 14.**17**   A 58-year-old patient with known bronchial carcinoma, who complained of severe and intractable low back pain for 8 weeks. A radiographic examination of the sacrum was without evidence of a destructive osseous lesion. The T_2^*-weighted image (TR = 125 msec, TE = 12 msec, flip angle = 30 degrees) shows a high signal space-occupying lesion involving first and second sacral elements, left lateral mass, left sacroiliac joint and left ilium and breaking through the cortex into the left iliopsoas (arrowheads). The left sacral plexus and left femoral nerves show metastatic infiltration.

thritis, which has to be considered in the differential diagnosis, shows neither sequestration nor extra-articular extension with muscular involvement.

Traumatic Changes

Involvement of the SI joints after trauma to the pelvis is adequately evaluated by conventional radiography and CT. MRI is indispensable for the detection of occult and stress fractures (Fig. 14.**16**).

Tumors and Tumor-Like Conditions of the Joint

The role of MRI in determining the type of tumor or tumor-like conditions found at or around the sacroiliac joints has not yet been established (93). Since neoplastic involvement of the sacroiliac joints might mimic 'inflammatory back pain,' MRI, or, alternatively, CT plays a role in excluding a tumor, in addition to differentiating any inflammatory rheumatoid changes. MRI can visualize neoplastic infiltrations of the sacral nerve roots of the femoral and ischial nerves (Figs. 14.**17** and 14.**18**). MRI is also capable of visualizing inflammatory changes of the sacroiliac joints due to direct invasion of the articular cartilage by a pagetic process (50) in the joint-forming bones (Fig. 14.**19**).

Pitfalls

A profound knowledge of the normal MRI anatomy of the sacroiliac joints is needed to avoid misinterpretations, in particular, in cases with asymmetry of the pelvis and lumbosacral junction. The most frequent normal variant is the unilateral or bilateral 'iliac hump or bulge' (Fig. 14.**20**), which can be quite pronounced. Other normal variants, occurring in about 10% of cases (87), are transitional lumbosacral vertebrae (lumbarization or hemilumbarization of S1, sacralization or hemisacralization of L5), which can be complete (Fig. 14.**21**) or partial (Figs. 14.**22** and 14.**23**). These anomalies can mimic sclerosis. Accessory articular facets (Fig. 14.**24**) can be found between the posterior inferior iliac spine and sacral crest or between the iliac tuberosity and sacral tuberosity. They can be unilateral or bilateral.

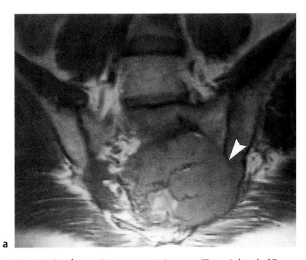

a

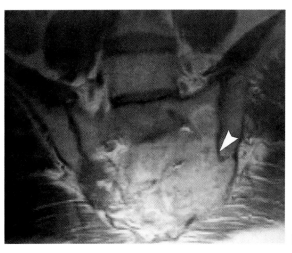

b

Fig. 14.**18a, b** **a** Pre-contrast image (T₁-weighted SE sequence, TR = 500 msec, TE = 15 msec, flip angle = 90 degrees) and **b** post-contrast image (T₁-weighted SE sequence, TR = 500 msec, TE = 15 msec, flip angle = 90 degrees) of a 30-year-old patient with histologically documented mesenchymal chon-drosarcoma of the sacrum. Tumor infiltration of the left sacroiliac joint (arrowheads), left sacral plexus, left piriform, and left gluteus maximus. After administration of contrast medium, intense enhancement of the hypervascular tumor.

Fig. 14.**19a–c** **a** A 57-year-old patient with histologically ▶ proven Paget's disease. CT shows areas of osseous sclerosis (asterisks) and anterior cortical thickening (arrowhead) with generalized enlargement of the left ilium. The left iliopsoas is thickened. The left sacroiliac joint is indistinctly outlined and narrowed. **b** T₁-weighted SE sequence (TR = 500 msec, TE = 50 msec, flip angle = 90 degrees) and c T₂*-weighted GRE sequence (TR = 125 msec, TE = 12 msec, flip angle = 30 degrees): The sclerotic areas of the ilium (asterisk) show a low signal intensity on both sequences. The middle third of the left sacroiliac joint is markedly narrowed (arrow) and exhibits a subchondral sclerosis. The periarticular sacral bone marrow shows fat accumulation (f). These findings are reminiscent of chronic inflammatory rheumatoid sacroiliitis, supporting the hypothesis of an inflammatory pathogenesis of Paget's disease.

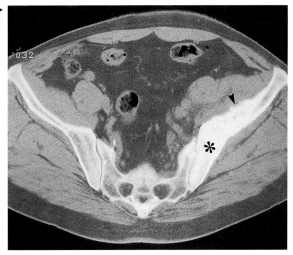

a

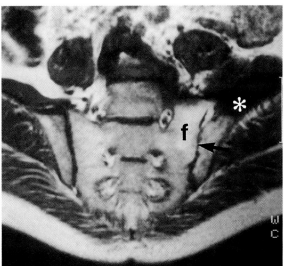

b

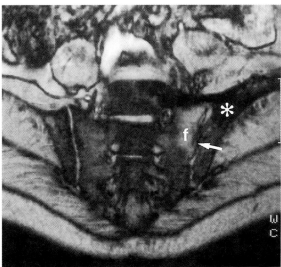

c

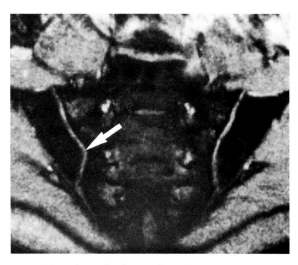

Fig. 14.**20** T₂*-weighted image (TR = 125 msec, TE = 12 msec, flip angle = 30 degrees) of a 38-year-old healthy person. Bulging of the right ilium is a normal variant (arrow). The sacroiliac joints are smoothly outlined and normal in width.

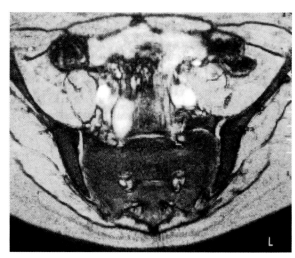

Fig. 14.**21** T₂*-weighted image (TR = 125 msec, TE = 12 msec, flip angle = 30 degrees) of a 15-year-old girl. Complete absence of a lateral apophysis of the first sacral element on the right as a manifestation of hemilumbalization. While the caudal sacral apophysis are ossified, the left apophysis of the first sacral element still contains residual cartilage tissue.

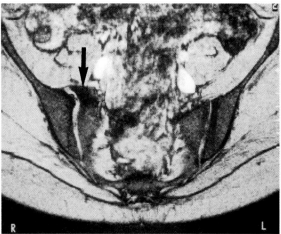

14.**22**

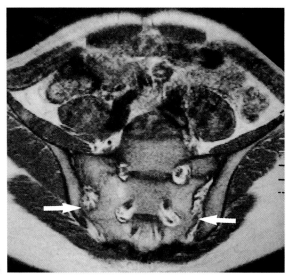

14.**24**

Fig. 14.**22** T₂*-weighted image (TR = 125 msec, TE = 12 msec, flip angle = 30 degrees) of a 15-year-old girl with a partial hemisacralization of the L5 vertebra on the right. This normal variant can mimic a pathologic sclerosis (arrow). The pelvic asymmetry secondary to this transitional anomaly causes an apparent narrowing of the left sacroiliac joint.

Fig. 14.**23** T₂*-weighted image (TR = 125 msec, TE = 12 msec, flip angle = 30 degrees) of a 14-year-old girl with a partial sacralization of the 5th lumbar vertebrae bilaterally, resulting in an apparent sclerosis adjacent to the anterior aspect of the joint.

Fig. 14.**24** T₁-weighted image (TR = 500 msec, TE = 15 msec, flip angle = 90 degrees) of a 13-year-old girl with bilateral accessory joint facets between the iliac tuberosity and sacral tuberosity (arrows).

References

1 Ahlström, H., N. Feltelius, R. Nyman, R. Hällgren: Magnetic Resonance Imaging of sacroiliac joint inflammation. Arthr. u. Rheuma. 33 (1990) 1763–1769

2 Ailsby, R. L., L. T. Staheli: Pyogneic infections of the sacroiliac joint in children. Clin. Orthop. 100 (1974) 96–100

3 Aufdermaur, M.: Die pathologische Anatomie der Spondylitis ankylopoetica. Docum. rheumatol. 2 (1953)

4 Avila, L.: Primary pyognic infection of the sacro-iliac articulation. A new approach to the joint. J. Bone Jt Surg. 23 (1941) 922–928

5 Bankoff, M. S., R. C. Sarno, B. L. Barter: CT scanning in septic sacroiliac arthritis or periarticular osteomyelitis. Comput. Radiol. 8 (1984) 165–170

6 Bellamy, N., W. Park, P. J. Rooney: What do we know about the sacroiliac joint? Semin. Arthr. Rheum. 12 (1983) 282–313

7 Biedermann, K., K. T. M. Schneider, B. Kleinert, A. Huch: Pyogene Sakroiliitis. Kasuistik und Review einer seltenen Komplikation im Wochenbett. Gynäkol. Rdsch. 24 (1984) 145–152

8 Bollow, M., H. König, C. Hoffmann, A. Schilling, K. J. Wolf: Erste Erfahrungen mit der dynamischen Kernspintomographie in der Diagnostik entzündlicher Erkrankungen der Sakroiliakalgelenke. Fortschr. Röntgenstr. 159 (1993) 315–324

9 Bollow, M., J. Braun, H. König, A. Schilling, F. Wacker, V. F. Seyrekbasan, U. Eggens, K. J. Wolf: Dynamische Magnetresonanztomographie der Sakroiliakalgelenke: Erkennung von Frühstadien einer Sakroiliitis. Röntgenpraxis 47 (1994) 70–77

10 Bollow, M., J. Braun, B. Hamm, U. Eggens, A. Schilling, H. König, K. J. Wolf: Early sacroiliitis in patients with spondyloarthropathy: evaluation with dynamic gadolinium-enhanced MR Imaging. Radiology 194 (1995) 529–536

11 Bollow, M., J. Braun, M. Taupitz, J. Häberle, B. H. Reißhauer, S. Paris, S. Mutze, V. F. Seyrekbasan, K. J. Wolf, B. Hamm: Intraarticular corticosteroid injection into the sacroiliac joints using CT guidance in patients with spondyloarthropathy: indication and follow-up with contrast-enhanced MR Imaging. J. Comput. assist. Tomogr. 20 (1996) 512–521

12 Bollow, M., W. Knauf, A. Korfel, M. Taupitz, K. J. Wolf, B. Hamm: Initial experience with dynamic Magnetic Resonance Imaging in evaluation of normal bone marrow versus malignant bone marrow infiltrations in human. Magn. Reson. Imag. (1997) in press

13 Borlaza, G. S., R. Seigel, L. R. Kuhns, A. E. Good, R. Rupp, W. Martel: Computed tomography in the evaluation of sacroiliac arthritis. Radiology 139 (1981) 437–440

14 Braun, J., M. Bollow, L. Neure, E. Seipelt, F. Seyrekbasan, H. Herbst, U. Eggens, A. Distler, J. Sieper: Use of immunohistologic and in situ hybridization techniques in the examination of sacroiliac joint biopsy specimens from patients with ankylosing spondylitits. Arthr. a. Rheum. 38 (1995) 499–505

15 Burgos-Vargas, R., J. Vazquez-Mellado: The early clinical recognition of juvenile-onset ankylosing spondylitis and its differentiation from juvenile rheumotoid arthritis. Arthr. and Rheum. 38 (1995) 835–844

16 Carrera, G. F., W. D. Foley, F. Kozin, L. Ryan, T. L. Lawson: CT of sacroiliitis. Amer. J. Roentgenol. 136 (1981) 41–46

17 Cassidy, J. T., J. E. Levinson, J. C. Bass, J. Baum, E. J. Brewer, C. W. Fink, V. Hanson, J. C. Jacobs, A. T. Masi, J. G. Schaller, J. F. Fries, D. McShane, D. Young: A study of classification criteria for a diagnosis of juvenile rheumatoid arthritis. Arthr. a. Rheum. 29 (1986) 274–281

18 Chevalley, P., J. Garcia: Imagerie des sacro-iliites infectieuses. J. Radiol. 72 (1991) 1–10

19 Cohn, S. M., D. J. Schoetz: Pyogenic sacroiliitis. Another imitator of the acute abdomen Surgery 100 (1986) 95–98

20 Coppola, J., N. M. Muller, G. D. Connel: Computed tomography of musculoskeletal tuberculosis. J. Canad. Ass. Radiol. 8 (1987) 199–203

21 Coy, J. T., C. R. Wolf, T. D. Brower, W. G. Winter: Pyogenic arthritis of the sacro-iliac joint: long-term follow-up. J. Bone Jt Surg. 58 (1976) 845–849

22 Dahlqvist, S. R., L. G. Nordmark, A. Bjelle: HLA-B27 and involvement of sacroiliac joints in rheumatoid arthritis. J. Rheumatol. 11 (1984) 27–32

23 Dale, K.: Radiograph grading of sacroliits in Bechterew's syndrome and allied disorders. Scand. J. Rheumatol. 100, Suppl 32 (1980) 692–697

24 Dale, K., O. Vinje: Radiography of the spine and sacroiliac joints in ankylosing spondylitis and psoriasis. Acta radiol., Diagn. 26 (1985) 145–159

25 Delbarre, F., J. Rondier, F. Delrieu: Pyogenic infection of the sacro-iliac joint. J. Bone Jt Surg. 57 (1975) 818–825

26 Deqeker, J., T. Goddeeris, M. Walravens, M. DeRoo: Evaluation of sacroiliitis: comparison of radiological and radionuclide techniques. Radiology 128 (1978) 687–689

27 De Smet, A. A., J. D. Gardner, H. B. Lindley, J. E. Goin, S. L. Fritz: Tomography for evaluation of sacroiliitis. Amer. J. Roentgenol. 139 (1982) 577–581

28 Dihlmann, W.: Röntgendiagnostik der Sakroiliakalgelenke und ihrer nahen Umgebung. Thieme, Stuttgart 1978

29 Dihlmann, W.: Röntgendiagnostik bei der Spondylosis hyperostotica. In Ott, V. R.: Spondylosis hyperostotica. Enke, Stuttgart 1982

30 Dihlmann, W., J. Bandick: Die Gelenksilhouette. Springer, Berlin 1995

31 Dihlmann, W., R. Lindenfelser, W. Selberg: Sakroiliakale Histomorphologie der ankylosierenden Spondylitis als Beitrag zur Therapie. Dtsch. med. Wschr. 102 (1977) 129–132

32 Dihlmann, W., K. F. Gürtler, M. Heller: Sakroiliakale Computertomographie. Fortschr. Röntgenstr. 130 (1979) 659–665

33 Dougados, M., S. von der Linden, R. Juhlin et al.: The European Spondyloarthropathy Study Group preliminary criteria for the classification of spondyloarthropathy. Arthr. a. Rheum. 34 (1991) 1218–1227

34 Duda, S. H., M. Laniado, F. Schick, M. Strayle, C. D. Claussen: Normal bone marrow in the sacrum of young adults: differences between the sexes seen on chemical-chift MR Imaging. Amer. J. Roentgenol. 164 (1995) 935–940

35 Dunn, E. J., D. M. Bryan, J. T. Nugent, R. A. Robinson: Pyogenic infections of the sacroiliac joint. Clin. Orthop. 118 (1976) 113–117

36 Dunn, N. A., B. H. Mahida, M. V. Merrick, G. Nuki: Quantitative sacroiliac scintiscanning: a sensitive and objective method for assessing efficacy of nonsteroidal, anti-inflammatory drugs in patiens with sacroiliitis. Ann. rheum. Dis. 43 (1984) 157–159

37 Esdaile, J. M., L. Rosenthall, R. Terkeltaub, R. Kloiber: Prospective evaluation of sacroiliac scintigraphy in chronic inflammatory back pain. Arthr. a. Rheum. 23 (1980) 998–1003

38 Fam, A. G., J. D. Rubenstein, H. Chin-Sang, F. Y. K. Leung: Computed tomography in the diagnosis of early ankylosing spondylitis. Arthr. a. Rheum. 28 (1985) 930–937

39 Feldmann, J. L., C. J. Menkés, B. Weill, F. Delrieu, F. Delbarre: Les sacro-iliites infectieuses. Etude mulicentrique sur 214 observations. Rev. Rhum. 48 (1981) 83–91

40 Forrester, D. M.: Imaging of sacroiliac joints. Radiol. Clin. N. Amer. 28 (1990) 1055–1072

41 D. M. Forrester, P. N. Hollingsworth, R. L. Dawkin: Difficulties in the radiographic diagnosis of sacroiliitis. Clin. rheum. Dis. 9 (1983) 323–332

42 Friedburg, H., S. Meske, J. Hennig, P. Billmann, H. H. Peter, W. Wenz: Die Kernspintomographie des Sakroiliakalgelenkes. Radiologe 27 (1987) 130–134

43 Gifford, D. B., M. Patzakis, D. Ivler: Septic arthritis due to pseudomonas in heroin addicts. J. Bone Jt Surg. 57 (1975) 631–635

44 Gillepsie, H. W., G. Lloyd-Roberts: Osteitis condensans. Brit. J. Radiol. 26 (1953) 16–21

45 Goldberg, R. P., R. K. Genant, R. Shimshak, D. Shames: Applications and limitations of quantitative sacroiliac joint scintigraphy. Radiology 128 (1978) 683–686

46 Gordon, G., S. A. Kabins: Pogenic sacroiliitis. Amer. J. Med. 69 (1980) 50–56

47 Grob, K. R., W. L. Neuhuber, R. O. Kissling: Die Innervation des Sacroiliacalgelenkes beim Menschen. Z. Rheumatol. 54 (1995) 117–122

48 Guyot, D. R., A. Manoli, G. A. Kling: Pyogenic sacroiliitis in IV drug abusers. Amer. J. Roentgenol. 149 (1987) 1209–1211

49 Häfner, R.: Die juvenile Spondarthritis. Retrospektive Untersuchung an 71 Patienten. Mschr. Kinderheilk. 135 (1987) 41–46

50 Hadjipavlou, A., P. Lander, H. Srolovitz: Pagetic arthritis. Pathophysiology and management. Clin. Orthop. 208 (1986) 15–19

51 Haliloglu, M., M. B. Kleinmann, A. R. Siddiqui, M. D. Cohen: Osteomyelitis and pyogenic infection of the sacroiliac joint. MR findings and review. Pediat. Radiol. 24 (1994) 333–335

52 Hare, H. F., G. E. Haggart: Oteitis condensans ilii. J. Amer. med. Ass. 128 (1945) 723–727

53 Ho, G., N. Sadovnikoff, C. M. Malhotra, B. C. Claunch: Quantitative sacroiliac joint scintigraphy: a critical assessment. Arthr. a. Rheum. 22 (1979) 827–844

54 Hollingsworth, P. N., P. S. Cheak, R. L. Dawkons, E. T. Owen, A. Calin, P. H. N. Wood: Observer variation in grading sacroiliac radiographs in HLA B27 positive individuals. J. Rheumatol. 10 (1983) 247–254

55 Hudson, O. C.: Acute suppurative arthritis of the sacroiliac joint. Med. Tms 63 (1935) 342–345

56 Huppertz, H. I.: Die undifferenzierte juvenile Spondylarthropathie. Kinderarzt 25 (1994) 455–465

57 Huppertz, H. I., H. J. Suschke: Chronisch entzündliche Gelenkerkrankungen im Kindes- und Jugendalter. Mschr. Kinderheilk. 142 (1994) 367–382

58 Hussein, A.: Das Spektrum der postenteritischen reaktiven Arthritiden im Kindesalter. Mschr. Kinderheilk. 135 (1987 a) 93–98

59 Hussein, A.: Die HLA-B27-assoziierten Spondyloarthritiden im Kindesalter. Mschr. Kinderheilk. 135 (1987 b) 185–194

60 Hussein, A., H. Abdul-Khaliq, H. von der Hardt: Atypical spondyloarthritis in children: proposed diagnostic criteria. Europ. J. Pediat. 148 (1989) 513–517

61 Hutton, C. F.: Osteitis condensans ilii. Brit. J. Radiol. 26 (1953) 490–493

61 a Segal, G., D. S. Kellogg: Osteitis condensans ilii. Amer. J. Roentgenol. 71 (1954) 643–649

62 Jelk, W.: Wie lautet Ihre Diagnose? Arthritis psoriatica. Schweiz. Rdsch. Med. Prax. 83 (1994) 319–321

63 Kaufmann, H. J.: Röntgenbefunde am kindlichen Becken bei angeborenen Skelettaffektionen und chromosomalen Aberrationen. Thieme, Stuttgart 1964

64 Khan, M. A.: An overview of clinical spectrum and heterogeneity of spondylarthropathies. In Khan, M. A.: Spondyloarthropathies. Rheum. Dis. Clin. N. Amer. 18 (1992) 1–10

65 Klein, M. A., C. S. Winalski, M. R. Wax, D. R. Piwnica-Worms: Mr imaging of septic sacroiliitis. J. Comput. assist. Tomogr. 15 (1991) 126–132

66 Knutsson, F.: Changes in the sacroiliac joints in morbus Bechterew and osteitis condensans. Acta radiol. 33 (1950) 557–569

67 Le Breton, C., I. Frey, M. F. Carette, J. Rischaud, A. Kujas, J. Korzee, J. M. Bigot: Infectious sacroiliitis: value of computed tomography and magnetic resonance imaging. Europ. J. Radiol. 2 (1992) 233–239

68 L'Episcopo, J. B.: Suppurative arthritis of the sacroiliac joint. Ann. Surg. 104 (1936) 289–303

69 van der Linden, S., H. A. Valkenburg, A. Cats: Evaluation of diagnotic criteria for ankylosing spondylitis. Arthr. a. Rheum. 27 (1984) 361–368

70 Mau, W., H. Zeidler, R. Mau, A. Majewski, J. Freyschmidt, H. Deicher: Clinical features and prognosis of patients with possible ankylosing spondylitis: results of a 10-year follow up. J. Rheumatol. 15 (1988) 1109–1114

71 Mielants, H., E. M. Veys, R. Joos, C. Cuvelier, M. De Vos, F. Proot: Late onset pauciarticular juvenile chronic arthritis: relation to gut inflammation. J. Rheumatol. 14 (1987) 459–465

72 Miller, J. H., G. F. Gates: Scintigraphy of sacroiliac pyarthrosis in children. J. Amer. med. Ass. 238 (1977) 2701–2704

73 Morgan, J. C., J. G. Schlegelmilch, P. K. Spiegel: Early diagnosis of septic arthritis of the sacro-iliac joint by use of computed tomography. J. Rheumatol. 8 (1981) 979–982

74 Moritz, J. D., H. Ganter, C. Winter: Vergleich von konventioneller Tomographie und Computertomographie bei Erkrankungen der Sakroiliakalgelenke. Röntgen-Bl. 43 (1990) 439–443

75 Murphey, M. D., L. H. Wetzel, J. M. Bramble, E. Levine, K. M. Simpson, H. B. Lindsley: Sacroiliitis: MR Imaging findings. Radiology 180 (1991) 239–244

76 Murphy, M. E.: Primary pyogenic infection of sacroiliac joint. N. Y. St. J. Med. 77 (1977) 1309–1311

77 Namey, T. C., J. McIntyre, M. Buse, E. C. LeRoy: Nucleographic studies of axial sponarthritides. I. Quantitative sacroiliac scintigraphy in early HLA-B27-associated sacroiliitis. Arthr. a. Rheum. 20 (1977) 1058–1064

78 Numaguchi, Y.: Osteitis condensans ilii, including its resolution. Radiology 98 (1971) 1–8

79 Olivieri, I., G. Gemignani, E. Camerini: Differential diagnosis between osteitis condensans ilii and sacroiliitis. J. Rheumatol. 17 (1990) 1504–1512

80 Olivieri, I., G. Gemignani, E. Cemerini, R. Semeria, G. Pasero: Computed tomography of the sacroiliac joints in four patients with Behçet's syndrome – confirmation of sacroiliitis. Brit. J. Rheum. 29 (1990) 264–267

81 Pollack, M., A. Gurman, J. G. Salis: Pyogenic infection of the sacro-iliac joint. Orthop. Grand Rounds 3 (1986) 2–9

82 Raffi, M., H. Firooznia, C. Golimbu: Computed tomography of septic joints. Comput. Tomogr. 9 (1985) 51–60

83 Rosenberg, D., A. M. Baskies, P. J. Deckers, B. E. Leiter, J. I. Ordia, I. G. Yablon: Pyogenic sacroiliitis. An absolute indication for computed tomographic scanning. Clin. Orthop. 184 (1984) 128–132

84 Russell, A. S., B. C. Lentle, J. S. Percy: Investigation of sacroiliac disease: comparative evaluation of radiological and radionuclide techniques. J. Rheumatol. 2 (1975) 45–51

85 Sandrasegaran, K., A. Saifuddin, A. Coral, W. P. Butt: Magnetic Resonance Imaging of septic sacroiliitis. Skelet. Radiol. 23 (1994) 289–292

86 Sashin, D.: A critical analysis of the anatomy and the pathologic changes of the sacro-iliac joints. J. Bone Jt Surg. 12 (1930) 891–910

87 Schmorl, G., H. Junghanns: Die gesunde und die kranke Wirbelsäule in Röntgenbild und Klinik. Thieme, Stuttgart 1968

88 Scott, W. W., E. K. Fishman, J. E. Kuhlman, C. I. Caskey, J. J. O'Brien, G. S. Walia, T. M. Bayless: Computed tomography evaluation of the sacroiliac joints in Crohn disease. Radiologic/clinical correlation. Scelet. Radiol. 19 (1990) 207–210

89 Shannahan, M. D. G., C. E. Ackroyd: Pyogenic infection of the sacro-iliac joint. a report of 11 cases. J. Bone Jt Surg. 67 (1985) 605–608

90 Shichikawa, K., M. Tsujimoto, J. Nishioka, Y. Nishibayashi, K. Matsumoto: Histopathology of early sacroiliitis and enthesis in ankylosing spondylitis. In Ziff, M., S. B. Cohen: Advances in Inflammation Research. Vol. 9. The Spondylarthropathies. Raven, New York 1985 (pp. 15–24)

91 Shipp, F. L., G. E. Haggart: Further experience in the management of osteitis condensanns ilii. J. Bone Jt Surg. 32 (1950) 841–847

92 Sicard, J. A., L. Gally, J. Haguenau: Ostéitis condensantes, a étiologie inconnue. J. Radiol. Électrol. 10 (1926) 503–507

93 Silberstein, M., O. Hennessy, L. Lau: Neoplastic involvement of the sacroiliac joint: MR and CT features. Austr. Radiol. 36 (1992) 334–338

94 Singal, D. P., P. de Bosset, D. A. Gordon, H. A. Smythe, M. B. Urowitz, B. E. Koehler: HLA antigens in osteitis condensans ilii and ankylosing spondylitis. J. Rheumatol. 4 Suppl. 3 (1977) 105–108

95 Solonen, K. A.: The sacroiliac joint in the light of anatomical, roentgenological and clinical studies. Acta orthop. scand. 28, Suppl. (1957) 1–127

96 Spoendlin, M., W. Zimmerli: Pyogene Sakroiliitis. Schweiz med. Wschr. 118 (1988) 799–805

97 Steere, A. C., S. E. Mlawista, D. R. Snydman: Lyme arthritis: an epidemic of oligoarticular arthritis in children and adults in three Connecticut communities. Arthr. a. Rheum. 20 (1977) 7–17

98 Ström, H., N. Lindvall, B. Hellstrom, L. Rosenthal: Clinical, HLA, and roentgenological follow up study of patients with juvenile arthritis: comparison between the long term outcome of transient and persistent arthritis in children. Ann. rheum. Dis. 48 (1989) 918–923

99 Taggart, A. J., S. M. Desai, J. M. Iveson, P. W. Verow: Computerized tomography of the sacro-iliac joints in the diagnosis of sacro-iliitis. Brit. J. Rheum. 23 (1984) 258–266

100 Thompson, M.: Osteitis condensans ilii and its differentiation from ankylosing spondylitis. Amer. rheum. Dis. 13 (1954) 147–156

101 Truckenbrodt, H., R. Hafner: Die Psoriasisarthritis im Kindesalter. Ein Vergleich mit den Subgruppen der juvenilen chronischen Arthritis. Z. Rheumatol. 49 (1990) 88–94

102 Vogler, J. B., W. H. Brown, C. A. Helms, H. K. Genant: The normal sacroiliac joint: a CT study of asymptomatic patients. Radiology 151 (1984) 433–437

103 Yazici, H., M. Turunc, H. Özdogan, S. Yurdakul, A. Akinci, C. G. Barnes: Observer variation in grading sacroiliac radiographs might be a cause of sacroiliitis in certain disease states. Ann. rheum. Dis. 46 (1987) 139–145

104 Wilbur, A. C., B. G. Langer, D. G. Spigos: Diagnosis of sacroiliac joint infection in pregnancy by Magnetic Resonance Imaging – case report. Magn. Reson. Imag. 6 (1988) 341–343

105 Wilkinson, M., J. A. Meikle: Tomography of the sacroiliac joints. Ann. rheum. Dis. 25 (1966) 433–440

106 Withrington, R. H., R. A. Sturge, N. Mitchell: Osteitis condensans ilii or sacro-iliitis? Scand. J. Rheumatol. 14 (1985) 163–166

107 Zeidler, H., W. Mau, M. A. Khan: Undifferentiated spondyloarthropathies. Rheum. Dis. Clin. N. Amer. 18 (1992) 187–202

Appendix

M. Vahlensieck

1 Differential Diagnosis of the Swollen Extremity by MRI

A diffuse swelling of one or several extremities can cause differential diagnostic problems. After clinical evaluation, invasive diagnostic modalities, such as venography, play an important role in the evaluation. MRI allows a non-invasive evaluation (4).

Venous edema. This is caused by venous stasis secondary to thrombophlebitis, chronic venous insufficiency, cardiac decompensation, etc, and can be unilateral or bilateral. It is compressible and detectable as pitting edema. Edema of long duration might no longer pit on pressure because of fibrotic induration of the skin. The MRI shows:

- diffuse muscle edema with increased signal intensity on the T_2-weighted images,
- increased signal intensity in the subcutaneous layers also,
- enhancement of the muscle compartment after administration of contrast medium,
- cross-sectional enlargement of the muscle compartment.

Lymphedema. This is caused by obstruction of lymphatic channels with physical signs indistinguishable from edema caused by other mechanisms. It is usually unilateral. The primary form is distinguishable from the secondary form at various stages (reversible swelling, irreversible swelling, elephantiasis). The T_2 weighted images show:

- definite increase in signal intensity in the subcutaneous tissues with accentuation of the subcutaneous connective tissue (honeycomb pattern) (Fig. 15.**1**),

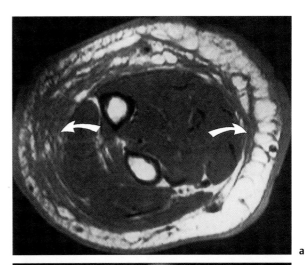

a

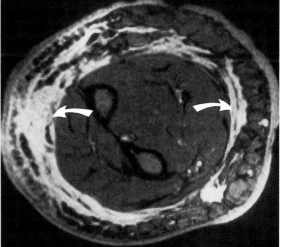

b

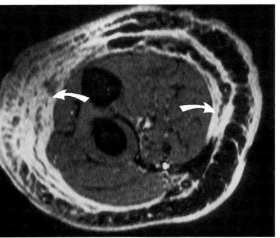

c

Fig. 15.**1a–c**   Female patient with breast carcinoma and massive lymphedema of the left forearm. Axial MRI. **a** T_1-weighted SE image. **b** T_2*-weighted GRE image, **c** Fat-suppressed STIR image. Marked thickening of the skin and subcutaneous tissues due to fluid accumulation (arrows; honeycomb pattern). The fluid has a low signal intensity on the T_1-weighted image and a high signal intensity on the T_2*-weighted and fat-suppressed images. No abnormal fluid accumulation in the musculature.

- normal signal intensity of the musculature,
- marked thickening of the subcutis in the presence of a normal cross-section of the muscle compartment,
- subcutaneous enhancement after application of contrast medium.

Lipoid edema. This causes a non-compressible bilateral swelling without pitting on pressure. It is not gravity dependent and spares hands and feet. It is a lipomatous hypertrophy and usually observed in obese women above the age of 20 years. MRI shows:

- massive increase in subcutaneous fat with normal visualization of the muscle compartment,
- normal signal intensities.

Mixed forms can be found and show various manifestations of the pattern described. Other causes of a swollen extremity, such as angiomas or Sudeck disease, can be

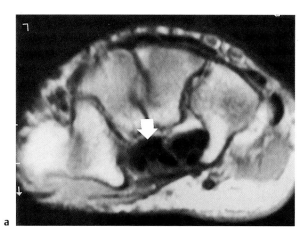

a

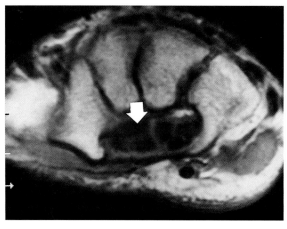

b

Fig. 15.**2a, b** Magic angle phenomenon. Wrist, axial plane. Identical parameters (proton-density weighted SE sequence, TR = 1800 msec, TE = 20 msec), same window setting, comparable section levels through the carpal tunnel. **a** The hand is flat and parallel to the main magnetic field (longitudinal axis of the unit). **b** Flexion of the elbow with the forearm 40–50 degrees angled relative to the axis of the main magnetic field, with an increase in the signal intensity in the flexor tendon due to the magic angle phenomenon (arrows).

usually excluded by history, clinical evaluation, and morphologic criteria.

2 Magic-Angle Phenomenon

A particular orientation of the tissue relative to the orientation of the main magnetic field induces an anisotropic signal pattern in certain tissues, such as cartilage and tendon. This is related to the dependence of the T_2 relaxation time on the spatial orientation of the tissue (1, 2, 6). The particular spatial arrangement of the collagenous fibers in tendon and cartilage affects the spin-spin coupling of the protons through the orientation of the magnetic fields by means of dipole interaction according to the following equation:

$$3 \cos^2 \theta - 1$$

with θ representing the angle formed by the main magnetic field (B_0) and a vector of neighboring protons. A decrease in the spin-spin coupling prolongs the T_2 relaxation time. The spin-spin coupling is minimal for $3 \cos^2\theta - 1 = 0$, which occurs for $\theta = 55$ degrees and 125 degrees. These angles are called the magic angle. The orientation of the collagenous fibers does not influence the T_1 and T_2^* (effective T_2) relaxation times. Higher field strengths exert a stronger effect on the T_2 relaxation time.

The prolongation of the T_2 relaxation time of a tendon can be quite pronounced. The tendon oriented longitudinally ($\theta = 0$ degrees) has a T_2 relaxation time of 250 μsec. If the tendon is positioned 55 degrees relative to the main magnetic field, the T_2 relaxation time increases and can last as long as 22 msec (6). As a result, tendons running at an angle of 55 degrees to the main magnetic field have an artificial increase in signal intensity on sequences with relatively short echo times (5). This effect is most apparent on proton-density weighted images. Sequences with echo times exceeding 22 msec are free from this effect and visualize the tendons as low-signal intensity structures irrespective of their orientation.

This phenomenon has important clinical implications since inflammation, hemorrhage, and partial tear of the tendon are diagnosed by the increased signal intensities that these conditions induce in the tendon. If the nature of an increased signal intensity is uncertain, increased intensity that is induced by the magic angle phenomenon can be excluded by obtaining supplemental heavy T_2-weighted sequences or by applying an MTC pulse. The MTC pulse can suppress the anisotropic effect. The sites affected by this phenomenon are the rotator cuff insertion in the shoulder, the flexor tendons of the ankle and the tendons of the wrist (Fig. 15.**2**) (5). Variations of the signal intensity induced by the collagen orientation have also been observed in the hyaline articular cartilage (11), but do not play an important role in clinical applications since, at most, the normally discernible layering of the cartilage is obliterated in certain orientations. Other tissues, such as kidneys, muscles or white matter, are not subject to any anisotropy of the relaxation times relative to the various orientations of the magnetic field.

3 Use of Dedicated MRI Systems

Dedicated MRI systems refer to MRI units that are designed to image only portions of the body, such as extremities, without enclosing the entire body. They are based on permanent (resistive) magnet technology and operate with relatively low field strengths of about 0.02 to 0.3 T. The open design of these units provides easy access to the body part in the unit, adding the capability of intervention and cinetic studies. Other advantages of dedicated MRI units in comparison with the superconductive high-field units are the lower purchasing price and operating cost, as well as the smaller size, generally requiring no remodeling of the room for installation. Disadvantages are the lower signal-to-noise ratio and the inability of to image the whole body (12). The lower signal-to-noise ratio leads to images with either a lower spatial resolution or a higher noise level, which, if unacceptable, can be overcome by longer acquisition times.

About 90% of knee examinations can be adequately performed with a dedicated extremity MRI system (3, 8). Promising results have been reported in the diagnostic evaluation of the wrist (9) and ankle, elbow, and peripheral tubular bones (7).

4 Examination Protocols (Tables)

The examination protocols listed here for the 0.5 and 1.5 Tesla MRI systems are based on the experience of the authors and summarize the examination techniques described in the respective chapters. The protocols are to be taken as recommendations for a comprehensive evaluation of a joint region. Modifications might be necessary for specific clinical questions. The tabulated format should make it easy to compare the protocols for the different regions and to find specific parameters when planning an examination. Values for other field strengths can be extrapolated from the values listed under the 0.5 T and 1.5 T field strengths.

• Temporomandibular joint

A. .5 T:

Plane	Sequence	TR	TE	TI	Flip	FOV	Matrix	Section	SA	Phase	Remarks
TRA	SE	Short	20			100	256 × 128	5/1.0	2	cc	Scout, body coil
O-SAG	SE	425	30			100	256 × 192	4/0.3	4	cc	Mouth open
S-SAG	SE	425	30			100	256 × 192	4/0.3	4	cc	Mouth closed
S-COR	SE	425	30			100	256 × 192	4/0.3	4	cc	

B. .1.5 T:

Plane	Sequence	TR	TE	TI	Flip	FOV	Matrix	Section	SA	Phase	Remarks
TRA	SE	Short	20			100	256 × 128	5/1.0	2	cc	Scout, body coil
O-SAG	SE	600	20			100	256 × 256	3/0.1	4	cc	Mouth open
S-SAG	SE	600	20			100	256 × 256	3/0.1	4	cc	Mouth closed
S-COR	SE	600	20			100	256 × 256	3/0.1	4	cc	
Option	SS-GRE	300	10		40	100	256 × 256	4/0.1	1	cc	

• Shoulder

A. .5 T:

Plane	Sequence	TR	TE	TI	Flip	FOV	Matrix	Section	SA	Phase	Remarks
COR	SE	Short	20			400	256 × 128	5/1.0	2	cc	Scout, body coil
TRA	SS-GRE	600	14/34		25	180	256 × 192	4/0.4	4	a.-p.	Ring coil
O-COR	SE	600	20			180	256 × 192	4/0.4	4	cc	Ring coil
O-COR	SS-GRE	600	14/34		25	180	256 × 192	4/0.4	4	cc	Ring coil
O-SAG	SS-GRE	600	14/34		25	180	256 × 192	4/0.4	4	cc	Ring coil
Option	Fast-STIR	1000	20	100		200	256 × 128	4/0.8	2	op	Ring coil

B. .1.5 T:

Plane	Sequence	TR	TE	TI	Flip	FOV	Matrix	Section	SA	Phase	Remarks
COR	SE	Short	20			400	256 × 128	5/1.0	2	cc	Scout, body coil
TRA	SS-GRE	600	9/28		30	160	256 × 192	4/0.4	4	a.-p.	Ring coil
O-COR	SE	600	20			160	256 × 192	4/0.4	2	cc	Ring coil
O-COR	SS-GRE	600	9/28		30	160	256 × 192	4/0.4	4	cc	Ring coil
O-SAG	SS-GRE	600	9/28		30	160	256 × 192	4/0.4	4	cc	Ring coil
Option	Fast-STIR	1200	20	140		200	256 × 128	4/0.8	2	op	Ring coil

• Ankle

A. .5 T:

Plane	Sequence	TR	TE	TI	Flip	FOV	Matrix	Section	SA	Phase	Remarks
TRA	SE	Short	15			400	256 × 128	5/1.0	1	a.-p.	Scout, body coil
COR	SE	600	15			160	256 × 192	4/0.4	4	cc	Head coil
COR	SE	2000	100			160	256 × 192	4/0.4	1	rl	Head coil
SAG	SS-GRE	600	14/34		25	160	256 × 192	4/0.4	4	cc	Head coil
TRA	SE	2000	100			160	256 × 192	4/0.4	1	a.-p.	Head coil
Option	Fast-STIR	1000	20	100		200	256 × 128	4/0.8	2	op	Head coil

B. .1.5 T:

Plane	Sequence	TR	TE	TI	Flip	FOV	Matrix	Section	SA	Phase	Remarks
TRA	SE	Short	15			400	256 × 128	5/1.0	2	a.-p.	Scout, body coil
COR	SE	600	15			140	256 × 192	4/0.4	2	cc	Head coil
COR	SE	2000	100			140	256 × 192	4/0.4	1	rl	Head coil
SAG	SS-GRE	600	9/28		30	140	256 × 192	4/0.4	2	cc	Head coil
TRA	SE	2000	100			140	256 × 192	4/0.4	1	a.-p.	Head coil
Option	Fast-STIR	1200	20	140		200	256 × 128	4/0.8	2	op	Head coil

• Knee

A. .5 T:

Plane	Sequence	TR	TE	TI	Flip	FOV	Matrix	Section	SA	Phase	Remarks
TRA	SE	Short	15			400	256 × 128	5/1.0	1	a.-p.	Scout, body coil
COR	SE	600	15			160	256 × 192	4/0.4	4	cc	Knee coil
COR	SE	2000	100			160	256 × 192	4/0.4	1	rl	Knee coil
SAG	SS-GRE	600	14/34		25	160	256 × 192	4/0.4	4	cc	Knee coil
TRA	SE	2000	100			160	256 × 192	4/0.4	1	a.-p.	Knee coil
Option	Fast-STIR	1000	20	100		160	256 × 128	4/0.8	2	op	Knee coil

B. .1.5 T:

Plane	Sequence	TR	TE	TI	Flip	FOV	Matrix	Section	SA	Phase	Remarks
TRA	SE	Short	15			400	256 × 128	5/1.0	2	a.-p.	Scout, body coil
COR	SE	600	15			160	256 × 192	4/0.4	2	cc	Knee coil
COR	SE	2000	100			160	256 × 192	4/0.4	1	rl	Knee coil
SAG	SS-GRE	600	9/28		30	160	256 × 192	4/0.4	2	cc	Knee coil
TRA	SE	2000	100			160	256 × 192	4/0.4	1	a.-p.	Knee coil
Option	Fast-STIR	1200	20	140		160	256 × 128	4/0.8	2	op	Knee coil
TRA	SS-GRE-3-D	30	8		45	160	256 × 192	0.6	1	a.-p.	Meniscus

• Hip

A. .5 T:

Plane	Sequence	TR	TE	TI	Flip	FOV	Matrix	Section	SA	Phase	Remarks
TRA	SE	Short	15			400	256 × 128	5/1.0	1	a.-p.	Scout, body coil
COR	SE	600	15			375	256 × 192	4/0.4	2	cc	body coil
O-COR	SS-GRE	600	14/34		25	180	256 × 192	4/0.4	4	cc	Ring coil
TRA	SS-GRE	600	14/34		25	180	256 × 192	4/0.4	4	a.-p.	Ring coil
Option	Fast-STIR	1000	20	100		200	256 × 128	4/0.8	2	op	Ring coil
O-SAG	SS-GRE	600	14/34		25	180	256 × 192	4/0.4	4	cc	Ring coil

B. .1.5 T:

Plane	Sequence	TR	TE	TI	Flip	FOV	Matrix	Section	SA	Phase	Remarks
TRA	SE	Short	15			400	256 × 128	5/1.0	1	a.-p.	Scout, body coil
COR	SE	600	15			375	256 × 192	4/0.4	2	cc	Körper coil
O-COR	SS-GRE	600	9/28		30	180	256 × 192	4/0.4	2	cc	Ring coil
TRA	SS-GRE	600	9/28		30	180	256 × 192	4/0.4	2	a.-p.	Ring coil
Option	Fast-STIR	1200	20	140		200	256 × 128	4/0.8	2	op	Ring coil
O-SAG	SS-GRE	600	9/28		30	180	256 × 192	4/0.4	2	cc	Ring coil

- ## Wrist

A. .5 T:

Plane	Sequence	TR	TE	TI	Flip	FOV	Matrix	Section	SA	Phase	Remarks
TRA	SE	Short	15			400	256 × 128	5/1.0	1	a.-p.	Scout, body coil
COR	SE	600	15			140	256 × 192	4/0.4	4	cc	Small ring coil
COR	SE	2000	100			140	256 × 192	4/0.4	1	rl	Small ring coil
SAG	SS-GRE	600	14/34		25	140	256 × 192	4/0.4	4	cc	Small ring coil
TRA	SE	2000	100			140	256 × 192	4/0.4	1	a.-p.	Small ring coil
Option	Fast-STIR	1000	20	100		160	256 × 128	4/0.8	2	op	Small ring coil

B. .1.5 T:

Plane	Sequence	TR	TE	TI	Flip	FOV	Matrix	Section	SA	Phase	Remarks
TRA	SE	short	15			400	256 × 128	5/1.0	2	a.-p.	Scout, body coil
COR	SE	600	15			120	256 × 192	3/0.4	2	cc	Small ring coil
COR	SE	2000	100			120	256 × 192	3/0.4	1	rl	Small ring coil
SAG	SS-GRE	600	9/28		30	120	256 × 192	3/0.4	2	cc	Small ring coil
TRA	SE	2000	100			120	256 × 192	3/0.4	1	a.-p.	Small ring coil
Option	Fast-STIR	1200	20	140		140	256 × 128	4/0.8	2	op	Small ring coil

- ## Elbow

A. .5 T:

Plane	Sequence	TR	TE	TI	Flip	FOV	Matrix	Section	SA	Phase	Remarks
TRA	SE	Short	15			400	256 × 128	5/1.0	1	a.-p.	Scout, body coil
SAG	SE	600	15			160	256 × 192	4/0.4	4	cc	Ring coil, rectangular coil
SAG	SE	2000	100			160	256 × 192	4/0.4	1	a.-p.	Ring coil, rectangular coil
COR	SS-GRE	600	14/34		25	160	256 × 192	4/0.4	4	cc	Ring coil, rectangular coil
TRA	SE	2000	100			160	256 × 192	4/0.4	1	a.-p.	Ring coil, rectangular coil
Option	Fast-STIR	1000	20	100		180	256 × 128	4/0.8	2	op	Ring coil, rectangular coil

B. .1.5 T:

Plane	Sequence	TR	TE	TI	Flip	FOV	Matrix	Section	SA	Phase	Remarks
TRA	SE	Short	15			400	256 × 128	5/1.0	2	a.-p.	Scout, body coil
SAG	SE	600	15			140	256 × 192	4/0.4	2	cc	Ring coil, rectangular coil
SAG	SE	2000	100			140	256 × 192	4/0.4	1	a.-p.	Ring coil, rectangular coil
COR	SS-GRE	600	9/28		30	140	256 × 192	4/0.4	2	cc	Ring coil, rectangular coil
TRA	SE	2000	100			140	256 × 192	4/0.4	1	a.-p.	Ring coil, rectangular coil
Option	Fast-STIR	1200	20	140		160	256 × 128	4/0.8	2	op	Ring coil, rectangular coil

Abbreviations:

a.-p.	= anterior-posterior
COR	= coronal
cc	= craniocaudal
Fast-STIR	= fast-short-tau-inversion recovery
Flip	= flip angle
FOV	= field of view
GRE	= gradient echo
Matrix	= matrix
O-COR	= oblique coronal
op	= optional
O-SAG	= oblique sagittal
phase	= direction of phase-encoding gradient
rl	= right – left
SA	= signal averaging
SAG	= sagittal
Section	= section thickness and distance
SE	= spin echo
SS-GRE	= steady state gradient echo
TE	= echo time
TI	= inversion time
TR	= repetition time
TRA	= transverse

References

1 Berendsen, H. J. C.: Nuclear Magnetic Resonance study of collagen hydration. J. chem. Phys. 36 (1962) 3297–3305

2 Berendsen, H. J. C., C. Migchelsen: Hydration structure of fibrous macromolecules. Ann. N. Y. Acad. Sci. 125 (1965) 365–379

3 Brennpunkt: 76. Deutscher Röntgenkongreß – bleibt die MRT in der Radiologie. Fortschr. Röntgenstr. 163 (1995) IX–X

4 Duewell, S., K. D. Hagspiel, J. Zuber, G. K. von Schulthess, A. Bollinger, W. A. Fuchs: Swollen lower extremity: role of MR Imaging. Radiology 184 (1992) 227–231

5 Erickson, S. J., I. H. Cox, J. S. Hyde, G. F. Carrera, J. A. Strandt, L. D. Estkowski: Effect of tendon orientation on MR Imaging signal intensity: a manifestation of the „magic angle" phenomenon. Radiology 181 (1991) 389–392

6 Fullerton, G. D., I. L. Cameron, V. A. Ord: Orientation of tendons in the magnetic field and its effect on T_2 relaxation times. Radiology 155 (1985) 433–435

7 Gehardt, P., W. Golder, B. Kersting-Sommerhoff, N. Hof: MR-Tomographie der Extremitäten mit dem Teilkörpersystem ARTOSCAN. Röntgenpraxis 47 (1994) 4–13

8 Kersting-Sommerhoff, B., P. Gerhardt, W. Golder, N. Hof, K. A. Riel, H. Helmberger, M. Lenz, K. Lehner: MRT des Kniegelenkes: Erste Ergebnisse eines Vergleichs von 0,2-T-Spezialsystem mit 1,5-T-Hochfeldmagnet. Fortschr. Röntgenstr. 162 (1995 a) 390–395

9 Kersting-Sommerhoff, B., N. Hof, W. Golder, K. Becker, K. D. Werber: MRT des Handgelenks: „Granulomatöse Tendovaginitis vom Sarkoidosetyp" – eine seltene Ursache des Karpaltunnelsyndroms. Röntgenpraxis 48 (1995 b) 206–208

10 Podiumsdiskussion: Dedizierte Systeme in der Magnetresonanztomographie. BVDRN – Info 6 –7 (1995) 6–7

11 Rubenstein, J. D., J. K. Kim, I. Morava-Protzner, P. L. Stanchev, R. M. Henkelman: Effects of collagen orientation on MR Imaging characteristics of bovine articular cartilage. Radiology 188 (1993) 219–226

12 Young, S. W.: Economic views on technical devices. Europ. J. Radiol. 3 (1993) 190–195

Index

Page numbers in **bold** refer to illustrations.